Nursing Care of the Aging Client

Promoting Healthy Adaptation

Evelynn Clark Gioiella, R.N., Ph.D.
Dean, Hunter-Bellevue School of Nursing
Hunter College of the City University of New York
New York, New York

Catherine Waechter Bevil, R.N., Ed.D.
Assistant Professor, School of Nursing
The City College of the City University of New York
New York, New York

Contributors

Anne J. Doyle, R.N., M.S.
Associate Professor, School of Nursing
The City College of the City University of New York
New York, New York

Elisabeth A. Pennington, R.N., Ed.D.
Consultant to the National League for Nursing
New York, New York

562905

APPLETON-CENTURY-CROFTS/Norwalk, Connecticut

JACKSON LIBRARY
WITHDRAWN
LANDER COLLEGE
GREENWOOD, S.C. 29646

ISBN 0-8385-7014-3

85 86 87 88 89 90/10 9 8 7 6 5 4 3 2 1

Prentice-Hall International, Inc., London
Prentice-Hall of Australia, Pty. Ltd., Sydney
Prentice-Hall of Canada, Inc.
Prentice-Hall of India Private Limited, New Delhi
Prentice-Hall of Japan, Inc., Tokyo
Prentice-Hall of Southeast Asia (Pte.) Ltd., Singapore
Whitehall Books Ltd., Wellington, New Zealand
Editora Prentice-Hall do Brasil Ltda., Rio de Janeiro

Library of Congress Cataloging in Publication Data

Gioiella, Evelynn Clark.
  Nursing care of the aging client.

  Includes bibliographies and index.
  1. Geriatric nursing. 2. Aging. 3. Adaptation (Physiology) I. Bevil, Catherine Waechter. II. Title.
  [DNLM: 1. Adaptation, Physiological—in old age—nurses' instruction. 2. Geriatric Nursing. WY 152 G495n]
  RC954.G56 1985   610.73′65   84-14574
  ISBN 0-8385-7014-3

Design: Lynn Luchetti
Cover: Mary Martylewski

PRINTED IN THE UNITED STATES OF AMERICA

Contents

Preface

The nursing profession has recognized only recently its important role in the health care of the aging. As a result, nursing faculty on the baccalaureate and graduate levels are only now beginning to alter their courses to ensure that graduates have the necessary educational preparation to provide high-level health care for this segment of the population. As the number of aging persons in our population continues to grow, it can be expected that even greater numbers of professional nurses will be prepared to work with the aging.

The authors wrote this book to enable practicing professional nurses, students, and faculty to understand the aging process and the unique responses of aging persons to the health problems that most commonly affect them. This understanding provides the intellectual base for nursing practice and the delivery of quality health care to our growing elderly population. Nursing approaches specifically designed or adapted for the aging client at any point along the health–illness continuum are presented. Since 95 percent of America's aging population is independent—healthy, chronically ill, or otherwise—a strong emphasis is placed on the nurse's role with this group.

This textbook presents information needed by the professional nurse providing health care to clients who are over the age of fifty-five. Since aging begins with conception, the decision designating an age to begin discussion of problems associated with aging is an arbitrary one. Age fifty-five was chosen in order to include the preretirement period, a decade that should be a time of preparation for aging and a decade during which many adults first experience problems associated with aging.

The philosophy permeating this book is one of evolving man. This philosophy underlies an optimistic view of aging, a view the authors believe is long overdue in Western society. The life process is characterized by a unidirectional becoming, and aging is part of that process. Aging is not a negative process but rather an achievement, the culmination of the life process and the point at which diversity is most apparent. The authors hope to stimulate a more positive view of aging by introducing this philosophical approach early in the book and using it throughout as a rationale for developing the nursing role.

The authors believe that the elderly should be full, active participants in making health care decisions and implementing a plan of care. Consequently, the word "client" has been chosen to express the relationship that exists between the nurse and the recipient of nursing services.

Stress and adaptation make up the organizational framework of the book. This framework was developed and used by the authors at The City College of The City University of New York School of Nursing as a curriculum framework. As an organizational framework it allows emphasis on the care of the healthy as well as the sick. It also facilitates integration of material from the physical, psychological, and social sciences, as well as from nursing subspecialties.

Stresses are factors that precipitate adaptive behavior changes in clients. These behavior changes may be both physical and psychosocial. As clients become less healthy, previous adaptations may become additional stresses for them. For example, a client whose stress is osteoporosis associated with aging may develop a pathological fracture as an adaptation. This adaptation is now an additional stress, leading to a variety of other adaptations, including immobility, which may also become stresses. Nursing interventions are aimed at preventing or interrupting this cascading effect and assisting clients to adapt in the most effective ways.

The stress and adaptation framework allows the nurse to provide appropriate care for clients at all points along the health–illness continuum, that is, at all levels of adaptation. The level of adaptation is determined by identifying and assessing the client's stresses and adaptations. At each level of adaptation client goals and nursing interventions are indicated.

Level One Adaptation includes all clients adapting effectively and in an optimal state of health. This is the level of adaptation the nurse aims to promote in all clients. Level Two Adaptation includes clients who are healthy but at a higher than normal risk to experience a sudden change in their health status. With these clients the nurse seeks to support any effective adaptations and limit those that are less effective. Clients at Level Three Adaptation have a chronic illness or other diagnosed health problem. They are able to adapt effectively and can independently perform the activities of living expected at their developmental stage with limited, but ongoing, nursing support. Clients at Level Four are those with acute health problems. Because some of their adaptations are ineffective and have become additional stresses for them, they are dependent on nursing care to meet many basic demands of daily living. At Level Five Adaptation are clients whose adaptations are so ineffective that they are totally dependent upon nursing care for survival.

Major nursing goals and basic nursing intervention modes are identified as appropriate for clients at each level of adaptation. The nurse can use these as guidelines when individualizing nursing care for clients.

The authors use the stress and adaptation framework in a simple, straightforward manner, without elaborate explanations or justifications. It is the vehicle to facilitate presentation of an integrated approach to both the processes and problems of aging and related nursing care.

The stress and adaptation framework is the basis for organizing this text. Following the introductory chapters, which include the nurse's roles with today's aging population, each level of adaptation is used successively to present nursing interventions with healthy clients, clients at risk, clients with chronic health problems, clients with acute health problems, and, finally, those who are facing death.

The intended audience for this book includes students and faculty in baccalaureate and higher degree programs, community health nurses, geriatric nurse practitioners, and professional nurses working in geriatric settings or with aging clients in other institutional settings. As an integrated textbook based on a holistic view of man, it should have wide appeal to baccalaureate and post-baccalaureate nursing programs, particularly those with an integrated curriculum.

The book is not intended to replace or substitute for a fundamentals of nursing or other basic nursing text. It is designed to be a primary textbook dealing with the end of the life span just as a pediatric nursing textbook deals with the beginning of the life process. In areas where a thorough discussion of the major health problem can be found in well-known basic textbooks, a less detailed discussion is included. In these instances the emphasis is specifically on the unique responses of the aging client experiencing that particular health problem and the implications for nursing assessment and care.

The subject is treated at an advanced level to provide the reader not only with an understanding of concepts basic to care of the elderly but with enough depth and detail to allow the professional nurse to apply these concepts in complex situations. In addition, discussion of health problems and nursing care is related to theory and research findings, thus providing the nurse with sound rationales for the recommended interventions. For those who would like further reading on a topic, extensive reference lists are included at the end of each chapter.

The authors strongly believe that there is a need for a sophisticated body of knowledge as a base for nursing practice and that this book contributes to that body of knowledge.

Acknowledgments

The authors are deeply grateful to Marion Kalstein, our acquisition editor, for her support, advice, and strongly communicated belief in this book. We are also very grateful to Daniel Payne, our production editor, for his expert assistance in all phases of editing and production of this text.

We wish to acknowledge the skill, cooperation, and cheerful efforts of our typist Kathy Fallon, who labored with us through multiple rewrites.

Finally, we want to express our thanks and appreciation to our faculty colleagues who participated in the development of the stress and adaptation framework used in this book, and to the friends, students, and family members who have supported our, at times, intense involvement in this project.

Nursing and the Aging Client

1

Aging:
An Appraisal

DEMOGRAPHIC PERSPECTIVES

The age distribution of the population of the United States has changed markedly in the twentieth century. Increased longevity and decreased fertility have led to a sevenfold increase since 1900 in the number of persons over the age of 65. In 1980, 11.3 percent of the population was in this age group as compared to 4.1 percent in 1900 (Table 1). This trend is expected to continue with the percentage of population over 65 projected to increase to 16 percent in the next 50 years (*Our Future Selves,* NIH, 1978). The 1980 census data clearly demonstrate this trend. In 1970 there were 20,065,502 people over 65. In 1980 this figure had risen to 25,544,133, a 28 percent increase in ten years (Fig. 1). The median age of the population rose from 28 to 30 in this decade due to the increase in elderly and a decrease in the number of children under 15.

Life expectancy after the age of 65 has also increased. The average 65-year-old male can now expect to live to 78 and the female to 82. The longer life expectancy of women has resulted in six million more females than males in the population as a whole and three women for every two men over the age of 65 (Table 2). The gain in life expectancy means that there are large numbers of young-old in their sixties and seventies, who are retired, vigorous, and relatively healthy. This group must find meaningful ways to utilize their time and talents. There are also increasing numbers of old-old in their eighties and nineties, who are often frail and

need a wide range of support services. This latter group is apt to be economically disadvantaged as many of them are immigrants who spent their working lives in low-paying jobs and were unable to save enough to see them through 20 years of retirement.

Distribution of the over-65 population is not equal across the United States. Florida has the highest median age, reflecting the continued popularity of the state as a retirement community. The northeast in general has a higher median age than the rest of the country. Utah, Wyoming, New Mexico, and Alaska have low median ages, probably related to recent rapid population growth of younger people attracted by the expanding mining, manufacturing, and recreation industries.

The 1980 census showed 83.2 percent of the U.S. population reports itself as white, 11.7 percent black, 1.5 percent Asian and Pacific Islander, 0.6 percent Native American, Eskimo, and Aleut. Those of Spanish origin comprised 6.4 percent of the population. The ethnic distribution for the over-65 age group is in Table 3.

Health statistics for the over-65 population indicate that less than 5 percent resides in institutions (Siegel, 1976). Fourteen percent of the non-institutionalized population is restricted in mobility, 12 percent has major restrictions in self-care, and 26 percent spent some time in bed due to illness in the past year (Shanas, 1980). The percentage of elderly reporting problems of mobility, self-care, and illness increases with the age of the population. These

TABLE 1. PERCENTAGE OF POPULATION OVER 65 IN THE UNITED STATES— 1900–2000

Year	Percent
1900	4.1
1940	6.8
1960	9.0
1970	9.8
1980	11.3
2000	12.2*

*Projected by U.S. Bureau of the Census Population Reports Series P-25, 704, 1977. (Source: 1980 Census of Population. Washingtion, D.C., U.S. Department of Commerce, 1981.)

data indicate that in general the elderly are relatively healthy, with 95 percent living in the community, 86 percent of this group able to go out daily, 88 percent able to manage most of their own care, and 79 percent experiencing no illness serious enough to require bed rest.

Major causes of death in this age group reflect the major causes of death for the total population. Most of the causes of death are related to chronic diseases developed over the years (Table 4).

HISTORICAL PERSPECTIVES

The present generation of people over the age of 65 were born in the late 1890s and early 1900s. Born to parents who experienced the Victorian Era's oppressive attitudes towards sexuality and women, this cohort has experienced enormous societal changes during its lifetime.

World events, including World War I, the great depression, World War II, the Cold War, and the development of the Third World, have all had an impact. Major shifts in attitude toward women, sexuality, race, and family structure have taken place.

Technological changes have encompassed the automobile, airplane, spaceship, telephone, electricity, computers, mass production, antibiotics, and life-support systems, to name only a few.

The over-65 age group in the United States may have themselves immigrated to this country or may be the children of the waves of immigrants of the last century. Formal education levels are likely to be lower than in younger groups. These two patterns, however, are rapidly changing. People turning 65 in the late 1980s will be much more likely to be native born and to have formal education, including high school.

Nurses should keep in mind how different the experiences of their aging clients have been from their own. Important differences in attitudes, values, and knowledge between the client and caregiver must be recognized and considered in implementing care.

CULTURAL PERSPECTIVES

Developmental tasks are universal. Adaptive tasks, however, are culturally determined. These tasks in the elderly involve behavior related to living within and accepting physical changes, contracting of life space, seeking new sources of need satisfaction, developing new criteria for self-evaluation, and creating new roles for oneself in life (Clark and Anderson, 1967). Different cultural groups approach these tasks differently.

Culture also influences more general kinds of behavior including:

- Time perception
- Use of space
- Body language
- Kinship behaviors
- Diet
- Rituals
- Health protective behaviors
- Dress
- Hygiene
- Modesty
- Expression of emotion including pain
- Language
- Role behavior
- Perception of illness and health
- Sexuality
- Life-style
- Attitudes toward aging

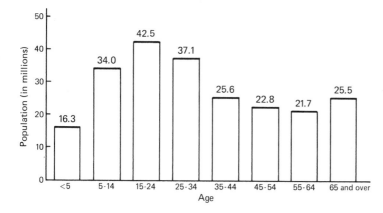

Figure 1. Population distribution by age in the United States in 1980. *From 1980 Census of Population. Washington, D.C., U.S. Department of Commerce, 1981.*

Studies of the elderly in different cultural groups often focus on socioeconomic status as well. Socioeconomic status comprises an important set of variables, including income and education; however, it is separate from culture. Cultural influences are learned and passed on from generation to generation. It is important for the nurse to assess the degree to which an individual identifies with a specific culture. Generalizations and assumptions about the client's behavior based on superficial knowledge of race or ethnic background may lead the nurse to misinterpret the client's behavior or wishes. Factors that are most likely to affect the degree of cultural identification include family ties, length of time in the culture, language, and education.

Leininger (1978) points out that caring practices differ from culture to culture. Nurses need to modify their caring practices to suit the cultural values and beliefs of their clients. Self-care is often given limited value in cultures with strong kinship systems and group behavior. Self-care is much more important in cultures that stress individualism. How, where, and what kind of help is sought when clients are ill or protecting their own health is related to culture. Some clients may seek professional advice from the medical establishment; some will use healers; some seek help to promote health; some seek help only when incapacitated. Certain systems are more important in different cultures. The Irish-American is more concerned with ENT symptoms whereas the Italian is more concerned with gastrointestinal symptoms (Spector, 1979).

Information about different cultural groups and their health practices is growing. A brief summary

TABLE 2. U.S. POPULATION DISTRIBUTION BY SEX 65 YEARS AND OLDER—1980

Age	Male	Female	Both Sexes
65–69	3,902,083	4,878,761	8,780,844
70–74	2,853,116	3,943,626	6,796,742
75–79	1,847,115	2,945,482	4,792,597
80–84	1,018,859	1,915,370	2,934,229
85+	681,428	1,558,293	2,239,721
Total	10,302,601	15,241,532	25,554,113

Source: 1980 Census of Population. Washington, D.C., U.S. Department of Commerce, 1981.

TABLE 3. U.S. POPULATION DISTRIBUTION BY ETHNIC/RACIAL GROUP 65 YEARS AND OLDER—1980

Ethnic/Racial Group	Number
White	22,944,033
Black	1,698,595
Native American	74,788
Eskimo, Aleut, Asian, Pacific Islander	211,834
Spanish origin	708,785

Source: 1980 Census of Population. Washington, D.C., U.S. Department of Commerce, 1981.

TABLE 4.   DEATHS AND DEATH RATES FOR THE TEN LEADING CAUSES OF DEATH IN SPECIFIED
AGE AND SEX GROUPS—1976

Rank	Age, Sex, Cause of Death, and Category Numbers*	Number	Rate per 100,000 Population in Specified Group
	65 Years and Over, Both Sexes		
All causes		*1,245,118*	*5,428.9*
1	Diseases of heart ---------------------- (390–398, 402, 404, 410–429)	548,956	2,393.5
2	Malignant neoplasms, including neoplasms of lymphatic and hematopoietic tissues ---(140–209)	224,543	979.0
3	Cerebrovascular diseases -------------------------------------(430–438)	159,304	694.6
4	Influenza and pneumonia ----------------------- (470–474, 480–486)	48,405	211.1
5	Arteriosclerosis ---(440)	28,032	122.2
6	Diabetes mellitus--(250)	24,797	108.1
7	Accidents--- (E800–E949)	23,961	104.5
8	Bronchitis, emphysema, and asthma ----------------------(490–493)	17,623	76.8
9	Cirrhosis of liver--(571)	8,378	36.5
10	Nephritis and nephrosis --------------------------------------(580–584)	5,732	25.0
	65 Years and Over, Male		
All causes		*624,778*	*6,672.1*
1	Diseases of heart ----------------------- (390–398, 402, 404, 410–429)	272,205	2,906.9
2	Malignant neoplasms, including neoplasms of lymphatic and hematopoietic tissues ---(140–209)	123,983	1,324.0
3	Cerebrovascular diseases -------------------------------------(430–438)	65,052	694.7
4	Influenza and pneumonia ----------------------- (470–472, 480–486)	24,307	259.6
5	Bronchitis, emphysema, and asthma ----------------------(490, 493)	13,315	142.2
6	Accidents--- (E800–E949)	12,527	133.8
7	Arteriosclerosis ---(440)	10,963	117.1
8	Diabetes mellitus--(250)	9,273	99.0
9	Cirrhosis of liver--(571)	5,297	56.6
10	Suicide -- (E950–E959)	3,489	37.3
	65 Years and Over, Female		
All causes		*620,340*	*4,571.1*
1	Diseases of heart ----------------------- (390–398, 402, 404, 410–429)	276,751	2,039.3
2	Malignant neoplasms, including neoplasms of lymphatic and hematopoietic tissues ---(140–209)	100,560	741.0
3	Cerebrovascular diseases -------------------------------------(430, 438)	94,252	694.5
4	Influenza and pneumonia ----------------------- (470–474, 480–486)	24,098	177.6
5	Arteriosclerosis ---(440)	17,069	125.8
6	Diabetes mellitus--(250)	15,524	114.4
7	Accidents--- (E800–E949)	11,434	84.3
8	Bronchitis, emphysema, and asthma ----------------------(490–493)	4,308	31.7
9	Cirrhosis of liver--(571)	3,081	22.7
10	Nephritis and nephrosis --------------------------------------(580–584)	2,763	20.4

*As specified in the Eighth Revision International Classification of Diseases, adopted 1965. *(Source: Facts of Life and Death, PHS Publication 79-1222, 1978.)*

of current knowledge about the more common groups found in the United States follows.

Black Americans

Black Americans represent several cultural groups. The population descended from Africans brought to the United States as slaves is different from the more recent immigrants from Africa and the Carribean Islands. Not all studies differentiate among these groups. In general, the black American reports more illness than white Americans and puts off getting care, especially care of the teeth and eyes (Weeks and Darsky, 1968). The black American equates health or wellness with being able to labor productively. Aging and death are viewed as natural processes leading to "crossing over." Among segments of the population, harmony with nature is sought, and demons and bad spirits are thought to disrupt this harmony (Branch and Paxton, 1976). Folk remedies, diet, prayer, healers, and voodoo are used to deal with disharmony by some (Spector, 1979).

A study of dietary patterns of urban elderly revealed that blacks had significantly poorer nutrition. Males had a significantly poorer diet than females regardless of race (Hunter and Linn, 1979). The same researchers also studied psychosocial adjustment in the elderly, finding black elderly to be the best adjusted. Whites in this study had a lower self-esteem than blacks (Linn et al., 1979). A study of the double jeopardy hypothesis compared a sample of black, white, and Mexican-Americans. Blacks were found to have poorer health and lower income than whites, as were Mexican-Americans. However, *no* differences in measurements of life satisfaction were found (Dowd and Bengtson, 1978). A study by Shanas (1980) on physical function in white and black elderly revealed that blacks had greater decreases in mobility and self-care capacity than whites. Black women had more limitations than black men. Blacks also had twice as much time spent in bed due to illness than the white subjects.

Hispanics

This cultural group includes both Mexican-Americans and Puerto Ricans. Many values and beliefs are similar in both cultures. Some Hispanics view illness as having social, spiritual, and physical origins

and wellness as a holistic balance and equilibrium between the individual and the universe. Illness may be due to fright, a punishment, or supernatural influences. Rituals, prayers, and magic to deal with the evil eye are used in healing by the *espiritualista* or the *curandero*.

The Hispanic may also use herbs, massage, and warm baths to restore balance between hot and cold, dry and moist. Illnesses, foods, and treatments are described as hot, cold, dry, or moist and must be combined appropriately by the care-giver.

The grandparent or godparent role is important in the Hispanic culture and often is an important role for the elderly family member. The extended family is also more common in this group, although erosion of this family structure is a growing phenomenon in younger generations of Hispanics.

Chinese-Americans

The Chinese and to some degree other Asians have a system of beliefs about health, illness, and the practice of medicine that differs greatly from Western beliefs and practices. Emphasis in the East is on prevention, maintaining a balance between energy systems, between the Yang and the Yin.

The Chinese have their own diagnostic techniques, avoid intrusive procedures that they believe affect the wholeness of the system and avoid drawing blood if possible. Herbs, acupuncture, meditation, massage, and diet are all used to treat illness. Healers play an important role in health care.

The elderly have an important role and great respect in Asian cultures. Children are expected to care for their elders. Some of this tradition is present in Asian immigrants in the United States. However, the elderly may expect more than their more Westernized children or grandchildren are prepared to give.

Native Americans

Health beliefs and practices of Native Americans vary from tribe to tribe. Healers are important in many, especially if the tribe relates illness to evil spirits. In general, Native Americans believe that health is God-given and reflects living in harmony with the universe. Many traditional treatments including diet, massage, herbs, and rituals are used.

In some Native American tribes the elderly are

considered a source of wisdom for the younger generation. Direct questioning or asking the individual to repeat information is considered a mark of disrespect.

White Ethnic Americans

Very little is known about health beliefs and practices of the elderly who continue to identify with Irish, Italian, Polish, German, or other European cultures. Cross-cultural studies do reveal differences in expression of pain; differences in diet; differences in life-style; and differences in perception of importance of certain symptoms.

One study examined personality change in late life in Irish-, Italian-, and Polish-American men and women. Increasing interiority occurred, as predicted, except in Irish-American men and to a lesser extent in Irish-American women (Cohler and Lieberman, 1979). Whether this result is a cultural phenomenon is very difficult to evaluate since the degree to which the subjects identify with their European origins is not known.

Another study looked at use of formal social support systems by white ethnic aged. It found that use in this group was generally low. Family, friends, and church groups were more likely to be used for assistance (Guttman, 1979).

Implications of Culture

Many clients may retain health folk practices as links to their cultural heritage in an effort to maintain identity. Most nurses in the United States are socialized into the scientific model of health care. A conflict of beliefs and practices may, therefore, arise between client and nurse. Certainly nurses should not abandon their own respect for science; however, respect for alternative healing methods and traditional health practices should be maintained.

To overcome cultural barriers to health care use of ethnic health providers, ethnic organizations, native languages, and foods should be considered by the nurse in providing care.

RELIGIOUS PERSPECTIVES

A review of the literature by Devine (1980) on studies of attitudes of the elderly toward religion found conflicting data. Whether religion becomes more important as an individual ages is probably idiosyncratic to the client. Attendance at a place of worship does decrease with age; however, this is usually linked to decreased mobility. Clients who have always held strong religious convictions are likely to continue to do so. Practices of a lifetime are likely to be continued as long as possible.

Nurses frequently involve the clergy in care of the elderly, often without consulting the client first. Although for many clients religion may be a significant source of support, studies show this is not universally true. Careful assessment, which goes beyond asking the client's religion, will provide the nurse with the data necessary for individualized care. The client who adheres to strict religious practices may require a special diet and observance of certain rituals. As with culture the nurse should not assume a given client will exhibit a particular attitude or behavior related to religion.

PHILOSOPHICAL PERSPECTIVES

The United States is a highly youth-oriented culture, valuing productivity, physical performance, and physical appearance. The society is fast paced, highly technological, and has little patience with machines or people who slow down, need repair, or are inefficient. For generations emphasis has been on the importance of the individual, independence, self-reliance, the development of the young into responsible, healthy citizens. Use of resources and research has been directed by these values. The result has been a society that devalues the elderly and neglects their needs, often viewing them as obsolete and expendable. In such a society the elderly are often roleless and experience feelings of worthlessness.

The roots of Western society's negative views toward aging and the aged are deep and complex. Society's attitudes have been influenced by the Puritan work ethic, which emphasizes productivity, the pioneering individualism that required good health and stamina to explore new worlds, the mechanistic view of man governed by the laws of entropy derived from Newtonian physics, and a dualistic view of mind and body as separate entities dating from Descartes. The rugged individual—hard working, productive, functioning smoothly, strong body controlled by a well disciplined mind—has emerged as the ideal. This ideal may have been appropriate to times when life spans were shorter and few people lived to experience the changes in functioning that accompany the later years of life. In the 1980s, however, this ideal is no longer relevant.

Newly, again as the result of many diverse factors, values and attitudes related to aging and the aged are being reappraised. The explosion of knowledge and theory related to the nature of human beings and the universe has stimulated the development of a philosophy of becoming. Darwin's evolutionary theory clearly established the human being's natural place in the universe, one species among many, constantly evolving. Humanism focused attention on obligations to others and the development of the self. Field theory in physics and its application to living systems led to an organismic model of the human: holistic, open, evolving, characterized by increasing order, complexity, and heterogeneity. The development of the theory of relativity, the whole field of psychology, and a new application for Eastern philosophy have contributed to this reappraisal of aging. Aging is part of a developmental process that is unidirectional. The individual is always becoming. One grows old to grow beyond. Old age is the culmination of the life process.

Reappraisal of Western society's attitudes and values regarding aging is not only logical and congruent with modern scientific thought; it is also inevitable. The growing number of aged in the population is focusing attention on the needs and problems of the elderly. Research on the aging process and the growing number of healthy aged, reinforced by changing values, is creating an environment for the development of new roles and a sense of worth for the aged. Because of its enlightened attitudes, modern nursing is in an excellent position to contribute to this emerging positive and optimistic reappraisal of aging.

REFERENCES

Branch MF, Paxton PP: Providing Safe Nursing Care for Ethnic People of Color. New York, Appleton-Century-Crofts, 1976

1980 Census of Population. Washington, D.C., U.S. Dept. of Commerce, Bureau of the Census, 1981

Clark M, Anderson B: Culture and Aging. Springfield, IL, Thomas, 1967

Cohler BJ, Lieberman MA: Personality change across the second half of life: Findings from a study of Irish, Italian and Polish-American men and women, in Gelfand DC, Kutzik AJ (eds), Ethnicity and Aging. New York, Springer, 1979

Cowgill D: A theory of aging in cross-cultural perspective, in Cogwill D, Holmes L (eds), Aging and Modernization. New York, Appleton-Century-Crofts, 1972

Crandall RE: Gerontology: A Behavioral Science Approach. Reading, MA, Addison-Wesley, 1980

Davitz L, Yasuko S, Davitz J: Suffering as viewed in six different cultures. American Journal of Nursing 76(8):1296, 1976

Devine BA: Attitudes of the elderly toward religion. Journal of Gerontological Nursing 6(11):679, 1980

Dowd JJ, Bengston VL: Aging in minority populations, an examination of the double jeopardy hypothesis. Journal of Gerontology, 33(3):427, 1978

Ebersole P, Hess P: Toward Healthy Aging. St. Louis, Mosby, 1981

Facts of Life and Death. Washington D.C., PHS Publication 79, 1978, p 1122

Gelfand DE, Kutzik AJ (eds): Ethnicity and Aging. New York, Springer, 1979

Gilson P, Coats S: A study of morale in low income blacks. Journal of Gerontological Nursing 6(7):385, 1980

Gioiella EC: Aging: A reappraisal. Nursing Forum 17(4):395, 1978

Guttman D: Use of informal and formal supports by white ethnic aged, in Gelfand DE, Kutzik AJ (eds), Ethnicity and Aging. New York, Springer, 1979

Harwood A (ed): Ethnicity and Medical Care. Cambridge, MA, Harvard University Press, 1981

Hunter KI, Linn MW: Cultural and sex differences in dietary patterns of the urban elderly. Journal of the American Geriatrics Society 27(8):359, 1979

Leininger M: Transcultural Nursing. New York, Wiley, 1978

Linn MW, Hunter KI, Perry PR: Differences by sex and ethnicity in psychological adjustment of the elderly. Journal of Health and Social Behavior 20(3):273, 1979

Martinez RA (ed): Hispanic Culture and Health Care: Fact, Fiction, Folklore. St. Louis, Mosby, 1978

Moriwaki SY: Ethnicity and aging, in Burnside IM (ed), Nursing and the Aged. New York, McGraw-Hill, 1981

Meyerhoff BG, Simic A (eds): Life's Career—Aging: Cultural Variations in Growing Old. Beverly Hills, CA, Sage, 1978

Our Future Selves. Washington D.C., NIH Publication 78, 1978, p 1143

Palmore E (ed): International Handbook of Aging. West-port, CT, Greenwood, 1980

Shanas E: Self-assessment of physical function in white and black elderly of the United States. Epidemiology of Aging. Washington D.C., NIH Publication 80, July, 1980, p 969

Siegel JS: Demographic aspects of aging and the older population in the U.S. Current Population Reports. Washington, D.C., U.S. Bureau of the Census, 1976

Spector RE: Cultural Diversity in Health and Illness. New York, Appleton-Century-Crofts, 1979

Spicker S, Woodward K, Van Tassel D (eds): Aging and the Elderly. Atlantic Highlands, NY, Humanities Press, 1978

Weeks HA, Darsky BJ: The Urban Aged: Race and Medical Care. Ann Arbor, University of Michigan Press, 1968

Wilson HS, Heinert J: Los viejatos, the old ones. Journal of Gerontological Nursing 3:19, 1977

2

An Organizing Framework for the Nursing Process

This book uses the concepts of stress and adaptation as the basis for defining health and illness, assessing health status, and determining nursing roles with the aging. Within the organizational framework of stress and adaptation the responses the aging exhibit in light of their health status and the factors most likely to precipitate changes in their health status can be discussed. The concepts of stress and adaptation also provide the basis for selecting nursing interventions appropriate for aging clients at all positions on the health continuum.

This chapter discusses the concepts of stress and adaptation as they are used throughout this text. It also incorporates these terms with the phases of the nursing process and demonstrates how the process is used to assist aging clients maintain or improve their functioning.

RATIONALE FOR USE OF A STRESS AND ADAPTATION FRAMEWORK

The Nature of Man

People have been described as energy fields, always striving to achieve higher levels of functioning as they interact with and exchange energy with their environment. Because people are unitary, with many different but related aspects, a change in just one aspect affects their entire energy field (Rogers, 1970).

Problems exist with almost any attempt to organize the various aspects of a person into different categories. Although such an arbitrary division is useful to assure completeness and clarity when studying people and their behaviors, categorization can result in both omission and overlap. Rogers (1970) has identified four dimensions of unitary man. Roy (1973) has identified four modes within which people change in response to environmental stimuli. Engel (1962) has divided man into biologic and physiologic systems and suggested that all behaviors are a product of processing by either the central nervous system or the mental apparatus.

Throughout this text, the person's many aspects as well as the behaviors that reflect those aspects will be categorized as either physical or psychosocial.

What Constitutes Health?

Repeated attempts to define health and illness throughout the years have resulted in some expansion of the scope of the definition. Health and illness have been viewed as two distinct and parallel entities. The 1949 definition of health by the World Health Organization reflects this view. Health and illness have also been described as different aspects of a single concept and represented as a continuum or as levels (Engel, 1962; Dubos, 1965). An adequate definition of health should consider that people are holistic, constantly interacting with their environment and continuously changing. It should also recognize that both health and illness are relative concepts. By virtue of their multiple aspects, people cannot be described as either completely healthy or totally ill.

In this text, *health is viewed as a dynamic state in the life cycle, during which the person is func-*

tioning at an optimum level. Health is dependent upon developmental, situational, and cultural factors. Health implies that the person is continuously adapting to stresses in the internal and external environments in ways which promote optimal functioning and movement toward achievement of full potential.

As people age, they grow in uniqueness and complexity. Elderly people cope with a great number of factors that may alter their health status and, in turn, their level of functioning. The diversity and complexity of this population make nursing's role with the aging particularly challenging.

The Nurse's Role in Promoting Optimal Functioning

The focus of nursing is on the whole human being in interaction with the environment (Fuller, 1978). Nursing has a role to play with people at all levels of functioning. In fact, the selection of nursing interventions will be influenced by the client's level of functioning. The goal of nursing is to assist clients to function at their highest level as they interact with the stimuli, or stresses, presented by their environment.

To achieve client goals, all professionals use the problem-solving process (Mauksch and David, 1972). It is an intentional and systematic process by which client problems are identified and solved. Nursing's unique way of using the problem-solving process is the nursing process. By allowing the nurse to consider the client's wholeness and uniqueness, it enables the nurse to provide comprehensive and individualized care. Four phases of the nursing process have been identified—assessment, planning, implementation, and evaluation (Yura and Walsh, 1973). These phases have been incorporated with the concepts of stress and adaptation and then used to provide appropriate nursing care to clients at all levels of functioning.

STRESS AND ADAPTATION

The concepts of stress and adaptation presented in this chapter do not reflect the thinking of one particular theorist. Instead, concepts developed by Hans Selye, George Engel, and Callista Roy have been drawn upon and modified for use. Although stress has been defined and used in several divergent ways, many writers have described stress as a stimulus or process with negative connotations. For these theorists, stress is to be avoided if people are to maintain either health or high level functioning. Some writers have used the term adaptation to indicate only those organism responses that suggest adjustment, promote health, or indicate optimal functioning (Goosen and Bush, 1979).

In this text, stress and adaptation have neither negative nor positive associations. Rather, they are a natural part of living. Stresses cannot be avoided. As people move through life, they constantly adapt to stresses. To do so is to live.

Stress

Definition of Stress. *Stress is defined as an input of energy into any system—individual, family, or group—that results in a repatterning of that system.* Stress includes factors that, by virtue of either their presence or absence, precipitate change in a system. Always present in our internal and external environments, stresses are the agents responsible for the constant changes occurring in individuals.

A stress serves as a stimulus. Its energy input produces a consequent energy expenditure by the person affected. Energy is exchanged but not necessarily used up. As a result, there is a modification in the person's pattern and organization that is manifested by behavior changes.

Because stress is a neutral factor, the changes it produces are not necessarily either beneficial or harmful. The changes people exhibit in response to a stress are highly individual, with differences depending not only on characteristics of the stress but on certain characteristics of the individual and the environment at the time the interaction occurs. Stresses serve as the stimuli people need in order to perform tasks appropriate to their developmental stage and reach optimal functioning and full potential. At times, however, people's responses to stress may place their well-being at risk or limit their level of functioning.

Categories of Stress. Four categories of stress— focal, contextual, residual, and potential—interact with the client at any point in time and precipitate behavior changes. This typology is a modification of that developed by Roy (1970). When assessing the client, the nurse should ascertain all four types of stress.

A focal stress is that immediately confronting the client and identified by either the nurse or client as the most important, or top priority, stress. This is the stress that requires immediate nursing intervention. At times, a client may be confronted simultaneously with two or more focal stresses. When this situation occurs, all focal stresses have equal priority and must be dealt with simultaneously.

A contextual stress is a stimulus presented to the client at the same time as the focal stress; however, it is of less importance than the focal stress. As a consequence of the complex nature of the client's internal and external environments, numerous contextual stresses are present simultaneously. Contextual stresses are important because they influence how the client responds to the focal stress. In addition, as the client adapts to the focal stress, contextual stresses may take on new importance and become focal stresses.

A residual stress includes any factor from the client's past that is relevant to the present situation. Residual stresses are an important source of data that can assist the nurse to predict the nature of the client's responses to the focal stress. The client's genetic background and family history form an important source of residual stresses. In addition, the client's previous positive or negative experiences with residual stresses relevant to the focal stress affect the nature of the responses to the focal stress.

A potential stress is any future stress that is predictable because of the client's focal, contextual, or residual stresses or responses to those stresses. For example, the nurse can predict that an elderly client with the stress of degeneration of the auditory nerve will experience a variety of future stresses, such as impaired group social activities. The goal of the nurse, in this case, is to intervene to alter the client's responses to potential stress.

Characteristics of Stress. Every stress, whether focal, contextual, residual, or potential, possesses certain qualitative and quantitative characteristics

that influence the nature of the client's responses. Gathering data about these characteristics adds to the nurse's ability to predict accurately how the client will respond to a stress.

Qualitatively, stresses are categorized as physical or psychosocial. Although clients respond holistically to stress, each stress impacts initially on one particular aspect of the client. Physical stresses include stimuli that interact initially with the client's physiologic aspects. Psychosocial stresses are generally processed first by the client's mental–emotional apparatus.

Physical stresses include factors from either the internal or external environment that may precipitate change whenever they interact with the person or only under certain conditions—by contacting one particular body part, by being present in excessive or deficient amounts, or by being absent altogether. Some physical stresses require an intermediary, such as an insect, animal, or another person, if they are to precipitate responses in people. Many parasites and microorganisms stimulate change in this fashion.

Examples of physical stresses include exposure to sun, heat, cold, radiation, or electricity. Medications, whether ingested in prescribed, insufficient, or excessive quantities, are physical stresses. Poisons, vitamins, and minerals are other physical stresses. Contact with mechanical forces, whether a back massage or head-on collision, serve as physical stresses. Gastric juice, whether present normally in the stomach, in insufficient amounts in an aging client, or in an inappropriate location such as the esophagus, is a physical stress. In each instance, it precipitates a unique set of responses.

Psychosocial stresses are those that precipitate change upon being perceived and experienced by the client and then represented at either the conscious or unconscious level. Psychosocial stresses need not be actually present to the client; they may be threatened or imagined. Three groups of psychosocial stresses are loss, injury, and frustration of drives or needs. Psychosocial stresses are a frequent source of stimulus to the aging. They often experience changes in or loss of certain body functions, loss of friends and loved ones, loss of status within their family group, and changes in long-time residence and life-style. Many aging people cling to old worn-out clothing or furniture or remain in a residence in a deteriorating neighborhood because these objects are invested with memories, and their loss would be far greater than the material value of the object. For some isolated elderly a pet can be their most important living object, and its loss is profoundly felt. The threat of injury is another stress experienced by many elderly, particularly in declining urban neighborhoods, and may be a stimulus for the aging to limit their social activities after dark. The aging also must deal with stresses that threaten to frustrate built-in biological drives that require satisfaction at all developmental stages. The current prohibition against sexual activity in most homes for the aged is an example of the conflict that can occur when external controls are imposed to inhibit or deflect drive impulses.

To demonstrate how the client responds holistically to stress, consider how an aging couple might respond to the psychosocial stress of loss of job and income when forced to retire. The husband might respond emotionally with changes in his self-image and feelings of depression. If the couple's retirement income is inadequate they may be required to reduce their social activities or participate in fewer or less costly leisure activities. In addition, if the loss of income requires them to limit the quantity and quality of foods they buy, the stress may affect the couple physically, producing vitamin deficiencies, weight loss, or malnutrition. On the other hand, loss of income might stimulate the couple to seek instruction on budget meal planning and result in an ultimate improvement in nutritional status.

Two quantitative characteristics of stress affect the nature of the client's responses. *The amount of stimulus provided by a stress should be considered.* Exposure to organisms in the measles vaccine stimulates a different response than would exposure to a person with measles. Elderly clients living in quarters without air conditioning respond differently to summer temperatures of 80°F than to ones of 100°F. *Quantity also has to do with the total number of stresses simultaneously impinging on a client.* Since responding to stress requires an energy expenditure by the client, the presence of numerous concurrent stresses may be a strain on the client's energy reserves and a reason why the client might respond to some or all the stresses in less than optimal ways.

Adaptation

Adaptation includes all those responses a system exhibits when it interacts with a stress. Because people, by nature, have numerous interrelated aspects and respond holistically, numerous adaptations occur simultaneously in response to a single stress. Some of these adaptations may be readily apparent. Others may be more subtle, more complex, and, hence, more difficult to identify. Adaptations encompass the universe of a client's responses to stress, not merely those indicative of disease. Adaptations may involve responses that improve, maintain, threaten, or reduce the client's level of functioning.

Adaptations have two separate but related components—a behavioral component and a process component. The behavioral component of adaptation includes all observable or measurable behaviors a system exhibits when responding to a stress. The nurse can readily gather data about the client's observable, measurable behaviors by performing a health history and physical assessment. The behavioral component of adaptation includes any client behaviors the nurse ascertains through one of the senses. Client laboratory data are also included.

The second component of adaptation involves all the unseen processes—physiologic, pathophysiologic, intrapsychic, or psychosocial—a system exhibits in response to stress. The processes serve as the scientific explanation linking each of the client's stresses to the corresponding behavior. The process component of adaptation explains how and why the behavioral component occurs.

For example, the nurse may observe that following the death of her spouse, a previously vivacious and happy woman weeps often, talks about her husband frequently, and complains of loss of appetite and poor sleeping habits. These constitute the behavioral component of adaptation. Depression might be the process component, the psychodynamics that link the death of her spouse to the changed behaviors observed in the client.

When adaptations are less than optimal they may become stresses that precipitate additional adaptations. For example, in response to the stress of aging, the size of the pupil decreases, allowing less light into the eye. This adaptation may be an additional stress to the person leading to a variety of other adaptations. For example, the person may use a brighter light for reading, may discontinue nighttime driving, and, because of shadows, dim light, and other factors, may fall at night when going to the bathroom (Hayter, 1974). The fall is an example of an adaptation that becomes a stress because it precipitates a fracture and a variety of adaptations including the changes involved with reduced mobility. Nursing interventions are aimed at interrupting this cascading effect and assisting clients to adapt in the most optimal ways. For example, in order to prevent the stress of fracture and its resulting adaptations related to immobility, the nurse could help the client arrange a route to the bathroom that was uncluttered and assure that the client has a light that can be reached from bed at night.

Characteristics of Adaptation. Like stress, numerous characteristics of adaptation can be useful in predicting the nature of the client's adaptation to a particular stress. When gathering data about the client's adaptation, the nurse should consider each of the following characteristics.

1. Because individuals are holistic, they can be expected to exhibit numerous adaptations in response to a single stress. In consideration of the client's physical and psychosocial aspects, the nurse should identify both physical and psychosocial adaptations. Physical adaptations generally involve the physical structure and function of the client. Psychosocial adaptations may involve the client's intrapsychic responses or relationships with other individuals, groups, or society. For example, in response to the stress of swollen joints, an arthritic client may experience physical adaptations such as pain and limited joint mobility and psychosocial adaptations such as depression or social isolation.

2. Since individuals are constantly changing, the adaptations they exhibit also change. In order to maintain an accurate and correct assessment of the client, the nurse must observe for changes in adaptation frequently and regularly.

3. Because their aim is to achieve their highest level of functioning, people adapt to stresses in the most effective way they can at any given point in time. Unfortunately, people are not always able to adapt in a fashion that will enhance or maintain their level of functioning. An important

goal for the nurse is to support, modify, or supplement clients' adaptations in a fashion that will assist them toward their goal of optimal functioning.

4. Adaptation involves the expenditure of energy. When a person adapts optimally, energy is conserved and the amount expended is minimal. When people adapt in less than optimal ways, they may do so either because their energy reserves have been depleted as a result of interaction with multiple stresses or because they are expending their energy in inefficient or ineffective ways. Nursing care is aimed at assisting clients to conserve their energy and expend it more efficiently or effectively. The nurse does this by offering the client alternative ways of adapting, thus increasing the options for energy expenditure.

5. Health status influences the nature of adaptation to stress. By depleting the client's energy reserves and reducing the level of functioning, disease tends to reduce the client's ability to cope effectively with other stresses. For this reason, chronically ill people are much more vulnerable to the influences of microorganisms. This is the basis for recommending that the chronically ill be immunized prophylactically against influenza.

6. Developmental stage influences the nature of adaptation to stress. Because energy reserves vary at each developmental stage, so do the options for responding to stress. In general, the very young and the very old have less flexibility in adaptation. For example, response to loss varies widely according to the person's developmental stage. A 3-year-old child will adapt to the death of a mother or father much differently than the person of 55 who loses an aged parent. Physical stresses also affect people at different developmental stages in different ways. For example, the stiffening of the rib cage, loss of lung elasticity, and weakened cough in the aging are factors that influence how they will respond to the stress of respiratory microorganisms.

7. Adaptations vary according to the amount of time the person has to prepare for a stress. In many cases, having time to prepare for interaction with a stress aids people to respond in beneficial ways. When certain stresses impinge without warning upon people, the capacity to adapt optimally may be affected.

8. Adaptations are influenced by the amount of time the person spends in interaction with a stress.

Often, the longer a stress interacts wtih the person, the more complex the adaptations become.

9. The person's environment influences the nature of adaptation to stress. For example, responses of an aging client with arthritis whose apartment is accessible by elevator will be different from those of a client who must climb several flights of stairs.

LEVELS OF ADAPTATION

Data regarding the client's stresses and adaptations are used to make an assessment of the client's overall level of functioning, referred to as the level of adaptation. The levels of adaptation form a continuum. Each level indicates the way the client is adapting to stresses, the degree of independent functioning possible, and the nature of nursing intervention required. Clients move from one level of adaptation to another as a function of changing stresses, adaptations, and nursing interventions.

Five levels of adaptation have been identified.

Level One—Maintenance of Optimal Functioning

Individuals at Level One function as integrated wholes within the context of their situation, culture, and developmental stage. People strive toward this ideal level of adaptation, which represents optimal functioning and self-actualization.

Level Two—Maintenance of Optimal Functioning with Potential Threat

Individuals at Level Two function independently as integrated wholes within the context of their society, but they fall into a "high risk" group. Due to their stresses or adaptations, these people are at risk for a change in health status and thus a change in level of adaptation.

Certain occupations, such as coal mining, place individuals at risk for adaptations that affect health status. The increased number of losses faced by the aging place them at risk for adaptations such as depression. Previous life patterns, such as smoking, excessive drinking, or limited exercise, are other factors that place the aging at risk for changes in health status.

Level Three—Maintenance of Optimal Functioning with an Aid Required

Individuals at Level Three have an identified health problem that is managed with the aid of structural, physiologic, or psychosocial supports. Such people are able to live independently within the community performing activities expected at their particular developmental stage provided they continue to utilize certain supports. Examples of physiologic supports include false teeth, eyeglasses, hearing aids, wheelchairs, home hemodialysis, and daily medication or special diet and exercise regimens. Psychosocial supports would include attendance at group therapy sessions, or regular appointments with a nurse mental-health clinician.

Level Four—Less Than Optimal Functioning: Adaptations Become Stresses

Individuals at Level Four exhibit adaptations that produce a separate and additional stress that impairs their structure or ability to function. People are unable to function independently in society and are no longer in complete control of the adaptations they exhibit. They are partially dependent on intervention by nurses and others, such as social workers or physicians, in order to perform activities of daily living or meet basic human needs. People at Level Four usually require hospitalization.

Any person requiring surgical intervention to alter an adaptation is at Level Four. So too would be the man who responded to the death of his spouse by developing a psychotic depression. If he failed to eat, drink or care for his basic needs, these adaptations would be eventual stresses precipitating additional adaptations such as dehydration or malnutrition.

Level Five—Optimal Functioning Appears Impossible

As people move down the levels of adaptation, they become less able to function in society and more dependent upon direct nursing care. Individuals at Level Five lack the energy to respond to stress in an effective fashion. They are no longer in control of their own behaviors and are totally dependent on members of the health team to meet basic needs. They require ongoing nursing care for basic survival. People who are unconscious or require life-support systems, those with life-threatening illnesses, and the elderly with advanced cerebral vascular insufficiency are at Level Five.

STRESS, ADAPTATIONS, AND ASSESSMENT

Client assessment involves two phases—data gathering related to the client's stresses and adaptations and judgment concerning the level at which the client is adapting. The client's behavioral adaptations comprise the most accessible portion of the data base. Often, stresses cannot be directly observed but must be inferred from the client's behavioral adaptations. Clients may not have insight into the stresses precipitating their behavioral adaptations. The nurse uses data from the client and other sources, coupled with nursing knowledge, to hypothesize about the nature of the client's stresses. As the data base increases, the hypotheses may be confirmed, stated in more specific terms, or revised. Behavioral adaptations, stresses, and knowledge from nursing science and physical, psychological, and social sciences are all used to make inferences regarding the process component of the client's adaptations.

The nurse then compares the data base with the levels of adaptation and makes a judgment regarding the client's level of adaptation. This judgment would be revised to reflect ongoing data collection as well as changes in the client's stresses and adaptations.

If the nurse is assessing an 80-year-old woman who has just been admitted to the emergency room, behavioral adaptations such as displacement of bones in the right forearm, swelling and discoloration on the right arm and other extremities, rapid pulse, weeping, and moaning can be ascertained immediately. Based on these data, the nurse could hypothesize that the client's focal stress is trauma. Later, after gathering more data, the nurse might further specify the stress as "a fall" or "a mugging." Information related to this stress and its behavioral adaptations would lead the nurse to infer that pain, anxiety, and the inflammatory process comprised a portion of the process component of this client's

adaptations. The nurse would identify this client's level of adaptation as Level Four.

NURSING INTERVENTION AT FIVE LEVELS OF ADAPTATION

The levels of adaptation provide the nurse with guidelines for selecting goals and nursing actions appropriate for each client. In the planning phase of the nursing process, the nurse sets goals aimed at promoting the client's optimal level of functioning.

Goals
Setting client goals is a process that should involve active participation by the client as well as the nurse. Mutual decisions should be reached regarding which stresses and adaptations take priority and what approaches would be best.

Both stresses and adaptations are targets for setting client goals. If the client is functioning at Level One, it is likely that many of the stresses impinging on the client are precipitating beneficial adaptations; thus, they would not require modification. However, if the client is functioning at a lower level of adaptation, altering one or more of the client's stresses may be desirable.

It is often possible to alter the client's contextual stresses, thus providing the client with an environment more conducive to optimal adaptation. There are fewer opportunities for the nurse to alter the client's focal stress. The nurse cannot heal a fracture, stimulate a pancreas to produce insulin, or bring a dead spouse back to life.

Goals aimed at the client's adaptations are often more realistic and achievable than are those aimed at stresses. The nurse may choose to reinforce, supplement, modify, or replace adaptations. If the client is functioning at Level One, the client's adaptations may require only reinforcement. At Level Two, however, clients may require new, more beneficial adaptations or a modification of current adaptations in order to slow movement toward a lower level of function. Goals for clients at Level Three, who often have chronic health problems, should be aimed at supporting those beneficial adaptations preventing clients from moving to a lower level of function.

Since clients at Levels Four and Five are exhibiting adaptations that are reducing their ability to function independently, goals are aimed at modifying or replacing client adaptations with ones that are more likely to promote optimal functioning.

Nursing Actions

Each level of adaptation provides guidelines for choosing broad nursing actions. These should be modified to reflect each client's individuality.

Level One.   At this level, nursing actions to maintain high-level function are appropriate. These include research and publication activities, health education, health assessment, and health-related legislative activities.

Level Two.   Nursing actions at this level are preventive in nature and include physical assessment, health screening, case finding, supportive care during diagnostic testing, preventative health teaching and counseling, and referral. Nurses who work with clients at this level often work as change agents and client advocates.

Level Three.   In order to maintain their independence, clients at this level require both supportive and preventative actions. Important actions include teaching proper use of aids and supports and ongoing counseling to assure continued adaptation at Level Three. Periodic reassessment and reevaluation as well as referral are other appropriate nursing actions. Nurses who work with clients at Level Three often function as part of complex interdisciplinary teams utilizing both collaborative and leadership skills.

Level Four.   Since people at this level have few energy reserves available, the nurse must assist clients to conserve them. Providing safety measures, comfort and treatment measures, and direct assistance with hygiene and other activities of daily living are frequent nursing actions with clients at Level Four. Ongoing assessment and client teaching are also appropriate.

Level Five.   Clients at this level are totally dependent upon nursing care for maintenance of function. Use of sophisticated technology for treatment, provision of comfort and safety, and rapid reassessment and reevaluation are among the nursing actions employed. Supportive nursing care for dying clients is also essential here.

Evaluation

Cyclical by nature, the nursing process terminates with the evaluation phase. Here, the nurse once again utilizes the stress and adaptation framework to assess effectiveness of nursing actions in reaching client goals. Data generated in this phase reflect changes in client stresses and adaptations and serve as the basis for revisions in nursing interventions.

Using the Stress and Adaptation Framework

In this book, the information about aging and the nurse's role with older people has been organized according to levels of adaptation. Part II of the text focuses on the healthy older person who is functioning optimally at Level One. The aging process is viewed as a stress that precipitates a complex series of normal, predictable physical and psychosocial adaptations. Nursing interventions are aimed at supporting and reinforcing clients who are adapting in an optimal fashion.

Part III identifies common stresses, such as loss, retirement, and loneliness, that affect the majority of older people. Although these stresses need not impair the ability of an older person to function independently, they may negatively affect the ability to adapt in optimal ways. Nursing interventions for older clients at Level Two are aimed at using techniques such as screening and casefinding to identify clients at risk and then preventing these clients from moving to a lower level of adaptation through strategies such as group work and crisis intervention.

Part IV discusses common health problems among older people that usually place them on Level Three. In most cases, these are lifelong problems, such as diabetes mellitus, osteoporosis, arthritis, or hearing loss. Each health problem is viewed as a stress that has the potential to stimulate a predictable series of adaptations in the older person. However, with appropriate intervention, many clients with these health problems are able to function independently most of the time. Nursing interventions discussed here include helping older clients manage medication, exercise regimens, therapeutic diets, and activities of daily living so that they can continue to maintain their independence. Older clients who have chronic health problems but continue to function independently with the help of such support systems exhibit an optimal level of adaptation.

In contrast to the health problems in Part IV that place older clients at Level Three, those selected for Part V are stresses to which older clients are usually unable to adapt in an optimal way. For this reason, the older client moves to Level Four. Again, while adaptations can be predicted, they often become additional stresses that simply deplete the client's limited resources. Among the health problems discussed here are myocardial infarction, cerebrovascular accident, fractures, and cancer. Often the older client requires hospitalization or surgery. Active nursing intervention on a temporary or long-term basis is required to help these clients meet basic needs. With appropriate nursing intervention many older clients at Level Four recover partially or completely and move to a higher level of adaptation.

Renal disease is the example used in Part VI to discuss how health problems may be stresses to which the older client is unable to adapt. Older clients at Level Five depend completely on the health care system and the nurse to meet all their needs. Although some clients who move to Level Five regain the ability to adapt, others do not. The nurse's role then involves helping the client and significant others to cope with death. Part VI discusses this important nursing intervention.

REFERENCES

Brower TF, Baker BJ: The Roy adaptation model using the adaptation model in a practitioner curriculum. Nursing Outlook 24(11):686, 1976

Cannon WB: The Wisdom of the Body, revised and enlarged edition. New York, Norton, 1939

Dubos R: Man Adapting. New Haven, CT, Yale University Press, 1965

Dunn HL: High Level Wellness. Arlington, VA, Beatty, 1961

Engel GL: Psychological Development in Health and Disease. Philadelphia, Saunders Company, 1962

Erikson E: Childhood and Society. New York, Norton, 1950

Fuller SS: Holistic man and the science and practice of nursing. Nursing Outlook 26(11):700, 1978

Goosen GA, Bush HA: Adaptation: A feedback process. Advances in Nursing Science 1(4):51, 1979

Gunter LM, Miller JC: Toward a nursing gerontology. Nursing Research 26(3):208, 1977

Guzzetia CC: Relationship between stress and learning. Advances in Nursing Science 1(4):35, 1979

Hayter J: Biologic changes of aging. Nursing Forum XIII (3):289, 1974

Helson H: Adaptation Level Theory. New York, Harper and Row, 1964

Jacox A: Theory construction in nursing: An overview. Nursing Research 23(1):4, 1974

Jones PS: An adaptation model for nursing practice. American Journal of Nursing 78(11):1900, 1978

Lawton MP: Social ecology and the health of older people. American Journal of Public Health 64(3):257, 1974

Mauksch IG, David ML: Prescription for survival. American Journal of Nursing 72(12):2189, 1972

Porth CM: Physiological coping: A model for teaching pathophysiology. Nursing Outlook 25(12):781, 1977

Riehl JP, Roy Sister C: Conceptual Models for Nursing Practice. New York, Appleton-Century-Crofts, 1974

Rogers ME: An Introduction to the Theoretical Basis of Nursing Practice. Philadelphia, Davis, 1970

Roy Sister C: Adaptation: A conceptual framework for nursing. Nursing Outlook 18(3):42, 1970

Roy Sister C: Adaptation: A basis for nursing practice. Nursing Outlook 19(4):254, 1971

Roy Sister C: Adaptation: Implications for curriculum change. Nursing Outlook 21(3):163, 1973

Roy Sister C: Introduction to Nursing: An Adaptation Model. Englewood Cliffs, NJ, Prentice-Hall, 1976

Roy Sister C: The Roy adaptation model. Comment. Nursing Outlook 24(11):690, 1976

Roy Sister C: Relating nursing theory to eduction: A new era. Nurse Educator IV(2):16, 1979

Roy Sister C, Obloy Sister M: The practitioner movement—Toward a science of nursing. American Journal of Nursing 78(10):1698, 1978

Selye H: The Stress of Life, revised edition. New York, McGraw-Hill, 1976

Selye H: The stress syndrome. American Journal of Nursing 65(3):97, 1965

Selye H: Stress Without Distress. Philadelphia, Lippincott, 1974

Selye H: A code for coping with stress. AORN Journal 25(1):35, 1977

Toffler A: Future Shock. New York, Random House, 1970

Wayner P: The Roy adaptation model—testing the adaptation model in practice. Nursing Outlook 24(11):682, 1976

Yura H, Walsh MB: The Nursing Process: Assessment, Planning, Implementing, Evaluating. New York, Appleton-Century-Crofts, 1973

3

Aging: Prospective Roles for the Nurse

PROFESSIONAL NURSING TODAY

Modern professional nursing is a humanistic applied science that encompasses knowledge and behavior that influence the health status of clients. The goal of nursing is to facilitate optimal adaptation through promotion, prevention, care, and restoration activities. These activities include improving health care services and enhancing the quality of life by removing barriers to health throughout the life span.

Professional nursing in the 1980s is moving forward in several dimensions. Increasing autonomy and accountability as well as scope characterize nursing practice. Growing public acceptance of expanding roles is developing. A theoretical base for practice is being built through empirical research. Pressures from inside and outside the profession to clarify preparation for practice issues and to meet health care needs in cost-effective ways are stimulating change. The development of gerontological nursing as a specialty area of nursing practice reflects all of these growing dimensions.

THE EVOLUTION OF GERONTOLOGICAL NURSING

Gerontology, the study of the normal aging process, is a young science. Some research on aging was conducted in the early part of the twentieth century but major investment of energy in this field did not occur until the 1950s. The delay in the development of this science is probably related to the emphasis

on youth in our culture as well as to anxiety provoked when examining the years leading to death. However, the growing numbers and influence of elderly people in Western society stimulated increased interest and resources devoted to gerontology following World War II.

A related area of growing interest, geriatrics, is the study of diseases associated with aging and their medical treatment. The difference between these two areas is significant. Gerontology studies the nature of the older organism, how it changes over time. It uses controlled inquiry into the differences between old and young that reflect the aging process. The importance of distinguishing the effects of disease, history, and society from the effects of aging per se is crucial to this science. Methodological problems are enormous but gradually yielding to sophisticated design and analysis. Developments in gerontology will have a profound influence on geriatrics. Geriatricians often do not know which adaptations they are treating are the result of illness or aging, which are normal or abnormal, which are reversible or evolving. As gerontological knowledge expands more sophisticated geriatric practice will develop.

The development of a specialized field of interest related to care of the elderly in nursing reflects the evolution of nursing as an independent health-oriented profession. The establishment of an ANA Division of Geriatric Nursing Practice in 1966 recognized that treatment of illness in elderly clients differed from care of the ill in younger age groups. In 1976 the name of the division was changed to

Division of Gerontological Nursing Practice, thus acknowledging the importance of nursing care of the healthy elderly. Nursing is concerned with normal aging and illnesses related to the aging process. Nurses must distinguish adaptations that are a normal part of aging from those related to illness in the elderly.

A modern definition of nursing gerontology was stated by Gunter and Miller (1977) as ". . . the scientific study of nursing care of the elderly. It is characterized as an applied science, since its aim is to use knowledge of the aging process to design nursing care and services which provide for health, longevity, and independence—on highest level of functioning possible—in the aging and the aged." Gerontological nursing practice is characterized by application of knowledge of age-related changes, care of clients experiencing chronic illnesses and multiple pathologies, use of a myriad of uncoordinated health and social services, and the most diverse and complex client population in nursing.

The ANA Division of Gerontological Nursing has agreed that gerontological nursing practice involves the ability to incorporate an understanding of the following into nursing practice:

• The ramifications of normal aging that may be supported through health promotion
• The different rates at which people age
• The variable characteristics of the older population
• The interrelationship between the cultural, social, spiritual, economic, psychological, and biological factors
• The multiplicity and collectiveness of an older person's losses
• The grief work necessary in accepting multiple overlapping losses
• The frequently atypical response of the older adult to disease and to the treatment of disease
• The accumulated, often disabling effects of multiple chronic illnesses or degenerative processes
• The cultural values associated with aging and social attitudes toward the older adult

Many nurses in general practice care for elderly clients. These nurses may or may not be gerontological nurses. The gerontological nurse has acquired the specialized knowledge of nursing ger-

ontology and has selected to practice with, or teach or study about, the elderly client. Gerontological nurses may work in a variety of settings but the focus of their practice is the aged and aging. Gerontological nurse practitioners have advanced skills in assessment, are graduates of certificate or master's degree programs, and are capable of providing primary care for elderly clients. The gerontological clinical nurse specialist is prepared as a highly skilled clinician at the master's level of education. Nurses may also apply for certification as gerontological nurses. Certification is based on examination and practice credentials and is handled by the American Nurses' Association.

Despite the development of gerontological nursing as a specialty, few professional nurses choose this field of practice. Working conditions, salary, and status of nurses working with this population, especially in nursing homes, are frequently lower than for nurses in other fields of practice (Burnside, 1981). Nurses caring for the elderly expressed the highest level of job dissatisfaction in a survey done in 1977 (Godfrey, 1978). Unsafe practices, poor leadership, and poor communication were cited as the major causes of job dissatisfaction in that study. Those conditions that lead to job dissatisfaction tend to be worse in agencies caring for elderly clients. For some time researchers have hypothesized that negative myths, stereotypes, and attitudes have also contributed to the low preference for gerontological nursing practice.

Attitudes vary with age, self-concept, past experience, and sociocultural and religious values. The elderly are the most stereotyped of any age group. Beliefs influence attitudes, which in turn influence feelings. Negative presentation of the elderly in literature, on television, and in jokes all contribute to negative beliefs. Fear of the changes associated with aging such as wrinkles, loss of muscle tone, slowness, dependence, and approaching death also contributes to negative attitudes. Poor parental relationships or negative childhood experiences with elderly persons also may influence beliefs.

Several studies of attitudes of health care workers and students toward the elderly have been done. Results have been mixed. A study by Campbell (1971) on attitudes of nursing personnel toward geriatric clients showed that 50 percent of registered nurses and 60 percent of practical nurses and aides held stereotyped attitudes about the elderly. She concluded that increased education correlated with decreased stereotyping. Another study, this one by Gunter (1971), examined attitudes of nursing students before and after a course on healthy aging. Attitudes showed little change while interest in working with the elderly decreased after the lectures on normal aging. The opposite results were obtained by Hart et al. (1976) when a course that included clinical experience with the aged was presented. In this instance attitudes became less stereotyped and more positive and interest in working with the elderly increased. Wilhite and Johnson (1976) also found that students' attitudes became less stereotyped after a course on aging; they related this change to positive faculty attitude as much as to exposure to the course content. A study reported in 1978 by Taylor and Harned using a different attitude measuring instrument showed that registered nurses working with the elderly had neutral to slightly positive attitudes toward the aged. A more recent attitude study using the same instrument reported a significant relationship between attitude of nurses and the type of agency in which they worked (Brower, 1981).

Studies of physicians' attitudes have also been done. Miller et al. (1976) found a general disinterest among physicians surveyed in care of the ill aged. Another study of physicians, nurses, and nonprofessional staff showed that physicians and nurses had slightly positive attitudes whereas nonprofessional staff had slightly negative attitudes toward the elderly (Holtzman et al., 1977). These studies along with others not cited that examine physician attitudes have severe methodological limitations and small sample sizes.

Methodological problems have also been evident in the nursing studies on attitudes. Neither of the tools most commonly used by the researchers controls for responses made because they are socially desirable. Further, none of these studies distinguishes between attitudes (beliefs) and intention to behave in a certain way. If the purpose of measuring attitudes is to determine how the person will behave with the elderly, then a link between attitude and behavior must be demonstrated. Some recent studies have attempted to address these issues.

A very small exploratory study reported by

Hatton (1977) showed a correlation between positive behavior and positive attitude. Another study by Chaissen (1980) demonstrated that an educational program resulted in more positive attitudes but no change in behavior. For a study of nursing students, Robb (1979) developed a new instrument to measure intention and to control for socially desirable responses. This study demonstrated that positive behavioral intention increased after a course on aging, although attitudes did not change significantly. Further work on linking behavior to attitude is needed before any conclusions should be drawn from the studies done on attitudes toward the elderly.

The issue for gerontological nursing practice is one of quality of care provided. If negative attitudes interfere with providing good care then attitudes must be changed. However, some feel that professional behavior can be taught and internalized despite negative attitudes toward aging (Strumpf and Mezey, 1980). The negative attitude is linked to aging, not always to the elderly clients themselves. Nurses who are aware that they share society's negative views toward aging may be more apt to be consciously aware if this attitude affects their behavior. Attitude awareness workshops for nursing students and staff of agencies caring for the elderly may not change attitudes. However, these sessions might improve care by changing behavior. This educational technique needs to be tested, as do other means of improving care for the elderly.

THE GERONTOLOGICAL NURSE PRACTITIONER

The nurse practitioner is a registered nurse who has specialized education in the provision of primary health care to individuals and families. This expanded role was first recognized and formalized as a part of nursing practice in 1965 with the establishment of the first educational program for nurse practitioners (Mauksch, 1978). Since that time the role has gained wide acceptance by nursing and to a large degree by the public (Levine et al., 1978). The development of the role has stimulated vast discussion within nursing and change in health care delivery. Not all nurses agree that the nurse practitioner is an expanded or new role for nursing.

Some are concerned that the role overemphasizes the skills of physical diagnosis and functions of physicians. Others see the nurse practitioner as an opportunity to return the nurse to clinical rather than management status while increasing the prestige of the profession (Mauksch and Rogers, 1975). The nurse practitioner who uses a nursing model (conceptual framework) for practice should be in no danger of being confused with the physician's assistant.

Mauksch (1978), one of the principle advocates for this role, claims that 80 percent of primary care can be done by nurse practitioners, thus providing more health care to more people. Studies of nurse practitioners reveal that they are more apt to be found in publicly financed inner city or rural settings, and have more contacts with clients for prevention than for illness. They have also been found to provide high quality, cost-effective care (Pesznecker and Draye, 1978; Henry, 1978). These data support the position that the nurse practitioner provides more health care to more people.

Despite the increasing acceptance of the nurse practitioner, barriers to utilization of this individual exist. These barriers, identified in a survey of practitioners (Sullivan et al., 1978), include the following five areas:

1. Psychology of the nurse
2. Attitudes of other providers
3. Legal status
4. Organization of the health care system
5. Reimbursement.

The psychological barriers include fear of incompetence, conflicts regarding independence, and male–female role conflicts. Nurse practitioners must resolve these internal barriers themselves. Nurses in general need to be more supportive of their peers who are evolving this role.

Attitudes of other providers will be changed only over an extended time period. Conflict with physicians cannot be avoided, as a new division of labor is being sought. Physicians, in general, are not taught to delegate and are not prepared to recognize nurses as peers. Steele (1978) points out that role negotiation between nurses and physicians is essential for the nurse practitioner to function ef-

fectively. With the number of physicians increasing, relationships between the two types of providers may worsen as a competition for clients and funds develops.

Legal status is still a barrier to practice in some areas. In many states nurse practice legislation has been amended to allow a broad scope of independent nursing practice. Conservative, narrow legislation that restricts the scope of nurses' practice remains in place in some areas. Administrative statutes that broaden practice for particular types of nurse practitioners exist in some states (Trandel-Kovenchuk, 1978). The nurse should determine the law in any state before beginning practice in that state. Activities aimed at diagnosis, prescription, and treatment may be acceptable in one area and illegal in another.

Issuing of credentials to nurse practitioners is important to the legal status issue. The public has a right to expect competent performance of licensed professionals. Certification for advanced practice as a practitioner and accreditation of programs preparing nurse practitioners adds to the credibility of this role. The ANA has assumed a leadership role in offering these services. Recent studies on the issuing of credentials to nurses, done under the auspices of the American Nurses' Foundation, may lead to changes in the current systems and to more inclusive and uniform policies and procedures.

The organization of the health care system can be a barrier to utilization of the nurse practitioner in institutions or communities that do not value the skills nurses bring to this role. Limits may be put on the role. Some institutions will not create positions for the nurse practitioner. In a system still dominated by medicine, change that encourages independence and increased responsibility will be slow in coming. Companies providing malpractice and liability insurance may also pressure institutions to limit nurse practitioner functioning even without real evidence that such practice is illegal in a given situation.

Reimbursement is a major barrier to utilization of the nurse practitioner. Insurance carriers are reluctant to reimburse the nurse practitioner on a fee-for-service basis or to reimburse institutions for care provided by nurse practitioners. Again, medical domination of the reimbursement process is evident. Some progress has been made in obtaining reimbursement in special settings such as rural clinics. Nurses across the country are pursuing this issue at all levels of government.

The gerontological or geriatric nurse practitioner shares the same problems as other nurse practitioners. Preparation for this role is in certificate or master's degree programs. Content in these programs includes adaptations of normal aging, health assessment skills, communication skills, and health maintenance skills, all modified for use with the elderly client.

The gerontological nurse practitioner works in many settings. One growing area for this role is the nursing home. Traditionally underserved by physicians, the nurse practitioner's special preparation may dramatically improve the quality of health care in the nursing home (Kellogg Foundation, 1981). The nurse practitioner may conduct preadmission physical examinations and ongoing health assessments, order diagnostic tests, handle some medical procedures, counsel patients and families, arrange discharge planning, and provide in-service education for staff.

Another setting employing the gerontological nurse practitioner is the housing development clinic. Nurses in these units may provide primary health care for elderly clients living in the complex. Health maintenance, frequently including home visits, is the focus of care in these units. Independent functioning can often be prolonged for clients living at home with this on-site health care.

The gerontological nurse practitioner may also practice in a group practice setting such as a hospital clinic or private physician's office. Functions in these situations vary; however, counseling and teaching are primary activities for the nurse in any group practice. Regardless of setting, the gerontological nurse practitioner is a change agent in the health care delivery system. Whether involved in enrollment of clients in the health care system, health maintenance, long-term management, or sick care, the practitioner has the opportunity to improve the quality of health care for the elderly (Heppler, 1976).

Advanced preparation in gerontological nursing can involve roles other than the practitioner role. Preparation for education, administration, or clinical specialization is also available in master's level programs. Administrators in long-term care or am-

bulatory care settings that serve the aged need expert knowledge in gerontological nursing. Faculty in nursing programs and in-service education also need this preparation. Clinical specialists in gerontological nursing are needed in every setting where elderly clients need care to direct and supervise this care.

THE NURSE RESEARCHER

Nursing practice should reflect tested theory and new knowledge developed through rigorous research. The nurse researcher is a relative newcomer to the research arena. The gerontological nurse researcher is an even more recent arrival on the research scene. Rigorous research done by nurses in gerontological nursing is therefore sparse. Nurses in practice at this time must continue to look to related sciences for tested theory and knowledge as a base for nursing decisions. The practicing nurse, however, should also stay alert to the developing body of nursing research findings.

The nurse researcher in gerontological nursing confronts problems shared by all nurse researchers as well as problems unique to studying the elderly. The number of nurses prepared to do rigorous research is small. Young nurse researchers have few role models in the profession. All nurses can and should serve as data collectors for research projects. However, recognition that research is not problem solving on a day-to-day basis is still not well understood by nurses. The ability to evaluate research for use in practice is a critical skill for all nurses. Research textbooks provide the information required to critique research reports. In general, the nurse should consider the following areas:

1. The problem
2. Related literature review
3. Conceptual framework
4. Hypotheses
5. Methodology
6. Sample
7. Analysis
8. Findings
9. Interpretation of the findings
10. Recommendations

Problems confronting the nurse researcher in all areas include difficulty in obtaining money for research. This often leads to small sample sizes, less sophisticated design and analysis, and lack of replication of studies. The paucity of theory and knowledge in nursing science means that many studies are exploratory or descriptive rather than tests of theory or experimental in nature. Lack of access to subjects in clinical settings has hampered controlled research related to nursing interventions. The profession's focus on individualized care has emphasized a succession of untested interventions with a given client rather than more generalized interventions tested in groups of clients.

Problems that are unique to gerontological nurse researchers involve several factors. The newness of gerontology as a field of study means that the body of knowledge available for building sound theoretical frameworks is small. Measurement instruments tested on elderly populations are not commonly available. Illness and death often interrupt a study, decreasing the sample size or introducing a confounding variable. The diversity of the elderly population is a methodological challenge both in terms of developing reliable instruments and in establishing control over extraneous variables. Separating the effects of an individual subject's life history from the effects of aging makes cross-sectional studies suspect. Longitudinal studies, however, are very time consuming. Determining what age range is appropriate when studying variables important in aging or the elderly is a problem for researchers, as is determining whether chronological or functional age is the appropriate variable for the study. If functional age is to be studied then establishing an operational definition of this variable becomes a challenge.

Despite the problems of conducting research on gerontological nursing, more is being done now than ever before. Recent reviews of the literature reveal that a wide scope of studies relating to characteristics of the aged, nursing care, attitudes of nurses, institutionalization, and curriculum have been reported in nursing journals in the past 20 years (Kayser-Jones, 1981). The importance of reporting research in the journals so that it is available to the practicing nurse cannot be emphasized enough. Nursing research will be utilized in practice only if it is communicated effectively. Conferences, work-

shops, consultation and continuing education are all avenues for communicating research which gerontological nurses should use to transfer research to practice (Krueger, 1978). Defining a practice problem through observation and analysis, seeking out the related research findings, trying new solutions based on the research, evaluating the results of the new solutions, and communicating the effects is the process by which a body of knowledge in gerontological nursing is gradually built.

Robert Butler (1981), formerly of the National Institute on Aging, recently wrote that without new knowledge developed through research we will have nothing more 50 years from now than the same partial cures and inadequate services we now offer the elderly. Nurse researchers can and should contribute to the development of the new knowledge needed to improve the quality of life for the growing elderly population.

THE CLIENT ADVOCATE ROLE

Ethics and Accountability

Professional nurses are frequently required to act as client advocates. Advocacy may encompass a variety of actions. These actions are determined by the needs of the client, individual, family, or group. All advocacy actions are based on the basic assumption that the nurse's obligation is to protect the client. The ANA Code of Ethics for Nurses states that it is the right and duty of the nurse to act on the patient's behalf. Further, all recent discussions of client's rights emphasize the client's right to information (Table 1). Informed consent is now clearly understood to mean that the client understands the information provided and that the information is adequate and accurate.

Fulfilling these obligations may present ethical dilemmas for the nurse. The knowledge explosion has made decisions about what to explain and how to advise clients difficult for health professionals in general, and nurses in particular. Technical advances in diagnostic techniques, including electron microscopy, positron emission tomography, and improved methods of biopsy, culture, and analysis, have greatly increased the data base for decision making. However, these techniques may carry risks to the client's health status and all are costly. There

---

TABLE 1. NATIONAL LEAGUE FOR NURSING'S LIST OF PATIENTS' RIGHTS

NLN believes the following are patients' rights which nurses have a responsibility to uphold:

People have the right to health care that is accessible and that meets professional standards, regardless of the setting.

Patients have the right to courteous and individualized health care that is equitable, humane, and given without discrimination as to race, color, creed, sex, national origin, source of payment, or ethical or political beliefs.

Patients have the right to information about their diagnosis, prognosis, and treatment—including alternatives to care and risks involved—in terms they and their families can readily understand, so that they can give their informed consent.

Patients have the legal right to informed participation in all decisions concerning their health care.

Patients have the right to information about the qualifications, names and titles of personnel responsible for providing their health care.

Patients have the right to refuse observation by those not directly involved in their care.

Patients have the right to privacy during interview, examination, and treatment.

Patients have the right to privacy in communicating and visiting with persons of their choice.

Patients have the right to refuse treatments, medications, or participation in research and experimentation, without punitive action being taken against them.

Patients have the right to coordination and continuity of health care.

Patients have the right to appropriate instruction or education from health care personnel so that they can achieve an optimal level of wellness and an understanding of their basic health needs.

Patients have the right to confidentiality of all records (except as otherwise provided for by law or third-party payer contracts) and all communications, written or oral, between patients and health care providers.

Patients have the right of access to all health records pertaining to them, the right to challenge and to have their records corrected for accuracy, and the right to transfer of all such records in the case of continuing care.

Patients have the right to information on the charges for services, including the right to challenge these.

Above all, patients have the right to be fully informed as to all their rights in all health care settings.

Source: National League for Nursing, with permission.

has been a related growth in knowledge about treatment of health problems. Transplants, synthetic joints and other devices, cryosurgery, microsurgery, chemotherapy, and life-support techniques are only some of the recent advances in health problem management. Again, however, many of these techniques carry grave risk and large cost. Excessive exposure to radiation, extended suffering for client or family, and financial devastation are all potential outcomes of some of these advances. Expanded knowledge has given the health professional greater power to assist or to cause harm. Information and advice cannot be given haphazardly or lightly. The nurse as a professional is accountable for the results of meeting the obligation to inform the client. The client must be the ultimate decision maker; however, the physician and nurse are the primary source of information upon which the decision is made.

Since the nurse is in a position to control the flow of information both to the client and to the physician it is essential that the nurse exercise this control to protect the client. Determining what action is in the best interest of the client requires critical thinking and professional decision making. The nurse must assist clients to examine all the options available to them. This careful examination requires knowledge of the client's condition—past and present, physical and psychosocial. It involves information about all available treatment modes, their risks and benefits. It is based on predicted outcomes of treatment that take into account the interaction of multiple variables. In short, the nurse must assess, analyze, classify, and synthesize data in each client situation. A systematic, coherent system such as the stress/adaptation framework for use in the nursing process presented in this text is one method of organization. Other frameworks for organizing information are also useful. Selecting a framework is essential if a professional decision is to emerge.

The second essential element in professional decision making is an explicit moral philosophy. All nurses should be aware of their own moral principles. These principles will affect all decision making by the nurse and therefore should be explicit rather than unconscious. Moral principles are developed over a lifetime. Some derive from professional education and socialization. Science provides nurses with options. Moral principles or values assist nurses to determine what the outcomes of care should be. Some of the principles common to nurses are belief in the inherent worth and dignity of the individual, the client's right to self-determination, and belief in the validity of scientific truth. Situations may occur when moral principles are in conflict. When the client chooses to follow a diet that has no scientific validity does the nurse support self-determination or scientific validity? Should nurses withhold information to prevent clients from making decisions harmful to themselves? Is human dignity best preserved in terminal illness by limiting intrusive procedures? Answering these kinds of questions is a part of advocacy. Some authorities argue persuasively that the core of advocacy is client self-determination and the support of whatever decision the client makes (Kohnke, 1980). Not all agree that client wishes should be supported in every situation (Abrams, 1978). Ethical dilemmas are not easily solved. The nurse is accountable to the client for making the best decision possible in any given situation. Decisions that underlie advocacy are often much more critical than the general public or the nurse realizes. The nurse must also be sure that information is not distorted, that it is well presented at the right time, and that the client understands the explanations offered. Finally, the autonomy of the nursing profession is critical to effective advocacy. The nurse must have the right to make a professional decision involving the provision of information for informed client action. Client rights are served when nurses' rights are also respected.

Advocacy Actions

Providing information to clients and advising, counseling, and assisting them to make decisions is only one form of advocacy. The word advocacy also implies acting on the client's behalf and pleading for the client. Care must be taken when acting for the client, especially elderly clients, to avoid undermining independence. In caring for elderly, frail client situations arise that require nurses to act for the client. Helping a client to enter and negotiate the health care system is one example. Making a referral, making appointments, using contacts, manipulating schedules, coordinating care, telephoning, and filling out forms are all advocacy actions that may help the client or family obtain better care with minimal inconvenience. A client should be carefully evaluated to determine the degree of assistance needed. Confused clients, clients with limited mobility, loss of sight or hearing, or decreased self-esteem or depression, all common conditions in the elderly, may need more active intervention on their behalf. Illness alone compromises a client's ability to function independently. Illness plus aging will further undermine competence.

Supporting a client's decision once it has been made may involve being a spokesperson for the client with other health care workers or the family. Institutional or family dynamics may constrain the nurse's efforts to act on the client's decision if the decision is not acceptable to either. In these instances, the nurse must avoid undermining the client's decision, help the client to consider alternatives and evaluate the risks involved for client, nurse, family, and institution.

If a conflict arises between the health care system and the client the nurse may assume an ombudsman role, another form of advocacy. In this role the nurse represents the client's interests by facilitating open communication between client and staff. Interpreting client needs to staff and institutional regulations to clients may be necessary. Solving client problems through negotiated compromises may decrease client dissatisfaction. If staff or clients experience intense anger over a conflict of needs then the nurse should assist both parties to explore the reasons for the anger rather than trying to deal with the anger itself. The nurse may become an ombudsman in an individual situation or may be employed full-time in this role by an institution, agency, or community.

Advocacy may also involve actions aimed at improving the quality of care in an institution or community. The development of consumer rights groups has demonstrated this type of advocacy. Stimulating the public's awareness of poor quality care where it exists and then taking action to improve this care are basic to advocacy. Careful documentation of client care outcomes provides the data necessary to improve care. Via client records, observations, and reports of other health care workers, the nurse can gather evidence of poor care. In nursing homes especially, alertness to incidence of decubiti, pneumonia, urinary tract infections that developed after admission of the client, and the prevalence of confusion and immobility can lead the nurse to supporting documentation of poor care. High mortality rates, low ratios of professional staffing to patients, and underfinancing are other significant data. The nurse who gathers this kind of information should first attempt to bring about change by reporting it to the appropriate institutional authorities. This action itself may be dangerous for the nurse. If change does not occur, then going public may be necessary. The media, community action groups, politicians, agencies interested in the elderly, nursing groups, and official accrediting bodies are all potential bodies capable of exerting the pressure necessary to bring about change. Exerting pressure at this level carries even greater risk to the nurse than operating within the institution. It is also necessary to maintain accountability in some situations. A mechanism for anonymously reporting inadequate care to the Department of Health and Human Services exists, however. This may decrease the risk involved.

Every institution should have a mechanism for protecting client rights. A notice of the procedures for making a complaint should be given to every client. The staff should be aware of the protection mechanism and the complaint procedure. The client has a right to quality care and protection of personal liberties.

Finally, the nurse can act as a client advocate by joining local, state, and national organizations interested in health care. Sitting on boards of health care organizations and becoming politically active also permits advocacy. Supporting programs or initiating programs that address quality of care enhance advocacy. Supporting the hiring of appropriately prepared nurses, evaluating care continuously and regularly, and updating knowledge are also actions individual nurses can take that contribute to advocacy.

NURSING CONTRIBUTION TO HEALTH CARE OF THE ELDERLY

Because of its interest in health as well as illness, the nursing profession often assists older adults more effectively than other providers in the health care system. The nurse who views health as a relative state dependent on level of adaptation and function is able to focus on goals as well as problems. Nursing can help to reorient the health care system to a health model from the illness model developed as a result of the medically focused Medicare legislation. The modern nursing home particularly exemplifies the medical orientation. Instead of providing a homelike atmosphere, using the energies and talents of its residents, it has become an institution resembling a hospital run by physicians (American Nurses' Association, 1982). Long-term care of the elderly at home, in the community, or in an institution should focus on nursing needs and nursing interventions. The goal of care is health maintenance. Maximum use of self-care and self-help activities should be encouraged. Nursing can and should provide this type of health care service.

REFERENCES

Abrams N: A contrary view of the nurse as patient advocate. Nursing Forum 17(3):258, 1978

American Nurses' Association: A Challenge for Change: The Role of Gerontological Nursing. Kansas City, American Nurses' Association, 1982

Birren JE (ed): Handbook of Aging and the Individual. Chicago, University of Chicago Press, 1959

Borgatta EF, McCluskey NG (eds): Aging and Society. Beverly Hills, CA, Sage, 1980

Brill E, Kitts D: Foundations for Nursing. New York, Appleton-Century-Crofts, 1980

Brock AM: Gerontological nursing: Myth or science? Journal of the N.Y. State Nurses' Association 10(1):26, 1979

Brower HT: Social organization and nurses' attitudes toward older persons. Journal of Gerontological Nursing 7(5):293, 1981

Burkett GL, Parker-Harris M, et al: A comparative study of physicians' and nurses' conceptions of the role of the nurse practitioner. American Journal of Public Health 68(11):1090, 1978

Burnside IM (ed): Nursing and the Aged. New York, McGraw-Hill, 1981

Butler R: Research: The ultimate service. Geriatric Nursing 21(1):57, 1981

Campbell ME: Study of the attitudes of nursing personnel toward the geriatric patient. Nursing Research 20:147, 1971

Chaisson GM: Life-cycle: A social-stimulation game to improve attitudes and responses to the elderly. Journal of Gerontological Nursing 6(10):587, 1980

Conway ME: Clinical research: Instrument for change. Journal of Nursing Administration 8:27, 1978

Cuddihy JT: Clinical research. Translation into nursing practice. International Journal of Nursing Studies 16(1):65, 1979

Curtin L: The nurse as advocate: A philosophical foundation for nursing. Advances in Nursing Science 1(3):1, 1979

Davis AJ: To tell or not. American Journal of Nursing 81(1):156, 1981

DeWever MK: Nursing home patients' perception of nurses' affective touching. Journal of Psychology 96:163, 1977

Dracup KA, Brer CS: Using nursing research findings to meet the needs of grieving spouses. Nursing Research 27:212, 1978

Dwyer FM: A self-management health program for the elderly ill and disabled. Journal of Gerontological Nursing 4:53, 1978

Epstein C: Learning to Care for the Aged. Reston, VA, Reston, 1977

Feist JJ: A survey of accidental falls in a small home for the aged. Journal of Gerontological Nursing 4:15, 1978

Froome JH, Yeaworth RC: Master's level preparation in gerontological nursing. Journal of Gerontological Nursing 3:21, 1977

Gerdes JW, Pratt SC: In anticipation of the geriatric nurse practitioner. Nurse Practitioner 3:147, 1978

Godfrey M: Job satisfaction. Nursing 78, 8:89, 1978

Gunter LM: Students' attitudes toward geriatric nursing. Nursing Outlook 19:466, 1971

Gunter LM, Miller JC: Toward a nursing gerontology. Nursing Research 26(3):208, 1977

Hart LK, Freel MJ, Crowell CM: Changing attitudes toward the aged and interest in caring for the aged. Journal of Gerontological Nursing 2:17, 1976

Hatton J: Nurses' attitude toward the aged: Relationship to nursing care. Journal of Gerontological Nursing 3:21, 1977

Henry OM: Progress of the nurse practitioner movement. Nurse Practitioner 3:41, 1978

Heppler J: Gerontological nurse practitioner: Change agents in the health care delivery systems for the aged. Journal of Gerontological Nursing 2:38, 1976

Holtzman JM, Beck JD, et al: Geriatrics program for medical student and family practice resident. Journal of the American Geriatrics Society 25:531, 1977

Igoe JB: Nurse practitioners in primary health care systems, in Redman BK (ed): Patterns for Distribution of Patient Education. New York, Appleton-Century-Crofts, 1981

Jacox A, Prescott P: Determining a study's relevance for clinical practice. American Journal of Nursing 78(11):1882, 1978

Jordon J: A nurse practitioner in group practice. American Journal of Nursing 74(8):1447, 1974

Kayser-Jones J: A comparison of care in a Scottish and a U.S. facility. Geriatric Nursing 2(1):44, 1981

Kayser-Jones JS: Gerontological nursing research revisited. Journal of Gerontological Nursing 7(4):217, 1981

Kellogg Foundation. Physicians' boon and patients' blessing. PROFILES 4(1):2, 1981

Kohnke MF: Advocacy—Risk and reality. The Dean's List 1(2):1, 1980

Kohnke M: The nurse as advocate. American Journal of Nursing 80(11):2038, 1980

Krueger JC: Utilization of nursing research. The planning process. Journal of Nursing Administration 8:6, 1978

LaMonica EL: The nurse and the aging client: Positive attitude formation. Nurse Educator 4(6):23, 1979

Lester PB, Baltes MM: Functional interdependence of the social environment and the behavior of the institutionalized aged. Journal of Gerontological Nursing 4:23, 1978

Levine E: What do we know about nurse practitioners? American Journal of Nursing 77(11):1799, 1977

Levine JL, Orr ST, et al: The nurse practitioner's role, physician utilization, patient acceptance. Nursing Research 27(4):245, 1978

Martin RM: Ethical issues in present-day health care, in Ethical Issues in Nursing and Nursing Education. New York, National League for Nursing, 1980

Mauksch IG: Critical issues of the nurse practitioner movement. Nurse Practitioner 3:151, 1978

Mauksch IG: Nurse practitioner movement—Where does it go from here? American Journal of Public Health 68(11):1074, 1978

Mauksch IG, Rogers ME: Nursing is coming of age . . . through the practitioner movement. American Journal of Nursing 75(10):1834, 1975

Miller DB, Lowenstein R, Winston R: Physicians' attitudes toward the ill aged and nursing homes. Journal of the American Geriatrics Society 24:498, 1976

Nelson LJ: The nurse as advocate for whom? American Journal of Nursing 77(5):851, 1977

Olsen LP: A nurse administered long-term care unit. Journal of Gerontological Nursing 6(10):616, 1980

Olsen LP: Ombudsman for all. Geriatric Nursing 1(3):172, 1980

Pepper GA, Kane R, Teteberg B: Geriatric nurse practitioner in nursing homes. American Journal of Nursing 76(1):62, 1976

Pesznecker BL, Draye MA: Family nurse practitioners in primary care: A study of practice and patients. American Journal of Public Health 68(10):977, 1978

Polit D, Hungler B: Nursing Research: Principles and Methods. Philadelphia, Lippincott, 1978

Robb S: Advocacy for the aged. American Journal of Nursing 79(10):1736, 1979

Robb SS: Attitudes and interactions of baccalaureate nursing students toward the elderly. Nursing Research 28:43, 1979

Robb SS: Theories of aging and theory-related issues and attitudes and behavior in the environment of the aged, in Yurick AG, et al (eds), The Aged Person and the Nursing Process. New York, Appleton-Century-Crofts, 1980

Robb S, Yurick A, Spier B, Eberts N: Resources in the environment of the aged, in Yurick AG, et al (eds), The Aged Person and the Nursing Process. New York, Appleton-Century-Crofts, 1980

Robinson LD: Gerontological nursing research, in Burnside IM (ed), Nursing and the Aged. New York, McGraw-Hill, 1981

Roy C, Obloy M: The practitioner movement toward a science of nursing. American Journal of Nursing 78(10):1698, 1978.

Siegel H: Baccalaureate education and gerontology. Journal of Nursing Education 18:4, 1979

Sigman P: Ethical choice in nursing. Advances in Nursing Science 1(3):37, 1979

Smith JP: Is the nursing profession really research based? Journal of Advanced Nursing 4:319, 1979

Steele GE: Precepts for practitioners. Nursing Outlook 26:498, 1978

Strumpf HE, Mezey MK: A developmental approach to the teaching of aging. Nursing Outlook 28:730, 1980

Sullivan JA, Dachelet CZ, Sultz HA, Henry M: The rural nurse practitioner: A challenge and a response. American Journal of Public Health 68(10):972, 1978

Sullivan JA, Dachelet CZ, et al: Overcoming barriers to the employment and utilization of the nurse practitioner. American Journal of Public Health 68(11):1097, 1978

Taylor KH, Harned TL: Attitudes toward old people. Journal of Gerontological Nursing 4:43, 1978

Trandel-Kovenchuk DM, Trandel-Kovenchuk KM: How state laws recognize advanced nursing practice. Nursing Outlook 26:713, 1978

Wilhite MJ, Johnson DM: Changes in nursing students' stereotypic attitudes toward old people. Nursing Research 25:430, 1976

Williams MA, Holloway JR, et al: Nursing activities and acute confusional states in elderly hip-fractured patients. Nursing Research 28:35, 1979

Wolanin MO: Relocation of the elderly. Journal of Gerontological Nursing 4:47, 1978

II

Level One Adaptation: The Healthy Aging Client

4

Theories of Aging

Aging is a normal, lifelong process beginning at conception. Study of this process has produced a great deal of knowledge about the early years of growth and development but relatively little knowledge of changes associated with the latter years of life. Research has demonstrated changes in muscle composition, nervous system functioning, brain size, sensitivity to hormones, and numerous others. The causes of these changes, however, remain to a large degree an enigma. Information is largely descriptive, often disputed, frequently contradictory.

RESEARCH METHODOLOGY

Our understanding of the aging process and the fundamental causes of aging is still largely theoretical due to several factors. Lack of interest in basic research on aging until recent years and inadequate funding for research have played a role. However, even more significant is the problem of appropriate research methodology. Separating the effects of individual experience, environment, and pathology to determine what changes are a part of normal aging alone is very difficult.

Three research methods, each having strengths and weaknesses, are used in gerontological research. Cross-sectional studies of birth cohorts are the most common. In this method a group (cohort) of individuals of the same age is compared with a cohort of a different age. Thus subjects aged 30 to 40 may be compared with subjects aged 60 to 70, 80 to 90, and so on. This method will show differences, such as in learning abilities, present in different age groups. However, whether the differences are due to aging or due to the experience

(history) of the cohort is not known. The cohorts are not really comparable groups.

A second method used is the longitudinal study. This type of study looks at subjects as they age. A carefully controlled longitudinal study can minimize the effects of history. On the other hand, these studies require years to complete. Also, in studying very old groups it is likely that only the healthiest survive, thus distorting the results.

Research on aging using animals instead of human subjects is a third way of trying to obtain valid data. Animal studies can be highly controlled and completed in reasonable time periods since many animals have short life spans. However, applying results from the study of laboratory animals to humans presents all the problems of trying to generalize from one unlike species to another. Despite these methodological problems, basic research is being done and several biological and psychosocial theories of aging have been proposed.

BIOLOGICAL THEORIES

Biological theories of aging may be divided into two categories, extrinsic theories and intrinsic theories. Extrinsic theories propose that aging is due to factors in the environment that produce changes in the human organism. Intrinsic theories suggest that the changes arise from internal, predetermined causes. Behnke et al. (1978) discuss several extrinsic theories in their book *The Biology of Aging*. One is the "wear and tear" theory associated with the work of Hans Selye, in which body systems are viewed as wearing out due to the stress of life. Little evidence has been generated to support this view of aging. Another is the theory developed by Leo Szilard that hypothesizes that background radiation causes damage to chromosomes that result in aging over time. This theory has been refined by Leslie Orgel to attribute aging to an accumulation of errors in cell replication and repair. Recent research, however, shows that error rates are low and repair capacities amazingly high (Behnke et al., 1978). Other researchers theorized that a combination of spontaneous mutations, radiation-induced mutations, and mutations with a low level of repairability cause aging (Sinex, 1974). It has also been hypothesized that radiation, ozone, drugs, or other environmental stimuli cause the production of "free radicals" during biochemical cell activity. These free radicals may cause damage to cell membranes or other cell structures, resulting in changes associated with aging and death. This hypothesis has been derived from circumstantial evidence. No clear demonstration that this occurs as a part of the aging process exists (Finch and Hayflick, 1977).

Intrinsic theories point out that each species has a characteristic life span, which indicates some sort of internal genetic control of the aging process. Whether a biological clock that winds down over time exists is not known. Further, if it does exist, is it intrinsic to each cell or to the organism as a whole? Is it in the nucleus or the cytoplasm? The rate of aging appears to be different from system to system within the organism. Cells live longer than the organism itself. However, cells are not immortal. Hayflick and subsequent researchers have demonstrated that some cells will reproduce themselves in vitro about 50 times and no more. Also cells from an older donor die in the laboratory sooner than cells from younger donors (Schneider, 1979). Studies on identical twins indicate that 60 to 80 percent of an individual's longevity is inherited (Bierman and Brody, 1978). A large part of this may be due to age-related diseases. It is not clear how many or which genes account for normal aging. Chemical stability of DNA probably plays an important role in aging. Changes in RNA may underly changes in various tissues (Sinex, 1975).

Cells and Aging

Additional biological theories of aging have been proposed. It has been demonstrated that an array of changes in cell structure and composition occurs as the cell ages. Proliferating cells (blood, gut, skin) lose their capacity to divide over time. Cells that are reproduced in older organisms may not be as healthy as cells produced by younger organisms. Protein synthesis in cells becomes faulty in the aging organism. Age-associated alterations in chromatin composition have been noted in tissues. Waste materials are built up in interstitial spaces, which may interfere with functioning (Busse and Pfeiffer, 1977). Lipofuscin granules, also known as age pigment, accumulate, especially in cardiac muscle cells and neurons. Old cells appear swollen, with secondary lysosomes associated with breakdown of cell products. Senescent cells show an increase in lysosomal enzyme activity. The reasons for this accumulation are not known. Because the age pigment replaces functioning cell cytoplasm it may contribute to cell malfunction and death. An alternate view is that lipofuscin is an end product of a neutralized toxic substance and those cells without lipofuscin may have already died of the toxin's effect (Behnke et al., 1978). It is not known whether any of these cellular changes account for behavioral changes associated with aging of the organism as a whole.

The Immune System and Aging

Changes in the immune system occur with aging. Lymphoid tissue undergoes involution. T lymphocytes with suppressor activity increase and normal T cells decrease. It has been suggested that a decrease in cellular immune functioning is associated with an increase in the production of autoantibody. The appearance of autoantibody (antibodies specific to a person's own tissue or serum) in older individuals is common. Why the immune system declines in function is not known. The possibility of an internal clock in immune system stem cells has been suggested. Links between multiple viral infections during earlier life and the development of autoantibody are being investigated (Adler, 1974).

Collagen Tissue and Aging

As the organism ages changes in collagen tissue also occur. Collagen molecules form cross-links of several types as they age. This leads to stiffness and rigidity of tissue that may be related to changes in cardiac functioning and other physiological changes. It is known that cross-linking is sensitive to temperature and thyroid hormone changes. The role, if any, that these play is not known (Brash and Hart, 1978). It is known that certain chemicals interfere with formation of cross-links. Use of these chemicals in animal experiments has not increased life span (Shock, 1974). Thus, any theory that involves changes in collagen tissue as an explanation for aging is highly speculative.

Hormones and Aging

Alterations in tissue responsiveness to hormones are an important part of the aging process. Binding of hormones to target cell receptors is an initial requirement for action. Loss of these receptors occurs over age, thus decreasing the degree of response to hormones. Decrease in production of hormones themselves is not common, except for those produced by the ovary. There is a decrease in the production of insulin but only in relation to an elevation of blood sugar. Basal insulin secretion remains at the same level throughout normal aging (Davis, 1978).

The Aging Brain

Cerebral atrophy is a part of normal aging. This atrophy produces a decrease in blood flow. The 10 to 12 percent loss in brain weight that occurs as the organism ages is assumed to be due to a progressive loss of neurons. Research has demonstrated that the dendrite arbor shrinks and that neurofibrillary tangles and plaques develop. Changes in enzymes that affect synapses also occur. A depletion of dopamine as well as other catecholamines also occurs with age. How or if these changes are related to the development of senility is not known (Finch, 1978). Sleep patterns show pronounced changes with age. Percentage of time awake increases markedly from age 40 to 60. After 65, sleep is more fragmented, rapid-eye-movement (REM) sleep declines, and sleep is less intense. Changes in neurons or catecholamines may be responsible. Effect on functioning is not known. However, hormonal activities that take place during normal sleep may be impaired when sleep is disturbed over long time periods.

Slowing of Activity

A slowing of activity in the aging organism has been demonstrated. Reaction time studies show that response time for simple tasks decreases slightly while response time for complex or paced tasks slows more dramatically. This slowing appears to be related to central nervous system functioning rather than changes in cardiovascular or muscle tissue. It has also been hypothesized that changes in the hypothalamus, which regulates habitual activity in the organism, may produce a general slowing in older people (Shepard, 1978). There is a progressive loss of lean tissue and an infiltration of muscle with fat that compromises muscle strength over age. Both anaerobic and aerobic powers are decreased. This, along with changes in cardiac functioning, increases in subcutaneous fat that interfere with thermal regulation, lower glycogen reserves, and increased need for glycogen for exercise in older people, decreases tolerance for heavy work in the aged. Slowing of the organism for whatever reason is an important part of normal aging and has implications for many behavior changes seen in the elderly (Gioiella, 1978). Changes in psychomotor performance seen in the elderly can be simulated in younger subjects by lowering oxygen tension in inspired air. This has stimulated the development of a hypoxia theory of aging. This theory maintains that aging is a result of decreased oxygen tension in cells, especially in the brain. However, evidence indicates that oxygen tension of the blood remains uniform even in advanced age, making this theory seem unlikely (Shock, 1974).

Nutrition

Finally nutrition appears to affect aging. Animal studies indicate that severe underfeeding from birth extends the life span. However, side effects including increased infant mortality, stunted growth, and brain damage also occur. Data from animal studies are still too incomplete to serve as a model for nutrition in man. No long-term data in humans yet exist to assess the affect of diet on the life span. Diet does appear to be a factor in the emergence of age-linked disease. Research on the impact of nutrition on normal aging as well as age-related pathology is needed.

Summary

No particular biological theory of aging can be considered more powerful than any one of the others discussed. Most evidence at this time is descriptive and even contradictory in nature. Investigation is ongoing, adding new data that will eventually clarify some of the issues. It appears likely that aging is a multifaceted process affected by both extrinsic and intrinsic factors. Change occurs in all systems and involves cells, enzymes, hormones, and tissues. Changes are variable, occurring at different times and different places in each individual. To effect change in the aging process many theories must be considered. Each theory has potential for better understanding of life span and changes associated with aging (Shock, 1977).

PSYCHOSOCIAL THEORIES

The behavioral scientist studies the aging process from several perspectives. Theories that attempt to explain psychological or social changes associated with aging include changes in cognition, memory, perception, sensation, socialization, life satisfaction, environmental interaction, and attitudes. Some of these theories postulate a biological basis for psychosocial changes; others are independent of biological aging. All of the theories are still incomplete and are driven by the adherence of the researcher to a particular field of psychology.

Cognition and Aging

Changes in cognitive functioning over age have been examined by researchers for many years. The methodological problems of separating generational from autogenic change is critical in this area of study. Cognitive change may not reflect biological change in competence (Thompson and Marsh, 1973). Newer longitudinal studies are giving data that contradict earlier cross-sectional studies. Changes in cognitive functioning are not uniform in all areas. Motivation and relevance of material are important variables to be controlled in studies of learning and problem solving.

Research on intelligence shows no general decline with age. Studies in the 1960s indicated that older people did better than younger people on tests of crystallized intelligence. This type of intelligence is related to education and experience. Tests of fluid intelligence, nonverbal intelligence essentially independent of education and experience, demonstrated that elderly subjects did more poorly than younger subjects. Recent longitudinal studies that controlled for generational differences, however, showed decline in both types of intelligence only in the very old (Labouvie-Vief, 1979). One explanation for the decline in the very old is that research has demonstrated a significant drop in intelligence approximately 5 years prior to death in many people (Kleemeier, 1962). This phenomenon may be affecting the data obtained on subjects in late life.

Studies of age differences in memory show that the constructs of short-term and long-term memory are not valid. Rather, memory is better conceived as primary memory (PM) and secondary memory (SM). PM refers to material still in the mind and being processed. SM refers to material in storage that must be retrieved. Thus, immediate recall or short-term memory involves some PM and some SM functioning. There is no change in primary memory with age. There is decline in secondary memory among older normal subjects (Craik, 1977). Recall memory declines due to difficulty in retrieving material from storage. This may be related to slowing in the central nervous system that prolongs the search process of the memory store and to the increased scope of the research required as the individual ages (Arenberg, 1973). The widespread belief that elderly people have intact long-term memories is not supported by current research.

Research on learning and problem solving in the elderly has produced conflicting information. In general, both learning and problem-solving performance decline in later life. Why this occurs is not clear. Eisdorfer (1973) has demonstrated that arousal levels during and after learning are above optimal levels in older subjects. This results in increased errors in performance. If arousal is decreased through administration of a drug then performance is improved. Other research shows that resistance to learning new verbal associations is related to preexisting linguistic habits. Also, retention of learning decreases with age if the information is nonsense material. However, if the information is meaningful then retention is equal in young and old subjects (Arenberg, 1973). Some studies indicate that motivation is an important variable in learning in the aged. Some older subjects may show more caution in a test situation. Both increases and decreases in motivation affect performance (Neugarten and Maddox, 1978). Pacing is also critical. When time is not a factor and if problems are concrete and relevant, performance is less affected by age (Botwinick, 1973). Another factor that influences problem-solving ability in the aged is difficulty in ignoring redundant or irrelevant material (Hoyer et al., 1979). The role anxiety plays in performance is not clear. Investigators have hypothesized that anxiety is experienced by the elderly especially when learning or problem solving is paced. However, this has not been demonstrated by research.

Cognitive changes in aging, whether in registering, storing, and retrieving information or in learning or problem solving, may also be affected by the environment. Lack of stimulation, lowered expectations, and the adaptive utility of this behavior may all influence performance. At this time simplistic theories must be discarded and new research undertaken to augment the sparse literature in this area.

Personality and Aging

Research on personality changes in the elderly has produced markedly conflicting results. Again methodology is the main problem. Few longitudinal studies have been done and few tools have been developed to use with elderly subjects. Several theorists have postulated that psychosocial development is a dynamic, continuous process. Erik Erikson identifies a series of developmental stages characterized by various tasks. In this formulation, Stage VIII (the last stage) is described as Ego Integrity Versus Despair. Tasks involve accepting one's life course, defending the dignity of one's life-style, and emotional integration of one's life to prepare for death. Good adjustment implies a certain acceptance of aging and one's life. Some support for this view has been derived through testing but more is needed (Neugarten et al., 1964). The life review process in which older persons examine their lives may be a recognition that time ahead is limited and may serve to preserve identity. Some have identified it as a developmental task (Butler, 1963). The reinvestment of psychological attachments once associated with body image, occupation, sex, and the like is also a task of aging. This may involve a balancing between activity and withdrawal, a continual shifting of time orientation from engrossment

with the here and now to perspective on the past, present, and future (Kastenbaum, 1965). Other theorists agree that although one's past life is important there are still possibilities, whether in this life or through a legacy to people or society for the future.

Havighurst (1972) has elaborated developmental tasks as markers along the life span. Neugarten (1977) and others take this concept further by identifying life periods, including middle age, young-old, and old-old. Behavior appropriate for one period may not be appropriate in another. Continuity of behavioral patterns developed over the life span is the underlying theme of the developmental theorists. New tasks may emerge but radical shifts in behavior are unlikely (Neugarten et al., 1964). In his discussion of the aging family, Duvall (1977) also identifies tasks of aging. These include coping with bereavement, living alone, closing the family home, and adjusting to retirement.

One generalization that emerges from the research is that introversion or interiority increases in later life. Whether this change is intrinsic to the aging process or related to environmental transactions is not known. Social behaviorists view behavior as jointly determined by individual and society interaction. It is based on perception of expectations of others. Introversion may result from an internal need for self-actualization or from a lack of congruence between organism and environment expectations. It may be a developmental task or a coping behavior. Other personality changes that have been studied in the elderly may also develop as coping behaviors. Rigidity or reluctance to change has been noted in many elderly. However, research shows that this is not a unitary concept. Subjects may be rigid in some situations and not in others. Rigidity may be related to individual life experience or to slowing of the organism. Links to decreased ability to problem solve have also been demonstrated (Botwinick, 1973).

Older people tend to have less sense of mastery over their lives. They may accept less, expect less, see problems as inevitable, and seek palliative rather than curative or preventative measures. One recent study demonstrated in 150 subjects over 65 that subjects whose locus of control is internal (respond to internal cues more than external environmental cues) tend to see themselves as younger than their chronological age. This perception of self as younger correlated with improved psychological functioning (Lina and Hunter, 1979). Studies of cautiousness hypothesize that the elderly are uncomfortable in new, uncertain situations; they are less self-confident, tending to fear failure, loss, and rejection. Testing has not yet supported or refuted this hypothesis. Research has shown that aging men move from active to passive modes in dealing with the environment, whereas aging women move in the opposite direction (Neugarten et al., 1964). Some investigations show a reluctance to undertake risk-taking decisions in the elderly. However, other researchers have questioned the methodology of these studies (Botwinick, 1973). Some elderly hold negative views of themselves and of aging. This may be related to loss of roles and status, rejection, and being neglected. Since the young also view aging negatively this is not intrinsic to the aging process. However, low self-esteem may result in coping behaviors such as hostility, denial of aging, retreat, preoccupation with health, dependency, and an increase in preferred personal space (Knopf, 1975; Gioiella, 1978). Sensory and perceptual decline with age is well documented. This decline may contribute to behavior change such as the development of suspiciousness (Corso, 1971).

In summary, there is no convincing evidence of any universal developmental process associated with aging. The evidence shows that change in personality, values, and behavior may occur. These changes are rarely perceived by the individual, as they are integrated over time. Individuals tend to see themselves as being consistent even when trapped in certain behavior patterns. There is more stability than fundamental change in personality type or style over age. Current literature and research tend to neglect the wide range of behavior in the elderly and the increase in differentiation expected with aging (Usdin and Hofling, 1978). Differences observed are more likely to be related to individual history and social demand than to aging alone.

Social Interaction and Aging

No single theoretical framework organizes research on the social aspects of aging. Present knowledge indicates that age is not a good predictor of social behavior. A recent theory that should be further explored is social exchange theory, which is derived from economics and anthropology. This formulation looks at social behavior in terms of what is valued and rewarded in a society. Roles and kinship systems are studied in relationship to power. The heuristic value of this framework for studying aging and society has yet to be explored. Since the aged are often faced with decreasing resources and increasing dependence on family or other support systems they have less value and less power. This makes them apparent unequal contributors in social exchange situations. The implications of this hypothesis need to be investigated.

Roles are stratified by age in all societies. With advancing age there is a decline in the number of roles allocated by society. Retirement precipitates the loss of the worker role. In recent years the age of separating from the work force has decreased. The decision to retire is related to income, job satisfaction, and attitude toward work. About one-half of all workers retire earlier or later than expected (Foner, 1972). Less than 15 percent leave the work force due to health reasons. Satisfaction with retirement is related to income, health status, and whether or not the retirement was voluntary. Workers prefer to retire if the work is heavy or boring and if postretirement income will be adequate. Attitudes preretirement are important predictors of adjustment (Binstock and Shanas, 1976). Studies done at Duke University indicate that most individuals adapt surprisingly well and quickly to the impact of retirement (Maddox, 1978).

Other role changes associated with aging are completion of parental role and widowhood. Roles that are maintained or developed late in life are often related to volunteerism, friendship, and grandparenting. Studies indicate that older people tend to maintain involvement in voluntary associations if this has been a lifelong pattern. This involvement does not correlate with an increase in life satisfaction (Ward, 1979). Friendship patterns in the elderly are affected by loss of earlier friends due to death or because they were friends linked to a deceased spouse or to work. Friendships may be increased if based on shared new experiences such as leisure activities or movement to a retirement community. Maintenance of friendships is higher in high socioeconomic status groups, higher in women, and even higher in nonworking women. Proximity of similar people is a critical factor in maintaining a social network (Hess, 1972). Little is known about the impact of elderly people forced to change their pattern of socializing by circumstances whether it be to increase interaction or move toward isolation. One study has shown that having a confidant is more important than the degree of social interaction (Lowenthal, 1967).

One other important aspect of friendship in late life is the role a friend may play in socializing the older person to the norms of retirement, widowhood, disability, and the like. Socialization is a developmental age-related process. In the elderly it includes learning new roles, transferring energy and interest and gratification from one role to another, and relinquishing roles no longer available or appropriate. In the young, socialization is often anticipatory, that is, begun before a new role is assumed, assisted by adults and teachers. In the elderly it is usually tenancy socialization, socialization that occurs after the role is taken on often on a trial and error basis. Lack of age-superior models places the burden on peers, both friends and acquaintances, to socialize each other.

One's role as a family member also changes with age. Evidence indicates that families retain responsibility for elderly members but often in separate homes. Studies of stress and adaptation in later life have found that there is little or no change in physical or psychosocial adaptation after the death of a spouse in most people (Palmore et al., 1979). The need for intimacy and mutuality continues through old age. Women have a greater capacity to transfer this need to women friends after the death of a spouse. Men seem less able to develop intimate friendships in old age and tend to remarry instead (Lowenthal, 1975). Both men and women cite desire for companionship as the most frequent reason for remarriage. Extended family relationship studies show multiple factors that affect the quality but no one overriding factor of significance in predicting continuity or disruption of the extended family. There has been little or no study of the grandparenting role. In general there are many unanswered questions regarding relationships in later life. To what extent is one type a substitute for another? Does

increased commitment to one type require a decrease in commitment to another? Do past relationships continue to have symbolic meaning and thus compensate for decreased involvement in later life?

Activity and Aging

Change in activity level over age has been an area of interest to gerontologists for years. Cumming and Henry (1961) developed disengagement theory in the 1950s. This theory proposed that progressive social disengagement was a mutually acceptable state for the aging individual and society. Subsequent research has failed to support this theory. In contrast, Havighurst (1972), Maddox (1978), Carp (1966), and others proposed activity theory, which claims that successful aging depended on maintaining high levels of activity. Several studies have linked high activity levels with high life satisfaction. This has not been demonstrated to be generally true either (Lemon et al., 1972; Hoyt et al., 1980). However, longitudinal studies have developed evidence that decreased activity in one area results in increased activity in another (Palmore and Maddox, 1977).

Kastenbaum (1965) has suggested that degree of disengagement varies with individual personality and that level of activity is a lifelong pattern. This is supported by studies by Lehr (1969) that showed a consistency of social participation over time. Where patterns did change many variables, including health, income, and role change, were found to be important influencing factors. Activity level may be linked with energy levels. Rather than decrease level of activity as energy diminishes the aging individual may change types of activity, becoming more sedentary and doing more things at home. One study of nursing home residents found that most residents spent half their waking time apparently doing nothing (Gottesman and Boureston, 1974).

The relationship between decrease or change in activities and the development of social isolation and even sensory deprivation is not clear. Quality or meaningfulness of the activities to the individual may be more significant than the quantity of activity itself. Kleemeier (1961) has pointed out that attitude toward activity and use of leisure time is culture bound. The development of a leisure class of elderly people is a recent phenomenon in Western society.

Little research has been done on the psychological meaning attached to leisure time by the participant or by society. This should be a major area of investigation in the future.

Environment and Aging

A recent area of investigation in the elderly involves spatial behavior. There are two different types of spatial behavior that are being researched. One type of spatial behavior has been termed territoriality and may be specific to a species. It has been observed that animals will fight to maintain dominance or control over a particular geographic area. Some theorists have claimed that humans have the same need to control certain spaces. Studies of behavior in institutions such as schools, hospitals, and prisons have shown that people do identify seats or places as their own and will aggressively assert their right to this space. Sommer (1969) studied this type of behavior in elderly subjects in nursing homes. He found that the subjects marked their territory by routinely sitting in the same place or always putting their wheelchairs in the same position in a line of wheelchairs. In animals, hostility is the result of territorial invasion. It is not yet certain how humans react to territorial encroachment. It seems likely that identity, security, and sense of power may be compromised if territory is not respected (Sommer, 1969).

The second type of spatial behavior is called personal space. Personal space refers to the distance individuals maintain between themselves and others. It may be viewed as a bubble surrounding the person—a buffer zone between oneself and the environment. This space is dynamic. It decreases between intimate friends, increases during stress or if self-esteem is low. The study of behavior related to personal space or interpersonal distances is called proxemics. Hall has described four phases of personal space: 1. intimate, 6 to 18 inches; 2. personal, 1 and one-half to 4 feet; 3. social, 4 to 12 feet; and 4. public, 12 to 25 feet plus. Different cultures approach or use these distances differently (Hall, 1966). One study of personal space in the elderly has indicated that older people prefer more distance between themselves and others for the social phase (Gioiella, 1978).

Environment also includes housing for the elderly. Very little is known about the effects of var-

ious types of housing and living facilities on the aged. A move to new housing may be followed by an increase in feelings of well-being (Carp, 1966). Some investigators have postulated a need for age peers but no evidence has been developed for or against retirement communities. An overly complex, fast-paced environment may be difficult for the older person to negotiate. It has been suggested that many elderly people find their environment threatening, that they are more sensitive to environmental change, and may feel incompetent in dealing with it (Lawton, 1970). A balance between need and competence should be a goal of environmental planning.

Attitudes and Aging

A number of studies on attitudes toward the old have found that younger groups have a negative view of the aged. The elderly also tend to hold negative views of themselves, a reflection of the general society view. More recent data indicate that these negative attitudes are diminishing. In some segments of Western society the elderly are becoming a visible and contented leisure class (Harris and associates, 1975). The impact of negative attitudes toward the elderly on their self-esteem has been explored. Various surveys have found low self-esteem in older subjects. This has been attributed to a variety of factors, including society's attitudes, decrease in meaningful activity, social isolation, and loss of roles (Kutner, 1956; Kleemeier, 1961; Weiss, 1973; Zung, 1967; Gioiella, 1978). Studies of life satisfaction in the elderly have demonstrated many variables related to an individual's happiness. Health status, activity level, and income are the most important influencing factors assuming a significant role in feelings of life satisfaction (Markides and Martin, 1979).

Investigation of attitude change in old age has also been carried out. Recent studies indicate that older subjects change attitudes as readily as younger subjects. Older subjects were more susceptible to argument or persuasion; younger subjects had a higher rate of retention of information related to the subject being discussed (Herzog, 1979). Studies on voting in the elderly show that older people tend to participate more in political activity and tend to become more identified with a particular party. If issues are studied separately the older voter changes attitude from conservative to liberal depending on the issue. In general the elderly are more conservative than younger subjects. This may be a posture due to this generation's life experience (low educational levels, few women voting, the depression, Nazism, etc.). Future cohorts of older voters may change this picture (Foner, 1972).

Finally studies of the status of elderly in Western society indicate a fluid state. Status is related to several factors, including wealth, power, and recognition of success. Retirement does not decrease status unless income is drastically compromised. A decrease in status is more likely to occur if health is undermined, thus decreasing independence and power. Among the elderly today the low status group is likely to be over 75 (Binstock and Shanas, 1976).

Summary

As in biological aging there is no universal psychosocial theory that explains the aging process. Changes occur in cognition, especially memory. Introversion develops. Social interaction decreases. Whether those changes are intrinsic to the aging process or largely the result of social forces is not known. Again, as in biological aging, individual differences are great. Diversity among the aged, rather than similarity, may be the norm.

INTERRELATIONSHIPS AMONG THEORIES

Few investigators have attempted to examine the relationships between biological and psychosocial theories of aging. No theory that examines the holistic person has yet been applied to the normal aging process. Examining the human organism as a biological entity or a psychosocial entity will not lead to a true understanding of the aging process. Are changes in memory related to slowing in the central nervous system? Is the development of introversion also related to these two phenomenon? Are these three changes related to changes in activity levels? How important is the impact of societal–environmental circumstances on the total aging process?

Application of theory to practice in caring for aging clients requires caution on the part of the nurse. Exploration and cognizance of these unknown interactions must be continually kept in mind when planning interventions.

REFERENCES

Adler W: An autoimmune theory of aging, in Rockstein M (ed), Theoretical Aspects of Aging. New York, Acacemic Press, 1974

Andrey R: The Social Contract. New York, Atheneum, 1970

Arenberg D: Cognition and aging, in Eisdorfer C, Lawton MP (eds), The Psychology of Adult Development and Aging. Washington, American Psychological Association, 1973

Behnke J, Finch C, Moment G (eds): The Biology of Aging. New York, Plenum, 1978

Bierman E, Brody H: Our Future Selves: A Research Plan Toward Understanding Aging. Washington, NIH Publication, 1978

Binstock R, Shanas E (eds): Handbook of Aging and the Social Sciences. New York, Von Nostrand Reinhold, 1976

Birren J, Schaie KW (eds): Handbook of the Psychology of Aging. New York, Von Nostrand Reinhold, 1977

Birren J: The Psychology of Aging. Chicago, University of Chicago Press, 1969

Botwinick J: Aging and Behavior. New York, Springer, 1973

Brash D, Hart R: Molecular biology of aging, in Behnke J, et al (eds), The Biology of Aging. New York, Plenum, 1978

Busse EW, Pfeiffer E (eds): Behavior and Adaptation in Late Life, 2nd ed. Boston, Little Brown, 1977

Butler R, Lewis M: Aging and Mental Health, 2nd ed. St. Louis, Mosby, 1977

Butler R: The Life Review: An interpretation of reminiscence in the aging. Psychiatry 26:90, 1963

Carp F: A Future for the Aged. Austin, University of Texas Press, 1966

Corso J: Sensory processes and age effects in normal adults. Journal of Gerontology 26:90, 1971

Craik F: Age differences in human memory, in Birren J, Schaie KW (eds), Handbook of the Psychology of Aging. New York, Von Nostrand Reinhold, 1977

Cumming E, Henry W: Growing Old: The Process of Disengagement. New York, Basic, 1961

Davis P: Endocrinology and aging, in Behnke J, et al (eds), The Biology of Aging. New York, Plenum, 1978

Duvall EM: Marriage and Family Development, 5th ed. Philadelphia, Lippincott, 1977

Eisdorfer C, Lawton MP (eds): The Psychology of Adult Development and Aging. Washington, American Psychological Association, 1973

Finch C, Hayflick L (eds): Handbook of the Biology of Aging. New York, Von Nostrand Reinhold, 1977

Finch C: The brain and aging, in Behnke J, et al (eds), The Biology of Aging. New York, Plenum, 1978

Foner A: The polity, in Riley M, Johnson M, Foner A (eds), Aging and Society. New York, Russel Sage Foundation, 1972, vol. 3

Gioiella E: The relationships between slowness of response, state anxiety, social isolation, and self-esteem and preferred personal space in the elderly. Journal of Gerontological Nursing 4:140, 1978

Gottesman L, Boureston N: Why nursing homes do what they do. Gerontologist 14(6):501, 1974

Hall E: The Hidden Dimension. New York, Doubleday, 1966

Harris L, and associates: The Myth and Reality of Aging in America. Washington, National Council on Aging, 1975

Havighurst R: Developmental Tasks and Education. New York, David McKay, 1972

Herzog A: Attitude change in older age: An experimental study. Journal of Gerontology 34(5):697, 1979

Hess B: Friendship, in Riley M, et al (eds), Aging and Society. New York, Russel Sage Foundation, 1972, vol 3

Hoyer W, Rebok G, Sved S: Effects of varying irrelevant information on adult age differences in problem solving. Journal of Gerontology 34(4):553, 1979

Hoyt D, Kaiser M, Peters G, Bobchuk N: Life satisfaction and activity theory: A multidimensional approach. Journal of Gerontology 35(11):35, 1980

Kastenbaum R (ed): Psychobiology of Aging. New York, Springer, 1965

Kent S: Can dietary manipulation prolong life? Geriatrics 32(4):102, 1978

Kleemeier R (ed): Aging and Leisure. Oxford, Oxford University Press, 1961

Kleemeier R: Intellectual changes in The Senium: Proceedings of the Social Statistics Section of the American Statistical Association, 1962

Knopf O: Successful Aging. Boston, G.K. Hall, 1975

Kutner B: Five Hundred Over Sixty. New York, Russel Sage Foundation, 1956

Labouvie-Vief G: Does Intelligence Decline with Age? Washington, NIH Publication, 1979

Lawton MP: Ecology and aging, in Pastalan L, Carson D (eds), Spatial Behavior of Older People. Ann Arbor, University of Michigan Press, 1970

Lehr V: Consistency and change of social participation in old age. Human Development 12:255, 1969

Lemon B, Bengston V, Peterson J: An exploration of the activity theory of aging. Journal of Gerontology 27:511, 1972

Lina M, Hunter K: Perception of age in the elderly. Journal of Gerontology 34(1):36, 1979

Lowenthal M: Interpersonal relations, in Loether H (ed), Problems of Aging. Belmont, CA, Dickenson, 1967

Lowenthal M: Psychosocial variations across the adult life course: Frontiers for research and policy. Gerontologist, 15(1):6, 1975

Maddox G: The social and cultural context of aging, in Usdin G, Hofling CK (eds), Aging: The Process and the People. New York, Brunner/Mazel, 1978

Markides K, Martin H: A causal model of life satisfaction among the elderly. Journal of Gerontology 34:86, 1979

Neugarten B, Maddox G: Our Future Selves: A Research Plan Toward Understanding Aging. Washington, NIH Publication, 1978

Neugarten B, Crotley W, Tobin S: Personality in Middle and Late Life. New York, Atherton, 1964

Neugarten B: Personality and aging, in Birren J, Schaie KW (eds), Handbook of the Psychology of Aging. New York, Van Nostrand Reinhold, 1977

Palmore E, Cleveland W, et al: Stress and adaptation in later life. Journal of Gerontology 34(6):841, 1979

Palmore E, Maddox G: Sociological aspects of aging, in Busse EW, Pfeiffer E (eds), Behavioral Adaptation in Late Life, 2nd ed. Boston, Little Brown, 1977

Palmore E (ed): Normal Aging I and II. Durham, Duke University Press, 1970, 1974

Pastalen L, Carson D: Spatial Behavior of Older People. Ann Arbor, University of Michigan Press, 1970

Rose A: Older People and Their Social World. Philadelphia, F.A. Davis, 1965

Ross MH: Nutrition and longevity in experimental animals, in Winick M (ed), Nutrition and Aging. New York, Wiley, 1976

Schneider E: Cells and Aging. Washington, NIH Publication, 1979

Shepard R: Exercise and aging, in Behnke J, et al (eds), The Biology of Aging. New York, Plenum, 1978

Shock N: Biological theories of aging, in Birren J, Schaie KW (eds), Handbook of the Psychology of Aging. New York, Von Nostrand Reinhold, 1977

Shock N: Physiological theories of aging, in Rockstein M (ed), Theoretical Aspects of Aging. New York, Academic, 1974

Sinex FM: The mutation theory of aging, in Rockstein M (ed), Theoretical Aspects of Aging. New York, Academic, 1974

Sinex FM: The biochemistry of aging, in Spencer MG, Dorr CJ (eds), Understanding of Aging: A Multidisciplinary Approach. New York, Appleton-Century-Crofts, 1975

Sommer R: Personal Space: The Behavioral Basis for Design. Englewood Cliffs, New Jersey, Prentice-Hall, 1969

Sommer R: Studies in personal space. Sociometry 22:260, 1959

Thompson L, Marsh G: Psychophysiological studies of aging, in Eisdorfer C, Lawton MP (eds), The Psychology of Adult Development and Aging. Washington, American Psychological Association, 1973

Usdin G, Hofling C (eds): Aging: The Process and the People. New York, Brunner/Mazel, 1978

Ward R: The meaning of voluntary association participation to older people. Journal of Gerontology 34(3):438, 1979

Weiss R: Lonliness: The Experience of Emotional and Social Isolation. Cambridge, MA, M.I.T. Press, 1973

Zung W: Depression in the normal aged. Psychosomatics 8(10):287, 1967

5

The Aging Process— Physical Adaptations

The aging process occurs in all creatures, from the simplest invertebrate to man himself. Although it is a universal phenomenon, aging manifests itself in many different ways in different species. No single aging process is common to all species. No one theory can explain the myriad changes in structure and function that occur with aging (Finch, 1971).

Maturity occurs when growth of long bones is completed. At this point, the incremental processes associated with growth and development slow down or stop and aging processes accelerate. Although some aging processes begin prior to maturity, the resulting adaptations generally do not become obvious until after maturity. To determine those adaptations that occur as a consequence of aging, it is important to identify only those changes that take place after maturity. Comparisons between immature and old individuals would be misleading (Kohn, 1977).

Because aging is an inevitable process, it is considered normal. Although inevitable, aging progresses at different rates in different individuals, depending upon a variety of factors, including genetic background, environment, activity pattern and nutritional status. Aging is intrinsic to cells, organs, organ systems, and body functions. However, not all organs or organ systems age in the same way, at the same rate, or to the same extent in a given individual.

The aging process is progressive and physiologically irreversible (Kohn, 1977). It leads to a decreased ability to adapt to the environment and therefore to an increase in the mortality rate among the aged (Rockstein et al., 1977). Consequently, aging changes are viewed as decremental.

For most people, however, senescence is not the cause of death. Although the human life span seems to be genetically determined, the percentage of a person's life span that is ultimately realized usually depends upon stresses in the environment that affect the individual's physical and psychosocial adaptation. True aging is usually complicated by several pathological conditions. These make it more difficult to determine whether the adaptations seen in older people are a consequence of normal aging or pathology (Rockstein et al., 1977).

The events of normal aging can be classified in one of four ways:

1. *Growth and hyperplastic changes*. These changes include such events as the thickening of the cranial vault, suture closure, thickening of the lens of the eye, enlargement of cartilaginous portions of the nose and ear, and an increase in the diameter of many bones.

2. *Use-related changes*. These are inevitable changes that occur as a consequence of motion or use. Use-related changes include cartilaginous changes in the vertebral spine and knee joints and some skin wrinkles.

3. *Passage of time events*. These are passive processes that leave their mark over time, such as arcus senilis.

4. *Regressive events*. These are atrophic changes and include the shrinkage of cells, tissues, and organs such as the skin, subcutaneous tissues such as the fatty deposits, muscles, and areas of the central nervous system (Rossman, 1977).

CELLS

A cardinal feature of age-related regression is a progressive decline in the number of cells in most organs. Cell loss appears to be the most distinctive and universal of the multiple changes that occur with aging (Rossman, 1977). Loss of cells has been confirmed by changes in organ weights and total cell counts and by changes in the amount of potassium, DNA, intracellular water, and nitrogen in the aged as compared with the young. Atrophy of the musculature, brain, lungs, spleen, kidneys, and liver occurs. These aging tissues are characterized by an increase in fatty infiltration and a decrease in the number of cells (Goldman, 1979).

Structural changes in the remaining cells occur with age. Postmitotic cells are nondividing cells, destined to die without further cell division. They are found in the nervous system, musculoskeletal system, and heart. Certain endocrine and kidney cells are also postmitotic. They are present throughout an individual's lifetime and the organs they comprise exhibit "true" postmaturational aging. These cells must repair or replace most of their intracellular structural elements and enzymatic machinery on a regular basis to prevent the accumulation of damaged molecular elements over time. These cells and the tissues they comprise are the most probable sites for the accumulation of defects with age that could cause reduced functioning that eventually becomes life-limiting (Latham and Johnson, 1979).

Remaining postmitotic cells exhibit some structural changes in ribosomes, nuclei, lysosomes, and mitochondria. Mitochondria are much less able to adapt to changes in their environment as cells age. Cell membranes are also altered structurally, possibly by cross-linkage or oxidation. The structural changes could alter the permeability of the cell to ions and other substances, thereby producing major alterations in the intracellular environment of aging cells. Postmitotic cells show an increase in lipofuscin, also known as aging pigment or "wear and tear" pigment. Lipofuscin consists of brown, autofluorescent intracellular granules composed of protein, steroids, and phospholipids. It has been found in the cytoplasm of cells in the myocardium and other muscles, spleen, liver, adrenal glands, nervous system, prostate, corpus luteum, and other organs. It is currently believed that lipofuscin is a waste product that originates from incomplete digestion by the lysosomes of membranes from an intracellular organelle or other cellular components. The effects of lipofuscin accumulation on cells is unknown. It is not known whether the pigment accumulates as a fundamental part of the aging process or whether it is the result of various types of stress (Sanadi, 1977; Balazs, 1977).

Mitotic cells are somatic cells that are capable of reproduction. These cells also undergo changes with age. It was once believed that mitotic cells had an infinite capacity for reproduction and replacement. Hayflick and Moorhead (1971) demonstrated that normal human diploid cells in tissue culture underwent a finite number of doublings and then died. After about 50 doublings the cells exhibited a sharp decline in proliferative power. During the period of decline, aging cells are characterized by an increase in doubling time, accumulation of cellular debris, a gradual cessation of mitotic activity, and eventually complete degeneration (Hayflick, 1977). Normal cells in vitro are also limited in their growth potential. This has been confirmed by studying the growth of cells from human transplants. It was found that cells from older human donors had a decreased potential for cell division (Latham and Johnson, 1979). The period of decline that aging cells undergo is called the Phase III phenomenon. Cessation of cellular function and cell division capacity is believed to be an expression of aging at the cellular level. The causes of the Phase III phenomenon are not known and are the focus of intensive research (Hayflick, 1977).

BODY COMPOSITION

With age, the major body components are redistributed (Fig. 1). Fat is the body tissue that undergoes the widest fluctuations throughout the life span. As aging progresses, there is an overall increment in body fat. Skin fold measurements have documented that fatty subcutaneous tissue in the aged is decreased. Subcutaneous fat is lost earlier and to a greater degree from the extremities and is maintained longer on the trunk (Rossman, 1977). Therefore, the fat increment occurs elsewhere in and around the viscera and muscles. The increase in body fat equals or exceeds the decrease in tissue cell mass

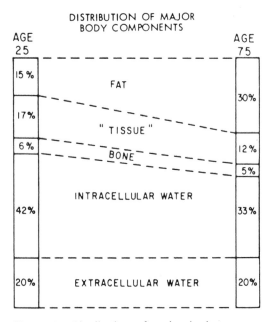

Figure 1. Distribution of major body components with age. *From Goldman R: Speculations of vascular changes with age. Journal of the American Geriatric Society 18:765, 1970, with permission.*

the subsequent increase in fat, basal heat production falls progressively with age from age 30 to age 90, resulting in a total loss of 15 percent over the life span. The fall reflects the loss of metabolizing tissue. Remaining metabolizing tissue produces heat at the same rate as in the young (Shock, 1977).

Total body water also drops with age when calculated as a percent of body weight. This decline is due to the decline in lean body mass and the rise in body fat. Adipose tissue is low in water. The decline in the ratio of total body water to body weight in the aged mirrors the rise in proportion of fat to lean body mass. Although total body water decreases, there is no change in extracellular water. Few changes have been noted in the solute content of the extracellular fluid (Rossman, 1977). Only the amount of intracellular water drops, reflecting the change in cell mass.

Body weight fluctuates with age and mirrors the changes in body composition (Table 1). In general, after age 55 males experience a steady decline in weight of more than 20 pounds. In normal females, weight increases until the sixth decade, plateaus, and then gradually declines. Weight in aging

discussed above. Therefore, these changes in body composition may be obscured.

In most bones, loss of bone protein matrix and minerals outpaces appositional growth. As a result, the bone becomes more porous, and the risk of fractures increases. Changes in bone with age are discussed in detail later. As a result of the characteristic loss of bone and cells and the gain in fat, which is the only tissue lighter than water, the specific gravity of the human body diminishes progressively into advanced age.

Lean body mass is the name given to fat-free body tissues such as skeletal muscles, organ parenchyma, and nerves. These organs are called the "engine of the body" because they use oxygen and burn calories. Lean body mass tends to remain stable during maturity. Then, as the aging process advances, lean body mass slowly, progressively diminishes with age. This decline begins earlier and is more marked in aging men.

As a result of the loss of lean body mass and

TABLE 1. AVERAGE HEIGHTS AND WEIGHTS BY AGE AND SEX: U.S. HEALTH EXAMINATION STUDY 1960–62*

	Males		Females	
Age	Height (in.)	Weight (lbs.)	Height (in.)	Weight (lbs.)
18–24	68.7	160	63.8	129
25–34	69.1	171	63.7	136
35–44	68.5	172	63.5	144
45–54	68.2	172	62.9	147
55–64	67.4	166	62.4	152
65–74	66.9	160	61.5	146
75–79	65.9	150	61.1	138

*Based on a nationwide probability sample of 7,710 persons. Averages and fiftieth percentiles were quite equal. Both secular trends and aging changes are mirrored by such measures as the three-inch difference in height of younger and older males. *(From Stoudt HW, Damon A, et al: Weight, height and selected body measurements of adults–U.S., 1960–62. Public Health Service Publication 1000, Series 11, No. 8. Washington, D.C., U.S. Government Printing Office, 1965.)*

females is approximately the same in age groups 25 to 34 and 75 to 79. The weight decline in women is proportionately less than that in men (Rossman, 1979; Rossman, 1977).

MATRIX OF CONNECTIVE TISSUE

The intercellular matrix of connective tissue, which is responsible for the solid structure of the body, undergoes important changes with age. This matrix helps compartmentalize cells with similar functions. Without it, the body would be nothing but a random distribution of cells packaged in an epithelial bag. The matrix consists of a macromolecular network, fluids and solutes enclosed in a basement membrane. The macromolecules include collagen, elastin, glycoproteins, proteoglycans, and hyaluronic acid molecules arranged in a highly ordered framework. The structure of connective tissue is highly specific and depends upon the specific tissues associated with it. Connective tissue produces and maintains the molecules that form the matrix.

Both collagen and elastin undergo changes with age. These two fibrous proteins normally play key roles in limiting deformation, transmitting forces and determining elastic properties of tissues (Kohn, 1977). With age, collagen fibers become more and more stable to external influences. The tissues become dense and less responsive to mechanical stress, losing flexibility. These changes are caused by the formation of intermolecular bonds called cross-links. Cross-links can include a variety of intermolecular bonds between two chemically identical or chemically different molecules. The nature of the mechanism of the formation of cross-links is not understood. The aggregated collagen molecules, reinforced with covalent cross-links, give collagen fibers unusual stability. The dense, cross-linked collagen molecules probably affect diffusion of nutrients and wastes and impair function. This would account for the reduced pulmonary compliance and vascular elasticity that occur with age. "Changes in the properties of collagen probably constitute the most definitive basic aging process that has been observed in mammals" (Kohn, 1977, p. 311).

The elastic fibers of the connective tissue are composed of the macromolecular complex elastin. With age, the elastic fibers undergo chemical mod-

ification resulting in the formation of cross-links. Fibers become yellow, brittle, frayed, and fragmented, and bind calcium salts. As a result, tissue elasticity is reduced. These changes have been documented in the elastic fiber of both skin and blood vessels. The matrices of cartilage, which contain both collagen and elastin, become brittle and more easily disrupted. These changes contribute to the increased incidence of arthritis in the elderly (Balazs, 1977; Tonn, 1977; and Goldman, 1979).

MUSCULOSKELETAL SYSTEM

After maturity, a series of complex changes related to use, growth, hyperplasia and regression occur in all parts of the bony skeleton. Atrophic changes take place in the muscles as well. These changes have profound consequences not only for the appearance but also for the function of the older person.

Bone

With aging, the bone undergoes complex changes, some of which are poorly understood. After age 45 in both men and women, there is a shift from an increase in bone mass to a progressive decrease. Aging bone loss is a universal phenomenon which parallels the atrophy of other tissues that occurs with age (Exton-Smith and Overstall, 1979).

Bone tissue consists of fibrogenic and osteogenic cell compartments, and age changes occur in both. Age changes occur in different ways and at different rates in endosteal and periosteal cells. Endosteal bone cells show higher activation than periosteal cells, and age changes appear much later in the endosteum than they do in the periosteum (Tonn, 1977).

Changes in many bones indicate that bone growth continues beyond the sixth decade. The process of apposition by which osteoblasts lay down new bone beneath the periosteum continues at least until advanced old age. Consequently, the circumference of bones is increased. Appositional bone growth has been demonstrated in the ribs, femur and metacarpals until the eighth decade. In addition, the pelvis continues to widen until the sixth decade, when growth stabilizes. The skull thickens. The sphenofrontal, mastoccipital, and parietomastoid sutures begin to close, a process that is not completed until the eighth decade. Changes in the cranial vault are particularly interesting because they cannot be related to weight bearing or stress (Rossman, 1977).

In spite of osteoblastic activity, reabsorption of the interior of long and flat bones occurs at a faster rate than bone growth. Both protein and minerals are lost from bone matrix. Trabecular bone is lost to a greater degree than cortical bone (Barrows and Roeder, 1977). Loss of bone mass, called osteoporosis, is a universal phenomenon but occurs to a greater extent in females. Bone loss in women is about 25 percent and in men about 12 percent (Goldman, 1979). Atrophy of cortical bone and demineralization of vertebral trabecular bone occur with greater frequency in women (Tonn, 1977). Loss of bone mass weakens the bone and places the older person at risk for fractures. Although a degree of osteoporosis is a normal concomitant of aging, a number of stresses, including immobilization, failure to absorb calcium, excessive calcium loss or endocrine disorders place older persons at risk for other types of osteoporosis. In Chapter 15 osteoporosis is discussed in more detail.

Joints

Progressive changes in both weight-bearing and non-weight-bearing joints begin as early as the second or third decade. After age 40, changes due to use are even more marked and increase each decade. Damage to joints may not be seen on roentgenograms, but it is obvious upon autopsy.

Cartilage, which surfaces joints, is particularly affected by the passage of time. The typical translucent, bluish appearance of articular cartilage is altered by age 20 to an opaque, yellowish structure. By age 30, the surface cracks, frays, and shreds. Eventually, deep vertical fissures form on the surface of the cartilage. Cartilage cells, called chondrocytes, cluster in large numbers in individual lacunae. Progressive cell death occurs and masses of irregular bodies are found. Slowly, cartilage layers are eroded and the bone makes direct contact with bone. Pain and crepitation can result. Gradually, the subchondral bone is rubbed smooth and becomes dense and hard. Subchondral bone marrow becomes hyperemic and extravasation of red blood cells and fibrosis occur (Tonn, 1977).

Depending upon the degree of stress and degradation of cartilage, osteophytes are formed at the margins of joints. This irregular growth of new bone is an attempt to buttress the joints and can eventually result in the formation of a bridge between the articular ends (Subbarao, 1979).

Synovial membranes exhibit numerous age changes, including fibrosis and shredding. The synovial fluid becomes more viscous (Subbarao, 1979).

The percent of water in the intervertebral discs decreases with age and contributes, in part, to the loss of height in the aged. Progressive degenerative changes occur in the cells and matrix of the nucleus pulposus. The number of cells decreases and metachromatic material is lost. As a result, the nucleus pulposus loses turgor and becomes increasingly friable with advancing age (Tonn, 1977). In addition, osteophyte formation on the vertebral column is so predictable that it is used as a criterion for age. This osteoarthritic change is especially marked in the mobile portions of the spine, particularly the cervical and lumbar spine. By age 50, 25 percent of persons have osteoarthritic changes in the cervical spine at the C6 or C7 level. By age 70, 75 percent of people exhibit osteoarthritic changes (Rossman, 1977).

Muscles

Muscles are composed of motor units. Each motor unit is composed of bundles of muscle fibers and is enervated by a single motor neuron. Each muscle fiber is a postmitotic cell, and as such, is not capable of replacing itself. The motor unit is dependent upon its neuron for structural and functional integrity. Without a nerve supply, muscle fibers atrophy. With age, changes occur at all levels—in muscle cells, motor units, and muscles.

Changes in muscle cells are not uniform and vary widely, depending upon the muscle's function. With age, muscle cells are lost. Those that remain atrophy, and the diameter of the fibers is reduced. The process of protein synthesis in aging muscle cells is changed and overall muscle cell activity is decreased.

Because of cellular atrophy, there is a decrease in muscle weight relative to body weight. In old age, muscles exhibit an increase in extracellular substances, including water, sodium, and chloride. Intracellular components, including potassium, are reduced. Fat and collagen are increased. The density of capillaries in aging muscle is decreased and may result in inadequate transfer of metabolites between capillaries and muscle cells.

The end result of changes in muscle cells and motor units is a decrease in muscle mass. With age, there is a progressive loss of muscle bulk. Muscle wasting may be masked somewhat by increased fat and collagen in muscles or it may be obvious. Wasting of the muscles on the dorsum of the hand is usually indicative of the amount of muscle wasting elsewhere (Gutmann, 1977).

Motor function undergoes a marked decline with age. Muscle strength declines slowly during maturity and at a somewhat faster rate after the fifth decade. At age 60 the total loss is about 10 to 20 percent of the maximum. Muscle endurance declines significantly and muscles are more quickly fatigued. Changes in overall cellular activity and protein synthesis may be partially responsible for the decline. Changes in nervous pathways, central synaptic mechanisms, receptors and effectors take place and also contribute to declining function. Motor nerve fibers, including their myelin sheath and Schwann cells, undergo degenerative changes. Segmental demyelination and remyelination of peripheral motor nerve fibers occur. Over time this process results in lesions that retard the ability of the nerve to conduct synchronous volleys of impulses (Brody and Vijayashanker, 1977). Although some swelling may occur on the longest axons, the axons in aging muscles remain intact. Consequently, there is a reduction in muscle fibers but no corresponding reduction in motor nerve fibers. Thus, there is a change in the overall pattern of enervation in aging muscles. There is a decrease in norepinephrine in aging muscles and a decrease in postsynaptic cholinesterase activity in aging muscle end plates. It is possible that the neuromuscular junction is less sensitive to acetylcholine. Apparently, declining function is attributable, in part, to the diminished sensitivity of aging muscle to neural input (Gutmann, 1977).

Motor function is a complex phenomenon that is affected by endocrine function, nutrition, activity level, and motivation. A number of hormones, including somatotropin and thyrotropin, are important in regulating protein metabolism. Changes in these hormones may affect development of senescent muscle atrophy. Testosterone and possibly other androgens play a role in muscle function, as does growth hormone. Changes in the circulating blood levels of these hormones may contribute to the decline in muscle function. Decreased mobilization of glucose in response to exercise may also be a factor. The rate of decline in muscle function is also affected by nutritional patterns. Inadequate nutrients accelerate the degenerative process. Disuse is also believed to be a factor in the rate of change in senescent muscles because both the diaphragm and the heart exhibit aging changes to a lesser extent than other muscles (Gutmann, 1977).

Body Measurements

Evidence of statural decline with age comes from studies of persons who were measured and then remeasured after a suitable interval. Loss of height begins earlier and is more marked in females. Because long bones do not undergo significant shortening with age, loss of height is due primarily to a loss of sitting height. The vertebral column shortens as a result of narrowing of the disks and loss of height of individual vertebrae. Thinning of vertebral disks is the main reason for declining stature in middle age. Diminution of the height of the vertebrae is the main reason for loss of height thereafter. Osteoporotic vertebral narrowing also contributes to loss of height, particularly in women. Data on people over age 80 are sparse but indicate that the decline in height is accelerated in the very old (Rossman, 1979).

Other measurements also change with age. At maturity, the span measurement is equal to height. After age 65, the span measurement in both men and women decreases by about 2 or 3 percent, an insignificant amount. Shoulder width declines because of a decrease in the deltoid muscles and the acromion. The chest increases in size and depth (Rossman, 1977).

THE INTEGUMENT

Because of its accessibility, the skin can be readily observed for changes that occur with age. All three layers of the epidermis undergo characteristic changes. The barrier efficiency of the stratum corneum in restricting penetration of water and chemicals is reduced. Cells throughout the epidermis become more varied in size and shape and in other cellular properties. Mitotic activity is reduced. As a consequence, epithelialization of open wounds takes more time. Exposure to the sun tends to further reduce mitosis.

In Caucasians the melanocytes in the inner layers of the epidermis undergo changes. In many areas of the body, including the buttocks and abdomen, the number of melanocytes decreases. Those that remain are unevenly distributed and are often larger in size, possibly as a result of functional hypertrophy. The function of remaining melanocytes is diminished, and they are no longer able to produce an even distribution of pigment when exposed to the sun (Selmanowitz et al., 1977).

Dermal changes, particularly in collagen, make the skin stiffer and less pliable. Collagen fibers make up about 75 percent of the dermis. With age, cross-links between the collagen molecules do not increase in number. Instead they become more stable and less soluble. The elastin content of the dermis increases and becomes irregular, calcified, and cross-linked. Changes in elastin and collagen are accentuated in sun-damaged skin. The number of capillary loops and blood vessels in the superficial dermis decreases and the vascular network flattens. Vessels become more fragile, resulting in small hemorrhages, called senile purpura (Selmanowitz et al., 1977). The subcutaneous fat below the dermis is markedly reduced, particularly on the extremities, and places the person at risk for decubiti. Fat loss is usually greater in men. As a result of degenerative changes in the epidermis and dermis, the skin becomes yellowish and leathery and loses its resiliency.

Wrinkling of skin is a hallmark of aging. Several factors are involved in the development of wrinkles. Changes in the dermis and loss of subcutaneous fat are partially responsible for wrinkle formation. As the skin becomes lax, it sags and drapes itself according to gravitational pull. Wrinkling is also enhanced where the skin is frequently folded. The repeated use of facial muscles acts as a mechancial stress responsible for the characteristic facial wrinkles observed in the aged. Factors such as toughness and elasticity of skin, amount of subcutaneous fat, exposure to the sun, and nutritional status also determine the extent of wrinkling (Selmanowitz et al., 1977).

Wrinkling normally begins on the forehead early in the second decade. Curvilinear wrinkles parallel to each eye are caused by muscle contraction. Wrinkles called "crow's feet" radiate laterally from each canthus. Other facial wrinkles develop by the root of the nose, on the upper and lower lids, around the mouth, and in the area adjacent to the mouth toward the chin. Individuals past 60 years of age develop multiple fine wrinkles of the upper and lower lips that radiate out from the vermilion border. Often, the neck undergoes shrinking and wrinkling that may be even more marked than facial wrinkles. A characteristic change that occurs in the fifth decade is the appearance of two prominent lines coursing up the neck on either side of the midline. In addition to the wrinkling, the lax skin drapes itself and produces a ptosis of lids, ears, jowls, and submental wrinkling (Rossman, 1979).

Many of the characteristic adaptations of the aging skin are due to regressive changes. However, there are also alterations of a hyperplastic and neoplastic character, such as the formation of senile keratoses, acrochordons, cherry angiomata, leukoplakia, and carcinomas. These changes point up some of the contradictory aspects of the aging process (Lombardo, 1979). They are discussed in detail in Chapter 7.

The sebaceous glands do not atrophy with age, but function decreases. Sebum production declines after the menopause in women but remains high in men until age 80. Diminished sebum production is believed to be due, in part, to reduced gonadal and adrenal androgen production (Selmanowitz et al., 1977).

Changes in the sweat glands result in drier skin and difficulty in regulating body temperature. Eccrine glands decrease in number. Most apocrine glands show no structural changes; however, function is reduced. These glands are influenced in part by hormone levels (Selmanowitz et al., 1977).

Sensory nerves in the skin, specifically Meissner's and pacinian corpuscles, are reduced in number. This adaptation is a reliable indication of advancing age (Selmanowitz et al., 1977).

In general, aging skin is characterized by diminishing function and reserve capacity. Wound healing is retarded. Trauma that might be insignificant for a younger person can result in serious adaptations, such as decubiti, for the older person.

Fortunately, the skin's diminished function rarely reduces the older person's longevity (Selmanowitz et al., 1977).

Nail growth progressively declines with age. The growth rate is influenced by activity, temperature, nutritional status, hormones, circulatory changes, and race. Longitudinal ridges, which develop on the nailplate as a result of localized injuries to the nail matrix, become more numerous and more prominent with age. Color changes of the nail plate also occur (Selmanowitz et al., 1977).

Hair follicle function in the aged is influenced by sex-linked endocrine and genetic factors. There are two types of baldness: sex-linked baldness and common baldness. Sex-linked baldness affects men. It is inherited from the mother and effectuated in the presence of testosterone. Sex-linked baldness involves several different patterns of hair loss and may begin when the man is in his 20s.

Common baldness is the hair loss that normally accompanies the aging process. A progressive diminution of the deep dermal blood vessels of the scalp accompanies common baldness (Selmanowitz et al., 1977). Hair follicles decrease in size, not number. The coarse, long, pigmented terminal hairs found on the head are replaced by fine, short, nonpigmented vellus hairs. As a result, the scalp hairs are lighter, thinner, and less numerous. Hair loss from common baldness is not patterned and is usually evident in both men and women after age 60.

Graying of hair usually precedes hair loss. It is influenced by hormonal and genetic factors (Rossman, 1979). Graying occurs because melanocytes at the base of the hair follicles are reduced in number. Because those that remain are less productive of pigment, graying results (Selmanowitz et al., 1977).

Patterns of body hair also change with age, but there are vast differences between the sexes and among various racial and ethnic groups. In Caucasian women, facial hirsutism frequently occurs after age 40, and in Caucasian men, terminal hairs may grow in the ears, particularly on the tragus or antitragus. Loss of axillary hair occurs gradually in both men and women, proceeding from the periphery to the center. Pubic hair is also lost. Remaining hairs are gray, thin and less kinky. Hormonal factors probably influence axillary and pubic hair loss.

Often leg hair may be scanty or absent in both men and women. In females, arm hair may also be thin. Some very old persons may be almost hairless (Rossman, 1979).

RESPIRATORY SYSTEM

Despite numerous age-related changes in the structure and function of the respiratory system, the aged retain the ability to maintain adequate oxygenation under conditions of health and moderate activity. In one way, respiratory status might even be said to improve. The frequency of colds declines in the aged from 2 per year in young adulthood to 1 per year in old age because immunities are built up (Goldman, 1979). However, intensive physical exertion or stresses such as infections, surgery, and prolonged bed rest compromise the respiratory function of the aged and may even threaten life.

With age, the anteroposterior diameter of the chest increases, giving the appearance of a "barrel chest." This condition has been called "postural emphysema" or "senile emphysema." Both terms are misleading because most of the elderly with this adaptation do not have the functional characteristics of emphysema (Klocke, 1977).

The chest wall includes the rib cage and diaphragm. With age, the rib cage becomes more rigid. Progressive kyphosis, osteoporosis, and calcification of costal cartilages further reduce the compliance of the chest wall and compromise lung function. The respiratory musculature atrophies and weakens. In the elderly, the rib cage plays a less important role in altering lung volume and the diaphragm becomes more important.

Although there is a decrease in chest wall compliance with age, there is a simultaneous increase in lung compliance. However, because the increase in lung compliance is less than the decrease in chest wall compliance, the work expenditure of breathing increases to overcome the elastic forces and move the chest wall. Between ages 20 and 70 the work of breathing increases by 20 percent. Because lung compliance is increased and elastic recoil is reduced with age, it is less likely that the lung will collapse when the chest cavity is opened (DeVries, 1975; Klocke, 1977).

Ciliary action, responsible for moving secretions, declines as a result of epithelial atrophy. The cough reflex may be less sensitive to stimuli and the cough itself is less effective because of decreased muscle strength and increased chest wall rigidity. These changes impair broncho-elimination and contribute to the increased incidence of pneumonia in the elderly. Bronchial mucous glands hypertrophy with age. There is no information about how this change affects lung function. No changes have been identified in pulmonary surfactant, an important factor in maintaining the stability of the air-tissue interface in the lungs (Klocke, 1977). Respiratory bronchioles enlarge and alveolar ducts dilate. These changes combine to reduce the overall alveolar volume and increase the pulmonary dead space.

Lung Volumes

There is a high correlation between lung volumes and age. While total lung capacity and inspiratory capacity remain constant, various other lung volumes are markedly influenced by age (Fig. 2). Vital capacity decreases with age in both men and women and consequently, both functional residual capacity

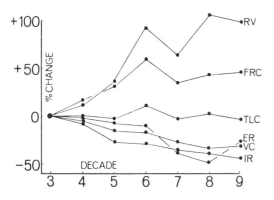

Figure 2. Percentage change in static lung volumes in normal subjects at various ages compared to values found in the third decade of life. All data are expressed as volume per square meter of body surface area. RV = residual volume, FRC = functional residual capacity, TLC = total lung capacity, ER = expiratory reserve, VC = vital capacity, IR = inspiratory reserve. *From Mithoefer JC, Karetzky MS: The cardiopulmonary system in the aged, in Powers JH (ed), Surgery of the Aged and Debilitated Patient. Philadelphia, Saunders, 1968, with permission.*

and residual volume increase. Elevation of the ribs and flattening of the diaphragm account for a 50 percent increase in functional residual capacity between ages 30 and 90. Residual volume increases by 100 percent and results in partial inflation of the lungs at rest. Expiratory reserve volume and inspiratory reserve volume also decline (Klocke, 1977). The maximum ventilation attained during exhausting work gradually declines by about 60 percent from the late teens to the eighth decade (DeVries, 1975).

Airflow

Indices of airflow also decline with advanced age. The maximum voluntary ventilation, maximal expiratory flow rate, maximal mid-expiratory flow, and the forced expiratory volume decrease by about 20 to 50 percent through the adult years. These tests depend on a variety of factors and there is controversy about why decreases in airflow occur. More work needs to be done to identify factors that result in reductions of airflow indices (Klocke, 1977).

Pulmonary Circulation

Pulmonary arterial walls thicken due to deposits of acellular material in the intima and thickening of the media (Klocke, 1977). Pulmonary blood flow is reduced subsequent to the decrease in cardiac output. The number of capillaries surrounding the alveoli decreases, and those that remain develop thickened walls due to excessive fibrous connective tissue. Consequently, the pulmonary diffusing capacity of oxygen decreases about 8 percent over the life span (Shock, 1977).

Pulmonary Oxygen

There is a progressive increase in the alveolar–arterial oxygen difference $(A - a)O_2$ with age. Alveolar oxygen tension remains constant, but arterial oxygen pressure declines with age. Because arterial Pa_{CO_2} remains normal in the aged, this difference is not believed to be due to alveolar hypotension. Instead, it is believed that the development of uneven distribution of inspired oxygen and pulmonary blood flow is responsible (Klocke, 1977). In young adults the basal portions of the lung are ventilated optimally and capillary blood flow to this area is greatest. The increasing lung rigidity that accompanies aging results in relative basal alveolar collapse and improved apical ventilation. However, capillary blood flow to these upper regions remains inadequate. As a result, a mismatch develops between areas of optimal ventilation and areas of optimal perfusion. The mismatch is reflected in the arterial Pao_2, which decreases progressively to approximately 70 to 85 mm Hg in the elderly (Elkowitz, 1981). The oxygen saturation declines by about 5 percent (Goldman, 1979).

Another factor that may contribute to the nonuniform ventilation and decline in Pao_2 has to do with the changes in closing volume and residual volume that accompany aging. Due to the diminished elastic recoil of the lungs, closing volume increases progressively with age (Wynne, 1979). This means that in the aged, small airways begin to close at a greater lung volume. When closing volume approaches functional residual capacity, the airways at the base of the lungs close and those at the apex remain open, contributing to nonuniform ventilation. Deep breathing minimizes premature airway closure in the aged and thus may raise the Pao_2 (Tichy and Malasanos, 1979a). Other factors that may contribute to the lower pressure of arterial oxygen in the aged include the increased dead space and reduced diffusing capacity (Goldman, 1979).

CARDIOVASCULAR SYSTEM

Changes involving the cardiovascular system are central to major questions about aging. Aging of the cardiovascular system may underlie, in part, the general decline in structure and function that characterizes the aging process. Differentiating primary and secondary age changes in the cardiovascular system is difficult because a change in one component of the cardiovascular system influences the properties and activity of other components. The major causes of death in the aging population are diseases of the cardiovascular system. Some of these diseases may represent the aging process itself and others are undoubtedly influenced by or dependent upon the aging process.

Because it is composed of postmitotic cells, the cardiovascular system is not designed to live forever. Smooth muscle and endothelial cells in blood vessels do not divide unless they receive some special stimulus, such as injury. Age-related changes take place in the chemical composition, cells, and tissues of the heart and blood vessels and affect many aspects of cardiovascular function (Kohn, 1977).

Heart

Data on age-related changes in heart size are inconclusive. Heart weight, expressed as a percent of body weight, increases in older age, particularly in males. However, this change is believed to be due to the age-related reduction in overall body weight (Kohn, 1977). According to Burch (1977) heart size in many healthy aging people remains normal or decreases slightly. On the other hand, studies have documented an increase in the thickness of the left ventricular wall in healthy individuals. Between ages 30 and 80, the thickness of the left ventricular wall increases by 25 percent (Sjögren, 1971; Exton-Smith and Overstall, 1979; Gerstenblith et al., 1977). Accumulated data suggest that while a small amount of cardiac enlargement may occur in a large portion of the aging population, significant cardiac hypertrophy is not inevitable and should not be considered a primary aging change.

A characteristic change in the myocardium is the deposition of lipofuscin pigment in cardiac cells. The amount present has not been related to any disease or abnormality in cardiac function, but its presence increases progressively with age (Kohn, 1977).

The atrial and ventricular myocardium differ somewhat in their aging changes. Muscle as a percentage of the heart decreases with age. In the ventricles, muscle fiber size gradually increases with age (McMillan and Lev, 1962). Fibrosis and sclerosis occur, particularly in the endocardium, which lines the cavities of the heart (Kohn, 1977). Fat infiltration occurs, particularly in the right atrium and ventricles (McMillan and Lev, 1962). The amount of connective tissues increases. Changes in the properties of the connective tissue are responsible for increased myocardial stiffness. Therefore, with age, there is reduced compliance, or reduced relaxation of tension. As a result, the heart functions less efficiently as a pump (Kohn, 1977).

Hemodynamic stresses alter the heart valves, particularly the mitral and aortic valves. Nodular thickening, calcification, and fibrosis cause them to become rigid (Exton-Smith and Overstall, 1979). Distortion of the aortic valve cusps occurs with age and may result in some blockage of flow to the coronary vessels. Rigidity and incomplete closure of heart valves in the aging may result in systolic murmurs.

Cardiac Function

Rate. The resting heart rate is essentially unchanged by age. The heart rate increase in response to stress is less effective with age and the time for the heart rate to return to normal is prolonged (Kohn, 1977). The increase in heart rate may be impaired because of increased connective tissue in the sino-atrial (S A) and atrioventricular (A V) nodes and in the bundle branches. The number of catecholamine receptors on muscle fibers may be decreased and influence the reduced rate. In addition, with age, the refractory interval between stimuli that cause a mechanical response increases even though there is no increase in the electric refractory interval. Other studies indicate that the isometric contraction and relaxation times are prolonged with age (Harrison et al., 1964; Landowne et al., 1955; Shock, 1977).

Rhythm. Because the myocardium becomes more irritable with age, extrasystoles may occur (Rodstein, 1977). Sinus arrhythmias and sinus bradycardias may also occur in the normal aging heart (Harris, 1976). Atrial arrhythmias, such as atrial fibrillation and atrial flutter, may develop due to changes in the myocardial fibers, particularly a decrease in the amount of muscle and an increase in fibrous tissue at the S A node and internodal atrial tracts (Harris, 1976).

Electrocardiogram. The normal electrocardiogram undergoes several changes as a result of the aging process. Because these changes occur so frequently they do not have diagnostic significance. P-wave notching, slurring, and loss of amplitude are common, and may reflect loss of myocardial tissue and fibrosis (Rodstein, 1977). The PR interval increases. The QRS complex may also reveal

slurring and notching with age. There is diminished QRS amplitude due to obesity, senile emphysema, and an increased anteroposterior diameter. The QRS axis shifts to the left as a result of left ventricular thickening, kyphoscoliosis, and a lowered diaphragm, or the increased anteroposterior diameter of the chest (Rodstein, 1977; Goldman, 1979). Early in the aging process, there may be a flattening of the ST segments and low T waves (Mihalich and Fisch, 1977). Notched T waves may occur and are attributed to changes in the chest and metabolism, and to myocardial atrophy (Rodstein, 1977).

Cardiac Output. There is evidence to indicate that stroke volume, heart work (stroke volume × mean systolic blood pressure), and resting cardiac output decrease with age. With age, as the total vascular resistance increases, more heart work must be done to overcome the pressure, so less useful work is done (Landowne et al., 1955). Determinations of stroke volume and cardiac output in the aging vary somewhat depending on whether or not the subjects were truly in the resting state (Goldman, 1979). Resting cardiac output appears to decrease about 1 percent each year after age 20. This agrees with estimates of the strength of the myocardium, which also declines at a rate of about 0.85 percent each year after age 20 (Brandfonbrener et al., 1955).

Circulation Time. Circulation time is believed to increase with age in both men and women. Because of differences in heart rate and height, there is a wide range of individual variation in circulation time, but the range of variability is even greater among the aged (Willems et al., 1971).

Oxygen Consumption. The heart extracts large amounts of oxygen from each unit of blood. The maximal oxygen consumption declines with age at about the same rate as cardiac output. Maximal oxygen consumption is a measure of the limit of performance capacity. Since oxygen uptake does not vary with age, the decline in maximal oxygen consumption indicates a decline in work capacity with age (Goldman, 1979).

Cardiac Function During Stress. As stated earlier, the maximal heart rate achieved during stress goes down with age. When maximally stressed, stroke volume is also reduced. Therefore cardiac output is reduced. In both men and women this decrease is about 40 percent between the ages of 30 and 80, or slightly less than 1 percent a year. Aging apparently has no effect on the relationship of ventricular end-diastolic volume and ventricular performance. This relationship is known as the Frank-Starling law and states that the length of muscle fibers is proportionate to end-diastolic volume. At maximal stress, the right and left ventricular and diastolic pressures and the pulmonary wedge pressure are significantly higher in the elderly (Goldman, 1979).

Blood Vessels

Arteries. The vascular system exhibits progressive structural changes that directly influence function. Large arteries, particularly the aorta, show characteristic aging changes. The intima of arteries thickens and there is progressive fibrosis of the media. Smooth muscle cells in arteries decrease in number. Extracellular materials and collagen accumulate in both the intima and media (Bourne, 1960). The absolute number of collagen fibers in arteries increases. The fibers cross-link and become more restrictive with age. Materials such as lipids and minerals become trapped in arterial walls, injure cells, and may stimulate low-grade inflammation. It is believed that trapping may be a characteristic property of aging collagen. The development of atherosclerotic plaques is a complication of the trapping process rather than an intrinsic part of the aging process. Aging, however, is the major risk factor in the development of atherosclerosis. Arterial dilation, vessel tortuosity, and rigidity are age-related changes due in part to changes in the molecular structure of collagen (Kohn, 1977).

The most striking change in arteries is the redistribution, thinning, and fragmentation of elastin. In young adults, elastin accounts for 30 percent of the weight of the arteries and gives arteries resilience. With age, elastin binds increasingly with calcium and the total concentration of elastin drops. One theory is that, with age, elastin is progressively

destroyed. These phenomena are thought to be an intrinsic part of the aging process (Kohn, 1977).

With age, elastin and smooth muscles play less important roles in the functioning of aging arteries, and collagen takes on an increasingly prominent role. The result is an age-related stiffness throughout the arterial system. Aged arteries have been described as having the "elastic properties of rigid tubes" (Kohn, 1977, p. 286). Stiffening is not due, as once thought, to the atherosclerotic process. Research indicates that arterial stiffening may be a characteristic of all mammalian aging. Age-related structural changes are particularly marked in the ascending aorta and arch due to hemodynamic events (Exton-Smith and Overstall, 1979).

Until age 60, the aortic volume increases to compensate for the stiffness of large arteries. However, the intraaortic systolic pressure rises abruptly as an increasing amount of blood is forced into the vessel. Arterial stiffness impairs the pulsatile flow of blood and increases the work load of the left ventricle.

Arterial stiffness also makes the baroreceptors sluggish. Baroreceptors are located in the carotid sinus, aorta, pulmonary arteries, and other large arteries of the chest region. The baroreceptors are less able to moderate blood pressure, particularly during postural change (Kohn, 1977).

Because of arterial rigidity, the pulse wave velocity increases. This is reflected in changes in the character of the aging individual's pulse, which becomes more forceful (Harrison et al., 1964).

Veins. Veins undergo many of the same changes as arteries, but to a lesser degree because of the lower stresses to which they are subjected. The intima thickens and the media fibroses. The veins dilate and stretch. Structural changes in the valves of the large leg veins contribute to inadequate venous return (Syzek, 1976). Increased tortuosity of veins and phlebosclerosis are so common that they are considered normal aging changes (Kohn, 1977).

Microvasculature. Recent studies have indicated important changes in microvasculature. Arteriole walls and capillary basement membranes thicken. Narrowing of the lumen and other deformities of capillaries have also been noted. It may be that these changes slow the exchange of nutrients and waste products across the capillary wall (Kohn, 1977).

Blood Pressure

Several longitudinal studies have been done to determine blood pressure changes with age. There is an increase in systolic pressure and a slower rate of increase in diastolic pressure up to age 70. In women, the systolic pressure may decline slightly after age 70. In old age, the diastolic pressure in both sexes levels off or decreases. Because the aorta becomes increasingly rigid with age, systolic pressure rises to a greater extent than diastolic. The result is a widening of the pulse pressure (Bender, 1965). Reduced compliance of blood vessels and increased peripheral vascular resistance account for the rise in blood pressure. The slight elevation in blood pressure associated with aging may help preserve brain function in the elderly.

There is some question about whether increased blood pressure is inevitable in the aging. Elevated blood pressure is characteristic of many aging populations, but it may not be irreversible. It appears that there are vascular changes that tend to raise blood pressure with age. However, some individuals and populations seem capable of compensating by bringing other factors into play (Kohn, 1977).

Exercise causes proportional increases in systolic blood pressure in people of all ages, but in people over age 60, it takes longer for the blood pressure to return to resting levels after exercise. When placed on tilt tables, it takes longer for the elderly to increase their diastolic pressure and pulse rate when tilted from horizontal to vertical. These findings suggest that, with age, cardiovascular reactivity becomes sluggish during postural changes and recovery from exercise. However, the vasomotor response during exercise does not appear to be affected (Kohn, 1977).

Peripheral Vascular Resistance

Total peripheral vascular resistance is determined by the ratio of mean arterial pressure to cardiac output. With age peripheral vascular resistance progressively increases. The change in peripheral vascular resistance tends to decrease blood flow to various body organs. However, the decrease is not uniform. There are differences between organs in the degree of change. In addition, compensatory mechanisms, such as increased vascularization and vasodilation, may be initiated and mask the alterations in total systemic blood flow. In the absence of arteriosclerosis, cerebral, coronary vessel, and muscle flow changes are minimal. Finger–hand and especially renal flow decrease significantly (Bender, 1965). The decrease in renal blood flow is 53 percent between the ages of 20 and 90 (Shenkin et al., 1953; Kohn, 1977).

BLOOD

A large number of studies have focused on age-related changes in the blood and its components. A comprehensive review of this research by Hyams (1978) points out that most of the findings are conflicting and that very little certain knowledge exists about age-related changes in the blood.

Red Cells

Structural differences between the red blood cells of the young and the old are so subtle that it is very difficult to differentiate between erythrocytes of the old and the young. The mean diameter of red cells may increase slightly after age 50. Changes in red cell enzymes occur with age, but their significance is uncertain. These changes may influence the life span of the red cell (Hyams, 1978).

Blood volume remains constant throughout the life span and erythrocyte values undergo very few changes. The values may be very slightly reduced, their distribution becomes wider, and differences between the sexes with age become less. It is well known that testosterone influences hematopoiesis. Hyposecretion of testosterone by elderly males may account for the narrowing of differences between male and female values that occurs with age (Hyams, 1978). Total red cell, hematocrit, and hemoglobin values remain in the same range throughout life in healthy elderly persons who live at home and are socially active. Many differences recorded in these values in the aged are a reflection of stresses associated with living conditions, life-style, and level of adaptation, not a consequence of normal aging (Maekawa, 1976). For these reasons, a hemoglobin value below 12 g/100 ml in an elderly person should not be considered normal. Although anemia is common among the elderly, it is not a normal consequence of aging (Clifford and Bewtra, 1979).

Sedimentation Rate

Because the erythrocyte sedimentation rate (ESR) is a nonspecific test used to establish the presence or absence of a number of organic diseases, it is important to know whether normal values change as a consequence of age. Perhaps because the ESR requires careful standardization and is influenced by a variety of environmental factors, there is no general agreement on the effect of age on ESR. According to the best available data, the ESR is often found to be raised in normal healthy aging people, but plasma viscosity remains normal (Shapleigh et al., 1952). Because the ESR rate depends on plasma constituents, its rise in older people is believed to be due to the rise in globulins and fall in albumin that accompanies aging (Exton-Smith and Overstall, 1979; Hyams, 1978).

White Cells

Only very minor changes have been reported in the number, distribution, and morphological characteristics of leukocytes. There is no significant increase or decrease in the total number of white cells. Changes in the differential leukocyte count are less certain. MacKinney (1978) found that the number of lymphocytes decreased significantly with age. The lymphocyte count remained stationary until age 40 and then declined to age 90. There was no change in the granulocyte count. It is believed that the decrease in blood lymphocytes represents a loss of T lymphocytes with age. It is believed that the leukocytosis of inflammation in the elderly may be delayed and slightly diminished. No changes in phagocytic ability occur (Maekawa, 1976).

Platelets

No morphological change with aging has been reported, and platelet count and function are considered to be normal in the elderly (Shapleigh et al., 1952). There is a wide variation in platelet adhesiveness in the elderly, and some increased platelet adhesiveness may be characteristic of aging (Hyams, 1978).

Hemostasis

A rise in plasma fibrinogen occurs in the coagulation system of the elderly. As a result, diminished clot retraction occurs with age. It appears that changes in the hemostatic mechanism are slight and there is no significant change in coagulation in the healthy aged person. In addition, there appears to be no change or tendency toward shortening of the bleeding time in the elderly (Maekawa, 1976).

Hematopoiesis

Active hematopoietic cells in bone marrow gradually diminish with age as the fat content increases. This process occurs first in long bones and is slower in flat bones. Vertebrae are the last bones to exhibit this change (Hyams, 1978). Some minor changes occur in the ratios of various hematopoietic cells. Cells of the reticuloendothelial system increase and tissue mast cells appear. The reasons for bone marrow changes are not well understood and may be due to disease processes rather than aging.

Changes in stem cells have not been investigated extensively. There is some evidence for a gradual depletion of the stem cell pool during senescence and a decrease in the ability of hematopoietic stem cells to recover from radiation damage. Whether the decrease in relative size of the stem cell pool during old age reflects impairment of hematopoiesis or some other process is unclear at this time. Hematopoiesis is regulated by erythropoietin, a humoral factor, but there is no information about age-related differences in this substance (Maekawa, 1976).

A fall in hematopoiesis following bleeding has been noted in the elderly, but it is believed to be due to iron depletion (Maekawa, 1976). Iron absorption from the gastrointestinal tract is reduced and plasma iron, iron-binding capacity, and the iron-binding protein transferrin are decreased in the elderly (Hyams, 1978).

The usual adaptation to reduced oxygen tension at high altitudes is also reduced. Usually, respiratory volume increases and in a few days the hemoglobin concentration of the blood is increased. This response requires more time in the aged, and the final increase in hemoglobin content in the blood is lower. In fact, some of the elderly actually exhibit a decline in hemoglobin in the first few days at high altitude, indicating an impairment of the response. Because this impairment is usually seen in the very old, the response is believed to get progressively worse with age (Shock, 1977).

IMMUNE SYSTEM

The immune system protects the body against foreign invasion by viruses, bacteria, fungi, and possibly one's own somatic cells that have undergone neoplastic changes. Any stress that can decrease the normal surveillance of the immune system will allow the growth of invasive antigens that can disrupt body functions. The immune system, therefore, plays a major role in preserving or shortening life.

The bone marrow, thymus, spleen, and lymph nodes are the major organs of the immune system. Immune cells include lymphocytes and macrophages. The B cells develop in the bone marrow and are responsible for humoral antibody response. After initial contact with an antigen, some B cells pass through several stages of development and form the gamma globulin antibodies that circulate throughout the body. The T cells develop in the thymus. They are responsible for cell-mediated responses such as delayed hypersensitivity, rejection of foreign cell tissues, and immunity against tumor cells. It is believed that T cells also act to mediate some or all of the antibody responses in B cells. The macrophages, also derived from bone marrow, are scavengers of foreign antigens and present foreign antigens to the B and T cells for antigenic recognition.

With age, certain anatomical changes that may affect immune functions take place, With the onset of sexual maturity the cortex of the thymus atrophies. As aging progresses, histological changes occur in the lymphatic tissues, and the lymph nodes and spleen diminish slightly in size. There is disagreement about whether the number of lymphocytes decreases or remains constant throughout life. Further disagreement exists over whether the number of B and T cells remains constant. There may be a reduction in the absolute number of T cells with age (Clifford and Bewtra, 1979). Alterations in circulating immunoglobulins in the aged are also uncertain (Hafercamp et al., 1966). A striking observation of one study was the increased variability

of serum immunoglobulin concentrations with age (Buckley and Dorsey, 1974).

Although the precise changes that occur in the immune system are poorly understood, we do know that normal immune function declines with age, beginning after sexual maturity, when the thymus begins to involute. At present, the strongest theory is that age affects the T cells, their ability to proliferate when antigenically stimulated and to promote B-cell function. Once the thymus involutes, the body must rely on what T cells are present for the remainder of the life span. Over time, these aged cells show a decline in function (Adler et al., 1978). There is no evidence that B cells change with age. However, their function, particularly their ability to proliferate, declines with age. This decline may occur because normal T cells are important for the optimal functioning of B cells (Makinodan, 1977).

Age-related immune dysfunction predisposes the aged to a variety of stresses. There is an age-related increase in the incidence of autoantibodies, and their preponderance in women in young adulthood alters to a more equal incidence in the sexes in old age (Hyams, 1978). A number of autoimmune disorders, including senile amyloidosis, adult-onset diabetes, certain hemolytic anemias, and forms of periarteritis, are found most often in the aged. The incidence of certain infectious diseases and cancers is also increased (Latham and Johnson, 1979). On the other hand, there is a decrease in delayed hypersensitivity reactions in old age and other forms of allergy may be less marked (Hyams, 1978).

GASTROINTESTINAL SYSTEM

The gastrointestinal system performs important activities, including secretion, motility, and absorption. For the aged, it is also the source of many complaints but is rarely responsible for death. Little substantial information is available on the effects of aging on the gastrointestinal system. Lack of information stems from the fact that the alimentary system has such an enormous reserve capacity that significant decrements in normal function can occur with little appreciable effect on physiological processes. Refinements in measuring techniques used to study the gastrointestinal system are needed to overcome this handicap. In addition, studies are needed to differentiate the effects of normal aging from the effects of diseases, diet, daily habits, and environmental factors.

Oral Cavity

Age-associated changes take place in the teeth, gums, taste buds, and saliva and compromise the ingestion and digestion of food. Teeth are gradually lost with advancing age. Those that remain show numerous changes. Attritional wear at the height of the cusps occurs and diminishes the height of the crown. The enamel may be completely penetrated and the underlying dentin exposed. Attrition occurs because of stresses such as wear and caries.

The dentin found in the teeth of the aging is called "secondary dentin," a calcified, tubular substance that is slowly, progressively laid down throughout life. Gradually, it replaces most of the volume of the dental pulp or "nerve" of the tooth. Though softer than enamel, secondary dentin is hard and fibrotic and less conductive of pain than young dentin. Eventually, secondary dentin occludes the pulp chamber, leaving residual pulp tissue confined to the root. This progressive walling in of the pulp is a universal sign of the aging process.

Throughout life, cementum continues to be deposited around the root. In addition, cementum calcifies. An almost universal relationship exists between age and cementum thickness.

With aging, a migration of gingival epithelial tissue in the direction of the apex occurs. This passive migration results in the visible elongation of the exposed tooth. The process involves the detachment of the epithelium from root cementum, lysis of gingival submucosal collagen, and atrophy and progressive lowering of the apical crest of supporting alveolar bone. There is some question about whether gingival migration is a normal aging change or a pathological process (Zack, 1979).

Beginning in middle age, the number of taste buds per papilla decreases. There is also an increase in the average taste threshold with age (Storandt, 1979).

Because saliva lubricates food, it facilitates chewing and swallowing and enhances the sensation of taste. Saliva contains ptylin, which initiates the breakdown of starches, particularly dextrin. With age there is a decline in the secretory rate of saliva, both stimulated and unstimulated. The aged produce only one-third of the saliva produced by young adults. Decreased saliva contributes to dry mouth and tongue and perhaps to diminished taste sensation (Goldman, 1979).

Esophagus

In the aged, columnar epithelia replace squamous epithelia in the lower esophagus, but it is not certain whether this is a normal aging change or a sign of pathology (Goldman, 1979). Normally, swallowing generates peristaltic waves that transport the food bolus to the stomach. Nonperistaltic waves are localized, ringlike, nonpropulsive contractions that occur normally in the lower esophagus after swallowing or spontaneously. Apparently, peristaltic waves often fail to occur in the elderly and nonperistaltic waves occur more often. In addition, researchers have found that the esophagus is often dilated and the lower esophageal sphincter often fails to relax (Hollis and Castell, 1974). Consequently, there is a delay in esophageal emptying. This phenomenon is called presbyesophagus. It is uncertain whether presbyesophagus is age related or a consequence of disease (Bhanthimnavis and Schuster, 1977; Hollis and Castell, 1974). Further research needs to be done to delineate normal esophageal changes with age. Esophageal disorders, including diffuse spasms, achalasia, scleroderma of the esophagus, and hiatal hernia occur with increasing frequency in the elderly (Bhanthimnavis and Schuster, 1977).

Stomach

After age 50 morphological changes are evident in 80 percent of the population and occur in all layers of the stomach. Adipose tissue accumulates and smooth muscle thins out. Loss of parietal and chief cells is reflected in hyposecretion of acid and pepsin (Schuster, 1976). Loss of surface epithelial cells results in a decreased secretion of alkaline viscid mucus, which serves to protect the stomach from autodigestion (Tichy and Malasanos, 1979b). Thinning of the gastric mucosa is sometimes accompanied by leukocyte infiltration and metaplasia of the glands of the fundus. The submucosa may be infiltrated with monocytes and elastic fibers. These changes increase the risk of polypoid and precancerous neoplasia (Schuster, 1976). The incidence of atrophic gastritis or gastric atony rises with age (Tichy and Malasanos, 1979b).

As a consequence of structural changes, the functional ability of the stomach declines. Diminished secretion of acid and pepsin, first noticed in the fifth decade, declines further in men over 60. Because diminution of free and total gastric acid is most marked in association with atrophic gastritis, it is uncertain whether this is a normal or pathological change (Bhanthimnavis and Schuster, 1977). The efficiency of pepsin is also reduced. The low acid environment of the aging stomach reduces the absorption of vitamin B_{12} and iron. Gastric atrophy also results in decreased production of intrinsic factor, but the decrease is not sufficient to result in pernicious anemia. Between ages 40 and 60, gastric secretions drop to about 20 percent of their earlier values and then become stable (Goldman, 1979). However, ample quantities of digestive enzymes remain available for digestive functions (Sklar et al., 1956).

Small Intestine

Data concerning age-related changes in the structure of the small intestine are meager. After age 40, the weight of the small intestine drops steadily. Fibrous tissue replaces parenchyma. The number of muscle fibers in all three layers of the small intestine decreases, and some of those that remain atrophy (Schuster, 1976). Peyer's patches are decreased in number and the number of lymphatic follicles in individual patches is reduced (Bhanthimnavis and Schuster, 1977).

Information on intestinal enzymes in the aged is scarce. It has been suggested that there is a decrease in enzymatic concentration, but that the enzyme structure remains the same.

There have been few studies of intestinal absorption in the aged. Absorption is a critical function of the gastrointestinal tract. A number of age-related factors could influence absorption, including the rate and degree of digestion, the integrity of absorbing surfaces, the efficiency of transport mechanisms, bowel motility, and vascular perfusion. Lipids are known to be absorbed more slowly, possibly because of a decreased production of lipase by the pancreas. However, there is a possibility that blood lipid levels in the aged may also be the result of impaired metabolism or distribution of fat, rather

than impaired absorption (Bender, 1968). Defects in amino acid absorption have also been noted and are believed to be due, in part, to a decrease in trypsin production by the pancreas (Goldman, 1979). There is also a decrease in the ability to absorb pentose and hexose sugars, such as glucose and galactose, from the jejunum by an active process that does not require bile salts or pancreatic enzymes (Guth, 1968). Passive transport processes also exhibit impaired absorption after age 65, possibly due to a reduction in the number of cells (Bender, 1965). Therefore, aging is associated with some small bowel mucosal dysfunction.

Both calcium and iron are absorbed in the proximal small intestine and depend upon gastric acid secretion. Absorption of calcium falls after age 60, and may contribute to osteoporosis. Nearly everyone over age 80 has significant malabsorption. Impairment of calcium absorption may be due to decreased active transport or to deficiencies in vitamin D (Bender, 1968; Goldman, 1979; Bhanthimnavis and Schuster, 1977). Although data are scanty, iron absorption may be diminished with age. Vitamin A absorption may be delayed but is otherwise unimpaired. Absorption of vitamins B_1 (thiamine) and B_{12} may be slightly diminished with age, but the level of absorption remains adequate to meet the body's needs (Bender, 1968).

In conclusion, studies on absorption of nutrients are meager, and more work needs to be done. Absorption of most nutrients seems to remain adequate throughout the life span, perhaps because of the enormous reserve capacity of the intestinal mucosa. Low serum levels may be due to reduced intake and poor food preparation rather than inadequate absorption.

Large Intestine

Little information is available about age-related changes in the structure and function of the large intestine. The functions of the colon are to receive ileal contents; absorb water, sodium, and chloride; secrete potassium, bicarbonate, and mucus into the lumen; process these modified contents; and store them until bowel evacuation.

In the vermiform appendix there is fibrous atrophy of large amounts of lymphoid tissue. The lumen of the appendix becomes progressively obliterated. The aging colon shows thickening of the muscularis, rather than thinning. It is speculated that segmental areas of the colon undergo spasms that increase intraluminal pressure and result in the mucosal expansion (Goldman, 1979).

Studies of stool specimens from the elderly show little evidence of undigested nutrients. This finding supports the notion that the digestive process is adequate in normal aging persons (Goldman, 1979).

Because the incidence of colon disorders is high among the aged, it is surprising that there has been so little research on this portion of the alimentary canal. It is believed that many of these disorders are the result of complex factors, including dietary changes, environmental influences, and medication, and are not inevitable consequences of the aging process (Bhanthimnavis and Schuster, 1977). Constipation is perhaps the most frequent complaint of the aged (Schuster, 1976). Diverticulosis of the sigmoid colon occurs in over 33 percent of all people over age 60. Fecal incontinence increases in frequency among the aged and may occur in 20 percent of hospitalized older persons. Although internal sphincter control seems to remain normal in the aged, the external sphincter reflex appears diminished. This factor may contribute to incontinence. Neurological changes and confusion have also been suggested as reasons for the incidence of incontinence among the aged (Goldman, 1979).

Liver

Liver weight decreases in relation to body weight after age 50, and it continues to decline until the tenth decade (Calloway et al., 1965). Data on structural changes in liver cells are limited. Some characteristic changes take place in both the size and the nuclei of parenchymal cells. Knowledge of hepatic enzymes in aged humans is particularly sparse. There is some reduction in hepatic enzyme concentrations and in enzyme responses to external stimuli. Enzymes located in the smooth endoplasmic reticulum of hepatic microsomes decrease markedly with age. These enzymes carry out many oxidation and reduction reactions, including drug metabolism and detoxification processes. A decrease in these enzymes has important implications for drug dosimetry and detoxification (Schuster, 1976; Bhanthimnavis and Schuster, 1977).

The status of hepatic blood flow is unclear due to conflicting information on changes in splanchnic blood flow with age. Hepatic blood flow does diminish, at least to some extent, but it is unclear whether the decline is more than the average decline in relation to the decrease in total cardiac output. Nevertheless, there do not seem to be any age-related changes in liver function attributable to changes in blood supply. The liver has a large reserve capacity. It is known that as much as 80 percent can be nonfunctional without evidence of hypofunction (Schuster, 1976).

Results of bromosulfophthalein (BSP) studies on young and aged subjects show no change (Schuster, 1976; Bhanthimnavis and Schuster, 1977). The clearance of bilirubin remains unchanged in the aged, as do the values for total serum bilirubin, SGOT and SGPT (Reed et al., 1972; Schuster, 1976; Hesch et al., 1976). Apparently alkaline phosphatase levels increase with age (Reed et al., 1972). With age, total serum protein remains constant or decreases slightly (Reed et al., 1972). Electrophoretic serum protein patterns in the aged show a decrease in albumin and an increase in the globulin fractions, particularly beta and gamma globulin (Bhanthimnavis and Schuster, 1977). A/G ratios decrease from 1.5 to 1.3 in the aged (Reed et al., 1972). The reasons for the decrease are unclear, but may be due to a decrease in the efficiency of liver function resulting in a diminished rate of albumin synthesis or to dietary patterns (Bhanthimnavis and Schuster, 1977).

Gallbladder

Age does not appear to alter the function of the gallbladder (Sklar et al., 1956). The mechanism of bile formation remains unchanged throughout the life span, but normal mechanisms of cholesterol stabilization and absorption may become less efficient. The incidence of gallstones is higher in the aged but is not the result of the aging process. In the United States, it is estimated that 10 percent of men and 20 percent of women between ages 55 and 65 years of age have gallstones (Bhanthimnavis and Schuster, 1977).

Pancreas

Due to rapid postmortem changes in the pancreas, information about changes in cellular structure is scanty. Microscopic and electron microscopic studies indicate changes in both ductile cells and parenchymal cells as well as in subcellular organelles. The volume and concentration of trypsin, amylase, and lipase appear to be reduced, but are still sufficient to maintain adequate digestive function (Goldman, 1979). There appears to be no difference in bicarbonate secretion between the young and the old (Bhanthimnavis and Schuster, 1977).

EXCRETORY SYSTEM

The aging excretory system undergoes structural and functional changes that in many ways are no different from most other systems. Some alterations reflect intrinsic aging processes, while others reflect degeneration of the cardiovascular system. In healthy aging people, the progressive loss of renal mass and function is of little significance. However, a number of stresses may challenge the aging excretory system's ability to function adequately and may jeopardize the older person's adaptation.

Kidney Structure
Aging changes in the kidney have been studied extensively. From birth to maturity, the kidney grows until it reaches a maximum mass. Although remaining nephrons hypertrophy, the kidney mass declines with increasing acceleration with age. The median weight of both kidneys declines from 250 g in individuals ages 40 to 49 to 200 g in individuals over age 70 (Goldman, 1977).

At birth, the kidney contains between 800,000 and 1,000,000 nephrons, which grow in size until maturity. After maturation, loss of nephrons accelerates. Between the ages of 40 and 70 years, the number of nephrons decreases by 33 to 50 percent (Moore, 1931). Cell mass decreases and extracellular fluid in the kidney increases with age (Timaras, 1972). The medulla of the kidney increases in collagen and intercellular material after age 50, but, apparently, these changes do not affect kidney function.

Each nephron contains a vascular component, the glomerulus, and a tubular segment. Progressive changes take place in the arterial tree, the glomeruli, and the tubules (Feinstein and Friedman, 1979). It is likely that reduction in the renal vascular bed is a major component of the normal aging process in the kidney (Rowe et al., 1976). After age 50, there

is a spiraling of renal afferent arterioles. This change is the result of interstitial fibrosis with shortening of vessels. Cortical arterioles not connected to glomeruli increase with age. These arterioles end blindly and are the result of glomerular degeneration. On the other hand, juxtamedullary arterioles associated with deteriorated glomeruli do not end blindly but serve as a shunt to maintain the continuity of the afferent and efferent arterioles. These vessels serve as the blood supply to the renal medulla. With age, the presence of aglomerular juxtamedullary arterioles increases. In the aging kidney, blood supply to the medullary region is somewhat better than to the cortical region, but the supply to both areas diminishes (Feinstein and Friedman, 1979).

Although changes in the renal parenchyma occur simultaneously with changes in the renal vasculature, parenchymal changes are not believed to be due directly to arteriolar changes. Basement membranes in renal tubules show age-related changes, and there is a gradual reduction in tubule length and volume. The proximal tubule exhibits atrophy, swelling, and either tubular collapse or dilation (Rosen, 1976). Interstitial fibrosis increases gradually, especially in the renal pyramid. The number of diverticula of the distal convoluted tubule rises progressively with age. Their etiology is unknown. Overall the decrease in the number of juxtamedullary nephrons is proportionately greater than the decrease in nephrons elsewhere (Feinstein and Friedman, 1979).

Kidney Function
Because the normal aging kidney undergoes gradual structural changes, functional changes would be expected. As the number of functional units declines, so does kidney function. The glomerular filtration rate as measured by inulin and creatinine clearance declines with age. Inulin clearance falls an average of 46 percent between ages 20 and 90 (Fig. 3) (Davies and Shock, 1950).

There is also a fall in creatinine clearance with age, beginning in the third decade, with the rate of decline accelerating after age 65. Rowe (1977) found the creatinine clearance in 30-year-old men to be 142 ml/min/m². It declined at a rate of about 8 ml/min each decade. Uncorrected laboratory measures of creatinine clearance in the aged, however, do not accurately reflect kidney function because

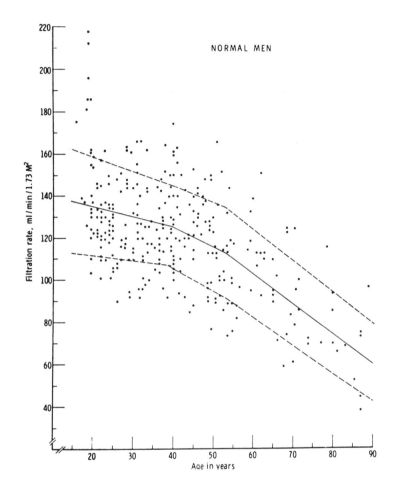

NORMAL MEN

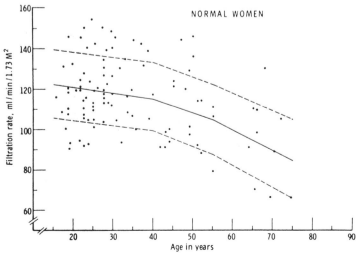

NORMAL WOMEN

Figure 3. Filtration rate (inulin clearance) per 1.73 M^2 in normal men and women. Solid and broken lines represent mean value and one standard deviation. *From Wesson LG, 1969, with permission.*

muscle mass is reduced with age and less creatinine is produced. Therefore, the uncorrected measure reflects the decline in both kidney function and muscle mass. Rowe et al. (1976) developed a nomogram that permits the determination of age-adjusted percentile ranks in creatinine clearance levels for individuals whose age and true creatinine clearance levels are known (Fig. 4). The decline in GFR is the key to understanding other nephron functions. The nephron acts as a unit and a decline in urine function at the glomerulus is reflected in a decline in other nephron functions (Bricker, 1969).

Mean serum creatinine rises slightly from 0.813

mg/dl (ages 25 to 34) to 0.837 mg/dl (ages 55 to 64) to 0.843 mg/dl (ages 75 to 84). Serum creatinine is a good indicator of renal function. The blood urea nitrogen (BUN) increases with age from 10 mg/dl in young adults to 20 to 30 mg/dl in the aged (Rowe et al., 1976).

The decline in GFR is due primarily to a decline in renal plasma flow (RPF), which, by age 80, declines by 53 percent. RPF is measured by studying the clearance of Diodrast (Fig. 5) (Wesson, 1969). The ratio of GFR to RPF is called the filtration fraction; in young adults, it is about 0.20. The filtration fraction represents the fraction of plasma extruded into the glomerular membrane as filtrate. With age, the filtration fraction rises. It was found to be 0.205 in individuals in the sixth decade and 0.2624 in individuals in the seventh decade (Davies and Shock, 1950). The factors responsible for decreased blood flow to the aging kidney are uncertain. The age-related decline in cardiac output and the regression of the vascular bed are not considered to be sufficient to explain the fall in perfusion (Rowe et al., 1976). Diminished renal blood flow may be related to cellular changes in the walls of the small vessels. A rise in vascular tone, however, is not believed to be a factor (Feinstein and Friedman, 1979).

Aging also impairs the ability of the kidney to respond to variations in sodium intake. Normally, increased sodium intake is accompanied by vasodilation, but this response is blunted in the aged. Age also impairs the sodium-conserving ability of the kidney. The time needed to achieve low urine sodium concentrations when salt intake is restricted is significantly longer in those over 60 than in younger persons. The decline in sodium-conserving ability involves both a decrease in nephron mass and a diminished aldosterone secretion rate in response to stimuli in the aged (Feinstein and Friedman, 1979).

Subsequent to filtration at the glomerulus, the filtrate undergoes many changes as it flows through the nephron. The reduced tubular mass with age is reflected by reduced tubular function. Tubular reabsorption and secretion decrease. Reabsorption of glucose from the filtrate (TmG) is a function of the proximal tubule. Its decline is 43 percent, about the same as that of the filtration rate. This reduction reflects a decrease in the number, not the function, of nephrons (Goldman, 1979).

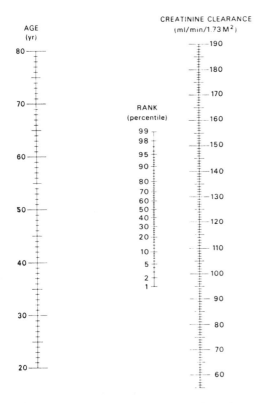

Figure 4. Nomogram for determination of age-adjusted percentile rank in true creatinine clearance. Clearance based on total chromogen creatinine determinations using AutoAnalyzer technique may be multiplied by 1.25 to obtain equivalent true creatinine clearance for use on the nomogram. *From Rowe JW et al., 1976, with permission.*

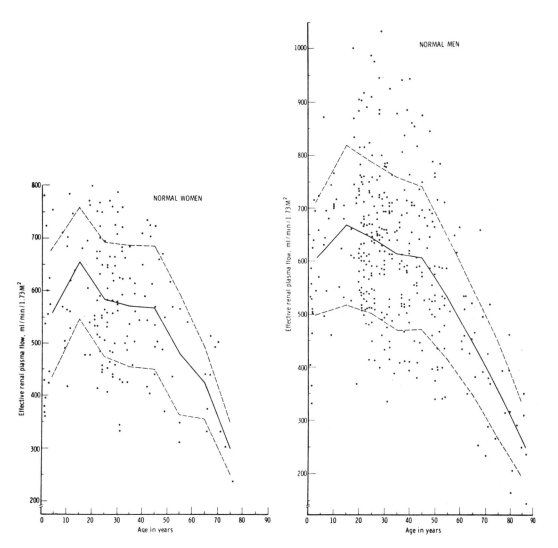

Figure 5. Effective renal plasma flow (PAH or diodrast clearances) per 1.73 M² in normal men and women. Solid and broken lines represent mean value and one standard deviation. *From Wesson LG, 1969, with permission.*

Concentrating Ability. Concentrating and diluting ability involve the loop of Henle, the distal convoluted tubule, and the collecting duct. In response to changes in extracellular volume, the kidney responds by alterations in glomerular filtration rate, urine flow, and vasopressin (ADH). With age, there is a decrease in minimal concentrating ability and diluting capacity. This decline occurs because as the number of functioning nephrons decreases,

the relative solute load to which the kidney must respond is increased. The maximum specific gravity decreases from 1.032 in youth to 1.024 at age 80. A similar decline in maximum osmolality occurs from 1040 mOs/L at age 20 to 750 mOs/L at age 80 (Goldman, 1979). Studies have shown that the tubular cells do not become less responsive to vasopressin (ADH) with age (Shock, 1977; Lindeman, 1975). The relatively greater blood flow through the medullary arterioles with age may impair the countercurrent mechanism and result in a more dilute urine (Feinstein and Friedman, 1979).

Acid–Base Regulation. The kidney participates in hydrogen balance by concentration of base and synthesis and excretion of acid ammonia. The elderly are able to readjust acid–base balance after it is disturbed, but they require more time to do so. The aging kidney responds more slowly and less effectively to an acid load. Young people excrete about 35 percent of an acid load, 72 percent of which is ammonia, in 8 hours. People over age 72 excrete only 18 percent of the acid load in 8 hours and only 59 percent of it is in the form of ammonia (Feinstein and Friedman, 1979). The response to base loads is also delayed and prolonged (Goldman, 1979). Overall, the aged need 3 times as long as the young to correct pH imbalances due to age-related changes in the GFR (Shock, 1977).

Ureters, Bladder, and Urethra

Because urinary incontinence is an important problem among the elderly, the aged bladder has been studied extensively, and anatomical and functional changes have been identified. The bladder demonstrates an increase in edema, round cell infiltration and occasional lymphoid follicles. The bladder muscle shows evidence of hypertrophy (trabeculation), and diverticula are often present. The bladder muscle weakens, but no changes in collagen or protein composition of bladder detrusor muscle have been found (Goldman, 1977).

Bladder size and capacity decrease with age, but the causes are not known. If the bladder is filled beyond capacity, there is either leakage or uninhibited bladder contractions and an urgent demand to urinate. The volume of residual urine increases, even in women for whom prostatic enlargement is not a factor. The source of the sensory stimulus for voiding is the intrinsic stretch receptors in the bladder wall. The sensation of needing to void occurs in youth when the bladder is about half full, but in the aged, the sensation is more variable. There may be no sensation to void even when the intravesicular pressure rises and the bladder is almost filled to capacity. These changes account for the increased precipitancy of urination with age (Goldman, 1977).

Ureteral and urethral muscle tone also diminish

with age. In women, mucosal prolapse at the external orifice is frequent. The urinary stream tends to be slower and at a lower pressure in old age (Feinstein and Friedman, 1979). In the normal bladder, there is no true internal sphincter. Competency is maintained by the tone of tissue and a concentration of elastic connective tissue surrounding the urethra at the bladder neck. Age-related changes in elastic tissues occur and may play a role in incontinence in the elderly (Goldman, 1977).

ENDOCRINE SYSTEM

The inevitability of hormone-mediated senescence in the ovary has focused attention on the possibility that hormones mediate the aging process. It was once hoped that simple hormonal replacement therapy would postpone aging. After all, nearly all organism responses directly involve or are somehow modulated by the action of hormones. Consequently, age-related changes in hormone actions have been extensively studied.

Aging affects many aspects of endocrine function, but it affects different organs in different ways (Fig. 6). Changes may occur in hormone secretion rates, secretion patterns or altered secretory responses to stimulation. In some cases, altered disposal rates are the reason for changes in secretion. Aging may also affect proteins that carry hormones in plasma, the amounts of chemically active hormones, or the sensitivity of target tissues to hormonal stimulation (Gregerman and Bierman, 1981). According to Roth (1978) the change in the body's responsiveness to hormones may be due to a loss of receptor sites from the target cells.

Research on normal endocrine function in the aged has been hampered because it is frequently altered by the multiple, chronic illnesses present in a large proportion of the aging population. Consequently, many of the research studies present conflicting data.

Pituitary

The pituitary secretes hormones that control the activity of nearly all other glands in the body, particularly the thyroid, adrenals, and gonads. The weight of the pituitary changes little with age, but structural

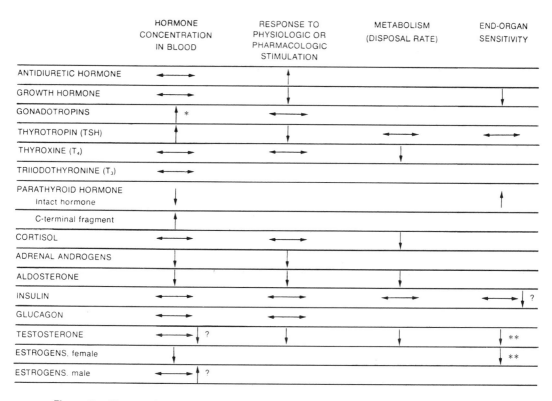

Figure 6. Changes in hormones during aging in man. Symbols: ↑ = increase, ↓ = decrease, ↔ = no change, * = post-menopausal, ** = hypothalamic. Blank spaces indicate no data currently available. *From Gregerman RI, Bierman EL, 1981, with permission.*

changes occur, particularly in the anterior pituitary and the cells that secrete the gonadotropins (Talbert, 1977). Pigment is deposited in the glandular elements, the amount of connective tissue increases, and there are changes in the relative proportion of certain cell types. The vascular network is reduced (Bourne, 1960; Goldman, 1979).

Adrenocorticotropic Hormone. The pituitary concentration and basal levels of adrenocorticotropic hormone (ACTH) do not appear to change with age. In addition, the circadian rhythm of ACTH, with peak values in the morning, remains intact (Andres and Tobin, 1977).

Recently, a few direct measurements of serum ACTH in relation to stress and age have been made (Gregerman and Bierman, 1981). It appears that the release of ACTH in response to stress and the neg-ative feedback mechanism involving plasma cortisol levels is intact in the aged (Davis, 1978; Andres and Tobin, 1977). It is believed that the hypothalamus–pituitary–adrenal axis is not significantly impaired with age.

Antidiuretic Hormone. Antidiuretic hormone (ADH), or vasopressin, is a water-conserving hormone whose target organ is the kidney. ADH has normal secretory dynamics in the elderly. The kidney's ability to concentrate urine declines with age, but this decline is believed to be due to the kidney's decline in GFR, not to a decreased sensitivity to ADH (Gregerman and Bierman, 1981).

Receptors in the brain and cardiovascular system are sensitive to blood osmolality and regulate ADH secretion. These receptors appear to become more sensitive as aging progresses (Davis, 1978).

Thyrotropin and Thyrotropin-Releasing Hormone. Studies of the response of the aging pituitary gland to thyrotropin-releasing hormone (TRH) have yielded conflicting data. The range of findings suggest that subtle genetic or environmental factors may influence pituitary function in aging. Plasma thyrotropin (TSH) levels increase with aging (Gregerman and Bierman, 1981).

Gonadotropins. The gonadotropins—follicle-stimulating hormone (FSH) and luteinizing hormone (LH)—are polypeptide trophic hormones whose target is the gonad. In women, serum levels of FSH and LH increase until at least the eighth decade, when secretion of FSH may decline (Davis, 1978). The level of FSH is 15 times that in young adults and the level of LH is 3 times that of the young. In addition, there is a marked rise in urinary gonadotropins in postmenopausal women (Andres and Tobin, 1977). In men, the increase in circulatory gonadotropins is smaller and occurs more gradually (Talbert, 1977). FSH and LH begin to rise in men in the fourth decade, with the rise becoming more conspicuous in later decades. There is no impairment of the pituitary's ability to secrete FSH and LH in menopausal and postmenopausal women. As estrogen wanes with menopause, FSH and LH production by the pituitary increase via a negative feedback loop.

It has been suggested that a primary hypothalamic or pituitary process involving FSH and LH secretion could initiate the menopause if changes took place in the negative feedback system, causing inappropriately high levels of FSH and LH and eventual ovarian failure. Although this may be the case in some animals, aging changes in the human pituitary are not responsible for cessation of ovarian activity.

Adrenals

The adrenal glands, located above the kidneys, produce a number of hormones that assist the body in coping with emergencies and maintaining the balance of salt and water. There are numerous microscopic changes in the adrenals, including vascular dilation and hemorrhages, loss of characteristic lipids, fragmentation of mitochondria, and accumulation of pigment (Andres and Tobin, 1977). Fibrous and connective tissues accumulate. A classic finding in the aging adrenal gland is the formation of tiny nodules in the cortex (Goldman, 1979; Bourne, 1960).

Glucocorticoids. Basal plasma levels of cortisol and corticosterone persist with age. The normal diurnal variation, high in the morning and low in the evening, is maintained as long as the elderly person is healthy. Diseases may alter the normal diurnal variation (Andres and Tobin, 1977). However, in the elderly the evening levels are somewhat higher than they are in the young. The secretion rate of cortisol is reduced and the degradation rate is prolonged, allowing the plasma level to remain constant with age. The half-life of cortisol is longer in the elderly, indicating that the metabolism of cortisol changes with age (Andres and Tobin, 1977). The ability of the adrenal cortex to increase the secretion of cortisol in response to ACTH is not clear.

Muggeo et al. (1975) studied the plasma cortisol response to hypoglycemic stress in subjects aged 53 to 84 and found no difference in cortisol responses. He suggested that adrenal and possibly ACTH secretion do not show any important modification with age. On the other hand, Andres and Tobin (1977) reported that adrenal secretion in response to ACTH is reduced, possibly due to diminished sensitivity of the adrenal glands to stimulation by ACTH. These findings imply that the aging adrenal gland may be less able to respond to stress.

Aldosterone. Secretion of aldosterone by the adrenal cortex is influenced by a complex variety of substances, including the end products of chemical reactions stimulated by renin, ACTH, and serum potassium. Both the blood levels and the urinary excretion of aldosterone are decreased by 50 percent by old age. The increase in urinary excretion following sodium depletion is only 30 to 40 percent that in young adults. Plasma renin levels also decline with age. Renin activity falls 30 to 50 percent, even when levels of renin substrate are normal (Rowe, 1977). The responsiveness of renin and consequently aldosterone to a variety of stimuli, including altered salt intake and changes in body posture, declines as age proceeds. The physiological consequences of changes in aldosterone are not known (Davis, 1978; Gregerman and Bierman, 1981).

Adrenal Androgens. Testosterone, androstenedione, dehydropriadrosterone, and epiandrosterone comprise the adrenal androgens. The quantity of adrenal androgens equals or exceeds that of all other adrenal steroids, but their functions are still unclear. The adrenal androgens, particularly dehydropriadrosterone, exhibit a striking decline with age, but the relationship of this decline to the aging process is not known (Goldman, 1979). In women, testosterone levels are slightly increased after menopause but the range of variability is wide (Greenblatt et al., 1976).

Adrenal androgens comprise about two-thirds of the 17-ketosteroids excreted in urine. The excretion of 17-ketosteroids decreases by 50 percent in the aged. This decrease may be due to a reduced rate of production rather than to a reduction in removal (Goldman, 1979).

Norepinephrine and Epinephrine. Few studies have been done on age-related changes in the urinary excretion of norepinephrine and epinephrine. No age differences have been found in these hormones (Goldman, 1979).

Gonads

The gonads are the target organs for FSH and LH. Although blood levels of these hormones increase with age, the testes and ovaries undergo numerous structural and functional changes. Consequently, secretion of gonadal hormones is significantly reduced.

The size and weight of the aging ovary decrease with age (Andres and Tobin, 1977). There is a decline in the number of ovarian follicles, the basic organizational unit of the ovary. Residual follicular units are insensitive to gonadotropins and do not mature or produce estrogen (Davis, 1978). Hilar and thecal cells, which produce androgens, remain active (Goldfarb, 1979). The postmenopausal ovary continues to secrete a considerable amount of testosterone, a moderate amount of androstenedione, and a minimal amount of estrogen. The ovary remains active, but in respect to androgen, not estrogen, production (Goldfarb, 1979).

The testes secrete both testosterone and estradiol. In the testes, the interstitial cells that produce testosterone, called Leydig cells, accumulate pigment (Bourne, 1960). The number of Leydig cells declines with age (Tichy and Malasanos, 1979b).

Estrogen. The production of ovarian estrogen ceases following ovarian atrophy at the time of menopause. Concurrently, there is a decrease in estrogen production from nonfollicular sources. It is believed that the remaining estrogen in postmenopausal women comes from peripheral conversion of androgens, particularly androstenedione to estrone. The extent of this conversion process varies widely among different women. The peak secretion of estrogens attained in the third and fourth decade drops precipitously with menopause and remains the same thereafter. In women in their 70s, estradiol and estrone drop to 10 and 30 percent of their earlier levels, respectively. The metabolic clearance rate of estradiol and estrone declines by 75 percent, indicating that the actual production rate of these hormones is even lower (Goldfarb, 1979). In men, estrogen levels remain constant throughout the life span (Greenblatt et al., 1976).

The reasons for cessation of ovarian activity have been widely discussed. In some animals, it appears that ovarian failure may be secondary to other changes in the ovary's environment. It has been speculated that changes in the hypothalamus and pituitary may stimulate ovarian changes. In humans, however, cessation of ovarian function is believed to be a primary event (Davis, 1978).

Testosterone. Although it had been believed that testicular testosterone levels in the blood remained constant throughout the life span, recent evidence indicates that testosterone levels in blood do decline in aging males after the age of 60 (Talbert, 1977). There are enormous individual variations in testicular androgen secretion capability at all ages. Therefore, some elderly men have higher testosterone levels than some young men (Davies and Shock, 1950). Both the metabolic clearance rate and the production rate of testosterone decline with age. In addition, free testosterone is further diminished because the capacity of testosterone-binding globulin increases with age (Goldman, 1979).

Progestin. Progesterone is secreted by the ovary and placenta and to a lesser degree by the testes and adrenal cortex. The rate of production declines by 60 percent in old age, dropping precipitously with the onset of menopause. The renal production of progesterone may be sustained because progesterone is a precursor of cortisol (Goldman, 1979).

Pancreas

In addition to its digestive functions, the pancreas secretes two hormones. Insulin is secreted from the beta cells, called Islets of Langerhans. It is believed that glucagon is secreted from the alpha cells. There is some evidence that the number and volume of Islets of Langerhans increase with age (Bourne, 1960). Other changes in the structure of the pancreas were discussed under the section of this chapter on the digestive system.

Insulin. Glucose tolerance, the ability to dispose of administered glucose efficiently, deteriorates with age beginning as early as the fourth decade. In both the oral and the intravenous glucose tolerance tests the rise in blood glucose levels is greater and the return to resting levels is slower in older people than in the young (Exton-Smith and Overstall, 1979).

Andres (1971) reviewed a number of studies reporting on changes in oral and intravenous glucose tolerance tests in the aging. After an oral glucose load of 50 g, the blood glucose after 1 hour rose 10 to 14 mg per decade of life. After 2 hours, the age differences in blood glucose levels were somewhat less. If criteria that are used for the diagnosis of diabetes mellitus are based on the results of glucose tolerance tests in young adults and then used for the elderly, a high proportion of older people will have "chemical diabetes." A nomogram has been developed to enable the clinician to rank a response to the oral glucose tolerance test against the response of other people of the same age (Fig. 7). A line extending from the subject's age to the 2-hour blood glucose concentration will intersect the percentile range line and indicate the percent of those who will outperform the subject and the percent with even lower tolerances (Andres, 1971).

Steroid hormone administration causes deterioration of tolerance in subjects of all ages, but the deterioration is greater in the elderly (Andres, 1971).

It is important to note that in normal older people, higher blood sugar elevations occur only after a glucose load and not in the fasting state. Fasting blood sugar levels are within the normal range, even in the very old (Shock, 1977). Basal insulin secretion, that is, insulin release after an overnight fast, is not influenced by age. One study has indicated that the insulin released by older people contains a greater proportion of proinsulin, a less active fraction of insulin (Duckworth and Kitabchi, 1972). The fate of insulin once it has been released into the circulation by the beta cells is known as insulin turnover. This is also unchanged with age (Davis, 1978).

More work needs to be done to identify the mechanism that underlies the deterioration in glucose tolerance in the aged. The change may be due to a decreased sensitivity of the pancreatic beta cells to hyperglycemia and consequent sluggish insulin release (Andres, 1973). Therefore a greater rise in blood sugar would be required before insulin was released (Shock, 1977). However, in another study, the glucoreceptors at the cell membrane exhibited a diminished responsiveness to insulin, indicating reduced tissue sensitivity (Soerjodibroto et al., 1979). It is also possible that the older person's diminished glucose tolerance may be due to increased levels of circulating insulin antagonists (Feldman and Plonk, 1976).

Glucagon. Glucagon is an important regulator of carbohydrate metabolism and may play a critical role in diabetes. Little research has been done on glucagon physiology in the aged. In one study, there was no difference either in fasting plasma levels of glucagon or in the glucagon response to intravenous arginine stimulation (Dudl and Ensinick, 1972). Goldman (1979) reports another study on the effect of glucagon that showed a delayed and diminished response with age.

Thyroid

The thyroid hormones thyroxine (T_4) and triiodothyronine (T_3) play roles in regulating the rate of metabolism and heat production. Secretion of T_3 and T_4 is dependent upon a complex feedback loop system, subject to the control of the hypothalamus. Thyrotropin-releasing hormone (TRH), produced

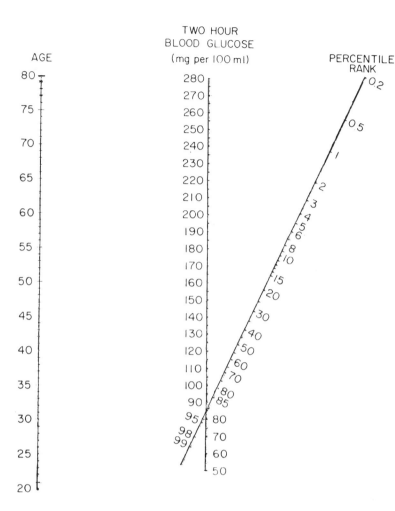

Figure 7. Oral glucose tolerance test nomogram. For example, a 51-year-old subject with a 2-hour glucose of 130 mg/100ml will have a rank of 50 percent, an exactly average performance. A 49-year-old man with a glucose of 190 mg/100ml will rank at 3 percent, a very poor performance. *From Andres R, 1971, with permission.*

by the hypothalamus, stimulates the pituitary gland to produce thyrotropin (TSH), which, in turn, stimulates the thyroid gland to release T_3 and T_4.

Because certain adaptations to thyroid hormone deficiency, including skin pallor, dry skin, thinning hair, and languor, are similar to adaptations to aging, substantial efforts have been made to implicate inadequate thyroid hormone action in the aging process. In fact, however, the thyroid gland in the aged appears to function normally and maintain its reserve capacity (Davis, 1978).

Although functional changes have not been identified, the thyroid gland undergoes numerous structural changes with age. Follicles become dis-

tended, contain large amounts of colloid, and exhibit some degeneration. Lipid material collects in the cells. Connective tissue increases between the lobules and in the follicles, and fibrosis occurs. Blood vessels in the gland also undergo changes (Bourne, 1960).

The bulk of circulating thyroid hormone does not exist in the free state but is bound to two plasma proteins. The major carrier is thyroxin-binding globulin (TBG) and the minor carrier is prealbumin. TBG rises slightly and thyroxine-binding prealbumin falls with age. Plasma thyroxin (T_4), both bound and free, does not change with age (Andres and Tobin, 1977). Plasma triiodothyronine (T_3), the more potent form of thyroid hormone, also remains unchanged with age (Gregerman and Bierman, 1981).

Changes occur in the physiology of thyroid hormone but do not appear to threaten the older person's adaptation. In fact, these changes appear to mirror other age-related changes in the body. Thyroid hormone synthesis and release by the thyroid gland decrease with age. The rate of hormone destruction is also decreased proportionately (Davis, 1978). The reduced rate of hormone disposal may be due to slowed hepatic metabolism or to reduced peripheral need or physical activity (Goldman, 1979). Because the rate of destruction is reduced, the slower rate of synthesis does not result in decreased plasma levels of thyroid hormone.

Although the serum concentration of TSH increases with age, the influence of age on the response of the thyroid to TSH is unclear. It is likely that responsiveness remains unchanged with age. The thyroid response to stress, such as fever, is also unchanged (Andres and Tobin, 1977).

The uptake of radioactive iodine by the thyroid gland, a test of thyroid function, decreases slightly with advancing age. This small change is not a sign of thyroid failure, but an adaptation made by the gland in response to the increased blood levels of iodine that characterize decreasing kidney function in the aged (Davis, 1978).

The basal metabolism rate (BMR) decreases with age, but it is not due to changes in the thyroid gland. The decreased BMR is the result of age-related increases in fat and decreases in metabolic mass. In fact, oxygen consumption per unit of metabolic mass does not decrease with age (Shock, 1977).

Parathyroid

Parathyroid hormone (PTH) is a calcium-mobilizing polypeptide with important actions on bone, on the kidney and on the metabolism of vitamin D. It is secreted by the parathyroid glands embedded in the thyroid gland. With age, changes occur in the parathyroid glands. They show an increase in colloidal material, interstitial connective tissue, and cellular strands that develop between the cells. The number of chief cells and oxyphil cells increases and intracellular granules increase in number and in size. However, the glands show very little evidence of atrophy or degeneration (Bourne, 1960).

The dynamics of PTH in the aged are of particular interest because of the loss of mineral and bone matrix that develops as a normal concomitant of aging. There is no evidence to implicate PTH in the loss of bone mass that accompanies normal aging. Although the inactive fragment of PTH (C-terminal fragment) appears to increase with age, changes in the active hormone are less well understood. There appears to be no significant change, or only a slight decline, in the level of active PTH with age (Davis, 1978). Active PTH levels are below normal in clients with osteoporosis (Gregerman and Bierman, 1981). Since estrogen is known to protect against the demineralizing effects of PTH, the postmenopausal decline in estrogen may sensitize older women to PTH (Goldman, 1979). Excessive PTH production in both the young and the old occurs in a variety of pathological conditions and results in excessive demineralization of the bone.

REPRODUCTIVE SYSTEM

The reproductive organs undergo many age-related changes similar to those in other aging organs and tissues. However, this system is uniquely dependent upon a complex interrelation of hormones secreted by the hypothalamus, pituitary, and gonads for continuing function (Talbert, 1977). Changes in hormone function were discussed earlier in this chapter. In both men and women, aging is characterized by a decline in fertility and reproductive activity.

Male Reproduction

Decline in male reproductive function is a gradual process influenced partially by the individual's general level of adaptation. In many instances, all elements of the system remain functional and reproduction is possible at least into the ninth decade. Some changes do occur in the reproductive act, and these are normal. Changes in sexual response are discussed in Chapter 7.

The rate and age of decline in function of the human testes is quite variable. In contrast to females, male germ cells are constantly replenished from puberty to old age. The time it takes to develop a mature spermatozoan in the testes is not influenced by age.

The testes decrease in size and cellular changes

occur. The basement membrane thickens, fibrosis of tubules occurs, connective tissue increases, particularly around the sperm-producing tubules, and the number of capillaries declines (Talbert, 1977). Active sperm-producing cells remain in the testes until old age, when the number may decline (Bourne, 1960). The number of seminiferous tubules with spermatids drops from 90 percent in men under age 40 to 50 percent in 50- to 70-year-old men and to 10 percent in men over 80. Spermatogenesis continues into old age. Spermatozoa in the ejaculate decline slightly, from about 69 percent in men in the sixth decade to about 48 percent in men in the eighth decade (Talbert, 1977).

From puberty until the fifth decade, the prostate gland exhibits secretory activity from the tubulo-alveolar glands, which make an important contribution to the ejaculate. Beginning at age 40, atrophic changes in the cells of the prostate occur (Talbert, 1977). Smooth muscle fibers atrophy and stromal connective tissue increases. Although the acini remain large, the papillae are reduced in size and the epithelium becomes cuboidal. Changes in Leydig cells were discussed in the section of this chapter on the endocrine system. These changes occur in patches, leaving certain areas of the gland unaffected (Brocklehurst, 1979).

After age 60, the atrophic process progresses until the entire gland is involved. Focal areas develop complete atrophy of acini and others develop secondary hyperplasia. Concentrations of secretions may develop and become calcified (Brocklehurst, 1979). Collagen accumulates while protein declines. The blood supply to the prostate also diminishes. Reasons for prostatic atrophy are unclear. It has been speculated that the process might be triggered by the high levels of testosterone in the mature male. The seminal vesicles also undergo cellular changes. Aging changes in the epididymis, which plays a major role in sperm maturation, are unclear (Talbert, 1977).

Involutional changes begin in the penis as early as the third or fourth decade, and by the sixth decade, these changes are generalized. Both arteries and veins undergo sclerotic changes. It is believed that sclerosis of the veins may be associated with the development of impotence in some aging males. Fibroelastic changes occur in the tissues of the penis, and the penis becomes smaller (Talbert, 1977).

Female Reproduction

Females lose the ability to reproduce well before they reach the normal life span. In addition, there is a variable period prior to ultimate cessation of reproduction in which the efficiency of the process declines. The incidence of abortions, stillbirths, and newborns with defects rises during this period.

With age, the ovaries become fibrotic and decrease in size. The ovary continues to be active in old age but in different ways. Changes in ovarian follicles occur and are described in the section of this chapter on the endocrine system. Atrophic changes occur in the uterine tubes after age 60. The uterus and cervix atrophy, decreasing in both size and secretory activity. The vagina also decreases in size and vaginal elastic fibers may fragment, reducing elasticity. The vaginal epithelium atrophies. Vascularity, glycogen, and mucopolysaccharide content of the vaginal mucosa decrease and the pH increases.

During the reproductive years, the breasts consist of glandular, stromal, and adipose tissue. Beginning as early as age 35, there is a gradual replacement of glands by fat, ducts decrease in size, and fibrosis and calcification of ducts occur (Talbert, 1977).

NERVOUS SYSTEM

The effect of the aging process on the nervous system is of particular concern because the nervous system influences every aspect of human functioning. In addition, because neurons are composed of postmitotic cells, the central nervous system ought to be particularly vulnerable to age changes.

Although a great deal of research has been done there are still many unanswered questions about neural structures, how the nervous system functions, and how it changes with age.

The Brain

The brain controls or influences most organ and cell functions in the body, either directly through nerves or indirectly through hormones. How aging affects the functions of the brain is of great interest, but surprisingly little is known. For obvious reasons, examination of the human brain is limited to autopsy and to a few special techniques such as radiographic studies and computerized axial tomography. Because of the complexity of the brain and limitations in methods to study it, information related to age-related changes is incomplete and at times conflicting.

Experts disagree about whether or not the brain weight decreases with age. Brain weight is influenced by body size. Most studies are cross sectional and fail to take into account that earlier generations, as a whole, were smaller in body size than the present generation. The best available information is that the human brain undergoes slowly accelerating shrinkage as it ages and undergoes a 10 to 12 percent weight loss by very old age. Both gray matter and white matter are lost. Shrinkage narrows the convolutions and widens the sulci between them. There is also some question about whether or not the size of the ventricles changes with age. Presumably, changes in the size of the brain result in modest enlargements of the ventricles, particularly the lateral ventricles. There is no obstruction to cerebrospinal fluid and its pressure remains unchanged with age (Terry, 1978).

Numerous changes take place at the cellular level. The extracellular space is believed to decrease slightly with age. Since significant movement of metabolic precursors and products takes place throughout this space, a decline in its size could have important implications. The brain does not exhibit significant changes in the amount of protein, RNA, or DNA (Finch, 1977).

The primary reason for the brain's loss of weight with age is a progressive loss of neurons. It is believed that neuronal attrition is not a daily occurrence but occurs in different parts of the brain at different times. For example, a greater decrease in cells in the superior frontal gyrus occurs in the fifth decade than at any other time (Brody and Vijayashanker, 1977). Not all parts of the brain lose the same proportion of cells and in some areas of the brain there is no loss at all. The vestibular nucleus, a sensory area for head posture, maintains a constant cell number throughout life, as does the inferior olive in the brainstem, which is involved with motor function. Other areas of the brainstem where cell loss does not occur include the ventral cochlear nucleus and the nuclei of facial, trochlear, and abducens nerves (Brody and Vijayashanker, 1977). In contrast to the brainstem, where cell loss is minimal, the cerebral cortex demonstrates a 20 percent loss of neurons, with some cell layers showing losses

as high as 50 percent (Terry, 1978; Brody and Vijayashanker, 1977). In the cerebellum, a 25 percent loss is evident by age 100, but the loss is not appreciable until age 60 (Brody and Vijayashanker, 1977). There is a 20 to 30 percent loss of cells in the locus coeruleus, a source of noradrenalin-containing neurons that play a role in regulating sleep, among other things (Finch, 1978).

It has long been thought that Alzheimer's disease, a form of senile dementia, was associated with the loss of inordinate numbers of neurons. However, cell counts in brain specimens indicate that patients with Alzheimer's disease have as many cell units as do normal individuals of the same age (Terry, 1978).

Cerebral Circulation

Cell function in the brain is acutely dependent upon blood supply. Little is known about age-related changes in microcirculation in the brain or the blood–brain barrier (Finch, 1977). Because blood flow to the brain can be measured in several different ways, it is known that blood flow is reduced with age. Oxygen utilization by the brain and cerebral vascular resistance also undergo changes (Shenkin et al., 1953).

It is believed that the reduced blood supply in the healthy aged is a consequence of atrophy of the brain, not a cause of neuronal loss and brain shrinkage. The normal brain effectively regulates blood supply and flow is reduced when metabolic needs are reduced (Terry, 1978).

Neurons

Neurons consist of cell bodies and processes called axons and dendrites. Many age-related changes have been documented at the cellular level. In the brain and to a lesser extent in the spinal cord, neurons atrophy and shrink. Lipofuscin is found increasingly in the cytoplasm of most neurons as they age. The amount of lipofuscin accumulation varies, depending upon the type of neuron; in some cells, lipofuscin does not appear at all. Lipofuscin is found in particularly large amounts in the inferior olive, an area of the brain where the number of nerve cells remains unchanged. This fact indicates that the presence of lipofuscin in some cells, at least, does not result in cell death (Terry, 1978).

Because lipofuscin ultimately occupies so much of cytoplasmic volume, it probably displaces significant quantities of cellular organelles. Concentrations of endoplasmic reticulum, called Nissl bodies, decrease. These contain RNA and are the protein synthesizing apparatus. The endoplasmic reticulum also becomes less organized.

Mitochondria, which are involved in energy metabolism, may decrease in number. Many changes have been reported in the nucleus and the nucleolus. The Golgi complex, an extensive membrane system, undergoes many changes, but there is no agreement about their significance (Brody and Vijayashanker, 1977).

Two microscopic structures not seen in young brain tissue have been found in aging brain cells: neurofibrillary tangles and senile or neuritic plaques. The tangle is an abnormal mass of fibrillar material found in the cytoplasm of some normal aging people after age 60 and in almost all people after age 80. Tangles are most often found in the hippocampal cortex, the area concerned with memory processes. Neuritic plaques have a core of amyloid material surrounded by abnormal neural structures. Small numbers of plaques are found between and among neurons in the cortex and hippocampus of normal elderly people. It is likely that plaques and tangles, with the other structural and chemical changes of aging brain tissue, could account for the functional changes so readily found to some degree in the normal elderly and to a greater degree in the senile (Terry, 1978). Both plaques and tangles are also found, but in larger numbers, in individuals with Alzheimer's disease (Goldman, 1979).

Nerve Fibers. With advancing age, the number of nerve fibers decreases and structural changes occur as well. Some fibers may show splitting or granular fragmentation (Bourne, 1960). The fibers of astrocytes in the cortex and subcortex of the cerebrum and cerebellum show degeneration; this becomes more extensive with advancing age (Brody and Vijayashanker, 1977). Astrocytes are neuroglial cells that form part of the supporting tissue of the brain. Changes in motor nerve fibers were described in the musculoskeletal system section of this chapter.

Axons. Axons in many areas of the brain, particularly the gracile nucleus, develop lesions called "neuroaxonal dystrophy." Spheroid or ovoid swellings appear on the terminal parts of the axons. These lesions have never been seen in individuals under age 10, but they are increasingly seen in later life and are almost universal after age 60. The functional consequences of neuroaxonal dystrophy are unknown (Brody and Vijayashanker, 1977).

Dendrites. In the aging cerebral cortex, the dendrites on remaining neurons shrink, reducing the number of fibers that receive synapses from other cells. Degeneration of this apparatus results in a reduction of the number and complexity of transmitted impulses and must have major effects on brain function. The cause of the degeneration of synapses is not known (Terry, 1978).

Neurotransmitters

The neurotransmitters are chemical agents released from nerve endings that activate various sorts of synapses and are essential to function. Secretion of these substances by nerve endings causes depolarization of the membrane on the other side. The neurotransmitters include catecholamines, such as epinephrine, norepinephrine, and dopamine; serotonin; and acetylcholine. Acetylcholine is released at the myoneural junction and norepinephrine is released by sympathetic nerves.

The catecholamines are of interest because it is believed that they participate in the regulation of certain hypothalamic hormones. Changes in these hormones may influence changes throughout the central nervous system. The catecholamines need steroid sex hormones for adequate functioning. It is possible that the abrupt drop in estrogen levels in aging females may stimulate many of the adaptations associated with menopause.

Catecholamines and serotonin are metabolized to biologically inactive products by monoamine oxidase (MAO). With age, MAO and serotonin increase in the brain, platelets, and blood plasma, while the level of norepinephrine, the precursor of epinephrine, decreases. It is possible that increased MAO and decreased norepinephrine may play a role in the depression and apathy experienced by some of the elderly. A currently accepted theory of depression relates its origin to the presence of decreased catecholamine levels in the brain and the associated treatment calls for the use of MAO inhibitors (Goldman, 1979).

Dopamine levels in the normal human brain are also depleted in the aging. The extent of change is proportionate to the length of life. Although depletion of catecholamines, including dopamine, is not as great in the aging as in individuals with Parkinson's disease, this suggests a reason for parkinsonism being more common in the elderly (Finch, 1978).

It is believed that the metabolism of neurotransmitters undergoes significant age-related changes (Brody and Vijayashanker, 1977). The enzymes that synthesize neurotransmitters, particularly the ones associated with the catecholamines, are important for normal neurological function. Abnormalities have been found in three classes of enzymes related to a number of neurotransmitters, including enzymes related to catecholamines. A decrease in the enzymes involved with cholinergic transmitters has been found in senile patients. Alterations in neurotransmitters may be related to the loss of dendrites and synapses that accompanies the aging process.

Nerve Conduction Velocity

Age-related slowing of motor neuron conduction has been demonstrated with the use of electromyography. Most studies have been made on the conduction of the ulnar nerve. Significant decreases in velocity begin in the fifth decade and continue thereafter. In young adults, conduction velocity is about 60 m/sec. By age 80 or 90, the conduction velocity declines to 50 m/sec, a decrease of about 15 percent. Conduction velocity is slightly greater in women than in men. No significant differences have been found between the dominant and non-dominant extremities. A significant decrease also occurs in the latent period of both motor and sensory nerves (Goldman, 1979). Slower reaction time in the elderly is believed to contribute to accidents and to a lowering in IQ scores when speed of response is a factor.

Autonomic Nervous System

An age-related decline in the function of the autonomic nervous system (ANS) occurs, altering performance in several body systems. It may be a factor in the development of heat stroke, disturbances of esophageal and gastrointestinal motility, urinary retention, incontinence, and other problems (Exton-Smith and Overstall, 1979).

Although impairment of blood pressure regulation in old age is a consequence of many age-related changes, a decline in the ANS is believed to be the underlying mechanism. As discussed earlier in the chapter, although systolic and diastolic blood pressure rise slightly with age, compensation when moving from the supine to the upright positions is much reduced. In the elderly, a decline of 20 mm Hg or more in systolic pressure may be associated with postural change. Unlike in young adults, even a small decline in blood pressure in the elderly will produce cerebral ischemia because of an impairment in cerebral circulatory autoregulation (Exton-Smith and Overstall, 1979). Because of deterioration in other body systems, postural hypotension may be a serious stress for the elderly that triggers a chain of adaptations, including falls, fractures, and immobility.

The mechanisms involved in the baroreceptor reflex are uncertain, but the ANS does play a role. It is believed that age-related changes in the afferent pathways from the baroreceptors to the brainstem and the sympathetic chain contribute to the development of postural hypotension. Age-related changes may also occur in the central structures or in the baroreceptors themselves. In addition, aging may be accompanied by changes in the peripheral neural receptors, reducing the responsiveness of blood vessels to the catecholamines (Finch, 1977). Failure of constriction in the systemic arteriolar beds and possibly in the venous reservoirs is believed to be involved. In addition, it is likely that failure to control the splanchnic vascular beds plays an important role in the development of postural hypotension (Exton-Smith and Overstall, 1979).

Age-related defects have also been documented in the ability of the hypothalamus to regulate heat production and heat loss. Normally the sympathetic nervous system responds to core body temperature and skin temperature and stimulates a series of responses. In the elderly, many of the thermoregulatory responses are sluggish and diminished in their intensity. For example, the shivering mechanism is diminished or absent and the response of the sweat glands becomes sluggish (Finch, 1977).

Sleep

Sleep patterns also change with age. Sleep is divided into two major categories, rapid-eye-movement (REM) sleep and nonrapid-eye-movement

(NREM) sleep. REM sleep is borderline in depth and characterized by dreams and numerous physiological changes. NREM sleep consists of four stages, each with different electroencephalographic (EEG) characteristics. Stages 3 and 4 are considered deep sleep. The number of sleep cycles and REM periods varies between four and six a night depending upon the length of sleep. Throughout the life span, REM sleep remains constant, constituting 20 to 25 percent of sleep time. Children have the highest levels of deep stages 3 and 4 sleep and have few arousal periods. Throughout life, there is a progressive de-

crease in stages 3 and 4 sleep. The elderly have little stage 3 and virtually no stage 4 sleep. Sleep is characterized by the less intense stages 1 and 2. In addition the elderly have frequent awakenings and a marked increase in total awake time (Fig. 8) (Kales and Kales, 1974).

Reasons for changes in sleep patterns are uncertain. The locus coeruleus, a source of noradrenalin-containing neurons that play a role in regulating sleep, undergoes a 20 to 30 percent loss of cells during the life span. How this affects the sleep cycle is not known (Finch, 1978).

THE SENSES

Vision

Structural changes in the eye, particularly in the lens, occur with age, and most of these changes markedly affect function. One exception is arcus senilis, a lipid deposit in the margin of the cornea that is nearly universal in individuals over age 80. This deposit does not impair vision. There have been numerous attempts to determine its clinical significance. Its appearance in old age does not seem to be related to hypercholesteremia or arteriosclerosis. A relationship between arcus senilis and retinal arteriosclerosis has been identified. There is also an increased incidence of electrocardiogram abnormalities in persons with arcus senilis (Rodstein, 1963).

The cytoplasm of cells that form the lens of the eye is crystalline and transparent. Throughout life, new cells continue to develop and surround the transparent nuclear region. The crystalline lens becomes discolored, opaque, and more rigid. Only the outer portion of the lens is soft and elastic enough to participate in accommodation. Relaxation of the suspensory ligament by the action of the ciliary muscle limits the increase in the anterior–posterior diameter of the lens required for the focusing of near objects. Gradually the lens becomes set in a flat, unaccommodated position and the near point of the focus of the lens recedes. This change, called presbyopia, occurs late in initially myopic and earlier in hypermetropic individuals. By age 50, corrective lenses are almost universally required for reading and close work (Botwinick, 1978).

Changes in the lens and the vitreous humor

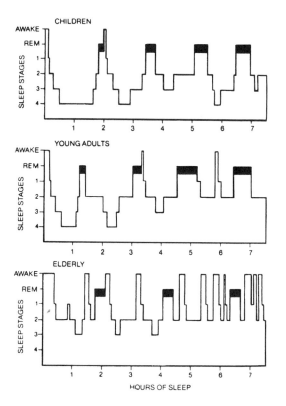

Figure 8. Changes in normal sleep cycles with age. REM sleep (darkened area) occurs cyclically throughout the night at intervals of approximately 90 minutes in all age groups. REM sleep shows little variation in the different age groups whereas stage 4 sleep decreases with age. In addition, the elderly have frequent awakenings and a marked increase in total awake time. *From Kales A, Kales JD, 1974, with permission.*

also cause a decline in visual acuity as measured by the Snellen Eye Chart. Before the fourth decade little change in acuity occurs, but after this time there is a marked decline. Although the extent of the decline is highly variable, by age 70, diminished visual acuity is almost universal (Botwinick, 1978). The extent of the visual fields also declines with age (Goldman, 1979). Other lens changes result in astigmatism with the major axis horizontal. As a person ages, the lens tilts above the vertical axis, increasing the power of the horizontal meridian. As the lens continues to grow, it moves toward the posterior surface of the cornea, reducing the depth of the anterior chamber and changing the optical nodal point. As a result, the refractive power of the lens increases, producing a relative myopia. Because the efficiency of the mechanism for reabsorption of intraocular fluid decreases with age, the decrease in the depth of the anterior chamber may contribute to the prevalence of glaucoma in the aged (Goldman, 1979).

As the lens hardens and becomes relatively opaque, the risk of cataract formation increases (Exton-Smith and Overstall, 1979). It is not known whether the complete opacification of the lens that occurs in cataract formation is a manifestation of normal aging or a pathological process (Goldman, 1979). Clouding of the lens also causes light rays to scatter as they make their way through the visual system. Scattered light rays create glare, which is not only uncomfortable but is also an obstacle to good vision (Botwinick, 1978).

The pupil becomes progressively smaller with age, probably due to increasing rigidity of the iris (Exton-Smith and Overstall, 1979). As a result, less light reaches the retina, making it harder for older people to see. There is a linear decrease in the amount of light reaching the retina from age 20 to age 60 (Botwinick, 1978).

There are two dimensions to dark adaptation: (1) the time needed to develop maximum seeing ability in dim light and (2) the level of vision eventually reached. Findings in studies of the rate at which older people achieve dark adaptation are contradictory. It is not known whether it takes the elderly longer to reach their maximum level of vision. There is, however, an almost linear relationship between age and the final level of dark adaptation, and the level achieved by the elderly is not nearly

as good as that reached by young adults (Botwinick, 1978).

Color vision also declines with age, but the reasons are not fully understood. The main reason seems to be related to age-related discoloration of the lens. As the lens yellows, it filters the blues and violets, which are the shorter waves of light. Although the decline in color vision occurs in the longer wavelengths, the reds and yellows, as well, it is greatest in the blue and green parts (Botwinick, 1978).

Brightness is a dimension of white and all other colors. There is evidence that various brightnesses are not as discernible to the elderly as they are to young adults. Increasing the level of illumination improves the older person's ability to discriminate different brightnesses (Botwinick, 1978).

Critical flicker fusion is a classic measure of visual efficiency. With age the threshold for flicker fusion is lowered. A flashing light is presented to the subject and the exact rate at which the flashing lights appear fused is determined. The rate depends upon a variety of factors, including the thickness of the lens, the size of the pupil, and the general efficiency of the central nervous system. With age, the stimulus persists and the flashing light is more readily perceived as fused (Botwinick, 1978).

Hearing

Hearing ability declines as a part of the normal aging process. However, the extent of the decline is difficult to measure because hearing ability is related to several nonsensory factors. The ability to concentrate and focus attention on sound plays an important role in hearing it. Older people are more likely than the young to be inattentive. In addition, during testing older people are more cautious about reporting hearing sounds and tend to report them only when they are quite sure they have heard them (Botwinick, 1978).

The normal human ear can hear sounds ranging in pitch from 20 to 20,000 vibrations per second, but the sounds at either end of the frequency must be louder than the middle frequencies to be heard. Speech frequencies range from 500 to 2000 Hz.

Hearing loss in old age is not equal across all frequencies. High pitches become progressively less audible for the elderly. Tones of lower pitch are better heard, but, eventually, even these are less audible. If sounds are to be heard, they must be made progressively louder as the frequency is increased.

This age-related decline in hearing is called presbycusis. Pure tone audiograms indicate that after age 50 in both sexes, some presbycusis is apparent in frequencies above 1000 Hz (Botwinick, 1978). By age 60 most people have lost serviceable hearing for frequencies above the speech range (above 4000 Hz). In the ninth decade, in men, there is little sensitivity for frequencies within the speech range (Goldman, 1979). In general, presbycusis affects men to a significantly greater degree than women (Botwinick, 1978). The prevalence of presbycusis is difficult to determine because hearing loss in older people is often the result of many factors. Noise pollution in the work place is one such factor that affects many men and produces adaptations similar to presbycusis.

Presbycusis is believed to be the result of structural changes that accompany aging. Multiple changes take place in the ear, from the auditory cortex to the inner ear, and are believed to contribute to hearing loss. Deterioration has been demonstrated in hair cells of the inner ear and in other parts of the cochlea, the auditory sense organ (Botwinick, 1978).

Older people also have difficulty discriminating among different pitches even when the tones are made as functionally loud for them as for young people. After age 55, the ability to discriminate decreases markedly, particularly in frequencies above 1000 Hz. Therefore, it seems that the age curve for pitch discrimination follows a trend similar to that of pitch threshold (Botwinick, 1978).

Presbycusis influences speech intelligibility as well as pure tone thresholds. Hearing levels for easy speech material are usually worse than expected from pure tone audiograms among the aged (Eisdorfer and Wilkie, 1974). Consonants such as s, z, t, f, and g, which are composed of high-frequency tones, may be indiscriminable. This may produce difficulties in the perception of normal conversation. The ability to perceive speech may be further hampered if background noise is present or if speech is distorted in some manner. A reduction in the ability of the higher brain centers to process information may also contribute to poor speech perception. The longer persistence of one word or sound

in a sentence interferes with the processing of the next word, and this makes speech less intelligible, particularly when it is rapid (Botwinick, 1978).

Taste and Smell

The four basic tastes are salty, sweet, sour, and bitter. Changes in the threshold for each of the tastes appear to be insignificant until after age 50, when sensitivity for all the basic tastes declines (Fig. 9) (Cooper et al., 1959). It is believed that the ability to detect sweet substances is particularly affected by age (Goldman, 1979). Pipe smoking further impairs taste sensation in the elderly, but cigarette smoking apparently has no effect (Hughes, 1969).

The decline in taste sensation is due at least in part to a decline in the average number of taste buds per papilla, from 248 in children to 88 in individuals from 74 to 85 years of age. Because many of the remaining taste buds atrophy, the decline in the number of functioning units is actually about 80 percent (Goldman, 1979). Taste is influenced by many other factors, including attitudes toward eating, the health of the oral cavity, and the sense of smell.

Data on the sense of smell are particularly sparse and the results of studies are conflicting. Most of the evidence of an age decline in smell is either indirect or of a clinical nature (Botwinick, 1978). In one study, only 22 percent of the aged subjects had a normal sense of smell, compared with 89 percent of younger subjects (Anand, 1964). A recent study suggests that smell sensitivity does not decline with age, particularly in healthy older people (Engen, 1977). Data must still be collected in this very difficult area of research. Hughes (1969) has suggested that taste, hearing, and smell are all appreciated in the parietal lobe of the inferior portion of the postcentral gyrus and that cellular degeneration in this area may be responsible for the losses in all three sensory modalities.

Somatic Sensations

Somatic sensations include touch, pressure, vibration, position, pain, and others. These sensations are perceived by receptors in the skin and beneath it, transmitted to nerve fibers and then to the spinal cord through the posterior root and to the brain. Touch, pressure, vibration, and position are trans-

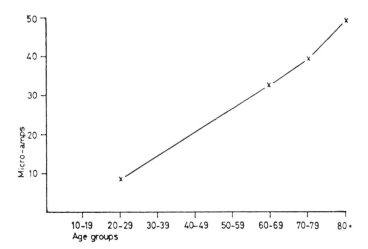

Figure 9. Increase in taste threshold level with advancing age. *From Hughes G, 1969, with permission.*

mitted in the dorsal column of the spinal tract. Pain sensations are transmitted in the spinothalamic tract. A decrease in the number and sensitivity of sensory receptors, dermatomes, and neurons in the central nervous system contributes to a general dulling of these sensations with age.

Touch and Pressure. Very little information is available about age effects on tactile and pressure sensitivity. The number of pacinian, Merkel's, and Meissner's corpuscles, receptor organs in the skin, decreases with age. Those that remain show a number of changes, including marked disorganization (Brody and Vijayashanker, 1977). Free nerve endings also serve as touch and pressure receptors but undergo very few changes. In one study, different parts of the body were stimulated with very fine bristles. It was found that touch sensitivity remains unchanged until the fifth decade, when a rise in the threshold occurs (Birren, 1964). The threshold of touch varies with the part of the body stimulated (Botwinick, 1978).

Vibratory Sensation. Vibratory sensation is caused by rapidly repetitive impulses from tactile or pressure receptors including the pacinian corpuscles. Sensitivity to vibration appears to diminish with age, particularly in the lower extremities. In old age, vibration sense in the malleolus may be lost completely (Corso, 1971; Carter, 1979).

Position Sense. Mechanoreceptors located in the joint capsules and ligaments detect joint move-

ment and the position of different body parts. Impulses move from the receptors to peripheral nerves and then to the spinal cord and cerebellum. With age, position sense is impaired or lost. Changes are particularly evident in the big toe (Carter, 1979).

Pain. Data on age-related changes in the sensation of pain are conflicting. Inconsistencies in research findings are due to the difficulty in measuring pain. Measurement of pain may be more a test of enduring it than the ability to perceive it. Also, older people may want to be more sure of the stimulus before reporting it (Botwinick, 1978). Both the feeling of pain and the reporting of it appear to be related to personality and to cultural influences.

There is much clinical evidence that old people do not feel pain as intensely as do younger people. Serious diseases often occur without the pain experienced by young adults, and minor surgery can often be performed without inflicting severe pain.

Although the ability to sense superficial pain may be relatively intact, the consensus is that the threshold for deep pain increases slightly up to age 60. After that age, the increase is progressively more noticeable (Schludermann and Zubek, 1962; Clark and Mehl, 1971). The threshold of pain varies with the part of the body touched. The increased pain threshold has been implicated as a factor in the incidence of accidents and burns experienced by the aged.

SYSTEM INTEGRATION

We have taken a systems approach to the discussion of the biological changes that accompany the aging process. Aging is accompanied by structural and functional adaptations at the cellular level, the tissue level, the organ level, and the system level of organization. Yet body systems do not exist in isolation or function alone. In holistic man, the functioning of one system is related to and dependent upon the others. Shock (1977) has proposed that the aging process may be more a function of the mechanisms that integrate the body's systems than of changes in individual systems, organs, tissues, or cells. The body's ability to adapt to stress requires an integrated effort on the part of the cardiovascular, pulmonary, muscular, nervous, endocrine, and other systems, and it is at these times that the results of the aging process on the person are most apparent.

Maintenance of Internal Homeodynamics
Age has little effect on the pH of the blood, its glucose and electrolyte content or its osmotic pressure. However, aging has a significant effect on the rate at which all of these parameters are returned to normal after they have been displaced. The aging body may be less sensitive to changes in homeodynamics and respond more sluggishly and less effectively to this stress. Ultimately, the aging person is able to return to resting levels. It would appear that, with age, the ability to maintain a state of homeodynamics is at risk when the individual is subjected to stress.

Response to Exercise
The performance of physical exercise involves the integrated activity and coordination of many organ systems if oxygen is to be delivered to muscles and wastes removed. The aging person's ability to perform light and moderate work is usually unchanged at least until age 65. To do so, however, the aging person expends at least twice the energy as a younger person. The increases in heart rate, blood pressure, and oxygen utilization are all greater in the aged, and the return to the resting level is slower.

Adaptation to strenuous exercise is much less effective in the old than in the young. The parameter most often used as an index of aerobic exercise capacity is the maximal oxygen uptake. It measures the capacity of the individual to perform sustained, strenuous work. The maximal amount of oxygen used during strenuous exercise peaks at age 20 and then declines with increasing age (Klocke, 1977). By age 80, maximum oxygen uptake is reduced by 50 percent. This parameter indicates an underutilization of oxygen already in the circulation. Because of ventilation–perfusion defects, the elderly require a higher ventilation volume than the young simply to achieve the same level of circulating oxygen (Shock, 1977).

Reasons for the decline in maximal oxygen uptake are complex and not fully understood. The pulse rate influences maximum oxygen uptake and, in the elderly, there is a progressive decline in the pulse rate that can be attained during exercise (Shock, 1977). Other possible causes include delayed oxygen diffusion or impaired utilization by the muscle.

Thermoregulation
There are many factors involved in thermoregulation, including neural, endocrine, and metabolic factors. Age-related defects have been documented in the ability to maintain a constant body temperature. Normally, a group of reflexes in the hypothalamus operates to maintain body temperature within a narrow range in spite of fluctuations in environmental temperature.

To maintain a uniform body temperature, a balance must be maintained between heat production and heat loss. Heat production is the result of the metabolic rate and muscle activity. Regulation of heat loss is effected primarily by changes in the amount of blood flowing to the skin. Changes in blood flow depend on the function of the nervous system. Receptors sensitive to slight changes in body temperature are located in the hypothalamus. Skin receptors also monitor peripheral body temperature. Impulses from the sympathetic nervous system respond to the sensory input and make appropriate changes in blood vessels, sweat glands, and muscles. Vasodilation and sweating promote heat loss. Vasoconstriction and shivering prevent heat loss and augment heat production (Shock, 1977). The hypothalamus can also activate caloric depots, such as fat cells and the liver, and can control appetite to help maintain body temperature (Brody and Vijayashanker, 1977).

Basal body temperature is the same for most of the elderly as for the young, ranging from 35.5°

to 37° C. In about 10 percent of those over age 65, deep body temperature is less than 35.5° C. With age, skin temperature, particularly in the fingers and toes, also may be reduced because it is influenced by the amount of vasodilation or vasoconstriction at any point in time. Circulation to the skin declines with age.

The elderly do not need to eliminate as much heat as younger adults. One reason for this change has to do with the fall in basal heat production that occurs over time as a result of a loss of metabolizing tissue. In addition, the decline in physical activity that accompanies aging results in a decline in heat production generated by muscle activity.

In spite of a decline in heat production, the elderly are usually able to maintain resting body temperature. After age 70, however, the elderly are progressively less able to adjust to changes in environmental temperature. Response to high or low environmental temperatures is less effective because the mechanisms involved in conserving and eliminating heat are not as effective.

Because the elderly are less sensitive to cold they are less aware of a cold environment. Consequently, they are less likely to take appropriate action when exposed to the cold (Shock, 1977). In addition, shivering is diminished or absent in the elderly (Exton-Smith and Overstall, 1979).

When exposed to heat, the normal response is vasodilation of peripheral vessels, sweating, and increased rates of pulse and respiration. In the elderly, pulse rate does not increase to the same extent as it does in the young, abnormal peripheral blood flow patterns occur, and sweat glands do not react or react much more sluggishly during warming periods. It is believed that a significantly higher body temperature is required to stimulate sweat glands in the elderly (Exton-Smith and Overstall, 1979). Heat loss from the hands is lower. The end result, reduced potential for heat loss, results in an increased number of deaths from heat stroke in persons after the sixth decade (Shock, 1977).

CONCLUSIONS

In this chapter, healthy aging has been viewed as a stress that stimulates normal and predictable adaptations. Structure and function at all levels from cells to organ systems are affected by aging, each in different ways and at different rates. Perhaps the

most significant changes are those that affect complex, intersystem processes responsible for maintaining normal homeodynamics when the body is presented with stress. Because normal aging changes impair the individual's ability to adapt optimally to stresses in the environment, they are viewed as decremental. Although the aging process is intrinsic, man's efforts to control and modify the environment should help future generations of older people to adapt in an optimal fashion.

Current information about healthy adaptations to aging remains incomplete. Not only is the topic complex, but efforts to gather data are hampered because adaptations to many pathological conditions that affect the elderly are confused with normal aging changes. As research into aging continues, it should help to clarify the real consequences of healthy aging.

REFERENCES

Adler H, Jones KH, Brock MA: Aging and immune function, in Behnke JA, Finch CE, Moment B (eds), The Biology of Aging. New York, Plenum, 1978

Anand MP: Accidents in the home, in Anderson WF, Isaacs B (eds), Current Achievements in Geriatrics. London, Cassel, 1964

Andres R: Aging and carbohydrate metabolism, in Carlson LA (ed), Nutrition and Old Age. Stockholm, Almquist and Wiksell, 1973

Andres R: Aging and diabetes. Medical Clinics of North America 55(4):835, 1971

Andres R, Tobin JD: Endocrine systems, in Finch CE, Hayflick L (eds): Handbook of the Biology of Aging. New York, Van Nostrand Reinhold, 1977

Balazs EA: Intracellular matrix of connective tissue, in Finch C, Hayflick L (eds), Handbook of the Biology of Aging. New York, Van Nostrand Reinhold, 1977

Barrows CH, Roeder LM: Nutrition, in Finch C, Hayflick L (eds), Handbook of the Biology of Aging. New York, Van Nostrand Reinhold, 1977

Bender AD: Effect of age on intestinal absorption. Implications for drug absorption in the elderly. Journal of American Geriatrics Society 16(2):1331, 1968

Bender AD: The effect of increasing age on the distribution of peripheral blood flow in man. Journal of American Geriatrics Society 13(3):192, 1965

Bhanthimnavis K, Schuster M: Aging and gastrointestinal function, in Finch C, Hayflick L (eds), Handbook of the Biology of Aging. New York, Van Nostrand Reinhold, 1977

Birren JE: The Psychology of Aging. Englewood Cliffs, NJ, Prentice-Hall, 1964

Botwinick J: Aging and Behavior: A Comprehensive Integration of Research Findings, 2nd ed. New York, Springer, 1978

Bourne G: Structural changes in aging, in Shock NW (ed), Aging: Some Social and Biological Aspects. Washington, D.C., American Association for the Advancement of Science, 1960

Brandfonbrener M, Landowne M, Shock NW: Changes in cardiac output with age. Circulation XII:557, 1955

Bricker NS: On the meaning of the intact nephron hypothesis. American Journal of Medicine 46(1):1, 1969

Brocklehurst JC: The urinary tract, in Rossman I (ed), Clinical Geriatrics, 2nd ed. Philadelphia, Lippincott, 1979

Brody H, Vijayashanker N: Anatomical changes in the nervous system, in Finch C, Hayflick L (eds), Handbook of the Biology of Aging. New York, Van Nostrand Reinhold, 1977

Buckley CE, Dorsey FC: The effects of aging on human serum immunoglobulin concentrations. Journal of Immunology 105(4):964, 1970

Buckley CE, Dorsey FC: Serum immunoglobulin concentrations, in Palmore E (ed), Normal Aging II: Reports from the Longitudinal Studies, 1970–1973. Durham, NC, Duke University Press, 1974

Burch E: The special problems of heart disease in old people. Geriatrics 31(2):51, 1977

Calloway NO, Foley CF, Lagerbloom P: Uncertainties in geriatric data. Part II. Organ Size. Journal of American Geriatrics Society 13(1):20, 1965

Carter AB: The neurologic aspects of aging, in Rossman I (ed), Clinical Geriatrics, 2nd ed. Philadelphia, Lippincott, 1979

Clark WC, Mehl L: A sensory decision theory analysis of the effect of age and sex on d', various response criteria, and 50% pain threshold. Journal of Abnormal Psychology 78(2):202, 1971

Clifford GO, Bewtra AK: Hematologic problems in the elderly, in Rossman I (ed), Clinical Geriatrics, 2nd ed. Philadelphia, Lippincott, 1979

Cooper RM, Bilash I, Zubek JP: The effect of age on taste sensitivity. Journal of Gerontology 14:56, 1959

Corso JF: Sensory processes and age effects in normal adults. Journal of Gerontology 26(1):90, 1971

Davies DF, Shock NW: Age changes in the glomerular filtration rate, effective renal plasma, and tubular excretory capacity in adult males. Journal of Clinical Investigation 29(5):496, 1950

Davis P: Endocrinology and aging, in Behnke JA, Finch CE, Moment GB (eds), The Biology of Aging. New York, Plenum, 1978

DeVries HA: Physiology of exercise and aging, in Woodruff DS, Birren JE (eds), Aging: Scientific Perspectives and Social Issues. New York, Van Nostrand Reinhold, 1975

Duckworth WC, Kitabchi AE: Direct measurement of plasma pro-insulin in normal and diabetic subjects. American Journal of Medicine 53(4):418, 1972

Dudl RJ, Ensinick JW: The role of insulin, glucagon and growth hormones in CHO homeostasis during aging. Diabetes 21(Suppl 1):357, 1972

Eisdorfer C, Wilkie F: Auditory changes, in Palmore, E (ed), Normal Aging II: Reports from the Longitudinal Studies, 1970–1973. Durham, NC, Duke University Press, 1974

Elkowitz EB: Geriatric Medicine for the Primary Care Practitioner. New York, Springer, 1981

Engen T: Taste and smell, in Birren JE, Schaie KW (eds), Handbook of the Psychology of Aging. New York, Van Nostrand Reinhold, 1977

Exton-Smith EN, Overstall PW: Geriatrics. Baltimore, University Park Press, 1979

Feinstein EI, Friedman EA: Renal disease in the elderly, in Rossman I (ed), Clinical Geriatrics, 2nd ed. Philadelphia, Lippincott, 1979

Feldman JM, Plonk JW: Effect of age on intravenous glucose tolerance and insulin secretion. Journal of the American Geriatrics Society 24(1):1, 1976

Finch C: Comparative biology of senescence: Some evolutionary and developmental questions, in Animal Models for Biomedical Research, VI. Washington, D.C., National Academy of Science, 1971

Finch C: Neuroendocrine and autonomic aspects of aging, in Finch C, Hayflick L (eds), Handbook of the Biology of Aging. New York, Van Nostrand Reinhold, 1977

Finch CE: The brain and aging, in Behnke JA, Finch CE, Moment GB (eds), The Biology of Aging. New York, Plenum, 1978

Gerstenblith G, Frederiksen J, et al: Echocardiographic assessment of a normal adult aging population. Circulation 56(2):273, 1977

Goldfarb AF: Geriatric gynecology, in Rossman I (ed), Clinical Geriatrics, 2nd ed. Philadelphia, Lippincott, 1979

Goldman R: Aging and the execretory system: Kidney and bladder, in Finch C, Hayflick L (eds), Handbook of the Biology of Aging. New York, Van Nostrand Reinhold, 1977

Goldman R: Decline in organ function with aging, in Rossman I (ed), Clinical Geriatrics, 2nd ed. Philadelphia, Lippincott, 1979

Greenblatt RB, Oettinger M, Bohler C: Estrogen–androgen levels in aging men and women: Therapeutic considerations. Journal of the American Geriatrics Society XXIV (4):173, 1976

Gregerman RI, Bierman EL: Hormones and aging, in Williams RH (ed), Textbook of Endocrinology. Philadelphia, Saunders, 1981

Guth PH: Physiologic alteration in small bowel function with age. The absorption of D-xylose. American Journal of Digestive Diseases 13(6):565, 1968

Gutmann E: Muscle, in Finch C, Hayflick L (eds), Handbook of the Biology of Aging. New York, Van Nostrand Reinhold, 1977

Haferkamp O, Schlettein-Gsell D, Schwick HG, Storiko K: Serum protein in an aging population with particular reference to evaluation of immune globulins and antibodies. Gerontologia 12(1):30, 1966

Harris R: Cardiac arrhythmias in the aged, in Caird FI, Dall JLC, Kennedy RD (eds), Cardiology in Old Age. New York, Plenum, 1976

Harrison TR, Dixon K, et al: The relation of age to the duration of contraction, ejection and relaxation of the normal human heart. American Heart Journal 67(2):189, 1964

Harvey AM, Johns RJ, et al (eds): The Principles and Practice of Medicine, 20th ed. New York, Appleton-Century-Crofts, 1980

Hayflick L, Moorhead PS: The serial cultivation of human diploid cell strains. Experimental Cell Research 25:585, 1971

Hayflick L: The cellular basis for biological aging, in Finch C, Hayflick L (eds), Handbook of the Biology of Aging. New York, Van Nostrand Reinhold, 1977

Hesch RD, Gatz J, et al: Total and free triiodothyronine and thyroid-binding globulin concentration in elderly human persons. European Journal of Clinical Investigation 6:134, 1976

Hollis JB, Castell DO: Esophageal function in elderly men—A new look at "Presbyesophagus." Annals of Internal Medicine 80(3):371, 1974

Hughes G: Changes in taste sensitivity with advancing age. Gerontologica Clinica 11(4):224, 1969

Hyams DE: The blood, in Brocklehurst JC (ed), Textbook of Geriatric Medicine and Gerontology, 2nd ed. New York, Churchill Livingstone, 1978

Kales A, Kales JD: Sleep disorders: Recent findings in the diagnosis and treatment of disturbed sleep. New England Journal of Medicine 290(9):487, 1974

Keating FR, Jones JD, Elevebach LR, Randall RV: The relation of age and sex to distribution of values in healthy adults of serum calcium, inorganic phosphorus, magnesium, alkaline phosphatase, total proteins, albumin and blood urea. Journal of Laboratory and Clinical Medicine 73(5):825, 1969

Kleinfield RG, Grieder MH, Fajola WJ: Electron microscopy of intra-nuclear inclusions found in human rat liver parenchyma cells. Journal of Biophysical Biochemical Cytology 2(4)(Suppl):435, 1956

Klocke RA: Influence of aging on the lung, in Finch C, Hayflick L (eds), Handbook of the Biology of Aging. New York, Van Nostrand Reinhold, 1977

Kohn RR: Heart and cardiovascular system, in Finch C, Hayflick L (eds), Handbook of the Biology of Aging. New York, Van Nostrand Reinhold, 1977

Landowne M, Brandfonbrener M, Shock NW: The relation of age to certain measures of performance of the heart and circulation. Circulation XII:567, 1955

Latham KR, Johnson LK: Aging at the cellular level, in Rossman I (ed), Clinical Geriatrics, 2nd ed. Philadelphia, Lippincott, 1979

Lindeman RD: Age changes in renal function, in Goldman R, Rockstein M (eds), The Physiology and Pathology of Human Aging. New York, Academic Press, 1975

Lombardo PC: Dermatologic disorders in the elderly, in Rossman I (ed), Clinical Geriatrics, 2nd ed. Philadelphia, Lippincott, 1979

MacKinney AA Jr: Effect of aging on the peripheral blood lymphocyte count. Journal of Gerontology 33(2):213, 1978

Maekawa T: Hematologic disease, in Steinberg FU (ed), Cowdry's The Care of the Geriatric Patient. St. Louis, Mosby, 1976

Makinodan T: Immunity and aging, in Finch C, Hayflick L (eds), Handbook of the Biology of Aging. New York, Van Nostrand Reinhold, 1977

McCormick D: The normal range for serum creatine phosphokinase. Irish Journal of Medical Science 145(3):86, 1976

McMillan JB, Lev M: The aging heart: Myocardium and epicardium, in Shock NW (ed), Biological Aspects of Aging. New York, Columbia University Press, 1962

Mihalich MJ, Fisch C: Should ECG criteria be modified for geriatric patients? Geriatrics 32(2):65, 1977

Moore RA: Total number of glomeruli in the normal human kidney. Anatomical Record 48:153, 1931

Muggeo M, Fedele D, et al: Human growth hormone and cortisol response to insulin stimulation in aging. Journal of Gerontology 30(5):546, 1975

O'Kell RT, Elliott JR: Development of normal values for use in multitest biochemical screening of sera. Clinical Chemistry 16(3):161, 1970

Piomelli S, Nathan DG, Cummens JF, Gardner FH: Red cell volume and body composition in aged men, in Shock NW (ed), Biological Aspects of Aging. New York, Columbia University Press, 1962

Reed AH, Cannon DC, et al: Estimation of normal ranges from a controlled sample survey. 1. Sex- and age-related influence on the SMA 12/60 screening group of tests. Clinical Chemistry 18(1):57, 1972

Rockstein M, Chesky J, Sussman M: Comparative biology and evolution of aging, in Finch C, Hayflick L (eds), Handbook of the Biology of Aging. New York, Van Nostrand Reinhold, 1977

Rodstein M, Zemen FD: Arcus senilis and arteriosclerosis in the aged. American Journal of Medical Science 245(1):70, 1963

Rodstein M: The ECG in old age: Implications for diagnosis, therapy and prognosis. Geriatrics 32(2):76, 1977

Rosen H: Renal disease in the elderly. Medical Clinics of North America 60(6):1105, 1976

Rossman I: Anatomic and body composition changes with aging, in Finch C, Hayflick L (eds), Handbook of the Biology of Aging. New York, Van Nostrand Reinhold, 1977

Rossman I: The anatomy of aging, in Rossman I (ed), Clinical Geriatrics, 2nd ed. Philadelphia, Lippincott, 1979

Roth GS: Altered biochemical responsiveness and hormone receptor changes during aging, in Behnke JA, Finch CE, Moment GB (eds), The Biology of Aging. New York, Plenum, 1978

Rowe JW: Clinical research on aging: Strategies and directions. New England Journal of Medicine 297(24):1332, 1977

Rowe JW, Andres R, et al: The effect of age on creatinine clearance in men: A cross-sectional and longitudinal study. Journal of Gerontology 31(2):155, 1976

Sanadi DR: Metabolic changes and their significance in aging, in Finch C, Hayflick L (eds), Handbook of the Biology of Aging. New York, Van Nostrand Reinhold, 1977

Schludermann E, Zubek JP: Effect of age on pain sensitivity. Perceptual and Motor Skills 14:295, 1962

Schuster M: Disorders of the aging GI system. Hospital Practice 11(9):95, 1976

Selmanowitz VJ, Rizer RL, Orentreich N: Aging of the skin and its appendages, in Finch C, Hayflick L (eds), Handbook of the Biology of Aging. New York, Van Nostrand Reinhold, 1977

Shapleigh JB, Mayes S, Moore CV: Hematologic values in the aged. Journal of Gerontology 7(2):207, 1952

Shenkin HA, Novak P, et al: The effects of aging, arteriosclerosis and hypertension upon the cerebral circulation. Journal of Clinical Investigation 32(6):459, 1953

Shock NW: System integration, in Finch C, Hayflick L (eds), Handbook of the Biology of Aging. New York, Van Nostrand Reinhold, 1977

Sjögren AL: Left ventricular wall thickness determined by ultrasound in 100 subjects with heart disease. Chest 60(4):341, 1971

Sklar M, Kirsner JB, Palmer WL: Gastrointestinal disease in the aged. Medical Clinics of North America 40 (1):223, 1956

Soerjodibroto WS, Hearn CR, Exton-Smith AN: Glucose tolerance, plasma insulin levels and insulin sensitivity in elderly patients. Age and Aging 8:65, 1979

Storandt M: Psychological aspects of aging, in Rossman I (ed), Clinical Geriatrics, 2nd ed. Philadelphia, Lippincott, 1979

Subbarao K: Radiological aspects of aging, in Rossman I (ed), Clinical Geriatrics, 2nd ed. Philadelphia, Lippincott, 1979

Syzek BJ: Cardiovascular changes in aging: Implications for nursing. Journal of Gerontological Nursing 2(1):28, 1976

Talbert GB: Aging of the reproductive system, in Finch C, Hayflick L (eds), Handbook of the Biology of Aging. New York, Van Nostrand Reinhold, 1977

Terry RD: Physical changes of the aging brain, in Behnke JA, Finch CE, Moment GB (eds), The Biology of Aging. New York, Plenum, 1978

Tichy AM, Malasanos LJ: Physiological parameters of aging. Part I. Journal of Gerontological Nursing 5(1):42, 1979a

Tichy AM, Malasanos LJ: Physiological parameters of aging. Part II. Journal of Gerontological Nursing 5(2):38, 1979b

Timaras PS: Developmental Physiology and Aging. New York, MacMillan, 1972

Tonn EA: Aging of skeletal-dental systems and supporting tissues, in Finch C, Hayflick L (eds), Handbook of the Biology of Aging. New York, Van Nostrand Reinhold, 1977

Wesson LG: Physiology of the Human Kidney. New York, Grune and Stratton, 1969

Willems JL, Roelandt JR, Van de Vel HR, Joossens JV: The circulation time in the aged. American Journal of Cardiology 27:155, 1971

Wynne JW: Pulmonary disease in the elderly, in Rossman I (ed), Clinical Geriatrics, 2nd ed. Philadelphia, Lippincott, 1979

Zach L: The oral cavity, in Rossman I (ed), Clinical Geriatrics, 2nd ed. Philadelphia, Lippincott, 1979

6

The Aging Process—
Psychosocial Adaptations

Many older people are convinced that deterioration in their mental functioning is an inevitable concomitant of the aging process. Expectation of a decline can, of course, become a self-fulfilling prophecy. So-called decline in mentation, however, is more mythical than real, growing out of societal caricatures and expectations. Although research does point to changing psychosocial adaptations in response to the aging process, it does not support the inevitable, steady decline so often taken for granted. What it does support is the tremendous diversity and the wide spectrum of abilities seen in elderly populations, a finding unlike that seen in younger populations, who show far less variance in their development.

PROBLEMS OF RESEARCH

Chown (1972) points out that there are problems with research techniques. Cross-sectional studies have a tendency to confound age changes with generational differences. The life-style, values, mores, and beliefs that stem from the generation and culture of the cohort under study may be misinterpreted as part of an age change. Even longitudinal testing fails to give an unbiased view of age changes, and, in fact, may underestimate them as a result of a greater sophistication that occurs with recurrent testing and the self-selection that is built-in with long-term study. Some of the more definitive studies have utilized a combination of longitudinal and cross-sectional design. Although the idea of following a

cross section over time is less subject to generational differences, it does tend to yield findings of a more stable population.

One factor that emerges from the research is the impact of health status on psychosocial adaptations. Sensory impairment, especially hearing loss, can lead to enhanced suspicion and outright paranoia. Decreased circulation and the atherosclerotic process can lead to severe impairment in mentation. Although it has been said that a healthy mental outlook is a better predictor of overall functioning than is good physical health, the two, like a double helix, are inextricably intertwined in producing a functioning older person.

In order to look more precisely at psychosocial adaptations normally occurring in a healthy aging population, these adaptations will be arbitrarily presented under three separate categories—cognitive abilities, personality and coping, and social functioning.

COGNITIVE ABILITY

Intelligence
Over the years studies have consistently demonstrated the correlation between intelligence and verbal abilities. Longitudinal studies have shown greater stability of intelligence with little or no decline in verbal abilities before age 70 and a relatively greater but not catastrophic loss after 70 (Zarit, 1980). Schaie and Labouvie-Vief (1974) followed three cohorts on a battery of tests and found that while the younger

cohort scored higher, attesting to a generational difference, there was no significant decline in any of the cohorts tested over time. Longitudinal studies conducted on college students (Owens, 1953; Cunningham and Birren, 1976) indicate the essential stability for arithmetic and verbal scores, with some decrement occurring in spatial relations (e.g., visualizing rotation of geometric objects).

Several studies (Riegel and Riegel, 1972; Blum et al., 1973) have identified what has been called "terminal decline," a drop in scores on various cognitive tests preceding a person's death. Jarvik (1975) found that subjects experiencing declines in vocabulary, block design, and digit symbol were less likely to survive the next 5-year interval.

In summary, many individuals in their seventies or eighties perform at levels found in the young. In the absence of major illnesses or a decline preceding death, there is considerable stability in intellectual performance.

Reaction Time

Speed of response declines with age on almost any performance measure (Welford, 1977). According to Birren (1974), a slowing in reaction time is a principal manifestation of neurological aging, related as it is to the slowing in the conduction of electrical impulses in the central nervous system. Slowed response can be aggravated by social deprivation or some pathological condition. Birren proposed that this slowed reaction time may account for the higher rate of accidents among the elderly and may, in addition, affect other cognitive and social behaviors like complex problem solving and information retrieval. Several recent studies suggest that test performance can be affected by manipulating reinforcement schedules. Hoyer et al. (1973) showed that the speed with which older adults performed on ability tests could be increased markedly by rewarding participants with trading stamps. Incentives have traditionally brought about an individual's "best" performance.

Memory

The tendency to exaggerate memory loss is common among the elderly (Lowenthal et al., 1967; Kahn et al., 1975). Half of Lowenthal's large community sample claimed memory difficulties that did not correlate with scores on memory tests. Investigators

have, however, found a correlation between impaired performance and measures of depression (Kahn et al., 1975; Gurland et al., 1976).

The capacity for primary memory (the amount of information that can be held for active processing) appears to be stable with increasing age, provided no reorganization of the material is required (Craik, 1977). Asking the client to process and remember digits is an example. Where it is required that the digits be recalled in reverse order, involving a reorganization, primary memory has been found to be poorer in the elderly.

Secondary memory requires primary memory to be transferred into a storage system and retrieved at a later time. This process has been studied by comparing performance under conditions of recall and recognition. Here the findings are mixed, with some studies reporting that the elderly perform at the same level as their younger counterparts on tests involving recognition (Schonfield, 1965) while others report decrements in both recognition and recall when compared with a sample of young people (Gordon and Clark, 1974; Perlmutter, 1978). Several factors emerge from the research. Older persons score better when tested with meaningful material than, for example, with nonsense syllables, which seems to suggest an unwillingness to expend energy on meaningless tasks (Botwinick, 1978). The elderly also do less well and show greater deficits on both memory and learning tests when there are distractions and a time pressure to respond (Canestrari, 1963).

There is some question whether recent versus remote memory is impaired in the elderly. Zarit (1980) raises the question of equivalency in the questions being asked. "When did you get married?," which signals a significant event can hardly be equated with "What did you have for breakfast?" Kahn et al. (1975) found that when equally significant questions were asked about the present and the past, older persons performed well on both recent and remote measures.

Problem Solving

The difficulties experienced by older people in problem solving seem to result from a combination of cognitive changes, including memory, learning, information processing rate, attention, and perceptual integration (Rabbitt, 1977). Evidence is clear that either stimuli deprivation or overload can cause a decrement in performance, whether for cognitive reasons or because of fear and anxiety. Shmavonian and Busse (1963) showed that both old and young tend to perform better on problem-solving tasks if the challenge is meaningful, although the elderly are disproportionately affected by meaningless tasks. Nonetheless, problem-solving abilities tend to hold up well in the elderly. From the sixties to mid-seventies there is a normal decline on some but not all abilities for some but not all individuals, once again attesting to the remarkable diversity and individuality of the aging population. Beyond the age of eighty, a decrement in problem solving is the rule for most individuals (Schaie, 1980).

In summary, given the increased variability from one person to the next during the aging process, measures of intelligence, memory, and problem solving show little decline until the seventies unless sensory deprivation or chronic ailments intervene. Reaction time, on the other hand, declines with age on almost any performance measure, but even here incentives can improve performance. The major effect of the aging process seems to be the attendant risk of illness, which may in turn bring about a deterioration in cognitive functioning.

PERSONALITY AND COPING BEHAVIORS

A second area of psychosocial adaptation relates to personality and its characteristics, namely the self-concept, traits, cognitive style, and coping behaviors. In this realm, there seems to be even greater stability during the aging process. More than 25 years ago, Busse and his colleagues at Duke University (Busse et al., 1954, 1955) indicated that if no organic damage occurred in the brain and nervous system, emotional states in later life were essentially similar to those of earlier periods. Emotional responses might intensify, but they remained fundamentally consistent with prior personality functioning. If, for example, a man has been hysterical or depressive, in all likelihood he will tend to remain so or perhaps become worse. If, on the other hand, he functioned reasonably well and appropriately, he will probably continue to do so. In other words, there is a basic continuity in the manner in which people cope with life events generally and with stress specifically that does not seem to change in old age.

Kimmel (1974) found the self-concept, that is, the ways in which individuals typically see themselves, relatively stable over time. Schwartz and Kleemeier (1965) asked subjects in good health and others with significant health problems to describe themselves using the Osgood Semantic Differential. Differences in the self-concept were found between healthy and ill but not between young and old. Once again, good health plays a significant role in psychosocial adaptation.

Woodruff and Birren (1972) did find generational differences occurring in the self-concept. In testing a group of undergraduates on measures of self-esteem, they found that scores achieved by an earlier cohort (tested at the same university 25 years before) were higher, indicating a higher degree of self-adjustment and social adjustment for students of that generation.

Cognitive Style

Cognitive style refers to the way in which people organize and interpret incoming stimuli. It has much to say about the character structure and consequent coping styles of people. Shapiro (1965) reviewed the impact of thinking and perception on the functioning of neurotics. He considered cognitive style an important psychological structure from which specific personality traits, defense mechanisms, and behaviors seem to flow.

Two major cognitive styles have been the subject of continuous study. Witkin and his associates (1962) proposed that persons are either field-dependent or field-independent in the way in which they respond to stimuli. Field-independent people tend to make internal judgments, avoiding environmental influences. Field-dependent persons are more likely to be swayed by environmental pressures. One recalls the now famous study of social pressure by Asch (1955) when one of six subjects in an experiment disagreed with the unanimous, though false, consensus given by the other five subjects and continued to maintain his own independent judgment.

Another style, locus of control, developed by Rotter (1966), assesses whether or not an individual feels he has control over events and the ability to extract reinforcement from the environment. Kuypers (1972) reported that subjects with an internal locus of control were more active and better adapted to their environments than externally oriented individuals. More recently, Wigdor and Yankofsky (1977) found that the elderly with an internal locus of control showed greater persistence when dealing with frustrating tasks and, generally, a greater life satisfaction. Since internal locus of control was also found to be associated with intelligence in the Kuypers study, it is not entirely clear whether internal locus or intelligence exerts more influence on adaptation. It is also not known whether locus of control shifts with aging.

Personality Traits

Constitutional factors, early environmental shaping, and a person's history of success and failure in trying to attain satisfaction all influence the development of personality traits. Although some personality traits may intensify with the aging process (cautiousness, rigidity, dependency, and conservatism), at any given time people tend to be more like they were at an earlier period of development than, for example, similar to their peers. Goldfarb (1969) proposed that dependency becomes more prominent in later life. Lancaster (1981) noted an increase in inner directedness or introversion, citing the older person's greater preoccupation with self—especially bodily functions, wants, and past reminiscences. She finds this introversion consistent with the conservatism and the general desire to avoid change seen in the elderly population. Botwinick (1978) found cautiousness increasing in the elderly. On tests involving right or wrong answers, they made more errors of omission than the young. There seems to be an unwillingness to take risks unless there is a high degree of certainty of success. Birkhill and Schaie (1975) found the elderly least cautious under conditions of low risk and low anxiety.

Rigidity has also received attention. In attempting to identify its components, Chown (1961) found that age and intelligence accounted for most of the variance, making it impossible to determine whether the aging process or low intelligence was the principal determinant of rigidity. Schaie and Labouvie-Vief (1974) studied age and its relationship to rigidity in a number of cohorts ranging in age from the twenties to the seventies who were tested at 7-year intervals. Under study were the ability to shift from one activity to another (motor-cognitive rigidity), self reports of adjustment to new surroundings, and the ability to change habits (personality–perceptual rigidity) and psychomotor speed. Using a cross-sectional analysis, they found more rigid behavior among the older subjects on all three measures. All three of the oldest cohorts (aged 53, 60, and 67 at the start of the study) showed a decline in psychomotor speed. The three oldest groups also showed an increase in personality–perceptual rigidity although only the oldest cohort showed a decrement in the ability to shift activities (cognitive-motor rigidity).

On a more positive note, Lehman (1953) demonstrated that creativity continues, subject, of course, to individual differences. Dennis (1966) examined creative productivity in subjects between the ages of 20 and 80 by reviewing the bibliographies of scholars who were found to be as productive in their seventies as in their forties. Scientists showed a slight decline during their fifties and sixties and a sharp decline in the seventies.

Finally, Schaie and Parham (1976) found an increase in humanitarian concerns with advancing age, a finding that was unrelated to any cohort difference.

Coping Behaviors

From what has already been said, it can be seen that coping behaviors tend to reflect the cognitive style and personality traits of the individual. Generally speaking, the larger the repertoire of behaviors one can muster to meet life situations, the more likely one is to adapt well to these situations. When coping behaviors fail to avert crisis situations, people are most susceptible to trying out new behaviors. This is discussed further in Chapter 13. It is sufficient to note here that the most effective copers tend to use fewer denial processes and are more likely to divert their attention deliberately from the ongoing irresolvable problems of aging. Golden (1980) found that denial was less likely to be used by those who perceived growing old and illness as separate problems.

Perception

"Perception refers to an individual's ability to receive, register, process, and respond to a stimulus"

(Lancaster, 1981, p. 38). It is determined as much by the past experiences that form our current beliefs and biases as it is by the quality of our sensory receptors. Weinberg (1976) points out that any given perceptual act is the result of many processes—sensory, cognitive, motor, conceptual, and affective. A change in perception will influence behavior more directly than any change in sensation (Debner, 1975).

One specific perceptual change that occurs in older people is difficulty in differentiating stimuli from their background. Older people need sufficient time to perceive complex or incomplete representations. Hurrying them may further diminish their perceptual acuity, since judgments tend to be made with more caution. What may sometimes appear as faulty reasoning may indeed be only faulty perception.

Motivation and Drive

Widgor (1980) in reviewing the literature finds a dearth of empirical research on drives and motivation, especially among the older population. She concludes that motivation and aging have a reciprocal influence on each other throughout the life span and that the interaction of the physiological condition and cognitive–perceptual processes over one's lifetime influences adaptation. Hebb (1955) described motivation as an energizer of behavior, the source of energy that provides continuity and direction to life. Energy, thus generated, finds its expression in basic drives, like hunger and thirst, the exploratory drive, and the sex drive.

Exploratory Drive

This drive regulates activity, exploration, and curiosity. If more energy is required to satisfy basic needs, there may be less available for the exploratory drive. Nevertheless, healthy individuals tend to seek activity and stimulation even when they grow older, and it results in better life satisfaction (Maddox, 1968). Mental health may be much more of a determinant than physical health in maintaining higher levels of activity, unless the physical condition is markedly incapacitating (Kral and Wigdor, 1957).

Sexual Drive amd Sexuality

In recent years a wide range of literature has been written about sexuality and the aging person (Sol-nick, 1978; Comfort, 1980; Yoselle, 1981). Some fifteen years earlier Masters and Johnson (1966), while documenting the physiological changes during sexual performance, reported that older individuals needed higher levels of stimulation to achieve arousal. Cameron and Biber (1973) have since amplified this by noting that fantasy, probably the most important determinant in sexual arousal, declines with age in both sexes. What has become apparent, however, is that individuals who have been active in early life and maintained high levels of interest show a tendency to maintain sexual activity longer and with greater frequency in their older years.

The major stumbling blocks to continuing sexual activity are loss of a partner, a disabling illness that interferes with performance, some emotional barrier, or societal convention. Of these, perhaps the greatest and most widespread handicap is misinformation and societal convention. Sexuality is closely linked to the aging process, so closely that how one feels about aging seems inextricably bound up with feelings about one's body, self-esteem and attractiveness, and even the sense of being wanted and needed. As Yoselle (1981) points out, American society is just as ambivalent in its outlook toward sexuality as it is toward the aging process itself.

Normally, sexual expression is subject to all the variability that one finds in an aging population. Some older people were never particularly interested in sex even as young people; for them the aging period, with cessation of sexual activities, may come as a relief. They may even rely on societal pressures as an excuse for withdrawal. The real problem exists for those who do enjoy sex and who see it as an opportunity to express tenderness, affection, and even loyalty. Butler and Lewis (1976) point out that loss of sexual activity results in a loss of the opportunity to grow and change in new directions.

With society continuing to downgrade the aging body and fostering the idea that sexual activity is or should be beyond the scope of interest for an aging person, it is not surprising to see older individuals comply with the message. When an aging actress on one of the long-extant soap operas had an affair written into her script, she fully expected disapproval for this fall from grace. In talking with members of her audience, however, she was surprised to hear herself commended for adding "spice" to their lives. Perhaps the spice was only vicariously enjoyed, but what had been provided was permission to continue enjoying an aging body. Since soap operas seem to reflect the culture and mores of our times, change may be on the way.

ROLES, TASKS, AND SUPPORT SYSTEMS

From the standpoint of adaptation, perhaps the greatest changes occur for the aging individual in the area of social adaptation. With retirement, widowhood, and other losses occurring, not only are role changes inevitable, but the changes frequently result in a loss of status. Aging persons find themselves stepping into a role vacuum, with few standards by which to judge themselves or their behavior.

In a very moving statement, Rosow (1973) points out that old age is the only stage of life with systematic status loss for an entire cohort. All other periods in the life cycle are marked by steady social growth, involving gains in competence, responsibility, authority, privilege, reward, and prestige. Since the roles people play identify them as social beings, role loss can deprive the aging person of social identity, together with its attendant self-esteem. A further stress is occasioned by the fact that these role losses (widowhood, retirement, death of friends) occur at a time when group support is critical yet difficult to come by. Group memberships tend to diminish by the age of 65 and certainly by age 75. Persons in this age bracket belong to fewer organizations, hold fewer offices, and participate less as members. They also have fewer friends and see them less often.

In view of the many social changes occurring, Clark and Anderson (1967) have outlined five adaptive tasks that present critical challenges to the aging client:

1. Acknowledging that some physical and mental limitations are inherent in the aging process, which necessitates an alteration in activity level in order to cope successfully and conserve finite energy resources.

2. Changing both the level and type of physical activities as well as social roles.

3. Finding new ways to fulfill physical, economic, and emotional needs.

4. Developing new criteria for self-evaluation by learning to relax, being tolerant of others, and experiencing happiness at seeing others succeed.

5. Establishing new values and goals by recognizing that some tasks will take longer than they previously took.

SUMMARY

Many psychosocial adaptations may be related to physical changes of aging. Decreasing reaction time, slowing of motor activity of all kinds, and decreasing sensory capacity, along with changes in memory, may contribute to the following common psychosocial adaptations:

1. Increased cautiousness
2. Increased rigidity
3. Increased introversion
4. Decreased interaction
5. Changes in learning motivation
6. Decreased self-esteem

Other adaptations may emerge as a result of new stages of development (see Chapter 4). Yet others may result from societal pressure and the losses that accumulate in late life.

REFERENCES

Asch SE: Opinions and social pressure. Scientific American 193:31, 1955

Birkhill WR, Schaie KW: The effect of differential reinforcement of cautiousness in intellectual performances among the elderly. Journal of Gerontology 30:578, 1975

Birren JE: Translations in gerontology—from lab to life: Psychophysiology and speed of response. American Psychologist 11:808, 1974

Blum JE, Clark ET, Jarvik LF: The New York State Psychiatric Institute Study of aging twins, in Jarvik LF, Eisdorfer C, Blum JE (eds), Intellectual Functioning in

Adults: Psychological and Biological Influences. New York, Springer, 1973

Botwinick J: Aging and Behavior, 2nd ed. New York, Springer, 1978

Busse EW, Barnes RH, et al: Studies of the aging process: Factors that influence the psyche of elderly persons. American Journal of Psychiatry 110:897, 1954

Busse EW, Barnes R, et al: Studies of the processes of aging: Strengths and weaknesses of psychiatric functioning in the aged. American Journal of Psychiatry 111:896, 1955

Butler R, Lewis M: Love and Sex after Sixty. New York, Harper and Row, 1976

Cameron P, Biber H: Sexual thought throughout the lifespan. Gerontologist 13:144, 1973

Canestrari RE: Paced and self-paced learning in young and elderly adults. Journal of Gerontology 18:165, 1963

Chown SM: Age and the rigidities. Journal of Gerontology 16:353, 1961

Chown SM: Intelligence, in Chown SM (ed), Human Ageing—Selected Readings. Baltimore, MD, Penguin, 1972

Clark M, Anderson B: Culture and Aging. Springfield, IL, Charles C. Thomas, 1967

Comfort A: Sexuality in later life, in Birren JE, Sloane RB (eds), Handbook of Mental Health and Aging. Englewood Cliffs, NJ, Prentice-Hall, 1980

Craik FIM: Age differences in human memory, in Birren JE, Schaie KW (eds), Handbook of the Psychology of Aging. New York, Van Nostrand Reinhold, 1977

Cunningham WR, Birren JE: Age changes in human abilities: A 28-year longitudinal study. Developmental Psychology 12:81, 1976

Debner AS: The psychology of normal aging, in Spencer MG, Dorr CJ (eds), Understanding Aging: A Multidisciplinary Approach. New York, Appleton-Century-Crofts, 1975

Dennis W: Creative productivity of persons engaged in scholarship, the sciences and the arts. Journal of Gerontology 21:1, 1966

Golden GY: The use of denial and denial-like processes in coping with problems of aging. Human Development and Aging Program, University of California, San Francisco. Paper presented at American Gerontological Society Annual Meeting, November, 1980

Goldfarb AI: The psychodynamics of dependency and the search for aid, in Kalish R (ed), The Dependencies of Old People. Ann Arbor, MI, Institute of Gerontology, 1969

Gordon SK, Clark WC: Application of signal detection theory to prose recall and recognition in elderly and young adults. Journal of Gerontology 29:64, 1974

Gurland BJ, Fleiss JL, et al : The geriatric mental state schedule: A factor analysis. International Journal of Aging and Human Development 7:303, 1976

Hebb DO: Drives and the CNS (conceptual nervous system). Psychological Review 62:243, 1955

Hoyer WJ, Labouvie-Vief G, Baltes PB: Modification of response speed deficits and intellectual performance in the elderly. Human Development 16:233, 1973

Jarvik LF: Thoughts on the psychobiology of aging. American Psychologist 30:567, 1975

Kahn RL, Zarit SH, Hilbert NM, Niederehe G: Memory complaint and impairment in the aged. Archives of General Psychiatry 32:1569, 1975

Kimmel DC: Adulthood and Aging: An Interdisciplinary, Developmental View. New York, Wiley, 1974

Kral VA, Wigdor BT: Psychiatric and psychological observations in a geriatric clinic. Canadian Psychiatric Association Journal 2:185, 1957

Kuypers JA: Internal–external locus of control, ego functioning and personality characteristics in old age. Gerontologist 12:168, 1972

Lancaster J: Maximizing psychological adaptation in an aging population. Topics in Clinical Nursing 3(1):31, 1981

Lehman HC: Age and Achievement. Princeton, NJ, Princeton University Press, 1953

Lowenthal MF, Berkman P, et al: Aging and Mental Disorder in San Francisco. San Francisco, Jossey-Bass, 1967

Maddox GL: Persistence of life-style among the elderly: A longitudinal study of patterns of social activity in relation to life satisfaction, in Neugarten BL (ed), Middle Age and Aging. Chicago, University of Chicago Press, 1968

Masters WH, Johnson VE: Human Sexual Response. Boston, Little, Brown, 1966

Owens WA Jr: Age and mental abilities: A longitudinal study. Genetic Psychology Monographs 48:3, 1953

Owens WA Jr: Age and mental abilities: A second adult follow-up. Journal of Educational Psychology 51:311, 1966

Perlmutter M: What is memory aging the aging of? Developmental Psychology 14:330, 1978

Rabbitt PSA: Changes in problem solving ability in old age, in Birren JE, and Schaie KW (eds), Handbook of the Psychology of Aging. New York, Van Nostrand Reinhold, 1977

Riegel KF, Riegel RM: Development, drop and death. Developmental Psychology 6:306, 1972

Rotter JB: Generalized expectancies for internal versus external control of reinforcement. Psychological Monographs 80(1):1, 1966

Rosow I: The social context of the aging self. Gerontologist 13:82, 1973

Schaie KW, Labouvie-Vief G: Generational versus ontogenetic components of change in adult cognitive behavior: A fourteen-year cross-sequential study. Developmental Psychology 10:305, 1974

Schaie KW, Parham IA: Stability of adult personality traits: Fact or fable. Journal of Personal Social Psychology 34:146, 1976

Schaie KW: Intelligence and problem solving, in Birren JE, Sloane RB (eds), Handbook of Mental Health and Aging. Englewood Cliffs, NJ, Prentice-Hall, 1980

Schonfield D: Memory changes with age. Nature 28:918, 1965

Schonfield AED: Learning, memory, and aging, in Birren JE, Sloane RB (eds), Handbook of Mental Health and Aging. Englewood Cliffs, NJ, Prentice-Hall, 1980

Schwartz AN, Kleemeier RW: The effects of illness and age upon some aspects of personality. Journal of Gerontology 20:85, 1965

Shapiro D: Neurotic Styles. New York, Basic Books, 1965

Shmavonian BM, Busse EW: The use of psychophysical techniques in the study of the aged, in Williams RH, Tibbetts C, Donahue W (eds), Process of Aging, Social and Psychological Perspectives. New York, Atherton, 1963

Solnick RL (ed): Sexuality and Aging. Ethel Percy Andrus Gerontology Center, University of Southern California Press, 1978

Weinberg J: On adding insight to injury. Gerontologist 16(1):4, 1976

Welford AT: Motor performance, in Birren JE, Schaie KW (eds), Handbook of the Psychology of Aging. New York, Van Nostrand Reinhold, 1977

Wigdor BT, Yankofsky L: Successful Adjustment to Old Age as a Function of Persistence and Effectence Coping and Locus of Control. Unpublished undergraduate thesis, McGill University, 1977

Wigdor B: Drives and motivations with aging, in Birren JE, Sloane RB (eds), Handbook of Mental Health and Aging. Englewood Cliffs, NJ, Prentice-Hall, 1980

Witkin HA, Dyk RB, et al : Psychological Differentiation. New York, Wiley, 1962

Woodruff DS, Birren JE: Age changes and cohort differences in personality. Developmental Psychology 6:252, 1972

Yoselle H: Sexuality in the later years. Topics in Clinical Nursing 3(1):59, 1981

Zarit SH: Aging and Mental Disorders: Psychological Approaches to Assessment and Treatment. New York, Free Press, 1980

7

Health Maintenance of the Aging Client

Historically, health care services for the aged have been illness or crisis oriented. Services to maintain high-level functioning in healthy aging persons have been few, despite statistics indicating that the aged who are ill are the exception, not the rule. Eighty-eight percent of the aging population in the United States are functionally healthy and active, living in the community and caring for themselves (Shanas, 1980).

According to the World Health Organization, health maintenance services for the aged should be aimed at allowing them to remain in their own homes for as long as they wish to do so. Health maintenance services include health assessment, teaching, counseling, and referral. For the aged, it is particularly important to obtain a comprehensive data base to serve as a base line against which to measure future adaptations that accompany the aging process. The professional nurse is uniquely qualified to provide health maintenance services to the aged wherever older people are located: clinics, community centers serving the aged, churches, apartment complexes, day care centers, social service agencies, and the client's own home.

Studies of healthy aging subjects have demonstrated that provision of regular and frequent health services is the key to maintenance of high-level functioning. Williamson et al. (1966) studied aging persons living at home and found that over half the stresses discovered during physical and psychological assessment had been unreported by the client. For the most part, older people do not report stresses or seek health care until adaptations are far advanced. The researchers concluded that if old people are assessed on a regular basis, stresses can be detected at an early stage, deterioration slowed, and independence maintained.

This chapter discusses the following elements of the health assessment:

- Nursing history
- Physical examination
- Laboratory data
- Psychosocial assessment, including home assessment.

HEALTH ASSESSMENT OF THE AGED

Health assessment of the aging client requires knowledge of multiple factors uniquely related to the aging process. An understanding of the adaptations normally associated with growing old and their functional implications is essential.

Assessment of the healthy aging client should achieve the following purposes: First, the client's overall level of adaptation should be identified. To do so, the nurse identifies normality and any deviations from it, then determines the effects of deviations on the client's ability to function. Second, the client's perception of and feelings about his or her level of adaptation should be explored. Last the nurse should identify those health-related practices that augment the client's current level of adaptation as well as additional practices that, if adopted, would improve adaptation. The emphasis of health assessment should be positive and should seek to identify and strengthen those practices that enhance functioning.

Scheduling the Health Assessment

The health assessment, particularly the health history, of the aging client may require more time than would be needed for a younger person. If only because of longevity, older people have longer and more complicated histories than do young adults. In addition, they may recount the history more slowly, reminiscing while doing so. A developmental task of aging involves the life review and integration of past experiences with the present situation. Consequently, one question by the nurse may prompt the client to relate a lengthy series of events. Since reminiscing is an excellent source of data, relevant to many aspects of the health history, it can be used as a means of obtaining data. Allowing reminiscence also helps to establish rapport and assures the client that the nurse is genuinely interested.

The length of the interview depends entirely upon the situation. A complete health history will take at least 1 hour. However, partial deafness or other communication barriers may prolong the interview. The client's need for socialization and reminiscence may also extend the interview, just as the client's fatigue may require that the interview be ended and resumed on another occasion.

At the beginning of the interview the nurse should orient the client to the topic and set a time limit. Doing so may assist those aging clients with a diminished perception of time to cope with the interview situation. If unable to complete the interview in the allotted time, the nurse should contract with the client for another session, again specifying the topic of the interview and the time. If the health history has been time consuming, it may be advisable to perform only the most relevant portions of the physical assessment at the same session. The complete physical assessment can be scheduled for a later date. Because some aging clients have decreased primary memory, it is best to write down the date, time, and place of the next appointment and leave this information with the client.

The time at which the interview is scheduled should take into account the adaptive patterns of the client. The interview should be held at a time when the client is fresh and not fatigued. For many of the aged, this is in the early morning. For others, who have become accustomed to sleeping later, midday or early afternoon may be a more convenient time. The time of the interview may affect the older client's mental status. If clients are oversedated with nighttime hypnotics, their mental status may be clouded in the early morning. Afternoon confusion (sundowning) may occur in mildly demented clients from the decrease in sensory stimuli that occurs as evening comes. Many elderly people, particularly those who reside in older urban areas, may be reluctant to schedule an interview during the late afternoon or evening in order to avoid being out of doors after dark. Older people who must rely on public transportation may also be reluctant to schedule appointments at times that require traveling during peak travel hours.

The Setting

Before beginning the interview the nurse should assure that the client is oriented to the setting and made as comfortable as possible. Some clients prefer the support offered by a sturdy, straight-backed chair to a large overstuffed chair. Clients who are not distracted by physical discomfort, such as joint pain or the need to void, will be able to cooperate more fully during the interview. If the client wears dentures, they should be in place before the interview begins to assure optimum communication.

Many aging clients have diminished sight, which requires modification of the environment. Of course, the client's own glasses or contact lenses should be in place. The use of several bright, contrasting colors to furnish the examining room may help the client to become oriented. The nurse should refer to these colors when giving directions: "Please look at the chart on the yellow wall." To compensate for visual deficiencies, the room should be well lit, but without bright lights or glare. The client should not be seated facing a sunny window. If the client's sight is severely impaired, the use of touch may enhance the nurse's contact with the client. In addition, it would be important to respond to the client vocally, since gestures and other nonverbal communication will not be effective.

Since nearly every individual over the age of 60 has some hearing impairment, the nurse should be alert to this adaptation. Since background noise can further impair the hearing ability of the client with presbycusis, the nurse should assure that the setting is quiet. Windows should be closed to shut out traffic sounds. Noisy air conditioners should be turned off. If the client is at home, televisions and radios should be turned off. Since the person with presbycusis has difficulty with the higher frequencies, the nurse should talk in a low-pitched voice and avoid shouting. Many clients with impaired hearing compensate by reading lips. The nurse should sit close to clients and face them directly, speak slowly, avoid covering the mouth, and use gestures that reinforce the content of the interview. Of course, if the client has a hearing aid, it should be used.

Privacy

Sensitivity is required when making the decision whether to interview the older client in private or in the presence of a family member or friend. In general, the older client should be interviewed alone. Having another person present during the interview implies that the client is incapable of relating the history. It may make it difficult or impossible for the older person to mention personal or private problems. Once the nurse and client are alone the nurse can ask if the older client would prefer to have the family member or friend who accompanied the client to the interview present. The nurse should not ask this question in front of the accompanying person because it places considerable pressure on the older client.

If the nurse discovers that the client is mentally impaired, the interview alone with the older client can be followed by an interview with the significant other included. The nurse can use this occasion to validate and expand on the information the client gave and to observe family dynamics and social interaction.

Interpretation of Data

Interpretation of data obtained from the health assessment of the aging client is complex and challenging. Body systems age at different rates and in different ways and this leads to variations in the level of functioning of these systems. Each aging client has spent a lifetime developing a unique pattern of behavior. Consequently, among the aging there is increasing divergence between one individual and another.

Data must be weighed uniquely for each client.

Criteria used to make judgments about the aging client's adaptation are different from those applied to children or younger adults. When acutely ill, many aging clients exhibit more subtle adaptations than do their younger counterparts with the same stress. Unless the nurse is aware of these differences, identification of serious, even life-threatening stresses, may be overlooked. For example, the aging client with a serious infection, such as pneumonia, may exhibit a mild, rather than a high, fever. The client with a perforated ulcer or appendicitis may experience little or no pain. The client with biliary colic may complain only of a dull ache. Myocardial infarction may be accompanied by mild discomfort or tenderness rather than crushing chest pain (Villaverde and MacMillan, 1980). However, because reserve function of circulatory, metabolic, and renal systems is usually diminished in the aged, they may not have the ability to adapt optimally to certain stresses. For example, because arteriosclerosis has compromised the circulation of many older people, minor amounts of cerebral insufficiency may result in adaptations usually indicative of massive cerebral injury (Lewis, 1979).

The health assessment provides an excellent opportunity to examine the client for evidence of those stresses for which the aging are at relatively high risk. These include illnesses of a chronic nature, diminished vision and hearing, poor nutrition, depression, and memory loss. Often, multiple stresses are present. However, generalizations about the aged must be applied with caution to the individual client. The ability to maintain independent functioning may be much greater than the nurse would expect, in view of the nature and the number of stresses an individual has (Sana and Judge, 1975).

THE NURSING HISTORY

As with clients of any age, gathering comprehensive data about the aging client begins with a detailed health history. The health history includes the following elements: reason for contact, demographic data, source and reliability, present health status, past health status, family history, personal and social history, and review of systems. Although the elements of the health history are the same for clients of any age, the emphasis placed on some aspects of the history will change as the client ages.

Conducting the Interview

When taking a health history from an aging client, it may be necessary to adapt some interviewing techniques to compensate for age-related changes. With advancing age, the voice may become softer and more difficult to understand. Consequently, the nurse will need to pay particular attention throughout the interview (Burnside, 1981).

As with any interview, the nurse should begin with a self-introduction. Using one's family name helps to establish the relationship as a professional one. In the initial stage of the interview, it is important for the nurse to establish rapport with the aging client. The nurse should determine how the client prefers to be addressed. Using the name the client prefers indicates respect and equality and helps to establish rapport. Calling the older person by an informal form of address, such as a first name or a pet name, serves to reinforce the stereotype of the older client as childlike, dependent, or senile and may be viewed by the client as demeaning or disrespectful (Sana and Judge, 1975; Mezey et al., 1980).

The nurse should conduct the interview in an unhurried manner. Response time to verbal stimuli is lengthened in aging clients, and their life experiences, accumulated over many years, may be difficult to recall in the detail required by the nurse (Sana and Judge, 1975). If the older client is rushed, the ability to respond in a cooperative, intelligent way may be impaired. The client will easily perceive nonverbal communication that indicates the nurse is hurried or short of time. As a consequence the client may become anxious or confused and unable to give complete answers.

The way questions are phrased is also important. Questions should be clearly stated, brief, and free of technical terminology and contemporary slang. Older clients are most likely to use the vocabulary and slang of their own time, not that of the nurse, who is usually younger. If the client has difficulty with abstract thinking, the nurse should consider using directive interviewing techniques. In order to assure validity of the data, the nurse should periodically clarify and summarize what the client has said.

Many of the current aging population have had limited contacts with modern health care institutions or with the expanded role of the nurse. They may not be familiar with the concept of health mainte-

nance or understand the importance of the health history. Therefore, they may be unwilling, at first, to invest the time and energy required to complete the health history. A small proportion of the aging population may be unwilling to share personal information with others and suspicious of a nurse who is a stranger to them (Mezey et al., 1980). The higher incidence of paranoia in the aging has been documented. With these individuals, establishing a trusting, empathetic relationship before taking the health history is important. About 5 percent of the population aged 65 and over are homebound and living in virtual isolation (U.S. Department of Commerce Current Population Reports, 1970 and 1974). Because they have limited opportunities to communicate with others, they may have difficulty at first talking at length with the nurse. Patience and the use of reinforcement are important with these clients.

During the interview many of the elderly engage in extensive life review, providing a great deal of information that is not relevant to the health history. Because reminiscing is time consuming, it may create pressures for the nurse who has many responsibilities. The nurse must deal sensitively with this situation and avoid cutting off the client. After allowing the client to talk for several minutes, the nurse should begin to focus the client's account on those areas that are relevant to the health history. By showing interest and facilitating discussion when the client focuses on these areas, relevant data can be obtained (Bates, 1979).

Some aging clients in the most advanced years have impairments of recent memory that may increase the difficulty in obtaining an accurate and complete history. Memory of past events may remain essentially intact. Associated with the memory loss may be a decreased ability to concentrate. Often the older client is aware of the memory deficit and will discuss it freely and without anxiety. Others may be embarrassed and compensate by focusing the discussion on past events. Assessment of memory is discussed in more detail later in this chapter.

Recording Data

Aging clients vary regarding their feelings about the nurse who takes notes during the interview. Obviously, notes must be taken if the nurse is to remember the large quantity of information the client is sharing. It is best to determine the client's preference regarding note taking. Some clients may find it distracting or feel that the nurse taking notes is not concentrating on what the client is saying at the moment. If this is the case, it is best to stop the interview at periodic intervals and jot down key information.

It is unlikely that the aging client will recount the history in a systematic fashion. Therefore, it will be necessary for the nurse to reorder the data according to appropriate categories at a later time when writing the complete client history.

Reason for Contact

Aging clients seek health care for many reasons. Some come for a regular checkup, while others are seeking assistance for a specific problem. Often they have multiple chief complaints. The use of an open-ended question is the most appropriate way of ascertaining the aging client's reason for seeking health care. If the client does have a problem, recording its nature, duration, and location in the client's own words is the best way to determine the client's perception and understanding of his or her health status. Beginning the interview by focusing on the client's main concern is an effective way for the nurse to communicate genuine concern for the client.

Demographic Data

Obtaining the client's "vital statistics" provides general information about the client as a person and about the client's background. Information about the client's ethnicity, place of birth, primary spoken language, and educational level has particular relevance for the current generation of aging, a large number of whom are foreign-born and have not completed high school. These data provide clues that will help the nurse individualize questions and explanations at a level appropriate for the client.

Source and Reliability

Early in the interview, the nurse should attempt to establish the reliability of the client. This is particularly important with the aging client, since persons in very advanced years may experience some secondary memory loss. As early as when collecting the demographic data, the nurse can ask questions to test the ability of the client to comprehend and respond reliably and validate the accuracy of the client's information. For example, the nurse can

ask both the client's age and the year of birth. When disorders of memory are apparent, the nurse should be alert to the need to use simple, familiar words and repeat questions, directions, and explanations. If the client seems confused and unable to give a clear history, the nurse should alter the focus of the history and begin a mental status assessment (discussed later in this chapter), to determine the client's orientation to time, place, and person.

If the client is mildly confused or is experiencing some memory loss, it is helpful to consult a family member or significant other in order to validate the client's reliability and supplement the health history. These individuals may be able to describe any recent changes in the client's behavior or physical and psychosocial adaptations. The nurse should bear in mind that, in general, mental functioning declines more slowly than physical functioning if it declines at all (Sana and Judge, 1975). Therefore, if the client is experiencing mental decline, the nurse should take care throughout the assessment process to search for physical adaptations that signal disease or decline.

Current Health Status

The current health status provides a general impression of the client's level of adaptation, perception of it, and degree of satisfaction with it. It includes a description of specific complaints, activities of daily living, and personal habits.

Although the meaning of being healthy varies greatly among the aging, most are realistic about their health status. Shanas (1968) found that the self-evaluation older people made of their health was highly correlated with their reports of restriction in mobility, their sensory impairments, and their overall incapacity. She concluded that if older people say their health is poor, there is a physical basis for this self-judgment.

There are a number of reasons, however, why many aging clients may be hesitant to discuss their health status or their complaints. Some may be reluctant because they believe the changes they are experiencing are a normal part of aging or of no interest to others. Some consider a new adaptation, such as pain, dizziness, or weakness, to be a part of a previously existing condition and thus fail to mention it. Some may minimize their complaints because they are concerned that illness may result in loss of independence or institutionalization. A few others who have not accepted the changes that accompany the developmental stage of aging may invent or exaggerate complaints or exhibit excessive preoccupation with their health status.

The nurse should ask the client to describe a typical day and determine if the daily activity pattern varies during a week or month. There is a positive correlation between an elderly person's day being varied and goal-directed and that person's survival into late life. The extent to which the client is able to carry out activities of daily living should be ascertained. In addition, the client should describe any recent changes in daily living patterns and the level of satisfaction with them. Assessing activities of daily living involves two areas: (1) capacity to take care of bodily functions, including eating, dressing and undressing, elimination, maintaining appearance, walking, getting in and out of bed, showering or bathing, and getting sufficient sleep; and (2) performance of activities required to maintain an independent household, including ability to use public transportation, shop, prepare meals, do routine housework, take prescribed medications properly, and handle personal finances.

A complete nutritional assessment, including a description of actual intake in a typical 24-hour interval, should also be obtained (see Chapter 10). Because complaints about bowel and bladder habits are frequent among the aging, a detailed history of elimination patterns should be made. The number and nature of stools per week should be determined as well as any difficulty or discomfort the client experiences during elimination. The nurse should ask about laxative usage, the level of fluid intake, exercise, and diet. The frequency and amount of urination should also be determined. The client should be questioned specifically about urgency, frequency, nocturia, difficulty starting the urinary stream, and incontinence.

Aging changes in musculoskeletal, integumentary, and cardiovascular systems should help the nurse to focus questions related to personal hygiene. Practices of bathing and grooming of nails and hair should be described. Mobility problems may make tub bathing dangerous or impossible for the aging. In addition the aging client may not know how to care for the feet and nails or may be unable

to do so. Elderly clients may not be aware that their drier skin necessitates changes in hygiene practices to avoid cracking, excoriation, or pruritus. They may be unable to bend over to wash the feet or cut the toenails. Failing eyesight may also cause difficulty, or the nails may be too thick or hard to cut.

Because of its relationship to health, the client's tobacco usage, including cigarettes, cigars, pipes, and marijuana, should be identified. Even if the client does not currently smoke, past practices should be described.

Sleep patterns vary greatly from one individual to another and undergo changes due to aging. Therefore, a complete sleep history should be taken, including number of hours of sleep per night, quality of sleep, difficulty falling asleep, cause and number of interruptions of sleep, and naps. The aging may report an increase in naps, but this is often related to inactivity or boredom. Research indicates that aging does create changes in sleep, but it should not significantly reduce the aging person's total sleep time. The older person may experience numerous brief arousals, which give the impression of sleeplessness. In most instances, sleep loss is minimal and the effectiveness of the total sleep period is not impaired. Other reasons for interruption of sleep in the aged include lack of physical exercise, pain, such as joint pain or the ischemic pain of peripheral vascular disease, and the need to urinate (Goldman, 1979; Agate, 1979).

Most aging clients take more than one medication. A detailed history of all medications, both over-the-counter and prescription, should be elicited. Name and dosage of all medications, as well as the frequency and times of day each medication is taken, should be ascertained. Clients should be queried regarding their knowledge of the actions and side effects of their medications and any difficulties they may have with their medication regimen. Because physiological changes of aging affect the absorption, metabolism, and excretion of drugs, baseline data about the client's medication regimen is important. In addition, certain aging changes, such as diminished vision, lapses in short-term memory, and joint changes, may contribute to the difficulties many aging individuals have in adhering to their medication regimen. A detailed medication history is described in Chapter 17.

Patterns of recreation and exercise, as well as

changes in these patterns, should be assessed. The nurse should determine whether clients' recreation and exercise patterns are consistent with their age. Ascertaining the time spent performing hygiene activities, the ability to perform household chores, and the frequency with which clients leave their house or apartment will provide cues to possible stresses in this area. Changes in the level of exercise over the years should also be determined. Although aging clients may not run five miles every day, it would be unusual for them to remain housebound because of fatigue or exertional dyspnea.

Past History

The past health history should include data about growth and development, health maintenance and preventive practices, interventions for health problems, allergies, occupational exposures, and travel. This part of the health history provides information about residual stresses and adaptations. In addition, data about the aging client's past health-related practices and encounters with the health care system provide valuable information about the client's attitudes toward health, health care personnel, and the health care system. Previous experiences and practices provide clues to how the older client will adapt to focal and potential stresses.

Because of the vast amount of data to be collected the nurse should not expect the client to provide information in chronological order. With increasing age, there is greater likelihood that the client will have experienced more medical and surgical events. Clients may not accurately recall events that occurred many years ago and are likely to be sketchy about such details as the names of communicable diseases they had, when they had them, and when they were immunized.

Collection of developmental data about an aging client requires particular skill. The nurse should elicit information related to the tasks of each stage of development. It is not reasonable to expect to collect a complete picture of the aging client at every developmental stage; however, significant events, particularly ones that affect current adaptations, should be noted. Late adulthood or old age is a time when clients should assess their lives, their accomplishments and disappointments. Determining how older people feel about their life and whether they have accepted their successes and failures is im-

portant. Physical and psychosocial adaptations may result in increasing dependence of the aging upon others. Changes in the client's level of independence should be identified. This is the stage in life when the person prepares to die. During the health history, clients should be given the opportunity to discuss their feelings about death and their preparedness for it.

Family History

The family history includes information about family composition, family relationships, the current health status of family members, and familial illnesses. It is likely that the client's role in the family has undergone major changes. The client may be a widow or widower, and although still a parent, contacts and relationships with children are likely to have undergone significant changes.

One role that may be altered by changes in family composition may be that of sexual partner. A sexual history should be a part of the health history, and may be elicited here, when discussing the past health history, during discussion of pregnancy or health problems related to the reproductive system, or during the review of systems. Sexual functioning is an area that many elderly clients find difficult to discuss. Many nurse interviewers find it more convenient to overlook this aspect of functioning when conducting the nursing history. However, omission of this important aspect of functioning constitutes a statement about it, namely, that older people should not be involved in sexual activities. The fact is that many elderly clients are sexually active and may have questions to raise about changes in sexual functioning that they perceive as abnormal. Because many of the aging were taught not to discuss matters related to sexuality or to ignore their sexual feelings, tact and sensitivity are required if information is to be elicited. A persistent problem in geriatric medicine has been the reticence of many elderly clients to complain about gynecological problems in the female and prostate problems in the male (Steffl, 1978). Nevertheless, fear of loss of sexual prowess is a common preoccupation for older men. It is likely that older women are also concerned about changes in sexual functioning. Data should be collected about the nature of the client's loving relationships, satisfaction with them, and, if applicable, feelings about the loss of those relationships. In addition, data should be obtained about the physical adaptations that occur with aging that may make sexual activity more difficult. Assessing sexual function is discussed in more detail later in this chapter.

Although physical separation of elderly clients from their adult children is common in Western societies, this is usually not accompanied by emotional abandonment. Normally at least one family member remains involved with the older client. The nurse should identify the client's attitudes toward the family and vice versa. The family's ability to assist the older client should also be determined. Factors such as jobs, travel time, and distance affect the family's ability to participate in the older client's care.

Particularly because of the diminished reserve capacity of the aging, it is important to determine if the client is caring for an ill spouse or child and the effect of this situation on the caretaker. In order to identify any health problems in the client, causes of death of parents, grandparents, and siblings or any illnesses before death should be noted. Although it is likely that the client may be unaware of specific causes of death and unable to provide complete information, the family history is important because survival patterns, longevity, and diagnoses are often related to parental and sibling history. Familial trends have been found for senile dementia, coronary artery disease, diabetes, glaucoma, neoplasms, and manic–depressive psychosis.

Personal and Social History

This part of the health history is important for identifying the client's social adjustment and the presence of potential psychosocial stresses in the environment. The extent of the social network that surrounds the client should be determined by gathering data about relationships outside the family, employment status, living arrangements, and the number and nature of social contacts. Is there a confidante in the social network whom the client can trust? Because the aged may fear increased dependence the nurse should identify whether the client has a relative or significant other who can be relied upon in an emergency. Is there someone who could provide ongoing care in the event of illness or disability (Duke-OARS, 1978)?

Although most aging clients will be retired, a past employment record can provide clues to current stresses or adaptations and may give valuable information about the client's sense of satisfaction with life. This component of the history also involves notation of significant hobbies and volunteer work.

Because of its relationship to occupational status, information about the client's financial situation should be obtained at this point. The client's financial status has bearing on every aspect of life and has a profound impact on the quality of life. Financial stresses may limit the aging client's social relationships, level of health care, nutritional status, and ability to maintain a livable home environment.

The nurse should be sensitive to the client's feelings, since many older clients find a discussion of economic resources intrusive. For many in this generation, finances were rarely discussed outside the family circle; moreover their steadfast independence makes the acknowledgment that help may be needed a difficult one at best. Clients are frequently asked if they have considered Medicaid assistance to procure needed services and very often the answer is, "No, I've always made ends meet. I prefer to pay for myself." Although most elderly clients seem convinced of their entitlement to Medicare, they still perceive other forms of assistance as welfare.

The purpose of the financial assessment is to determine whether or not clients are able to manage effectively on their income. The nurse should ask the client about employment status, current earnings, amount and sources of income, home or apartment ownership, and expenditures. The nurse should also ask the client for a subjective evaluation of his or her financial situation. Older people living on small pensions or social security have incomes that have been severely eroded by inflation. In view of escalating costs for basic necessities, they often have to make difficult choices. During the history, one older client admitted that she could only have meat once a week and still continue to afford her medications. It is important to find out if the budget can be stretched to include small luxuries like an occasional outing, a dinner at a restaurant, or a trip to a movie or the theatre.

Assessment of the client's home environment is described later in this chapter. Because of special needs related to mobility and safety, the home environment may have an enormous impact on the aging client's level of adaptation and satisfaction with it.

Review of Systems

The review of systems provides an opportunity to elicit data the client may have judged too insignificant to report. The purposes of a review of systems, to elicit forgotten information, validate data, and serve as a check that all relevant data have been obtained, take on increasing significance with the aged. Because of the quantity of data comprising the history of the aging client, the risk that relevant information will be forgotten is significant. The nurse should ask if the client has noted changes in structure or function of each system in the past 1, 5, or 10 years.

THE PHYSICAL ASSESSMENT: TECHNIQUES AND FINDINGS

This section focuses on the techniques and findings of the physical examination of the aging client who is adapting well and functioning independently. Adaptations found in the normal, healthy aging client are emphasized. Those adaptations that may not be intrinsic to healthy aging but that are nevertheless found in a large proportion of the aging population are described. Adaptations to stresses that constitute major health problems for the aging are presented in later chapters that deal with those specific stresses.

Procedures and techniques used during the physical assessment of the adult client are generally appropriate for the examination of the aging client. In some instances, techniques of inspection, palpation, percussion, and auscultation need to be modified to meet the specific needs and responses of the aging. In the sections that follow, those instances are pointed out.

Although the approach to the physical examination is generally the same, the examination will require more time than would examination of a younger person. The client must be given explanations of assessment activities to prevent anxiety. In addition, the aging client requires more time to respond to the instructions of the nurse. If hurried, the client may be unable to cooperate fully with the examination. As a result, adverse findings may be

inadvertently induced or intensified and may not be representative of the client's abilities (Sana and Judge, 1975). The aging client also needs more time to change from one position to another. As a consequence of age-related changes in the vasomotor reflex, compensation when turning around or standing upright after sitting is reduced (Brody and Vijayashanker, 1977).

The General Survey

Changes in height, weight, tissue distribution, and bony structure contribute to the characteristic appearance of the aging person. The aging client's height reflects the progressive statural decline that occurs with age. One way to determine the client's decline in stature is to use the client's span measurement. On the assumption that span and height are roughly equal in the fifth decade, the nurse can subtract the client's current height from the span measurement to determine what decline in stature has occurred. The average loss in height is 1.5 inches between ages 65 to 74, increasing to 3 inches between ages 85 to 94 (Goldman, 1979).

Changes in the client's weight may also be evident. In well nourished, healthy males, weight declines after age 55. In women, weight gains in the 50s are followed by the loss of weight in the mid-70s.

Observation of body contour reveals adaptations that accompany aging. There is a deposition of fat on the abdomen and hips. In persons in their 80s and 90s fat is lost from the periphery. Atrophy of subcutaneous fat in old age leads to an increase in the sharpness of body contours and a deepening of hollows, including the orbits of the eyes, axillae, supraclavicular and intercostal spaces, and pelvic contours. Bony landmarks become increasingly prominent and contribute to the bony appearance of very old persons. In advanced stages, some of the aged may appear cachectic. However, loss of subcutaneous fat in the aging is not related to nutritional status, and changes in dietary intake will not affect it (Rossman, 1979b). The neck shortens, resulting in a reduction in the occiput-to-shoulder distance. The width of the shoulders decreases, the chest depth increases, and the pelvis widens.

Changes in height, weight, and fat distribution may present difficulties for the client. Clothes may no longer fit—dresses may have become too tight and trousers too long. Expenditures for new clothing or even for alterations in the existing wardrobe may be a stress to the aging who have limited incomes.

The Integument

Skin. The aging skin should be systematically inspected and palpated. With advancing age, many changes are seen in the skin. The skin appears thinner as a result of a thinning of the cell layers of the epidermis, a flattening of the epidermal/dermal interface, and a loss of subcutaneous fat (Selmanowitz et al., 1977). Progressive wrinkling also occurs as fat is lost, as collagen and elastic fiber undergo changes, and as skin is repeatedly folded by continued use of facial muscles. The nurse should observe for characteristic wrinkles on the face, neck, and dorsa of the hands. In the very old, the nurse should observe for fine wrinkling of the face unrelated to the distribution of the major facial muscles. The wrinkling has an irregular or crisscross distribution, resembling that of crumpled paper (Rossman, 1977).

　Changes in pigmentation should also be noted. In Caucasians, changes occur in the number, distribution, and function of melanocytes. When exposed to the sun, the melanocytes are no longer able to produce an even distribution of pigment. Therefore, when exposed to the sun, tanning is reduced (Goldman, 1979). Clients should be instructed to use a sunscreen with a paraaminobenzoic acid derivative whenever they are in the sun (Lubowe, 1976). In addition, areas of brown, spotty pigmentation frequently occur. These macular lesions are most often located on exposed areas such as the hands, arms, face, neck and scalp. These are called liver spots, senile freckles, or lintigo. They may be the size of a pinpoint or slightly larger. Although they have no pathologic significance, they may be upsetting to the client for cosmetic reasons (Goldfarb, 1979; Kornzweig, 1979).

　The nurse should observe for areas of excoriation or trauma. As the skin becomes less elastic, it becomes more friable and is easily traumatized. Dermatitis, fungal infections, and bacterial infections occur with increased frequency among the aging (Lombardo, 1979). Hemorrhages, known as senile purpura, may also be visible. The skin be-

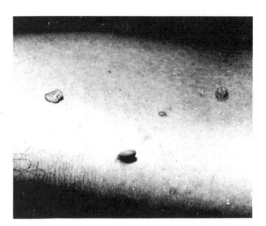

Figure 1. Acrochordons. *From Mezey MD, et al., 1980, with permission.*

comes less vascular and remaining vessels become more fragile. Reduced vascularity, coupled with the reduced rate of cell division of the epithelium, delays the healing process of open wounds.

Skin Lesions. With advancing age, many new growths appear on the aging skin. The development of dermatologic lesions is probably not an intrinsic part of the aging process. Instead, most lesions are actually a consequence of long-term environmental exposure or a reflection of an underlying circulatory, neurological, hormonal, or metabolic problem. It is important for the nurse to note the characteristics of dermatologic lesions and differentiate between benign lesions that do not threaten the client's adaptation and those that might be malignant or premalignant. Several benign lesions typically appear in clients over age 50. These are hallmarks of old age and are described below.

　ACROCHORDONS. Also called skin tags, these are soft, flesh-colored, pedunculated, irregular growths found on the neck, chest, upper back, axillae, and groin (Lombardo, 1979). They vary from the size of a pinhead to the size of a pea (Fig. 1) (Conrad, 1974).

　CHERRY ANGIOMATA. These are small collections of capillaries that appear as bright or ruby red papules, pinpoint or slightly larger in size. They are round, sometimes raised, and may be surrounded by a pale halo. They may blanch with external pressure. Cherry angiomata are usually found on the trunk and extremities and increase in size and number with age (Lombardo, 1979).

SEBORRHEIC KERATOSIS. This is perhaps the most common skin lesion found in the elderly. These small, discrete, raised, tan, brown, or brown-black greasy-looking lesions appear on the chest, back, neck, and face. They range in size from 1 to 4 cm (Fig. 2) (Conrad, 1974).

VASCULAR LESIONS. Abnormal vascular markings also occur frequently in the aged. *Senile purpura* are macular lesions less than 3 cm in diameter and often located on the exposed portions of the hands. They are caused by fragile blood vessels that lose their connective tissue support and result in spontaneous petechiae. *Venous lakes* are irregular, blue-black papules located on the face, ears, and neck. These nodules arise from small veins and usually occur after trauma. *Venous spiders* are vascular lesions often found on the legs. They result from increased pressure in the superficial veins. *Venous stars* are irregular, cascading, or spider-shaped blue lesions, a few centimeters in size.

All of these lesions are harmless. Usually, they do not require treatment unless they are injured by the client's clothing or jewelry. The older client is often uncomfortably aware of them, worried about their significance, or anxious or embarrassed about their appearance and asks that they be removed. If being free of lesions, even temporarily, provides the client with a psychological lift, this is a valid reason for their removal.

The skin of the aging foot becomes atrophic and delicate. Subcutaneous tissue is sparse. After age 65, the vascular supply to the feet is normally reduced, as a consequence of arteriosclerosis, and makes healing difficult (Jahss, 1979). Special attention should be given to examining the skin of the feet, since lesions in this area may limit the client's mobility. The feet should be clean and free of rash and localized red areas indicating pressure. The client should be instructed to seek treatment immediately if cuts, blisters, or fissures occur. In the aged, these may be easily infected. Fungus infections occur often and appear as fissures between the toes (Conrad, 1977). The cause of calluses and corns (clavus) should be determined. Calluses are acquired, superficial, circumscribed, yellow-white, flattened, thickened hyperkeratotic material. They serve a protective function in areas of irritation. Corns are circumscribed, horny thickenings with the apex pointing inward, seen over bony prominences. They produce pain when pressure is applied. Corns on the dorsal surfaces of the toes are hard and those between the toes are soft. To prevent corns, the nurse should check that shoes are properly fitted to avoid excessive pressure over bony prominences. If corns are present, the client should be referred to a podiatrist for treatment (Lombardo, 1979; King, 1978).

PREMALIGNANT AND MALIGNANT LESIONS. If the nurse suspects that a lesion is premalignant or malignant the client should be referred to a physician.

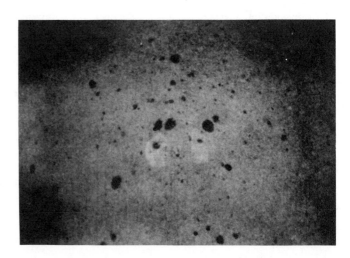

Figure 2. Scattered elevated pigmented seborrheic keratoses. *From Steinberg FU (ed): Cowdry's The Care of the Geriatric Patient. 5th ed., St. Louis, Mosby, 1976, with permission.*

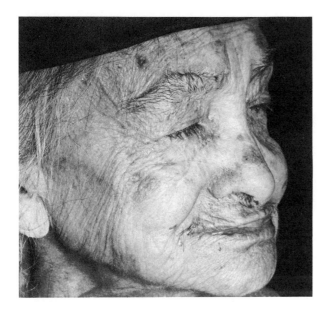

Figure 3. Actinic Keratosis. An erythematous, fairly well defined scaling lesion on the nose. Note suspicious raised nodular lesion on inner canthus of the right eye—basal cell epithelioma. *From Rossman I (ed): Clinical Geriatrics, 2nd ed. Philadelphia, Lippincott, 1979, with permission.*

ACTINIC KERATOSIS. Also called solar keratosis, this is the most common premalignant lesion (Fig. 3). Usually found on sun-exposed areas such as the forehead, nose, cheeks, or ears, these appear as reddened or light brown areas that are scaly and rough to the touch. When palpated, the client may experience slight discomfort. These lesions should be removed before they increase in size, a change that indicates squamous cell carcinoma.

LEUKOPLAKIA. This is another premalignant lesion seen in the elderly. If not removed it may evolve into a squamous cell carcinoma. Leukoplakia is usually seen on the lips, buccal mucosa, tongue and vaginal area (Fig. 4). Leukoplakia appears as a crusty, nontender whitish or grayish area (Lombardo, 1978; Zach, 1979). It is often precipitated by an irritant such as poorly fitting dentures, infection, or smoking.

BASAL CELL CARCINOMA. The most common malignancy of the skin, this is most often present on the face, but it can also be seen on the trunk or extremities. It has many appearances, but it usually presents as a skin-colored, raised, nodular lesion with fine telangiectasias. It appears waxy and shiny and may be ulcerated (Fig. 5) (Lubowe, 1976; Lombardo, 1979).

SQUAMOUS CELL CARCINOMA. This is most often seen in fair-skinned persons on sun-damaged areas

such as the face, ears, neck, hands, and forearm. Its lesions are of two types. One appears as discrete patches of erythema, which may be mistaken for eczema. The other is raised and nodular, with areas of erythema, inflammation, and frequently ulceration (Fig. 6) (Lombardo, 1979).

MALIGNANT MELANOMAS. These vary in size and may be nodular or flat. Nodular lesions often have a bluish color. Flat lesions have a typical rose-colored hue due to varying shades of color ranging from blue to red (Lombardo, 1979).

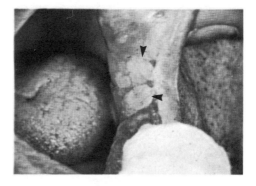

Figure 4. Leukoplakia. Seen here as white patches on buccal mucosa near the corner of the mouth (*arrows*). *From Shafer WG, Hine MK, Levy BM, 1974, with permission.*

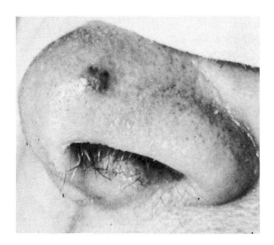

Figure 5. Basal cell epithelioma. Raised, well-marginated, 6 mm lesion with surface pigmentation, telangiectasia, and translucence. *From Rossman I (ed): Clinical Geriatrics, 2nd ed. Philadelphia, Lippincott, 1979, with permission.*

Dry Skin. Aging skin loses its emollience and softness and feels leathery and dry to the touch. Dryness is a result of decreased function of apocrine and sebaceous glands and a reduction in number and function of eccrine glands. One of the most frequent complaints of the aged is dry skin and itching. Dryness is accentuated in winter by cold, dry air outdoors and hot, dry air indoors. It is further increased by frequent bathing and the use of soap. If the client complains of itching, the skin should be examined closely for fine scaling and tiny fissures. It should be felt for flakiness. Some inflammation may be present. This condition is known as *xerosis* (Lombardo, 1979).

Skin Turgor. Aging skin is stiff and less pliable. When testing the skin for turgor, the nurse must interpret the findings with caution. Turgor may appear to be decreased in an adequately hydrated client. Elastic fibers, collagen, and total body water, largely responsible for skin turgor, undergo changes as a result of the normal aging process. Consequently, when skin is picked up between the examiner's fingers, it tends to remain heaped up rather than to snap back into its original shape (Lubowe, 1976). In older people, the skin of the sternum reflects turgor more accurately than that of the forearm.

Nails. The nails of the hands and feet should be carefully inspected. Longitudinal ridges on the nails of older people are a normal finding. In addition, nails appear dull and opaque and undergo color changes, turning yellowish, greenish, or gray. These changes are often more apparent in sun-damaged people. Aging nails also become increasingly thickened and brittle and are prone to peeling into layers (Selmanowitz et al., 1977). Peeling is complicated by the fact that nail growth slows with age. If indicated, the client should be taught how to cut the nails correctly.

Onychomycosis. This is a noninvasive fungal infection of the nails seen frequently in older people. The infection appears as white, silver, or yellow patches on the nailbeds and results in thickened nail plates and increased keratin under the nails (Fig. 7). It is painless unless irritated by pressure, such as tight-fitting shoes. Onychomycosis can be treated with antifungal agents (Lombardo, 1979; Pearson and Kotthoff, 1979). Ingrown toenails are another common problem in the elderly. Often infected, they occur as a result of poor toenail care and improper trimming (Jahss, 1979). Clients with problems requiring special care should be referred to a dermatologist or podiatrist.

Hair. Body and scalp hair should be thoroughly inspected and changes in the amount and nature of hair should be noted. Changes in amount and color of hair are influenced by many factors, including ethnicity. Loss of pigmentation of the hair shaft causes graying of the hair and usually precedes hair loss. In some persons, hair appears as unusual shades of yellow or yellow-green. Usually, the hair feels dry and appears thin and lifeless (Lubowe, 1976).

Hair loss should be noted. In women, and in men not subject to sex-linked baldness, scalp hairs are thinner and less numerous. If present, sex-linked baldness should be noted. It may begin either at the vertex or as an "M-shaped" pattern on either side of the midline. Eventually the two bald areas may coalesce.

Axillary hair in both men and women may be scanty. Eventually, women may no longer need to shave their armpits. In females, arm hair may be thin. Leg hair may be absent or scanty in both sexes.

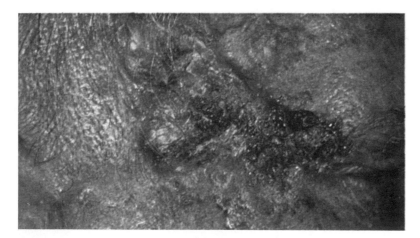

Figure 6. Squamous cell carcinomas, when arising from actinic keratoses, are not as aggressive or prone to metastasize as denova (new, arising from normal skin). The first clinical evidence of malignancy is induration, an abnormally hard spot or place, and resistance to pressure is much greater than that given by an inflammatory lesion. These are primarily found in sun-exposed areas. They can be removed surgically or by x-ray or chemical techniques. The areas should be checked at six-month intervals. *From Uhler DM: Common skin care changes in the elderly. American Journal of Nursing 78:1343, 1978, with permission.*

It is important to differentiate between normal hair loss and the abnormal findings associated with compromised peripheral vascular circulation; in the latter hair is scanty or absent, especially on the lower leg and dorsum of the foot.

The nurse should be alert for normal differences in hair patterns among the races. For example, many people of American Indian, Japanese, or Negro ancestry often have scant face and body hair throughout the age span. Among Caucasians, older women often grow hair on the upper lip and chin and men develop hairy ears (Rossman, 1979b; Goldman, 1979).

The Head and Neck

The Head. Inspection and palpation of the scalp usually reveals dryness. Flaking may also be present. Scalp dryness is due to the same factors responsible for the dry skin of the aged.

Characteristic changes are apparent in the face of aging persons. The nose and ears often appear larger in relation to the other structures of the face. The nurse may note an increased infolding of the mouth, and furrowed pockets at the corners of the mouth that give the mouth a "purse string" appearance. In addition, there may be a closing of the distance between the chin and nose. This adaptation is caused by resorption of the bone from the mandible and maxilla particularly in edentulous persons (Selmanowitz et al., 1977). Wrinkles are normally present on the forehead, at the lateral canthus of the eyes, on either side of the root of the nose, at the nasolabial groove extending toward the chin adjacent to the mouth, and on the upper and lower lids. Ptosis of lids and jowls and wrinkling beneath the chin occur as a consequence of gravitational pull.

When inspecting the face for symmetry the nurse should ensure that the edentulous client has dentures in place. Normally, the function of the seventh cranial nerve does not deteriorate with age. The edentulous state, however, may result in facial asymmetry that disappears once correctly fitted dentures are in place.

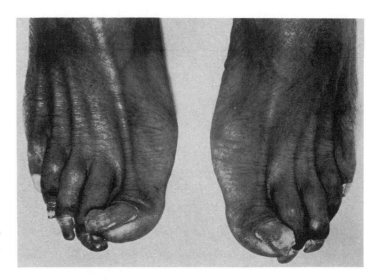

Figure 7. Onychomycosis of toenails. *From Prior JA, Silberstein JS, 1973, with permission.*

The Eye. Physical examination of the eye reveals numerous changes characteristic of the aging process. The eye should also be examined for a number of stresses that occur with increased frequency in the older age group.

In the absence of an opacity, tests for visual acuity and visual field assess the function of the second cranial nerve. When testing for visual acuity, the nurse should ensure that the area is well lit and the light source is placed behind the client. Visual acuity decreases with age, but the amount is highly variable. When testing visual acuity, the client's corrective lenses, if worn, should be in place. Each eye should be tested separately. Usually, the sight in one eye will remain good while that in the other eye diminishes (Kornzweig, 1979). The Snellen chart can be used for testing distant vision and newsprint may be used for near vision. A more useful tool for measuring near vision, particularly in clients who are beginning to experience presbyopia, is the Jaeger chart. Presbyopia, a loss of the eye's ability to focus on near objects, is the most common visual change in the aged. With age, changes in the crystalline lens impair the eye's ability to accommodate. As a result, older people discover they are less able to discriminate detail. They find they are holding reading material at arm's length. Between ages 40 and 45, most people need corrective lenses in order

to read and focus on objects near at hand (Goldfarb, 1979; Corso, 1971). Central field deficits do not occur normally with age and require further evaluation.

When testing visual fields, a loss of peripheral vision may be noted (Goldfarb, 1979). Although a peripheral field deficit may be a normal concomitant of aging, the nurse should consider the possibility that this adaptation may also be the result of increased intraocular pressure.

Other visual changes also occur with age. The size of the pupil becomes progressively smaller. This adaptation, called senile miosis, reduces the amount of light that reaches the retina and elevates the minimum threshold to light perception. Consequently, the aging client requires nearly three times as much light to see as do young adults (Corso, 1971; Wilson, 1971–1972).

With age, lens opacities also occur, causing light to scatter and increasing the older person's sensitivity to glare. When planning the client's care consideration must be given to achieving a balance between getting enough light into the eye and at the same time preventing glare. Aging persons also experience a decrease in dark adaptation and a greater proportional loss in visual acuity in dim illumination (Busech, 1976).

As the lens yellows, older people also expe-

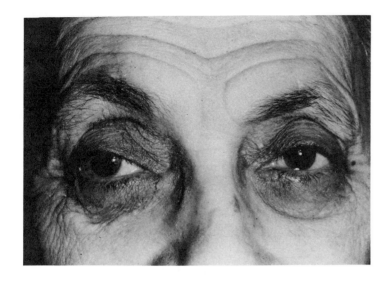

Figure 8. Senile pigmentation of both the upper and lower lids. *From Kornzweig AL: Lid affections of the aged. International Ophthalmology Clinics 4:55, 1964, with permission.*

rience a diminution of color discrimination, particularly of low tone colors, such as violets, blues, and greens. Reds, oranges, and yellows tend to be seen best. If not recognized, difficulty distinguishing between blues and greens can create problems and safety hazards. For the client, the ability to distinguish between levels of brightness also declines with age. Changes in visual acuity and peripheral vision, along with other aging changes such as elevation in the threshold to light, sensitivity to glare, decreased dark adaptation and reduced visual acuity in dim light, and diminution of color discrimination, increase the likelihood that the older client will need instruction in order to maintain safety. The physical examination provides an excellent opportunity for the nurse to teach the client.

Upon inspection, the skin of the eyelids appears thin. In many older persons, pigmentation covers the skin of the upper and lower lids (Fig. 8). Puffiness may occur around the lower lid due to a herniation of fat in the area. Atrophy of tissues of the upper lids results in the baggy lids often seen in older people (Fig. 9). There is wrinkling and elongation of the skin folds that may rest on the lashes. A partial ptosis results that, if severe, interferes with vision.

Tissue atrophy can result in several troublesome adaptations. If the relaxation of the tissue of the lower lid is severe, the lid may fall away from the eyeball. Tears cannot escape through the lower punctum and constant, excessive tearing results. Tears roll out of the eye, decreasing the lubrication

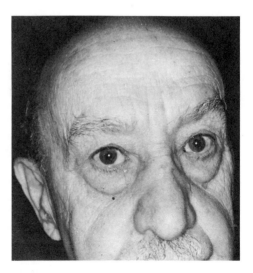

Figure 9. Atrophy of the skin of the lid and formation of large soft swellings of the lower lids (baggy lids). *From Kornzweig AL: Lid affections of the aged. International Ophthalmology Clinics 4:55, 1964, with permission.*

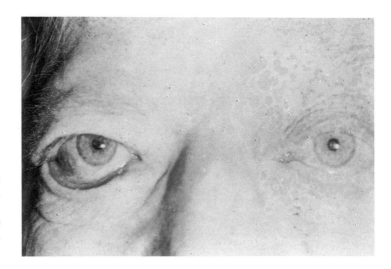

Figure 10. Senile ectropion of the lower lid. *From Kornzweig AL: Lid affections of the aged. International Ophthalmology Clinics 4:55, 1964, with permission.*

of the conjunctiva. This condition is called senile ectropion (Fig. 10). If the degree of ectropion is severe the exposed palpebral conjunctiva is no longer bathed in the tear film layer and the resulting chronic dryness leads to metaplasia and keratinization of the epithelium. The client should be taught to dry tears using an up-and-inward motion of the handkerchief, not the more usual down-and-outward motion. Simply by using lubricating medications in drop or ointment form, clients can partially relieve the drying effects of ectropion. Another adaptation resulting from tissue atrophy is senile entropion (Fig. 11). The lower lid margin becomes inverted, causing chronic irritation of the conjunctiva and the lower portion of the cornea. The client may complain of a sandy feeling or burning sensation. The action of the lashes against the cornea may lead to a breakdown of corneal epithelium and set the stage for viral or bacterial invasion. Clients with severe ectropion or entropion should be referred for palliative treatment or, if necessary, for corrective plastic surgery (Kornzweig, 1979).

The eyes of the aged may appear sunken due to a loss of fat from the orbit. This adaptation is called enophthalmos (Rossman, 1979b). The conjuctiva is pale or yellow, thin, and easily traumatized (Burnside, 1981). The eye may appear dry and lusterless and the client may complain of a burning sensation (Malasanos et al., 1977). There is a normal diminution of tear production with age.

Relief can usually be obtained by the use of artificial tears several times daily (Kornzweig, 1979). On the other hand, in some older people, exposure to cold, wind, dust, or air pollution results in excessive tearing. Applying cold compresses may give some relief (Busech, 1976). The sclera may be discolored or yellowish. The iris frequently appears pale, with brown discolorations (Carter, 1979).

Arcus senilis is visible in the eye of nearly everyone over age 80 (Fig. 12). It is more prominent in males. Initially, it is an arc-shaped deposit of gray matter. Eventually, it may become white or yellow and expand until it completely encircles the cornea. The arcus senilis is due to a deposit of a lipid substance in the margin of the cornea 1 to 2 mm from the limbus. Arcus senilis does not interfere with vision (Kornzweig, 1979; Rossman, 1979b; Rodstein, 1963).

Some irregularity and inequality of the pupils may be apparent (Carter, 1979). If the client has had surgery for removal of cataracts or for glaucoma, the pupil may have a keyhole shape. Pupillary reaction to light and accommodation tests the third cranial nerve. The response to light may become sluggish with age, but both eyes should respond equally. Accommodation slows with age, particularly pupillary constriction with near vision (Carter, 1979; Grob, 1978). Convergence also slows with age. By age 85, only one-third will respond to light and none will respond to accommodation.

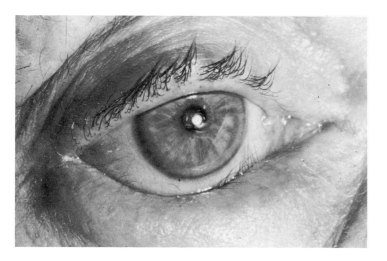

Figure 11. Marked senile entropion of the lower lid. *From Kornzweig AL: Lid affections of the aged. International Ophthalmology Clinics 4:55, 1964, with permission.*

Testing of cranial nerves III, IV, and VI may reveal a restriction of upward gaze due to changes in cranial nerve III. This is a normal variant in extraocular movement (Grob, 1978). Downward gaze (cranial nerve IV) and lateral gaze (cranial nerve VI) should be normal. The corneal reflex reflects the function of the fifth cranial nerve. A prolonged stimulus may be necessary to elicit a response. Once elicited, the response should be brisk and consensual (Mezey et al., 1980).

Ophthalmoscopic examination has particular significance for the aging because of the high incidence of diabetes, vascular disease, and other stresses that affect vision. Findings associated with specific stresses affecting vision are presented in Chapter 20. Because of pupillary changes, the ability to visualize the optic fundi becomes more difficult with age (Goldman, 1979). Therefore, if the client does not have glaucoma or adaptations suggesting glaucoma, the pupil may be dilated prior to fundoscopic examination.

As its transparency decreases with age, the lens may appear discolored (Sana and Judge, 1975). When using the ophthalmoscope, opacities of the lens may obstruct the red reflex. They may also make visualization of the fundus difficult. Cataract formation increases in frequency with age.

The aged fundus has less luster and a more yellow appearance. The retinal arteries become narrower, straighter, more opaque, and less regular than in adults (Gordon, 1971). The normal 2:3 ratio of arteries to veins may change to a 1:3 ratio, due to arterial narrowing. The optic disc may appear paler than in the young (Mezey et al., 1980). The examiner should look carefully for retinal hemorrhages and exudates. These are not normal findings in elderly clients but may be associated with diabetes or hypertension.

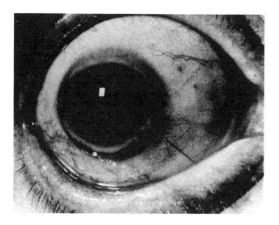

Figure 12. Arcus senilis totally encircling the cornea. *Courtesy of Malpica H, Department of Ophthalmology, Montefiore Hospital and Medical Center/Albert Einstein College of Medicine, New York.*

Examination of the eye should always include measurement of intraocular pressure with a tonometer. Elevations in pressure are indicative of glaucoma, the second most important visual stress in the aging (Rossman, 1979a). Tonometry should be a part of every eye examination for persons over age 40 (Sherman and Fields, 1976). Measuring ocular tension by palpating the globe may be useful in assessing dehydration, but it is not a reliable test for glaucoma (Lewis, 1979).

The Ear. The external ear appears large, since cartilage continues to be laid down throughout the life span (Rossman, 1979b). The lobe is elongated as a consequence of gravitational pull and wrinkled. The pinna of the ear should be carefully inspected because this area is a frequent site for squamous cell carcinoma (Keim, 1977). An increased number of terminal hairs may be visible in the ear, particularly in older men (Selmanowitz et al., 1979). Older men with hairy ear canals are at risk for cerumen impactions. The presence of coarse, stiff hair blocks normal cerumen extrusion and can result in a conductive hearing loss. The client should be referred to a physician for removal of wax with a cerumen spoon (Goodhill, 1979). Since atrophic skin changes also occur in the ear canal, the skin may appear dry. External otitis may develop, causing dry, scaling skin and itching. The client should be instructed not to clean the ears with cotton-tipped applicators or soapy wash cloths every day. Two or three drops of baby oil (mineral oil) in the ear on a daily or weekly basis should relieve the itching (Keim, 1977).

When examining the ear canal, the nurse should insert the otoscope with caution, since changes may occur in the cartilaginous portion of the ear canal. Upon otoscopic examination, the tympanic membranes may show some deviation in color from the normal pearly white. They may appear dull and retracted and there may be a slight diminution in the intensity of the light reflex (Mezey et al., 1980). Other landmarks should appear similar to those seen in younger adults.

Diminution of hearing is a frequent finding when testing the eighth cranial nerve. Tinnitus may accompany hearing loss. However, it is not a normal finding in the aging client and may signal the onset of a disease condition. Clients with tinnitus should be referred for further evaluation (Goodhill, 1979). A number of stresses place the elderly at risk for hearing loss: otosclerosis, eighth cranial nerve tumors, vascular lesions, ototoxic drugs, and environmental noise. Any of these may accompany the hearing loss that normally occurs with the aging process. The term presbycusis refers to the normal sensorineural hearing loss attributed to age alone. It usually affects both ears equally and does not lead to deafness (Keim, 1977). The ability to hear higher-frequency tones is lost first with losses progressing later to all frequencies. Although speech frequencies are relatively low, the client with presbycusis also has difficulty distinguishing spoken words, particularly when conversing in a noisy environment.

The Weber, Rinne, and Schwabach tests provide useful information about the older client's hearing sensitivity and the health of the auditory structures. When testing the older client, it is advised that three tuning forks with frequencies of 512, 1024, and 2048 Hz be used. Inclusion of these frequencies permits differentiation between normal and abnormal hearing sensitivity and conductive and sensorineural losses. These three frequencies constitute the "speech frequencies." If only the 512- and 1024-Hz tuning forks are used, a sensorineural impairment in the higher frequencies may be overlooked. Since early presbycusis involves a high-frequency hearing loss, the nurse who omits the 2048-Hz tuning fork risks overestimating the client's hearing sensitivity. The Weber test gives information about ears with unequal hearing sensitivity. If presbycusis is present in both ears, and if there is no conductive hearing loss, the tuning fork will lateralize to the most sensitive ear. If presbycusis is present equally in both ears, the tuning fork will not lateralize. In any case, more information is needed to clarify the findings. If presbycusis is present, the Rinne test will show a normal ratio (2:1) of air conduction to bone conduction. If the examiner's hearing is normal, the Schwabach test will indicate that the client's hearing is poorer than the nurse's at the given frequency (Pearson and Kotthoff, 1979).

Nearly everyone over age 60 has a diminution of hearing for frequencies above 4000 Hz. Because this adaptation occurs so often, clients in their 50s should be advised to undergo audiometric studies to obtain a baseline measurement against which to measure later losses. The aging client with a hearing loss should be advised to undergo radiographic as well as audiometric studies. Radiography can help distinguish between simple presbycusis and hearing loss due to lesions of the temporal bone or eighth cranial nerve (Goodhill, 1979).

Because presbycusis results in a gradual loss of hearing, many clients adapt by practicing lip-reading and limiting conversations to one or two persons in a quiet environment. The nurse might advise clients with mild presbycusis to purchase a telephone amplifier, a loud door buzzer, and radio and television ear phone attachments. "Ear cupping" is one technique that may improve the client's ability to communicate. Family members should be instructed about the social implications of hearing loss as well as techniques to improve communication with the client. Newer types of hearing aids are being developed and used successfully by persons with presbycusis. The nurse should refer clients to an otologist, working in collaboration with an audiologist and skilled hearing aid dispenser. Because many older people have limitations in manual dexterity, inserting the earmold and operating the controls of the hearing aid can be difficult. In order to obtain the greatest benefit from a hearing aid, the older client requires long-term instruction in its use and maintenance. Clients who expect a hearing aid to restore hearing to normal also require counseling regarding their expectations of the instrument (Goldman, 1979). Chapter 16 discusses the management of older clients with serious hearing impairments.

The Nose. Because cartilage continues to be formed, the nose of the older person becomes longer and broader. Often, examination with a nasal speculum reveals that nasal hairs are coarser and thicker. When testing the first cranial nerve, the nurse may find that the client experiences a diminished sense of smell. The effects of age on olfaction are still uncertain (Corso, 1971).

The Mouth. Physical examination of the mouth begins with inspection of the lips. In many aging persons, there is a blurring of the vermilion border of the lips. It may appear to merge with the perilabial skin (Fig. 13). This is a degenerative change of the lips that results from an increase in elastic tissues which normally decrease elsewhere on the

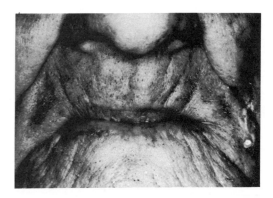

Figure 13. Lips. Changes associated with age and loss of teeth; note development of prominent lateral labial sulcus. *From Kerr DA, Ash MM, Millard HD: Oral Diagnosis, 3rd ed. St. Louis, Mosby, 1970, with permission.*

body with advancing age (Zach, 1979). The lips should be inspected for evidence of lesions, including leukoplakia or cancer. The lip angles should be assessed for angular cheilosis, or Perlèche (Fig. 14). Soggy white lesions, fissures, and yellow crusts appear in the lip angles. Perlèche usually occurs when teeth that supported the face and lip musculature are lost. As a result, there is an overclosure of the jaw, with a fold produced at the corner of the mouth, in which saliva collects. The client frequently licks the lesion to temporarily allay the burning pain and maceration eventually occurs (Langer, 1976). Often the lesion becomes infected with *Candida albicans* or other microorganisms. Perlèche is seen in older people without teeth and those with poorly fitting dentures. The nurse should refer the client to an orthodontist. Only when the underlying problem is corrected will the lesions heal permanently (Shafer et al., 1974).

Cancer of the lip usually involves the lower lip and is seen most often in men (Zach, 1979). It may appear as an ulcer, a thickened plaque, or a wartlike growth (Bates, 1979). A referral is indicated for any sore or crusting lesion on the lip that does not heal.

If the client is edentulous, dentures must be removed for a complete examination of the oral cavity. Since the presence of tooth roots is a major factor in the preservation of the bony structures of

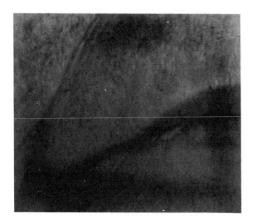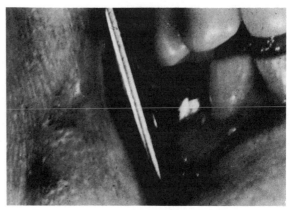

Figure 14. Perlèche associated with decreased intermaxillary space. Mouth closed (*left*), showing deep fissure at angle of mouth. Mouth opened (*right*), showing typical lesion. *From Schafer WG, Hine MK, Levy BM, 1974, with permission.*

the maxilla and mandible, facial dimensions in the edentulous person may be markedly changed. The area around the mouth will appear collapsed and sunken (Zach, 1979).

The number, location, and condition of remaining teeth should be noted. The teeth of the aged are different from those of the young. Remaining teeth are likely to show evidence of stains, chips, and dental caries. The teeth are worn down as a result of repetitive chewing and other stresses, such as night-grinding, abrasive foods, biting threads when sewing, clenching a pipe stem, or occupations where there is exposure to grit-laden air. Attrition may range from a minimal wear of the cusp to extreme loss of tooth enamel exposing underlying dentin (Fig. 15). The exposed dentin appears on the chewing surface of the tooth as a depressed area that is yellow, brown, or black in color (Zach, 1979).

The oral membranes appear thin and pale. The pallor is due to arteriosclerosis and a reduction in the capillary beds. The oral mucosa is at risk to break down when subjected to trauma or pressure. In some, the pressure of dentures creates a breakdown. The mucosa is also slower to heal (Zach, 1979).

Examination of the gums should be done with particular care. Normal gingival tissue in the elderly appears waxlike or glossy, and it loses its stippling (Langer, 1976). Periodontal disease is the major

factor responsible for the loss of teeth in the aged. With age, there appears to be a normal migration of the gingival epithelium surrounding remaining teeth. At the same time, atrophy of the alveolar bone occurs. This process results in a visible elongation of the tooth and a slow exposure of the root. Hence, the expression "long of tooth" (Fig. 16). If this process is combined with the additional stress of periodontitis, there is a gradual loss of the supporting structures of the root. Teeth loosen and eventually are lost. The client who is diabetic is at particular risk for this occurrence (Langer, 1976; Zach, 1979).

About 33 percent of denture wearers have lesions attributable to their dentures. These may be localized lesions, seen as ulcers with a raised and indurated border. Also common are fibrous overgrowths, called inflammatory hyperplasia, producing tissue flaps around the denture flange (Zach, 1979) (Fig. 17). The dentures may act as an irritant to the mouth. Generalized inflammation of the area beneath the denture may occur. Upper dentures may be a source of frictional irritation against the palate, resulting in papillary hyperplasia and the development of warty lesions (Langer, 1976) (Fig. 18). To detect the presence of growths, the oral cavity should be palpated.

The mouth and tongue may appear dry. Glandular activity is diminished, and the volume of

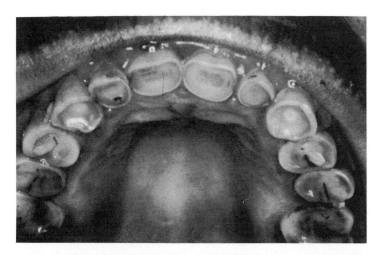

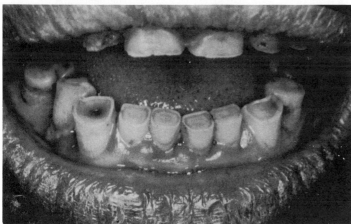

Figure 15. Advanced attrition. There is flattening of the incisal and occlusal surfaces and replacement of pulp chambers by secondary dentin. *From Shafer WG, Hine MK, Levy BM, 1974, with permission. Courtesy of Dr. Stephen F. Dachi.*

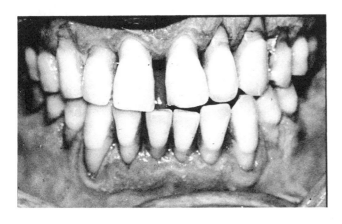

Figure 16. Advancing resorption of the alveolar bone leads to progressive root exposure and weakens the bony support. *From Langer A, 1976, with permission.*

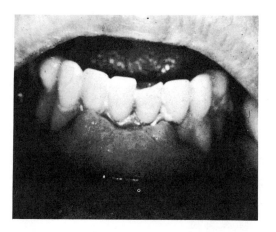

Figure 17. Inflammatory hyperplasia. Some cases of redundant tissue exhibit extremely large rolls of fibrous tissue around the denture. *From Shafer WG, Hine MK, Levy BM, 1974, with permission. Courtesy of Dr. Stephen F. Dachi.*

saliva produced by the elderly, on average, is one-third of that produced in youth (Goldman, 1979). Mouth breathing, dentures, the use of atropinelike drugs, and dehydration may also contribute to dryness. Dry mouth, called xerostoma, is the reason for numerous adverse adaptations in the aged. Because lubrication of the food bolus is reduced, the wear on teeth is increased (Zach, 1979). The saliva produces buffers that inhibit dental caries, and these are reduced. The risk of gingival and periodontal inflammation is increased. Some relief from dryness can be obtained by taking fluids or sucking lozenges. However, habitual use of lozenges places the client at risk for dental caries (Zach, 1979; Langer, 1976).

During inspection, atrophic changes may be noted in the papillae at the lateral edges of the tongue (Malasanos et al., 1977). Grapelike, tortuous vessels may be visible on the floor of the mouth and under the tongue. Called "caviar spots" these are varicosities that are an adaptation to increased venous pressure (Fig. 19). The client should be reassured that these are not a health risk and do not require treatment (Zach, 1979). The tongue should be inspected for evidence of carcinoma, which usually appears as an ulcer or nodule on the base or edges of the tongue (Bates, 1979). The twelfth cranial nerve remains intact with age; therefore when the client sticks out the tongue, no asymmetry, deviation, or atrophy should be noted.

Testing the sensory portion of the seventh cranial nerve will indicate a decline in the sense of taste after age 60. The threshold for sweet tastes is believed to be particularly affected. To test the four basic tastes, solutions of salt, sugar, lemon juice, and quinine are placed on the client's tongue (Corso, 1971). Stronger solutions are required for the elderly to recognize the substances than for the young. Diminution of taste sensation results from the age-related decrease in the number of taste buds, xerostoma, and a diminished sense of smell.

The gag reflex may be sluggish in the aging client in comparison with the young (Mezey et al., 1980). Palpation of the temporomandibular joint may reveal crepitation. The client may also complain of pain when chewing (Zach, 1979).

Because of its critical importance to the client's level of adaptation, assessment of the mouth and throat must be thorough. The nurse should obtain detailed information about the client's dental history. The aged are subject to a high rate of dental caries. Many factors contribute to their formation: the difficulty removing plaque from exposed roots, abraded dentin surfaces, clasps on partial dentures, bridgework, reduced saliva production, and changes in diet. Treatment of cavities is of particular importance for the aging client. Each remaining tooth assumes greater importance because it may be needed to secure a partial denture or bridge. The client's

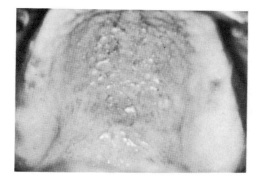

Figure 18. Papillary hyperplasia (papillomatosis). *From Shafer WG, Hine MK, Levy BM, 1974, with permission. Courtesy of Dr. Stephen F. Dachi.*

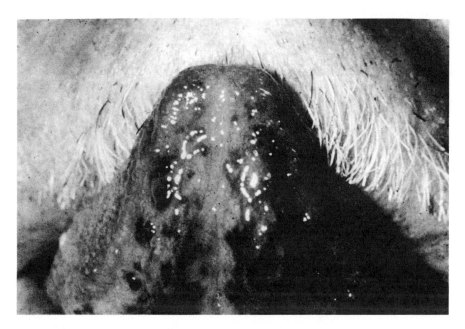

Figure 19. Varicosities occurring on the ventral surface of the tongue. *From Kamen S, Sherman FT: Oral and dental disorders, in Libow LS, Sherman FT (eds), The Core of Geriatric Medicine: A Guide for Students and Practitioners. St. Louis, CV Mosby Company, 1981, with permission.*

brushing habits should be identified. Instruction in correct brushing technique, regular flossing, and the use of oral irrigation devices may help the client prevent caries and periodontal disease (Zach, 1979).

Nearly one-half of persons over age 65 are edentulous. It is important that these people be fitted correctly for dentures. If the edentulous client delays obtaining dentures or fails to wear dentures, alveolar bone atrophy progresses more rapidly than when teeth are present. If bone loss is significant, the alveolar and basal bones may no longer be able to support dentures (Langer, 1976). Well-designed dentures correct the atrophy of the bones of the lower face and improve the client's appearance. They also allow the client to eat a more varied diet and improve the intelligibility of speech (Zach, 1979). It has been estimated that 25 percent of denture wearers do not wear them. The nurse needs to ascertain the client's satisfaction with the dentures as well as the length of time they have been worn, and their fit and comfort. It is important to encourage those clients who are not wearing their prosthesis

or are dissatisfied with it to go to the dentist. Edentulous clients who have not been fitted with dentures should be encouraged to obtain them before irreversible changes in the bones and gums make a proper fit impossible.

How often the client has visited the dentist, as well as the date of the last visit, should be ascertained. The elderly may postpone visits to the dentist on the assumption that the absence of tooth pain indicates an absence of problems. On the contrary, they have a diminished sensory level of pain originating in the teeth. As secondary dentin is produced, it replaces the dental pulp or "nerve" of the tooth, and is less efficient in conducting pain. One benefit of this process is that the aged experience less pain during manipulations such as drilling or grinding. Some dental procedures are more difficult in the aged. Cementum, which surrounds the root, is thickened with age and can make tooth extractions difficult. Assuring that the aging person visits a competent dentist on a regular basis is a service that can benefit the client's quality of life.

The Neck. Because the neck is shortened in many older people palpation of the thyroid may be more difficult. Because the thyroid gland may be lower in relation to the clavicles, its lower poles may be inaccessible (Rossman, 1979b). Findings noted when palpating lymph nodes and trachea should be similar to those of young adults.

The Thorax and Lungs

When inspecting the thorax of the aging client, the nurse should note an increase in the anteroposterior diameter of the chest. The ratio of the anteroposterior to lateral diameter increases from 1:2 in young adults to 1:1 in the normal aging adult (Bates, 1979). The barrel chest of the aging should not be presumed to be an adaptation to emphysema. Instead it is due to the degenerative changes in the intervertebral discs and increased spinal curvature that accompany the aging process (Goldman, 1979).

Changes in the thoracic spine are common in the elderly. If changes are present, the nurse should ascertain whether or not they influence the quality of respiration. Severe kyphosis interferes with the free movement of the ribs during ventilation. If it is observed, the nurse should measure the client's chest expansion to determine the degree of limitation of the chest wall. A scoliosis of significant degree will cause one side of the chest to be compressed and the other side to be abnormally expanded. This imbalance also interferes with respiratory motion (Sherman and Fields, 1976). A scoliosis of the upper part of the vertebral column may also result in tracheal deviation (Malasanos et al., 1977).

Bony landmarks on the chest, such as the sternum, vertebrae, and ribs, are more prominent, due to a decrease in subcutaneous fat. In addition, body hollows in the supraclavicular and intercostal spaces are accentuated.

The character of respirations at rest is unchanged with age. If the client is asked to breathe deeply, however, the older person may complain of some discomfort (Malasanos et al., 1977). During exercise, the older person's respirations are not as deep as those of the young. They are more rapid and return to normal less quickly. Impairment of respiratory excursion during exertion is due to a weakening of the respiratory musculature and reduced compliance of the chest wall.

Percussion of the healthy aging lung should produce either resonance or hyperresonance. With age, alveoli enlarge while alveolar walls remain intact. This adaptation has been named "senile emphysema." Percussion of lung fields affected by senile emphysema or percussion over areas affected by kyphosis produces hyperresonance (Wynne, 1979).

When auscultating the lungs of the older client, it may be necessary to provide encouragement to breathe deeply with the mouth open in order to obtain satisfactory respiratory excursion. Breath sounds are weaker in the aged due to diminished ventilatory airflow (Exton-Smith and Overstall, 1979). Some atelectic rales may be heard at the base of the lung during the first several respiratory cycles. These have been attributed to basal alveolar collapse. In the young, the basal portion of the lungs is better ventilated than the apical portion and a balance between ventilation and perfusion is achieved. With age the lungs become increasingly rigid, improving the ventilation at the apex and decreasing ventilation at the base. The balance between ventilation and perfusion is upset. Basal alveoli are underventilated and may collapse (Goldman, 1979). If the nurse learns to recognize the breath sounds that are normally present in the healthy client, identification of significant deviations from normal becomes less difficult.

Pulmonary function is altered with age. The residual volume and functional residual capacity are increased. These changes are due to the elevation of the ribs and flattening of the diaphragm that occur with age. As a result, the lungs remain partially inflated in comparison with those of the young. However, because dead space is increased with age, there is no change in total lung capacity or resting tidal volume. Because residual volume increases and total lung capacity remains essentially unchanged, vital capacity decreases with age.

At rest, changes in pulmonary function are not apparent. However, older persons do have a decreased capacity for exercise and alter their activities of daily living and their social patterns in order to compensate.

The functional changes of the aging lung resemble those found in emphysema. The healthy aging client, however, should not exhibit the same functional impairments as the client with emphysema. One way to assess the function of the aging lung is to ask the client to blow out a book match at 6 inches with the mouth wide open. Failure to do so suggests functional impairments other than the normal aging changes. The client should be referred for further evaluation (Goldman, 1979; Wynne, 1979).

Reduced cough efficiency, decreased ciliary activity, and increased dead space reduce the possibility that the aging client will adapt in an optimal way to such stresses as infectious agents, surgery, or immobility. In addition, the incidence of chronic obstructive lung disease, pulmonary tuberculosis, and cancer of the lung all increase with advanced age.

The Cardiovascular System

Blood Pressure. Assessing the older client's blood pressure must be done with great care. Many factors, including the stress of the health assessment itself, can temporarily elevate the older client's blood pressure. Blood pressure should be taken with the client lying and standing. There is a normal rise in both systolic and diastolic blood pressure up to age 70 in both men and women. After age 70, the systolic pressure may decline slightly in women (Rodstein, 1979). A widening pulse pressure is also present in the elderly. In spite of changes in both systolic and diastolic pressures, the blood pressure of the healthy aging client should be within the normal limits for any age (Babu et al., 1977).

A great deal of controversy still surrounds the definition and treatment of hypertension in the aging. Usually, the diagnosis of hypertension is made after the client's blood pressure has been elevated on three different occasions. Current data indicate that older people with blood pressures at or below 140/90 mm Hg have an increased longevity compared to those with higher blood pressures. The Framingham study found that elevations in systolic and diastolic blood pressure at any age were a potent cardiovascular risk factor (Kannel et al., 1971). Data on isolated systolic blood pressure elevations after age 65 also indicate that this is a potent risk factor for cardiovascular disease (Goldman, 1979). For these reasons, the nurse should refer any aging client with a blood pressure reading above 140/90 mm Hg for follow up.

A slowing of the vasomotor reflex involving the baroreceptors occurs with age. The baroreceptors are less able to prevent loss of blood pressure when the person moves from the supine to the upright position (Brody and Vijayashanker, 1977). Any aging client with a standing systolic blood pressure below 110 mm Hg should be referred for further evaluation. Postural hypotension occurs often in the elderly and may be the reason an older person has difficulty standing or walking or complains of dizziness (Caird, 1976).

Heart. Percussion of cardiac borders in the healthy aging client may show a heart of normal size or with a slight degree of cardiac enlargement. There is disagreement about the effects of aging on heart size. In many healthy aging people, heart size remains normal or decreases slightly (Burch, 1977). However, changes in left ventricular wall thickness may contribute to a small increase in overall heart size with age (Sjögren, 1971). Cardiac hypertrophy, however, is not a normal finding and requires further investigation.

The apical impulse or point of maximal impulse (PMI) is another indication of heart size. In the aging client, it should be palpable at approximately the fifth interspace but not outside the left midclavicular line if the spine is straight. If there is a thoracic cage or spinal deformity, such as kyphoscoliosis, the PMI is dislocated and loses its clinical significance. In the aging person, the apical impulse may appear less prominent and quick because of the reduced elasticity of the chest wall. However, chest wall rigidity allows the apical impulse to be palpated with ease, and the feel of the cardiac impulse is more significant than the sight of the apical beat as evidence of cardiac changes. During palpation, a powerful, hypertrophied left ventricle will be felt as a strong, sustained impulse. A dilated ventricle will feel less powerful but covers a wider area of the chest wall (Caird, 1976).

The resting pulse rate of the aging client should remain unchanged (Goldman, 1979). In response to physical activity, anxiety, and other stresses, the heart rate is not able to increase to the extent that it does in the young. For example, the aging client with an infection may not be able to exhibit the classic elevation in pulse rate. After activity, the heart rate takes more time to return to basal levels. Even a minimal increase in heart rate for the older person may be prolonged beyond the time normally expected for a young adult.

The rhythm of the aging heart should be regular. Irregular beats require further investigation (Caird and Dall, 1978). Apical and radial pulses should be taken simultaneously to ascertain any disparities. Certain irregularities of heart beat do occur with age and are believed to be a normal concomitant of aging. Extrasystoles increase with age. Atrial premature contractions occur in about 10 percent and ventricular premature contractions in about 6 percent of people over age 65. These are believed to result from the increase in irritability that characterizes the aging myocardium (Harris, 1976). In the absence of other cardiac adaptations, extrasystoles apparently have no adverse effects on mortality (Rodstein, 1977). Sinus arrhythmias that accelerate with inspiration and slow with expiration are also common (Harris, 1976). Sinus bradycardia with a heart rate below 60 may be physiological in healthy older people and is due to increased vagal tone (Harris, 1976). Atrial arrhythmias frequently occur when a person reaches 60 years of age. In one study of healthy aging persons, atrial fibrillation was the most common arrhythmia found, followed by atrial flutter. Supraventricular tachycardias are found frequently in the aging, but there is disagreement about whether or not these are normal aging changes. According to Harris (1976), supraventricular tachycardias in the aging were usually associated with heart disease.

Although some arrhythmias are believed to be a concomitant of normal aging, they are significant because the aging person has less cardiovascular reserve than the young. An arrhythmia in the aging client may be a signal of impending heart disease (Vaidya et al., 1976).

Auscultatory signs carry the same connotation for the aged as for the young. The first and second heart sounds can be clearly heard in normal clients. Many older people have difficulty in conducting the respiratory maneuvers necessary for proper identification of respiratory variation in splitting of the second heart sound (Caird and Dall, 1978). A fourth heart sound (S_4) may be heard in the normal older person. If there are no other cardiovascular adaptations, the S_4 can be considered a normal variant of aging. S_3 sounds are considered to be indicators of cardiovascular pathology (Luisada, 1977).

Basal systolic murmurs develop with advancing age in the healthy person without organic heart disease. An early or midsystolic ejection murmur, best heard at the base of the heart and often transmitted to the apex, may be heard in up to 60 percent of older persons (Caird and Dall, 1978). This systolic murmur is thought to be due to a slight dilatation of the ascending aorta or to minimal fibrotic fusion of one or more commissures of the aortic valve without significant narrowing of the opening. Unless other adverse cardiac adaptations are present, the murmur is considered innocent (Harris, 1978). This benign murmur can be distinguished from aortic stenosis, in which the peak of the murmur is usually heard at or after midsystole (Perez et al., 1976; Harris, 1977; Luisada, 1977). Other systolic murmurs heard in the normal aging person are regurgitant murmurs arising from the mitral or tricuspid valves (Caird and Dall, 1978). Diastolic murmurs in the elderly are always an adaptation to significant heart disease (Caird, 1976; Harris, 1978).

Normal blood pressure, heart rate, and heart size do not necessarily indicate normal cardiac function. Aging changes in the myocardium and vessels place the aging heart at a disadvantage and impair its ability to function efficiently (Harris, 1977). The nurse should look for signs of reduced cardiovascular function. Fluid retention should be determined. Pressure should be applied to the instep of the foot and the medial malleolus to determine the presence of pitting edema. Findings should be interpreted cautiously since many factors, including tight garters or prolonged sitting, can be associated with peripheral edema. The abdomen should be inspected for distention. The client should be questioned about recent weight gain or a change in the fit of rings, belts, or shoes. Recent changes in the client's activity level should be determined. The quality of the client's sleep should be determined. If the client is awakened by a need to urinate, or experiences paroxysmal nocturnal dyspnea or orthopnea, the nurse should refer the client for further evaluation.

Blood Vessels. The nurse must systematically examine the pulses in all locations. In many aging clients, arteries may be palpated more readily due to increased hardness, loss of surrounding connective tissue, and increased pulse wave velocity (Caird,

1976). However, in areas of decreased arterial perfusion, peripheral pulses may be diminished and thus more difficult to locate.

Age-related changes in blood vessels may be apparent in the neck. Atrophy of skin and subcutaneous tissues of the neck makes observation of venous pressure and pulses easier (Caird, 1976). In the aged, as in younger persons, the carotid pulses should never be palpated simultaneously. Cerebral circulation may already be compromised and any diminution of blood flow may result in syncope or stroke.

Because of the high incidence of cardiovascular disease in the aging, the physical examination should include auscultation of the carotid arteries at their bifurcation for the presence of bruits. The nurse will need to distinguish between a bruit and a murmur that radiates to the neck, such as occurs with calcified aortic stenosis (Rodstein, 1979). The abdominal aorta and renal arteries should also be auscultated for bruits. If a bruit is heard, the client should be referred for further evaluation.

The aorta elongates as a normal part of the aging process. In some cases, elongation produces buckling of the innominate or carotid artery, which is seen as a pulsating mass in the neck that can be mistaken for an aneurysm (Rossman, 1979b).

Age-related changes in both arteries and veins place the aging client at risk for arterial insufficiency and varicosities. The peripheral vascular examination should also include assessment of extremities for color, temperature, skin, hair and nail changes, edema, calf tenderness, ulceration, varicosities, and the presence of Homan's sign. When evaluating the findings, the nurse must keep in mind the skin, hair, and nail changes that normally accompany the aging process.

The Blood. With age few changes occur in the blood or its components. Anemia is not a normal concomitant of the aging process. However, because of nutritional deficiencies and blood loss from certain gastrointestinal stresses, the aging person is at risk for iron-deficiency anemia. A simple check for anemia can be made by observing the palmar creases for redness when the hand is stretched. Because the conjunctiva and oral mucosa of the aged often appear pale, their color is not a reliable indicator of anemia. The nurse should consider complaints of fatigue and weakness very carefully because these are not normal consequences of aging (Clifford and Bewtra, 1979).

The Breasts

Female. The breasts of the aging female become elongated, pendulous and flaccid due to glandular tissue atrophy and, in some, kyphosis (Rossman, 1979b). Because the breasts are an important symbol of sexuality, the aging woman may be very conscious of changes there (Rakoff and Nowroozi, 1978). If observation of pendulous breasts for size, symmetry, contour, and dimpling is to be accurate and complete, it is best accomplished with the client in a sitting position and leaning forward, so the breasts hang away from the chest wall. The technique of the breast examination may require further modification if the client has restricted joint mobility and is unable to raise the arms above the head while the breasts are inspected and palpated. If the client's breasts are large, palpation might be best accomplished by placing one hand on top and one hand beneath the breast so that simultaneous pressure from both hands will allow palpation of masses in the pendulous portion (Mezey et al., 1980).

The size of the aging female breast remains about the same throughout the life span. Nevertheless, atrophy of the muscular supports and breast tissue allows the breasts to sag and the nipples to drop far below the fourth intercostal space (Sana and Judge, 1975). Normal shrinkage and fibrotic changes may result in retraction of the nipple. Although this adaptation mimics that of cancer, if it is due to normal aging the nipple can usually be everted with gentle pressure and no associated tumor mass is palpable (Rossman, 1979b). Skin beneath pendulous breasts should be inspected for irritation or maceration.

Atrophy of fat and glandular tissue, fibrotic changes, and calcification occur, resulting in loss of fullness of breast tissue. Consequently, the breast tissue is more readily palpated. Breast masses may be detected more easily than in the younger woman (Rossman, 1979b). Unlike the younger woman, the borders of the breasts of the aging woman cannot be clearly identified. The aging breast develops an irregular consistency. The breasts may feel stringy, glandular, or nodular since nodules develop as the years go by (Prior and Silberstein, 1973). The linear strands of the terminal ducts gradually become firm as a result of fibrosis and calcification. Since this is a gradual process, it will be necessary to differentiate between normal changes in the terminal ducts and other suspicious lesions (Rossman, 1979b).

Older women should be taught that after menopause, regular breast examination remains as important as it is for women in the childbearing years. Whenever possible the older woman should be taught how to perform breast self-examination and encouraged to examine her breasts each month. The nurse needs to make a careful assessment of the client's mobility and tactile sensation in the fingertips to assure that the client can perform self-examination accurately. Because cystic mastitis is uncommon in the postmenopausal woman, any unusual mass in the breast takes on great significance. If a mass is detected, the nurse should refer the client promptly for follow up.

Male. Examination of the breasts should be a part of the examination of the aging male. Although the incidence is low, breast cancer may occur in the breasts of older men. Gynecomastia may also occur in later life, either spontaneously or as a result of several medications (Stern, 1964).

The Abdomen

Assessment of the abdomen should reveal few changes with age. Some aging clients may not be able to tolerate the supine position during this and later parts of the examination. If not, the client should be placed in the lowest semi-Fowler's position that can be tolerated.

With the client supine, the abdomen may appear convex in the area of the umbilicus. The aged frequently have a round abdomen due to a combination of factors: inactivity, reduced muscle tone, increased subcutaneous fat, or kyphosis of the dorsal segments of the spine (Sana and Judge, 1975).

Since there is a general loss of fibroconnective tissue as well as muscle wasting in the aging, the abdominal wall in the nonobese may be slacker and thinner. Consequently, palpation may be simpler and more accurate (Schouten, 1975). With age, the liver and kidneys decrease in size. In the older client with kyphoscoliosis or pulmonary emphysema, downward displacement of the liver may permit the liver edge to be felt (Harris, 1978). There is a dif-

ference in opinion about whether the size of the pancreas decreases or remains the same (Goldman, 1979; Feinstein and Friedman, 1979). According to Calloway et al. (1965) there is no decrease in the weight of the pancreas with age. Because normal aging changes in organ size are small, there should be no differences apparent upon palpation.

If abdominal masses are detected upon palpation, a knowledge of aging changes is important for evaluation. A distended bladder is a frequent occurrence in the aged and, therefore, the bladder may be palpable. A hard, movable mass in the lower left quadrant may indicate the presence of feces. This finding would be confirmed during the rectal examination. A mass, pulsating or nonpulsating, near the midportion of the abdomen may represent an aortic aneurysm (Straus, 1979).

The most comfortable position for the aged client during the rectal examination is the side lying, as opposed to knee-chest, position. The nurse should ask the client to bear down and palpate for a fixed, hard mass. A stool specimen for guaiac should be taken at the time of the rectal examination.

When evaluating the findings of the abdominal examination, the nurse must consider that the aging client's perception of abdominal pain is diminished. Even in acute abdominal emergencies the aging complain of less discomfort than do the young. In addition, because of muscle atrophy, the aging often fail to exhibit abdominal wall rigidity in the presence of peritoneal irritation (Schouten, 1975). For these reasons, stresses such as appendicitis or biliary colic may be difficult to recognize.

Genitourinary System

The Female. The vulva becomes thin and loses its contour due to reabsorption of fatty tissue (Brown, 1978). The skin of the vulva becomes atrophic and the hair becomes sparse and gray (Sherman and Fields, 1976). Because the mons pubis is prone to the same skin lesions found elsewhere on the body, it should be observed for irritation, redness, or scratch marks. If white, slightly raised plaques are present, they may be leukoplakia, a precursor of squamous cell carcinoma of the vulva (Straus, 1979; Sherman and Fields, 1975).

The labia majora become flattened and wrinkled as subcutaneous fat decreases. With age, the labia minora shrink and eventually become shriveled. The clitoris and prepuce decrease in size (Rakoff and Nowroozi, 1978). The vestibule between the labia minora and below the clitoris should be inspected for ulcerations, erythema, and swelling. This is a common site for malignant changes in the elderly. A common condition affecting postmenopausal women is kraurosis vulvae. The mucosa of the vestibule, urethral orifiace, vagina, and inner aspects of the labia majora appear dry, shiny, pallid, wrinkled, and inelastic (DeGowen and DeGowen, 1970; Brown, 1978).

The urethra should be examined for swelling, inflammation, or prolapsed outpouching of the urethral mucous membrane (Sherman and Fields, 1976). The postmenopausal woman is at risk for prolapsing of the urethral mucous membranes. If prolapsed, the membranes frequently become infected and are reddened and tender (Rakoff, 1978). The client should be asked to strain or bear down as the nurse observes for any loss of urine (Sana and Judge, 1975). As the client bears down, the vaginal orifice should also be observed for widening or protrusion, which indicates the presence of a cystocele, rectocele, or uterine prolapse. The fourchette should be observed for old tears and scarring.

The pelvic examination is a necessary part of the physical examination; however, because pelvic examination may be uncomfortable for the older woman, some women make efforts to avoid it. The nurse must reassure the older woman that gentleness will be used throughout the examination. Because of musculoskeletal or neurological stresses many aging women cannot tolerate the lithotomy position normally used for the pelvic examination. If so, a left lateral Sims' position or a modified lithotomy position may be necessary to make the examination possible and permit visualization of the cervix (Goldfarb, 1979; Mezey et al., 1980). Because the aging vagina is narrower, it may be necessary to use a smaller speculum (Gray, 1977). Before inserting the speculum, it is helpful to ascertain the size of the introitus by inserting one finger. In the postmenopausal virgin, tightness of the hymen may prevent passage of the speculum (Mezey et al., 1980). After the speculum is inserted and a specimen taken for a Papanicolaou smear, the vagina and cervix can be inspected.

The vaginal mucosa appears thin and fragile. The color is pale pink, rather than purple. Rugae are less prominent, and in the very old woman, the vaginal membrane is smooth. The vagina appears dry, as vaginal secretions diminish with age. The trauma of speculum insertion may stimulate bleeding of the vaginal epithelium. The nurse should observe for erosions, ulcerations, and adhesions (Rakoff and Nowroozi, 1978).

The cervix decreases in size, but not until some years after menopause (Rakoff and Nowroozi, 1978). It may be flush with the vault (Burnside, 1981). It may appear shrunken and its surface may be thick and glistening as a result of estrogen deficiency (Mezey et al., 1980). The os may be stenotic and obliterated (Burnside, 1981).

Changes in the vaginal epithelium and the acidity of vaginal secretions increase the susceptibility of the aging woman to irritation and infection (Rakoff and Nowroozi, 1978). A frequent finding in the postmenopausal woman is senile vaginitis. The vaginal mucosa appears yellowish and friable and there is an absence of vaginal rugae. In addition, the woman with senile vaginitis usually complains of urgency of urination, dyspareunia, itching, and bleeding. These clients should be referred for treatment with hormonal creams to restore the vaginal epithelium to a more normal state (Straus, 1979).

Weakening of the vaginal wall as well as the broad and round ligaments supporting the uterus may occur in the postmenopausal woman (Sana and Judge, 1975). When the speculum has been withdrawn to the midpoint, the nurse can evaluate the integrity of uterine supports and vaginal walls. The nurse should ask the woman to bear down and then observe for protrusion of the cervix or bulging of the anterior or posterior vaginal walls. If the uterine supports are relaxed, varying degrees of uterine prolapse may occur. The cervix may protrude into the open speculum and may follow it to the introitus. If there is relaxation of the anterior or posterior vaginal walls, a cystocele or rectocele may bulge into the vaginal cavity (Sana and Judge, 1975).

Because the vagina of the older woman is narrowed, it is often necessary to perform vaginal palpation using only one finger. Whenever possible, two fingers should be used. The vaginal walls should be palpated for tenderness, induration from scars, and adhesions (Sana and Judge, 1975). The client should be asked again to bear down while the examining fingers are in the vagina. Since the amount of relaxation of vaginal walls can be noted, vaginal palpation gives additional information about the presence of cystocele, rectocele, or prolapse of the uterus (Sana and Judge, 1975). With bimanual palpation, a shortened vagina will be felt (Rakoff and Nowroozi, 1978). Examination of the uterus and adnexa will reveal a smaller and firmer uterus and cervix, resulting from tissue hypoplasia. In the normal postmenopausal woman, ovaries and tubes should not be palpable. The ovaries of a woman age 60 are about half the size of a woman age 20 (Rakoff and Nowroozi, 1978). A palpable uterus is an indication of malignancy and the client should be referred for further evaluation (Goldfarb, 1979). The rectovaginal examination is an essential component of the gynecological appraisal of the older woman (Goldfarb, 1979).

The gynecological examination provides an opportunity for health teaching about appropriate health maintenance procedures following menopause. A discussion of perineal cleanliness measures may be pertinent, especially if the client experiences stress incontinence, pruritis, or vaginal infections. An annual pelvic and rectopelvic examination is essential. The incidence of cervical carcinoma, endometrial carcinoma, and endometrial polyps is highest in middle-aged women and uterine and ovarian cancers are leading causes of death in women over age 55 (Goldfarb, 1979). The aging woman should also be advised to have Papanicolaou smears annually or biannually.

The gynecological examination also provides an opportunity for the aging woman to discuss her feelings and concerns about the experiences of menopause and postmenopause. She may need the opportunity to discuss changes in her role in society, her perception of her femininity, her sexual experiences and satisfaction with them. In many situations, knowing that the changes she is experiencing are normal may be enough to allay a woman's apprehensions.

The Male. The aging male's pubic hair is sparse and gray. The penis decreases in size and shows progressive sclerosis of arteries and veins. The testes decrease in size and are less firm on palpation. The scrotum is elongated and flaccid and the rugae of the scrotum are diminished as a result of reduced muscle tone (Patient Assessment, 1979).

Palpation of the prostate gland by rectal examination is an essential component of the physical examination. Either the left lateral Sims' position or the standing elbow-knee position can be used when assessing the prostate of the aging male (DeGowen and DeGowen, 1970). Age is a major risk factor for benign prostatic hypertrophy. The highest frequency occurs between 60 and 70 years of age (Rossman, 1979). Carcinoma of the prostate is the third most common type of malignant disease causing death in males. It tends to occur about 10 years later than hyperplasia (Brocklehurst, 1979).

The prostate should be examined for size, consistency, and tenderness. The midline fissure should be palpable. If it is absent, the median lobe may be enlarged, a finding often associated with urinary retention. Benign prostatic hypertrophy produces a symmetrically enlarged gland that is smooth, firm, and rubbery (Patient Assessment, 1979; DeGowen and DeGowen, 1970). Carcinoma of the prostate is generally felt as a nodular, stony-hard mass (DeGowen and DeGowen, 1970). Enlargement is asymmetrical (Mezey et al., 1980). Both lateral sulci and the median sulcus may be obliterated (Patient Assessment, 1979). In the very old male, the prostate may be atrophied and will feel soft, mushy, or almost absent (Sherman and Fields, 1976).

As with the aging female, the genitourinary examination provides an opportunity for teaching and counseling about role changes, sexuality, and changing responses during sexual intercourse. A discussion of normal aging changes in sexual functioning is found later in this chapter. Stresses that may alter sexual functioning in the aging are discussed in Chapter 14.

Musculoskeletal System

The nurse should assess the muscles of the upper and lower extremities for size, tone and strength. With increasing age, muscle contours become more prominent. Muscle bundles and their tendinous points of attachment may be easily identified. Generalized, symmetrical muscle wasting is a normal concomitant of the aging process, as muscle tissue is lost and partially replaced with fat. Age, inactivity, and degenerative joint disease contribute to this process. The dorsum of the hand should be inspected for signs of fine muscle wasting. Usually, the muscles of the hand accurately reflect the extent of muscle wasting elsewhere (Carter, 1979).

Muscle strength should be tested against resistance. A progressive decrease in muscle strength is characteristic of normal aging and becomes noticeable at ages 65 to 70 (Pathy, 1978; Shock, 1977). Even if muscle wasting is extensive, the strength of the aging client's hand grip should not weaken (Carter, 1979). Stresses common to the aged, including inactivity, malnutrition and endocrine changes, contribute to muscle weakness. Muscle tone, assessed by palpating a muscle while putting a joint through passive range of motion, may be diminished but should remain symmetrical. The strength of the sternocleidomastoid and trapezius muscles (eleventh cranial nerve) remains strong.

The nurse should observe the client's posture for changes characteristic of the aging process (Fig. 20). These include a slight flexion of the knees and hips and a stooped posture. Postural changes are believed to be due to altered neuromuscular control, impaired muscle power and degenerative joint disease (Pathy, 1978). The spine should be assessed for alignment, curvature, and flexibility. Normal bone loss and narrowing of intervertebral discs and joint spaces result in loss of height and an accentuated bend of the thoracic spine. If osteoporosis is advanced, kyphosis may be apparent. When the aging client moves the spine through range of motion, the nurse should be positioned so as to protect the client from falling. Flexibility of the spine may be reduced in the aged.

The nurse should appraise joint function with particular gentleness. All joints should be put through their full range of motion. If possible, range of motion should be quantified and measurements recorded for noting later changes. Joints should be palpated as they are put through range of motion. Crepitation and stiffness on movement are common findings as a result of cartilage erosions (Rossman, 1979b).

Throughout the musculoskeletal appraisal, the nurse should observe for adaptations to osteoarthritis. In the past, osteoarthritis was believed to be a concomitant of normal aging, the result of "wear and tear" on joints. However, it is now thought that osteoarthritis is a process separate from normal aging. It involves the formation of osteophytes and bony overgrowths and is present, to some degree, in nearly everyone over age 65. When palpating the spinous processes, protrusion and lipping of the vertebrae may be noted. These bony overgrowths are called osteophytes and are found most often in the lower cervical spine (C_6 and C_7) and lumbar spine (Rossman, 1979a; 1979b). Nodules on the dorsolateral aspects of the distal interphalangeal joints, called Heberden's nodes, may be noted. These rarely result in pain or immobility. Similar nodules, called Bouchard's nodes, are sometimes evident on the proximal interphalangeal joints. Other joints, particularly the knee, are often involved (Habermann, 1979). Clients with osteoarthritis complain of varying degrees of discomfort and exhibit varying levels of immobility in the affected joints (Rossman, 1979a). A detailed discussion of osteoarthritis is presented in Chapter 15.

The incidence of musculoskeletal stresses increases with age. Many of these stresses were present at birth or as a result of childhood disease or trauma, but they caused troublesome adaptations only after the aging process had progressed. The foot is a significant source of problems, particularly for aging women (Shank and Conrad, 1977). The nurse should observe the feet for hallux valgus, bunions, and splay feet. If these problems were not corrected when the client was young, they may seriously hamper mobility in old age. Hammertoes, a congenital or acquired condition, is also frequent in the elderly. Hammering of the second toe often occurs with hallux valgus (Fig. 21). Often, surgery is deemed inappropriate for aging clients with these stresses either because of the client's age or the presence of contextual stresses that might hamper adaptation to surgery. Nevertheless, the nurse should refer the client to the podiatrist. If surgery is not feasible, appropriate shoes and protective padding may limit the problem and maintain the client's mobility (Jahss, 1979).

Neurological System

The aging client has difficulty cooperating with the many elements involved in a complete neurological examination. He or she is required to follow many complicated instructions and may need more time than a younger person to respond appropriately; retesting is often needed to validate findings. Because many clients will be fatigued by the physical examination, it may be necessary to schedule the neurological examination for a separate time (Mezey et al., 1980).

Motor Function. Motor function is tested by assessing muscle bulk, tone and strength, posture and gait, balance and coordination. Techniques and findings when assessing muscle bulk, tone, and

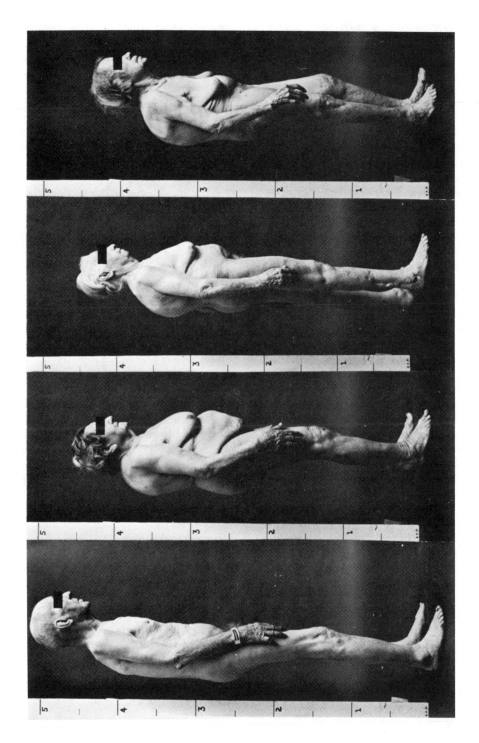

Figure 20. Four randomly selected patients from the ambulatory section of a nursing home, illustrating short stature, osteoporotic kyphosis, and relatively long extremities. *From left to right: T.H., age 82, L.B., age 78, A.I., age 79, and A.S., age 94. From Rossman I, 1979B, with permission.*

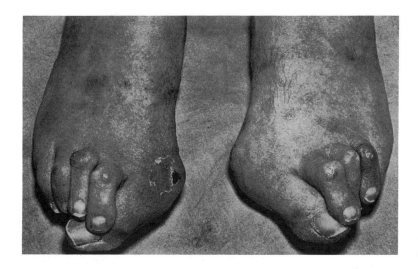

Figure 21. Bilateral hallux valgus. *From Prior JA, Silberstein JS, 1973, with permission.*

strength are described in the Musculoskeletal System section of this chapter. Atrophy and fasciculations that suggest lower motor neuron problems and involuntary movements should be noted. Older people may have fasciculations of the calves, hands and feet, and eyelids, especially if fatigued. If no undue muscle wasting or weakness is noted, these irregular, brief muscle twitchings are not indicative of central nervous system disease (Grob, 1978). Changes in muscle tone may suggest neurological disorders. Resistance to stretch is increased in Parkinson's disease and in upper motor neuron lesions. Resistance to stretch is decreased in the presence of lower motor neuron lesions or cerebellar lesions. In order to test for changes in muscle strength in the upper extremities due to neurological problems, such as cerebrovascular accident, clients should be asked to close their eyes and for 20 to 30 seconds hold the arms straight in front of them with palms up. This enables observation of downward and lateral drift of the hands in sensory loss, the presence of weakness of proximal or distal muscle groups, and the pronator sign characteristic of pyramidal lesions. If only one forearm pronates or drifts downward, mild hemiparesis is suggested. Muscle strength in the lower limbs is most easily tested by asking the client to lift the leg from the examining table and hold the heel off the bed.

The nurse has many opportunities during the history and physical examination to observe the client's gait. As a concomitant of the aging process, many people shuffle or take shortened steps, with a widening of the distance between the feet. Associated movements are reduced; for example, the aging person swings the arms less vigorously when walking (Pathy, 1978). Gait changes are related to changes in the extrapyramidal system, the vertebral column, intervertebral discs, tendons, and muscles. Many clients watch their feet as they move, an adaptation to the blunting of proprioception that occurs with aging (Sana and Judge, 1975). Stresses that occur frequently with age may also be responsible for abnormal gait patterns. Table 1 lists common stresses and the abnormal gait patterns that result. The aging client may have difficulty when performing tandem walking since this test reduces the base of support and accentuates abnormalities in coordination.

The Romberg test for proprioception and cerebellar function should be negative. The nurse should be prepared to support the client in case of loss of balance. Other tests for proprioception may be difficult to perform because of reduced coordination or musculoskeletal stresses that limit the client's mobility. These include touching the nose with the tip of the index finger of each hand, repeating the motion with increasing speed, and running the heel of each foot down the opposite shin.

Coordination is the synergistic action of muscles functioning in proper sequence to produce a

TABLE 1.   SOME ABNORMALITIES OF GAIT

Type	Characteristics	Examples
Parkinsonian	The body is held rigid, trunk and head bent forward. Short, mincing steps, sudden uncontrolled propulsive-like movements	Parkinson's disease
Ataxic	Staggering or reeling like an alcoholic	Cerebellar disease
Slapping	Feet wide apart, legs raised high and then feet slapped on the ground. Eyes fixed to the floor to help guide feet for placement	Disease of posterior column of spinal cord
Spastic	Jerking, uncoordinated movements	Cerebral palsy, multiple sclerosis
Dragging	Dragging of one leg around in a semicircle	Hemiplegia
Scissors	Thighs close together due to spasticity of adductor muscles	Spastic paraplegia

From Sherman JL, Fields SK, 1976, with permission.

smooth, purposeful movement. Loss of muscle coordination is a normal concomitant of the aging process and begins in the fourth decade. Muscles move less smoothly and more slowly (Grob, 1978). Changes will be noted first in loss of motor skills for more complex tasks and for activities demanding

precise, coordinated movements (Shock, 1977). The nurse has many opportunities to observe coordination during the physical examination, as the client removes shoes, arises from a standing position, walks, and climbs onto the examining table. The aging client should be asked to perform several simple tests involving rhythmic, alternating movements of hands and feet. It is best to have the client begin slowly, gradually increasing the tempo until discoordination occurs. Inability to perform rapid maneuvers is usually indicative of cerebellar disease, but it may be a normal finding in the aging.

Cranial Nerves.   Because reaction time decreases with age, the nurse should allow a longer time for response when testing cranial nerve function. Techniques for testing cranial nerve function and adaptations with aging were discussed earlier. Table 2 summarizes changes in examination techniques and common findings in aging clients.

Reflexes.   Eliciting tendon reflexes in the aged is more difficult because limb relaxation is more difficult for them. The use of reinforcement techniques, such as clenching the jaw, is essential to achieve adequate muscle relaxation. In general, reflex responses in older people are diminished. This change is due primarily to shrinkage and sclerosis of tendons and muscles, rather than to changes in the spinal reflex arc. Deep tendon reflexes of the arms, including supinator, biceps, and triceps, can be elicited, but are usually diminished in intensity. The deep tendon reflex of the knee is usually intact (Grob, 1978). Severe arthritis of the knee may require the nurse to locate the tendon by palpation and then tap the finger over it. The Achilles reflex is absent in as many as one-third of healthy aging clients (Carter, 1979). If possible, the client should kneel on a padded chair and clench the teeth when testing the Achilles reflex. In testing, it is important that the client's feet be warm (Mezey et al., 1980). Because hypothyroidism is an important health problem in the aged, the nurse should note the length of the relaxation phase of the Achilles reflex. If the client has foot problems, such as thick calluses or hallux valgus, the plantar reflex may be unobtainable (Grob, 1978).

In the aging adult, superficial reflexes are fre-

TABLE 2. DIFFERENCES IN CRANIAL NERVE ASSESSMENT TECHNIQUES AND ADAPTATIONS IN AGING ADULTS

Cranial Nerve	Common Adaptations with Aging	Changes in Testing Technique
I. Olfactory	No change or progressive loss of smell	No change
II. Optic	Reduced visual acuity Presbyopia Restricted visual field	Use bright light. Place light source behind client when testing visual acuity
III. Oculomotor	Reaction to light less brisk Accommodation less brisk (both pupillary constriction and convergence)	
III. Oculomotor IV. Trochlear VI. Abducens	Some restriction of upward gaze	No change
V. Trigeminal	No change	To elicit the corneal reflex, a prolongation of the stimulus may be required
VII. Facial	Sensory: Diminished perception of all taste modalities, especially sweet	Use more concentrated solution of sweet, salt, sour, and bitter
	Motor: No change in person with own teeth. Edentulous person may exhibit facial asymmetry unrelated to facial nerve function	No change
VIII. Auditory	Presbycusis: Initial loss of high frequencies; later losses in all frequencies	Test in quiet environment
IX. Glossopharyngeal X. Vagus	Gag reflex may be sluggish	No change
XI. Spinal accessory	No change	No change
XII. Hypoglossal	No change	No change

Adapted from Mezey MD, et al, 1980, with permission.

quently sluggish or absent. The abdominal reflex may be unobtainable by middle age, even in non-obese individuals. In aging women, absence of the abdominal reflex is due in part to muscles that have been overstretched, either by childbearing or obesity (Anderson, 1976; Grob, 1978).

Sensory Function. When testing sensory function, the aging client must be given sufficient time to respond to directions. If the client exhibits fatigue, poor concentration, or a negative attitude, the sensory examination should be rescheduled for a later time. If the client has mental status changes, testing sensory function may be difficult. Testing requires sustained attention to discriminate repeated stimuli (Mezey et al., 1980).

Because some reduction in the acuity of touch sensation occurs with age, stronger stimuli may be needed to test it. Diminished tactile sensation has important implications for the older person's safety. The sensation of superficial pain should be relatively intact, but the aging person's perception of deep pain may be severely diminished (Goldman, 1979). Perception of temperature is also blunted with age (Tichy and Malasanos, 1979). Although some sensory modalities are diminished with age, subjective sensory complaints, particularly paresthesias, increase with age (Pathy, 1978).

Position sense, particularly in the big toe, may be impaired or lost (Carter, 1979). When testing vibratory sense, the nurse must ensure that the client's limbs are warm. Appreciation of vibration decreases if the limbs are cold. The nurse should test vibration sense in both upper and lower limbs. Vibration sense remains intact until age 70. Thereafter, vibration sense appears to be diminished in the lower extremities to a greater extent than in the upper extremities. Eventually, vibration sense, particularly at the malleoli, may be lost altogether (Corso, 1971; Carter, 1979).

LABORATORY DATA: INTERPRETATION

In this technological age, clinicians rely heavily on laboratory values to determine whether the client is normal or different from normal. Age is known to have an important influence on a number of physiological variables, including laboratory values, which reflect declining organ function and changes in metabolic requirements. Consequently, standard laboratory values are required that are based on a healthy population similar to the client being tested.

A major problem that has confronted gerontologists is the lack of age-related standards with which to compare the aging client's values. When standards based on healthy young adults are used as criteria against which to measure the older client, there is uncertainty about whether deviations from

standard values represent normal aging or a disease process.

Normal values are usually determined by surveying a group of presumably healthy individuals, determining the mean of the results, and setting a normal range of two standard deviations on either side of that mean. A limited number of studies have been done to identify standard normal values for the aging client and the laboratory values cited in this section are based on those studies.

Not only has the number of studies that included an elderly population been small, but many of these studies had limited sample sizes. In addition, although some investigators performed physical examinations and did laboratory work to determine that the subjects in the study were in good health, others employed questionnaires. Even when great care is taken, it is always possible to overlook an underlying pathological process. The possibility of doing so in the elderly is even greater, as the incidence of disease increases with age. Some investigators included subjects who were institutionalized or taking medications, whereas others limited themselves to subjects who were living at home and were free of medication. Comparison among studies is complicated because several different acceptable methods and techniques of measurement were used to determine a number of the laboratory values.

Because of these limitations, standard laboratory values should be used with caution until more research data are available. Nevertheless, the nurse working with an older client should have age-related standard values available when making clinical judgments about the client's adaptations.

Hematology

Tables 3 and 4 present age-related erythrocyte values using data from a study by Shapleigh et al. (1952) of 50 men and 50 women, all deemed healthy, between the ages of 65 and 90. The results of this study agree with data from earlier studies and are believed to be an accurate reflection of the blood picture of a healthy older client. MacKinney's (1978) study, however, found that the lymphocyte count declines with age, reflecting a loss of T lymphocytes. This finding seems reasonable in light of the fact that immune functions are known to decline with age.

TABLE 3. ERYTHROCYTE VALUES

Variable		Young Adult Values[A] Range		Over-60 Values[B] Range	Mean	Expected Change with Normal Aging
RBC (millions/μl)	M	4.5–6.2	M	3.72–5.96	4.75	Remains within
	W	4.2–5.4	W	3.65–5.55	4.71	young adult range
HB (g%)	M	14–17	M	10.9–17.2	14.1	Remains within
	W	12.5–15.5	W	11.6–16.2	13.17	young adult range
Hematocrit (%)	M	40–52	M	38.12–42.1	46.08	Remains within
	W	35–47	W	37.91–40.8	43.69	young adult range
Reticulocytes (%)		0.1–2.0	M	0.2–4.2	2.01	Remains within
			W	0.4–3.6	1.16	young adult range
MCV (μm³)		82–105	M	74–110	89.2	Remains within
			W	78–101	87.3	young adult range
MCHb Gamma globulin (pg)		27–31	M	24–33	29.2	Remains within
			W	23–34	29.2	young adult range
MCHb concentration (%)		32–36	M	27–36	33.5	No change or slightly
			W	30–36	33.5	lower
Total WBC (μl)		4500–11,000	M	4250–16,000	7730	Remains within
			W	3150–10,350	6497	young adult range
White Cell Differential						
Basophils (%)		0–0.75	M	0–4	1.1	No change
			W	0.3	1.0	
Eosinophils (%)		1–3	M	0–9	4.4	No change
			W	0–17	4.7	
Myelocytes (%)		0	M	0–1	—	No change
			W	0–2	—	
Metamyelocytes (%)		occasional	M	0–1	—	No change
			W	0–1	—	
Bands or stabs (%)		3–5	M	0–5	1.4	No change
			W	0–8	1.5	
Polys or segs (%)		54–62	M	28–86	59.1	No change
			W	28–75	55.6	
Lymphocytes (%)		25–33	M	4–46	23.5	No change or
			W	11–62	27.7	decreased
Monocytes (%)		3–7	M	4–26	10.4	No change.[C]
			W	2–19	9.1	
Platelets (no./cm³)		400,000–800,000 (Dameshek method)	M	1,392,000–255,000	732,000	No change
			W	1,430,000–333,000	781,000	

[A]Harvey et al. (1980); Keopke (1979).
[B]Shapleigh et al. (1952).
[C]The higher levels reported here are due to the method of preparation used.
M = Men; W = Women

TABLE 4. ERYTHROCYTE SEDIMENTATION RATE (MM/HR; WINTROBE METHOD)

	Young Adult Value Range	Over-65 Value Range	Percent Above Young Adult Value
Men	<11 mm/hr	0–40+	92%
Women	<19 mm/hr	0–40+	84%

When evaluating the blood values of the elderly client, the nurse should expect the values to be close to or within the range established for young adults. If this is not the case, the nurse should look for stresses in the client's environment that might contribute to changes in the client's laboratory values. Does the client have the financial means to buy nutritious food? Is the client able to shop for food? Does the client eat well-balanced meals? Is the client taking medications that might interfere with the absorption of iron or vitamins or alter the hematology values of the elderly client? Might a subtle disease process be present?

Serum Chemistry

Table 5 presents data concerning serum chemistry values for the elderly. Available information on a number of values, including fasting glucose, inorganic phosphorus, potassium, sodium, creatinine, and total proteins, is conflicting. Nevertheless, when changes in these values have been noted, values have remained close to or within the normal ranges. Significant upward trends in cholesterol, urea nitrogen, and uric acid have been documented. After middle age, a significant decline in albumin occurs (Harnes, 1980; Reed et al., 1972). Although plasma potassium has been found to increase slightly in normal elderly subjects, hypokalemia is known to be common among the elderly as a consequence of diuretic therapy or dietary intake (Hyams, 1978; Wilding et al., 1972). Serum potassium levels do not accurately reflect potassium status in the body; red cell potassium levels are more reliable (Hyams, 1978). Plasma sodium levels have also been found

to remain constant or to decrease slightly as a result of diuretic therapy (Hyams, 1978; Wilding et al., 1972). Trends in the phosphate level have been difficult to pinpoint. With age, the level may fall slightly in men and rise slightly in women, so that the sex difference is more marked. Although more research is necessary to clarify normal serum chemistry values in the aged, it would appear that few, if any, values undergo significant changes.

Serum Enzymes

Because information about enzymes such as SCPK, LDH, SGOT, and SGPT are used to assess the status of the heart, liver, and muscles, the nurse should know whether any changes occur as a consequence of age alone. Information about serum enzyme values is displayed in Table 6. The upper limits of alkaline phosphatase levels gradually increase with age in both males and females, with females showing a more pronounced rise (Wilding et al., 1972; O'Kell and Elliott, 1970; Reed et al., 1972). No significant changes have been found in SGPT, SGOT, and SCPK (Reed et al., 1972; Hesch et al., 1976; McCormick, 1976). Stresses such as heavy exercise or an intramuscular injection may result in falsely high levels of SCPK in individuals at any age (McCormick, 1976). Data on LDH are equivocal. Although some studies indicate that LDH levels rise with age (O'Kell and Elliott, 1970), others indicate that no age-related change occurs (Reed et al., 1972; Hesch et al., 1976).

THE PSYCHOSOCIAL ASSESSMENT: TECHNIQUES AND FINDINGS

The psychosocial assessment of the healthy aging client can be as simple or as comprehensive as time and circumstance dictate. However, the more comprehensive the assessment, the more useful it will be in planning to meet the holistic needs of the client.

Much of the data needed for the psychosocial assessment is obtained from the health history, particularly the demographic data, current health status, family history, and personal and social history. Standardized assessment tools are also helpful in gathering data. To ensure that all the client's needs

TABLE 5. SERUM CHEMISTRY

		Young Adult Values[A]			Over Age 60 Values (Except Where Indicated)		
		Range	Median		Range	Median	Net Change
A/G ratio[B]	M	1.1–1.8	1.5	M	0.9–1.7	1.3	Decrease
	W	1.0–1.8	1.4	W	1.0–1.7	1.3	
Albumin[C] (g/dl)		3.5–5.0		M	3.5–4.8	4.1	Decrease; decline is more pronounced in men
				W	3.5–4.8	4.1	
Total bilirubin[B] (mg/dl)		0.3–1.00		M	0.1–1.0	0.4	No significant change
				W	0.2–0.7	0.3	
Calcium[B] (mEq/l)		4.6–5.6		M	4.6–5.6	5.0	Slight decrease; but fall is within normal values
				W	4.6–5.6	5.1	
Cholesterol[B] (mg/dl)		130–315		M	155–308	234	Increase
				W	182–353	250	
Creatinine[D] (mg/dl)		0.7–1.4			0.82–0.84	—	No significant change or slight rise
Glucose(fasting)[B] (mg/dl)		65–110		M	73–159	93	Data conflicting, no change or very slight increase
				W	58130	91	
					(ages 50 and over)		
Inorganic Phosphorus[B] (mg/dl)		2.5–4.5		M	2.0–4.4	3.1	No trend identified
				W	2.3–4.6	3.5	
Potassium[C] mmol/L		3.5–5.0		M	3.7–5.3	4.49	Data conflicting, slight increase
				W	3.5–5.6	4.55	
					(ages 60–69)		
Total Protein[B] (g/dl)		6.0–8.0		M	6.6–8.4	7.3	No change or slight decrease
				W	6.4–8.6	7.3	
Sodium[C] (mEq/L)		135–145		M	135.0–146.0	140.51	No change or slight decrease
				W	135.6–146.8	141.19	
Urea Nitrogen[B] mg/100 ml		8–19		M	10–38	18	Increase
				W	10–30	17	
Uric Acid[B] mg/100 ml	M	2.5–8.0		M	3.8–10.0	6.2	Slight increase
	W	2.5–6.4		W	3.3–7.8	4.9	

[A]All young adult values except A/G ratio from Koepke (1979); A/G ratio from Reed et al. (1972).
[B]Reed et al. (1972).
[C]Wilding et al. (1972).
[D]Rowe (1976).
M = Men; W = Women

TABLE 6. SERUM ENZYMES

		Young Adult Values (30–59)			Over Age 60 Values			
		Range	Median		Range	Median		Net Change
Alkaline[A]	M	5–16	7	M	5–21	8		Increase
Phosphatase	W	5–15	9	W	5–20	10		
(KAU/100 ml)								
LDH[A] (WU/1)	M	60–145	93	M	60–133	90		Conflicting data, no
	W	55–136	86	W	70–155	100		significant change or
								slight elevation
SGPT[B] (U/1)	M & W	1–35		M & W	0.74–12.5	6.60 (mean)		No significant change
SGOT[A] (KU/ml)	M	15–54	31	M	13–55	29		No significant change
	W	12–71	24	W	13–67	28		
SCPK[C] (U/L)	M	40–200		M	4.2–75	29.9		No significant change
	W	35–150		W	1.7–37.5	16.3		

[A]Reed et al. (1972).
[B]Hesch (1976).
[C]McCormick (1976).
M = Men; W = Women.

are met, the psychosocial assessment should involve the following elements:

- Mental status, focusing on cognitive and emotional adaptations
- Social adaptations, including social relationships and supports
- Sexual functioning
- Economic resources
- Functional status, especially the capacity to perform activities of daily living

Interviewing the Client

Unlike physical health assessment, which most clients are willing and anxious to undergo, aspects of the psychosocial assessment may be very threatening. Declining physical health is somehow easier to accept than the thought of a decline in mental functioning, which is often viewed as the final disintegration. Sexual functioning and economic resources are other areas that many elderly clients, unlike their younger cohorts, may find difficult to discuss.

Given the sensitive areas that must be ad-dressed in a thorough assessment it is necessary at the outset to instill confidence by conducting the interview in an empathetic manner. The older generation, unlike the much-tested students of today, approach any test situation with apprehension; moreover, the folklore that surrounds senility carries an added threat (Comfort, 1978). The more anxious clients are about memory loss, for example, the more likely they are to become cautious, vague, and inefficient during the interview. Consequently, it is wise to ask questions specific to mental functioning in the context of general health and social problems—as just one facet of the total person. It also helps to indicate that the questions asked are routinely asked of all clients to get a better perspective of the total life situation. Tests of intellectual functioning will be far less threatening if they are incorporated throughout the interview. For example, questions concerning remote memory ("What year were you born?") and recent memory ("What is your present address?" or "On what street is your food market located?") can be asked as part of the demographic data. Although excellent short forms of the mental status assessment (discussed later in this chapter) have been devised and thoroughly tested for their validity and reliability, the information they seek can be obtained without threatening the client, if the questions are interwoven within the nursing history.

Initially, clients should be encouraged to talk freely about any problems they are experiencing. The use of accepted interview techniques will assist both the flow and progression of the interview. Frequent restatement of what the nurse has heard indicates interest as an interviewer. The nurse should not allow the most anxiety-provoking issues (usually questions related to cognitive or sexual functioning) to be raised at the end of the interview. The end should be saved for the client's concerns. By allowing clients to have the last word, they can regain control over the interview situation. Complimenting them on how well they have handled the interview, for example, "You've really given me a good picture of yourself, your health, and your concerns," is another way of restoring control to clients.

Assessing Cognitive and Emotional Adaptations

In assessing mental status, several major areas take priority in the aging client. Among these are the client's appearance, cognitive status, including orientation, memory, and general intellectual level, emotional or affective state, and adaptive capacity.

Appearance. Overall appearance is a good indicator of health and well-being in the client. The client who is dressed appropriately for the occasion (weather and social situation), is clean in appearance, and well groomed provides an impression of health, vitality, and self-esteem. By the same token, evidence of deterioration, whether in mood, mentation, or functional ability, frequently shows up in the appearance of the individual. Clients who appear too old for their years or women who are too youthfully dressed for their age give one pause for consideration about underlying physical or emotional problems. The client who appears drably dressed in dark, colorless garb may be experiencing some degree of depression. The client who is unbathed, unshaven, or uncombed gives evidence of a general lack of self-interest, preoccupation, or perhaps a declining functional ability.

Motor Function. This is another key to health and vitality. Posture (whether erect or slouched) can also offer clues to mental outlook. (Some degree of stooping is encountered in the aging female client due to osteoporosis and subsequent Dowager's hump.) The grip of a handshake is another clue to vigor and outlook. Tremors, spastic movements, and weakness can be noted in the handshake. The nurse must keep in mind that cultural overlay, especially with the elderly woman, may preclude a vigorous handshake!

Overall Activity Level. Activity level can also be determined early in the interview. Clients who are overactive, for example, literally jumping out of the chair as words tumble out of their mouth, may well be experiencing severe anxiety; this can, in turn, interfere with thought processes and functional performance. The client who appears listless or underactive may be experiencing depression or an adaptation to the not uncommonly seen hypothyroidism.

Facial Expression. Facial expression is another clue to underlying problems. Tension, worry, sadness, anger, pain, or even suspicion can all be revealed in the client's expression. A wonderful film called "The Faces of Depression" produced many years ago by the Geigy pharmaceutical company illustrated the wide range of facial expressions that could be indicative of underlying depression. By the same token, it pointed up a number of other psychiatric conditions that could masquerade as depression if not more closely scrutinized.

Cognitive Status. Impairment of memory and intellectual function is a common concern of the elderly. The stereotype of forgetfulness, frequently presented as humorous in situation comedies, seems to have a brainwashing effect on the elderly. It makes the threat of memory loss and disorientation very real. One older client who was reciting events from the remote and more recent past, naming names and providing precise dates, kept interrupting her account to reassure herself and the listener, "You see, my mind is clear as a bell. I remember—I still have a good memory."

For a small percentage of the elderly, intellectual impairment does become a problem. Since

adaptations related to impaired mentation may be
the first sign of an acute but treatable brain syndrome, a careful assessment of mentation is desirable in every mental status exam. To assess orientation and memory (both remote and recent) a
battery of very simple questions can be used and,
for the most part, disguised as questions seeking
demographic information.

In assessing orientation, the client should be
tested for time, place, and person with questions
concerning the day of the week, the time of day,
the date, name of the agency, current address, and
names of familiar people in the surrounding. In
testing memory it is helpful to differentiate between
immediate retention and recall, memory for the recent past, and memory for the remote past. *Remote
past* can be tested by reviewing important events in
the client's life. Among the questions to be asked
are the time and place of birth, various schools
attended, occupational history, date of marriage,
and number of children. *Recent memory* can be
tested in a clinic situation by asking clients to review
the names and schedule of their medications. If at
home, clients might be asked about their last visit
to the clinic or health facility, or about the nurse's
last visit to their home. The nurse might also ask
for an update on health-related activities since the
last meeting. *Immediate retention and recall* can be
tested if the client is asked to repeat the nurse's
name several minutes after introductions have been
made. Here the attempt is to assess the client's
current ability to process and retain information.
Sometimes this test is conducted by giving the client
three digits to recall. This might be done more sub-
tly by giving clients the extension of the clinic telephone and asking them to repeat it.

General Intellectual Evaluation. An assessment
of overall intelligence and judgment can be made
by asking clients whether they have been following
some important issue of the day (a school strike,
an election, a threatened conflict) and asking for
their evaluation of the situation.

Emotional State. To evaluate a client's emotional
state it is necessary to ascertain both the subjective
aspect of the client's experience and its objective
expression. Objectively, the nurse can observe facial expression, motor behavior, tremors, respira-

tory irregularities, crying, and the general state of
excitement, fear, or depression. Subjective data are
best elicited through the use of nonleading questions: "How are you feeling?" or "How have you
been managing lately?" If clients respond with a
general term or phrase "Not too well," or "Nervous," they should be asked to describe in what
way things are not going well or how the nervousness shows itself and how it is affecting them. Nervousness may be the client's subjective way of pinpointing a problem with depression or anxiety, two
of the more commonly seen emotional problems in
the elderly.

Depression. Depression may be mild and represent a response to adverse factors such as isolation
or bereavement, but it is important to make an accurate diagnosis so that rational treatment can be
undertaken (Caird and Judge, 1974). To elicit the
depth, intensity, and persistence of the depression,
clients should be asked if they have been crying or
if they have felt like crying, if they feel discouraged,
and whether they have been troubled by thoughts
of hurting themselves.

Anxiety. Anxiety results in a number of observable adaptations. Affectively, the client will appear
worried, fearful or apprehensive. Cognitively, the
client will lack concentration and show decreased
memory. There may also be some perceptual defects. Most commonly, there will be a number of
somatic adaptations, including muscle tightness,
tremors, tension headaches, fatigue, palpitations,
hyperventilation, nausea and vomiting, urinary frequency, and flushing of the face. The client will
also complain of difficulty in falling asleep or fitful
sleep, sometimes with nightmares.

Adaptive Capacity. Another important aspect of
the assessment is to determine how elderly clients
have been able to cope with stressful events in their
life, especially events that have occurred within the
past year. At this stage of life, not only is more
stress likely to be encountered but its effects are
considered to be more deleterious to the aging system. Social stresses are generally viewed as significant precipitants of psychological impairment in
the elderly. Neugarten (1970) concluded that it was
not the expected event but rather those unexpected

events occurring "off time," such as the death of a spouse or loss of income, which were less well tolerated by the aging person. A study by Blazer (1980) suggests that although there is a correlation between stressful life events and health seeking behaviors (identified need for medication or counseling), the adaptive capacity of the elderly person is actually quite good. As Selye (1956) concluded years ago, older people may be at an advantage in adapting to the stress of life. The Blazer study also suggested that nonwhites, because of their increased experience with and exposure to stressful events, may have even more adaptive capacity when handling stressful events.

The kind of ego defenses and coping behaviors utilized by the client are an important indicator of adaptive capacity. In his study of ego defenses, Vaillant (1971) proposed that a hierarchy of defenses, ranging from mature to psychotic, exists. He found a correlation between predominant defenses used by his subjects and their overall life adjustment. Vaillant first examined the defensive system in use by his subjects as it was manifested behaviorally. He then had his subjects scored independently on the basis of adjustment. At the highest level of mature functioning, defenses such as altruism, humor, suppression, and sublimation were most commonly seen. At the next level were neurotic defenses like intellectualization, repression, displacement, reaction formation, and dissociation. At the "immature" level were defenses associated with character or affective disorders, such as acting out, passive aggressive behavior, and hypochondriasis. At the psychotic level of functioning, termed "narcissistic," were denial, delusion, projection, and distortion. Interestingly, over the course of three decades of study, Vaillant found that a given individual repeatedly used a certain defensive style. The adaptive behaviors of the aged apparently reflect an earlier coping style.

Assessing Social Adaptations

The social assessment includes elements of the family history and personal and social history discussed earlier. It appraises the client's interpersonal relationships within the supportive network of family, relatives, and friends. It also looks at the degree of involvement or isolation the client maintains with the outside world. This is often reflected in attendance at clubs, senior citizen centers, or services and socials sponsored by the client's place of worship. Many older clients rely heavily on the support and comfort provided by their association with their religion and place of worship, a fact that is too often overlooked by the younger professional. Often it is this association which provides the stimulation and sharing experiences that ward off isolation. An active religious affiliation may also be a viable source of strength and support in times of crisis.

Assessing Sexual Function

Changes associated with the sexual response in a healthy aging client appear in Table 7. The only age-determined change in male erectile physiology is the slowing of the general response cycle, combined with a less perfect regulation of inflow of blood in the corpora. As a result, erection in males often appears less firm than in youth, though it is fully adequate (Comfort, 1980). Though less fully documented in the literature, sexual function in women seems to persist even more effectively than in men. There is no evidence that the capacity for orgasm declines at any age. Comfort (1980) notes that women have been known to become orgasmic for the first time in ages in excess of eighty! Although coitus may be impaired by vaginal atrophy or a lack of lubrication, these conditions, as well as cystocele and uterine prolapse, are all remediable. It is even Comfort's belief that regular intercourse is as effective as exogenous estrogens in preventing secretory and atrophic changes.

Menopause, once considered synonymous with a decline in sexual function, is actually for many women a period of renewed sexual enjoyment untroubled by anxiety about conception. For the woman who perceives infertility as a loss of womanhood it may indeed have negative psychological overtones. The so-called male menopause inaccurately describes what is really a middle-age identity crisis that seems to affect the male sexual image but that has little effect on endocrine production. In the final analysis, the most important factors regarding continued sexual functioning in the later years seem to be the aging person's lifelong pattern of sexual expression, the availability of a partner, and a feeling of self-esteem.

A good psychosocial history should include a sexual history. Generally, physicians have ignored

TABLE 7. HUMAN SEXUAL RESPONSE: CHANGES ASSOCIATED WITH NORMAL AGING

Stages	Male	Female
Excitation	Longer arousal time Increased time for erection Penis not as firm due to decreased vasocongestion Decreased myotonia	Longer arousal time Increased time for lubrication Decreased lubrication due to decreased vasocongestion Decreased myotonia
Plateau	Can hold erection longer	Longer time needed for female orgasmic response
Orgasm	Less ejaculatory pressure May not always ejaculate Longer refractory period (may last 12–24 hours)	May be shorter in duration May be less intense
Resolution	Faster	Faster

this area, but this does not excuse the nurse. Steffl (1978) recommends that the sexual history be elicited in the context of other social relationships and other activities including religion. It may take time to broach the topic sensitively but there are ways of opening up this area for discussion. For example, the nurse can ask about early orientation to sexual behavior. How did the client first learn about sex? Children have many ingenious ways to satisfy their curiosity about the subject. The nurse should ask about masturbation as a child. Many of the current generation of older clients have residual feelings around this topic, since they were taught to believe that masturbation was the work of the devil. Alternatively, the nurse might ask if the client remembers a first sexual experience. The memory is usually quite vivid. If the client is currently widowed, the nurse can ask if the client has considered another relationship. If not, how are sexual feelings currently being handled?

Raising these questions within the context of an holistic social assessment gives the client permission to discuss current feelings and concerns about sexuality. It may also raise a number of questions that the nurse is unable to answer. However, the counseling role does not demand that the nurse provide all the answers (Steffl, 1978). What it does require is that the nurse help older clients to find their own answers. Many of these answers they already have; what they need is sanction and sup-port. By opening up the area for discussion, the nurse can lend that support and provide much needed information to dispel the ignorance and myth that surrounds the area.

Assessing Economic Resources
Another aspect of the social history is that of economic resources. It is a well-known fact that financial deprivation can impair social, mental, and physical functioning. Sufficient income, on the other hand, can greatly improve the client's life situation by making health-related resources available.

Assessing Activities of Daily Living
The client's functional ability in activities of daily living is a critical yet often neglected aspect of the psychosocial assessment. The ability to perform self-care activities can be crucial to the self-esteem of an aging client. The nurse should assess performance in two areas: capacity to care for bodily functions and ability to maintain an independent household (discussed earlier). Many clients will require some help with shopping, heavy housework, and laundry as they age, but this would be considered only a mild impairment in activities of daily living.

The Use of Assessment Tools
There are a variety of assessment tools that might be used in making a psychosocial assessment. Comprehensive tools, geared to a holistic assessment,

have also been devised and tested (Foley and Schneider, 1980; Duke-OARS, 1978). The advantage of a comprehensive tool is that, in addition to determining the client's mental and physical status, it includes social and economic determinants as well as functional data on activities of daily living.

The use of standardized tools for data collection has important implications for the nurse who works with an elderly population. Systematized, validated tools provide a common language for discussing the health problems and specific needs of the aging client. This aspect is especially critical if the nurse intends to communicate with a large system, i.e., at the regional, state, or federal level, where programs can be recommended based on identified needs. The use of standardized data collection tools will help develop the kind of data base that is needed to support such change. Should nurses feel limited by any particular standardized tool, they can always expand their data base by adding questions addressing their own area of research. Tools have been used by the U.S. Government Accounting office to provide information on the functional status of an aging client population from one year to the next. The kind of data generated from a standardized tool also allows for program evaluation, namely, whether current resources are adequate, misplaced, or are making a difference in the functional status of clients.

A problem in the use of assessment tools, recently brought to light in the research of Foley and Schneider (1980), was the great variation that exists in the application of standardized assessment tools. The researchers evaluated almost 700 clients using six different comprehensive tools and found that the level of care recommended differed markedly, depending on the tool used. Potentially negative consequences can result from this lack of uniformity in application. Clients can be made dependent by providing more assistance than is actually needed, or, perhaps worse, their care may be inadequate because insufficient assistance is being provided.

One example of a comprehensive assessment tool is the OARS Multidimensional Functional Assessment Questionnaire (MFAQ), developed by an interdisciplinary group at Duke University's Center for the Study of Aging and Human Development. The OARS instrument is designed for use with in-

dividuals and/or populations and measures a subject's current functional level in each of five areas: social resources, economic resources, mental health, physical health, and capacity for self-care (Pfeiffer, 1978). Information gathered can be compressed or summarized into a single functional rating. The best rating (1) represents outstanding functioning; the poorest (6) represents complete impairment. The same scale applies to each of the five areas evaluated. A rating of (5) on social resources means "severely socially impaired"; a rating of (5) on mental health means severe intellectual impairment.

A second part of the MFAQ seeks information about a variety of services that aging or impaired clients might require. A simple listing of basic maintenance, supportive, and remedial services is provided.

The major advantage of the OARS instrument (MFAQ) is that it is holistic in its approach to the person. Often the elderly client who is psychiatrically impaired will begin to show signs of impairment in the activities of daily living. A physically impaired client may become socially isolated, which, in turn, could result in depression. Today many disciplines who work with the elderly have become so specialized in their services that it is difficult for them to assess the total level of functioning of the client. Since the OARS tool has been thoroughly tested for validity and reliability, many agencies today are using all or part of the questionnaire for client assessment. The tool has the added advantage of requiring only 45 minutes for the total assessment, once some practice has been gained in its use.

Copies of the MFAQ can be obtained by writing to the Center for the Study of Aging and Human Development, Duke University Medical Center, Durham, North Carolina 27710. As of the present writing, cost of individual copies is $6.50.

Mental Status Assessment. One instrument that evaluates overall mental and social function as well as the parameters of judgment and emotional state was devised by Libow (1977) and is called by the acronym FROMAJE. The test is scored on a 3-point scale. A minimal score of 7 or 8 is indicative of adequate functioning; 9–10 indicates minimal dysfunction; 11–12, moderate dysfunction; and 13 and above indicates severe dysfunction. The areas assessed are as follows:

1. Function: ability to live at home and maintain oneself in the community.
   Score—(1) no support needed, (2) some home support, (3) 24-hour support.
2. Reasoning: ability to explain a proverb.
   Score—(1) well explained, (2) part explanation, (3) inability to explain or concrete.
3. Orientation: to time, place and person.
   Score—(1) no errors, (2) error in one area, (3) errors in two areas.
4. Memory: distant, recent, and immediate memory.
   Distant: "What was the name of the President of the United States during World War II?"
   Recent: "Have you had breakfast? lunch? supper?"
   Immediate: "What did I ask you about the President?"
   Score—(1) no errors, (2) error in one area, (3) error in two areas.
5. Arithmetic: counting from 1 to 10 and backwards to 1; subtracting 7 from 100 and continuing to subtract 7.
   Score—(1) complete accuracy, (2) one significant error, (3) two or more significant errors.
6. Judgment: "If you need help at night, how do you obtain it?" or "If you saw fire in your wastepaper basket, what action would you take?"
   Score—(1) generally sensible responses, (2) poor judgment, (3) extremely poor judgment.
7. Emotional state: client's manner is observed during interview. Client is asked about crying, sadness, depression, optimism, future plans, etc.
   Score—(1) reasonable, appropriate, (2) grandiose, anxious, depressed, paranoid, (3) inappropriate ideas, severe depression.

The Libow inventory offers a quick, easy to administer evaluation of major areas of the mental status exam. Many psychiatrists indicate that serial sevens (counting down by 7 from 100) is too difficult and suggest using serial threes instead, i.e., subtracting three from 100. The advantage of the Libow inventory is that it addresses three major areas of concern in the elderly client, namely the client's orientation, emotional status, and ability to function.

The Mental Status Questionnaire (MSQ) shown in Table 8 provides a simple yet valid test of cognitive impairment. Consisting of 10 items extracted by means of discriminant analysis from a pool of 31 items (Kahn et al., 1960), the MSQ utilizes a standardized format and quantifies responses of the client in terms of an error score.

In the Goldfarb–Kahn series of studies of the tool, it was found that only 6 percent of the clients who performed without error were later independently diagnosed by a geriatric psychiatrist as having a chronic brain syndrome. On the other hand, 95 percent of those who scored the maximum number of errors (ten) were diagnosed as having a chronic brain syndrome. The researchers also found a higher death rate (three times higher) in clients scoring nine or ten errors than in those scoring one or two errors (Gurland, 1980).

The MSQ has also been shown to correlate well with activities of daily living. In a study by Wilson et al. (1973), 100 female geriatric patients who were not unduly handicapped by their multiple physical problems were given simple tests, including serial sevens, proverb interpretation, and the MSQ. Their capacity for ADL was then rated independently by an occupational therapist. The MSQ correlated best with ADL performance. Surprisingly, levels of depression or anxiety had no bearing on ADL performance. The study indicates the importance of testing any person with a poor MSQ score on the ability to perform ADL.

There are many variations of the MSQ (Pfeiffer, 1975; Lawson et al. 1977) but all address essentially the same questions and are predictive of organic brain damage. There seems to be a basic orderliness in the sequence of abilities lost as the dementing process advances, and this is reflected in a worsening score on the MSQ. Although longer and more extensive testing might be more sensitive to minor changes in cognitive states, for most purposes the MSQ and its analogues provide an easy-to-use assessment tool for monitoring cognitive adaptations.

Another test of mentation frequently used is the Face–Hand Test (Goldfarb, 1964). The test involves a series of double simultaneous stimulations

TABLE 8.   MENTAL STATUS QUESTIONNAIRE (MSQ) AND RATING SCALE

MSQ

Question	Presumed Test Area
1. Where are we now?	Place
2. Where is this place located?	Place
3. What is today's date—day of month?	Time
4. What month is it?	Time
5. What year is it?	Time
6. How old are you?	Memory—recent or remote
7. What is your birthday?	Memory—recent or remote
8. What year were you born?	Memory—recent or remote
9. Who is the President of the United States?	General information—memory
10. Who was President before him?	General information—memory

Rating of MSQ

Number of Errors	Presumed Mental Status
0–2	Chronic brain syndrome, absent or mild
3–5	Chronic brain syndrome, mild to moderate
6–8	Chronic brain syndrome, moderate to severe
9–10	Chronic brain syndrome, severe
Nontestable	Chronic brain syndrome, severe

From Kahn RL, Goldfarb AI, et al.: Aging and organic brain syndrome (1960). From the program Aging and Organic Brain Syndrome, Frazier S (ed). Bloomfield New Jersey, Health Learning Systems, 1974, with permission.

of the face and hand. Any failure to correctly report the touch on the back of the hand is presumptive of loss of neurons from the cortex. The test results are highly correlated with the degree of brain syndrome measured by the MSQ and by psychiatric evaluation.

The Face–Hand test is conducted with the client seated facing the examiner with feet flat on the floor and hands resting on the knees. The client is touched or brushed simultaneously on one cheek and the dorsum of one hand, usually in a specified order. The test is first conducted with the client's eyes closed, then the series is repeated with eyes open. Eighty percent of persons who make errors with eyes closed will show no improvement with the eyes open.

In the four initial trials, the client becomes accustomed to the procedure. Trials 5 and 6 are teaching trials during which the examiner informs the client where he or she was touched. Trials 7–10 repeat the first four trials; any errors are considered presumptive of brain damage. Errors include the following: not reporting the touch to the hand (extinction), localizing the hand touch to the cheek, the knee, or elsewhere (displacement), pointing to the examiner's hand (projection); or pointing outside in space (exsomasthesia).

Measuring Depression. A number of scales are available to measure depression: The Hamilton Rating for Depression (Hamilton, 1960); Beck Depression Inventory (Beck et al., 1961); Depressive Scale by Cutler and Kurland (1961). One of the best and most practical is the Zung Self-Rating Scale (Zung, 1965), which is shown in Table 9. It is a brief, self-administered test that is balanced for positive and negative responses. It covers a wide variety of depressive adaptations (affective, somatic, and psychological) that are measured on a 4-point scale of severity. The Self-Rating Scale is constructed so

TABLE 9. SELF-RATING DEPRESSION SCALE

	A Little of the Time	Some of the Time	A Good Part of the Time	Most of the Time
1. I feel down-hearted and blue	1	2	3	4
2. Morning is when I feel the best	4	3	2	1
3. I have crying spells or feel like it	1	2	3	4
4. I have trouble sleeping at night	1	2	3	4
5. I eat as much as I used to	4	3	2	1
6. I still enjoy sex	4	3	2	1
7. I notice that I am losing weight	1	2	3	4
8. I have trouble with constipation	1	2	3	4
9. My heart beats faster than usual	1	2	3	4
10. I get tired for no reason	1	2	3	4
11. My mind is as clear as it used to be	4	3	2	1
12. I find it easy to do the things I used to	4	3	2	1
13. I am restless and can't keep still	1	2	3	4
14. I feel hopeful about the future	4	3	2	1
15. I am more irritable than usual	1	2	3	4
16. I find it easy to make decisions	4	3	2	1
17. I feel that I am useful and needed	4	3	2	1
18. My life is pretty full	4	3	2	1
19. I feel that others would be better off if I were dead	1	2	3	4
20. I still enjoy the things I used to do	4	3	2	1

From Zung W, 1965, with permission.

that lower scores correlate with lower levels of depression, higher scores with greater depression. A raw score of 50 and above was associated with depression requiring hospitalized treatment (Zung, 1965). However, any raw score above 30 would require a more extensive evaluation on the part of the nurse.

Where a self-administered test is not possible because of the client's frailty, perceptual problems, or lack of sophistication, a semistructured technique like the Geriatric Mental State Interview (Gurland et al., 1976) can be used. Whatever scale or interview technique is used, the assessment should include appraisal of the depressed mood, somatic adaptations (appetite, sleep pattern and other vegetative signs), the level of anxiety, motor retardation, and irritability. A good psychosocial history will also take note of any prior episodes of depression, including hospitalizations, and any recent stresses due to life-change events.

Measuring Anxiety. Karen Horney (1957, p 71) stated, "fear and anxiety are both proportionate reactions to danger but in the case of fear the danger is a transparent, objective one and in the case of anxiety it is hidden and subjective." As Freud linked anxiety to separation and the fear of castration, Horney links this feeling to repressed hostility. The person suffers a blow to self-esteem, but rather than fighting back, pretends that everything is all right. Such repression of anger generates a feeling of defenselessness. Repressed anger or hostility, traditionally viewed as the stresses that produce depression, may also, in Horney's view, produce anxiety.

Elderly clients have much to be anxious about in our society, beginning with the stigma of ageism and continuing with the insensitive treatment accorded by landlords, social agencies, and even health professionals—not to mention other segments of the society. The degree of anxiety evoked by a given stress can often be inferred from direct observations of the client's behavior. Such observations reflect cognitive, emotional, and somatic processes that are occurring simultaneously. As the level of anxiety increases and the sympathetic nervous system is fully activated, the perceptual field will narrow and the client will experience an increasing sense of threat and helplessness. At this point, signs of increasing disorganization will be observed directly in the behavior.

One of the tools used to assess anxiety is a self-administered scale devised by Zung (1971) (Table 10). The client is asked to rate each of 20 items to the degree that it applied within the past week. When the Zung scale was normed, using a control group of functioning professionals and a mixed diagnostic group of clients that included depressives,

schizophrenics, and patients suffering from anxiety disorders and personality disorders, the control group scored lowest and those in the patient group with an anxiety disorder scored highest. The average raw score for the control group was 27. For those with an anxiety disorder, the average score was 46. An alternate version of the SAS, known as the Anxiety Status Inventory, is designed for administration by the interviewer. Correlation between the Anxiety Status Interview and the Self-Rating Anxiety Scale is significant.

Making a Home Visit

The home visit has been advocated by Anderson (1978) as an essential component of health services for the aged. The home visit provides a way of

TABLE 10. SELF-RATING ANXIETY SCALE (SAS)

	None or a Little of the Time	Some of the Time	A Good Part of the Time	Most of the Time
1. I feel more nervous and anxious than usual	1	2	3	4
2. I feel afraid for no reason at all	1	2	3	4
3. I get upset easily or feel panicky	1	2	3	4
4. I feel like I'm falling apart and going to pieces	1	2	3	4
5. I feel that everything is all right and nothing bad will happen	4	3	2	1
6. My arms and legs shake and tremble	1	2	3	4
7. I am bothered by headaches, neck and back pains	1	2	3	4
8. I feel weak and get tired easily	1	2	3	4
9. I feel calm and can sit still easily	4	3	2	1
10. I can feel my heart beating fast	1	2	3	4
11. I am bothered by dizzy spells	1	2	3	4
12. I have fainting spells or feel like it	1	2	3	4
13. I can breathe in and out easily	4	3	2	1
14. I get feelings of numbness and tingling in my fingers, toes	1	2	3	4
15. I am bothered by stomach aches or indigestion	1	2	3	4
16. I have to empty my bladder often	1	2	3	4
17. My hands are usually dry and warm	4	3	2	1
18. My face gets hot and blushes	1	2	3	4
19. I fall asleep easily and get a good night's rest	4	3	2	1
20. I have nightmares	1	2	3	4

From Zung W, 1971, with permission.

contacting that portion of the aging population that is isolated or homebound. It allows for an assessment of the aging person's day-to-day environment where a few basic modifications may improve its safety and prolong the client's ability to live independently. The home visit also provides one of the best opportunities for assessing many aspects of the client's psychosocial functioning. On a single home visit, some assessment can be made of the client's activities of daily living, knowledge about medications and their administration, nutritional habits, and safety factors and health hazards within the client's home and in the surrounding community.

Community Resources.   On the way to the client's home, accessibility of public transportation, adequacy of shopping facilities and nearby health resources can all be assessed. Is there a bus or subway route nearby? Are shopping facilities located in the neighborhood? What type and variety of stores are available? The nurse can derive some idea of the range of prices for food and clothing in passing shop windows. Is the area densely or sparsely populated? Help for the client may be close at hand or at some distance. What health resources are located in the neighborhood? Is there a community hospital, a clinic, a roster of dentists, opticians, druggists, and podiatrists (some of the more frequently visited health resources of the elderly)? What about restaurants? Are there restaurants or cafeterias where reasonably priced meals can be taken?

Safety Factors.   Are sidewalks smooth and passable or are there broken, uprooted pavements that could be hazardous when walking? What about the traffic flow? Is it orderly? Are there stop signs at dangerous corners, and pedestrian crosswalks and crossing signals? Are the signs obeyed? What about litter in the streets or on sidewalks? Is refuse properly bagged? Is it piled high, indicating a lack of sanitation service to the area? Are animals allowed to run free or are they leashed and cared for? Are police evident on the streets? Is there a fire station nearby?

Social Resources.   Are there churches or other places of worship in the neighborhood? Are there other facilities for socialization—senior citizen clubs

or recreation centers? One New York bank provides three hours of piano music daily to local residents—most of them elderly people from the neighborhood. A suburban town with housing for the elderly has provided a nearby recreation facility offering daily programs to all elderly members of the community. A knowledge and understanding of the community will be helpful in suggesting resources to the client. Beyond that, it may contribute to a better understanding of the client's problems and more realistic planning with the client to resolve them.

The Client's Home.   Location is important. Is the client living in an elevated building, a fifth floor walk-up, a row house, or an isolated rural home? A fifth floor walk-up makes it difficult for all but the healthiest of clients to get out on a daily basis. Even if the client has no impairment in mobility, aging friends or children with young children of their own will find it difficult to visit. The nurse should look at the social atmosphere of the area. Are neighbors friendly? Do they drop in or call while the nurse is visiting? In an apartment building, do they seem to greet and talk with each other?

Home Safety.   Is there a phone within easy reach for emergency calls? Are emergency numbers of the police, fire department, medical doctor, and community hospital or ambulance service posted near the phone? Are there safety hazards in full view? Sometimes the clutter of accumulated treasures can be a safety hazard in itself. Many homes and apartments have become too crowded with memorabilia over the years. As visual acuity decreases, they can become a hazard. What about the physical condition of the interior? Is the paint chipping off?—it may contain a lead-based contaminant. Are the ceilings intact or is there danger from falling plaster due to plumbing leaks? Many elderly clients who live in rent-controlled apartments are afraid to complain to landlords about hazardous conditions in the apartment, knowing they may be subjected to harassment and pressure to vacate or be relocated. Relocation, even to better neighborhoods and improved housing, is not always in the interest of the client, who may have always lived in the same neighborhood.

What about cleanliness and orderliness in the home? Disorder is a lifelong adaptation for some people but for the person who is traditionally neat and well organized, disorder may be related to failing physical health or mental impairment. Vermin need not represent uncleanliness on the part of the client. For example, the first tenants of one luxury building with a riverside view moved in to find rats! Vermin may reflect what is happening in neighboring apartments or the inability of the client to confront the landlord for additional services.

Fastidiousness can also prove to be hazardous. Highly polished floors may cause loss of balance, falls, and fractures. Scatter rugs, although they lend a touch of warmth and charm, may also place the client at risk. Another risk factor encountered in older buildings is the uneven grading from room to room (the step-down living room, or the step-up bedroom). Although the client may have become quite accustomed to the split levels, there are times when night lighting or color coding are needed to call attention to these hazards.

Closets can also be a hazard, especially if heavy items are stored at the top. It may mean the use of step stools, which can be dangerous for the client, with the added danger that these items, if not securely stowed, could become dislodged during the client's attempts to reach other stored items.

The kitchen should also be assessed for safety. Poisonous cleaning materials should be stored away from food areas, so that they are not confused with cooking ingredients. Remembering that olfactory and visual cues are not as helpful to the aging client as they once were, other safety measures need to be considered. The stove should be checked. Is there a pilot light and is it glowing? Frequently pilot lights go out, emitting gas fumes; when jets are lighted, a minor explosion from accumulated gas may occur, possibly singeing the client or setting clothing afire. Is the stove located near a window? Frequently curtains will be blown close to gas jets, increasing the risk of a fire.

The bathroom is another area for safety checks. The aging client has diminished muscle strength to coordinate stepping in and out of the tub. If clients insist on maintaining established routines, they may be at risk for falls. If they do not, they may be at risk for reduced social interaction! Assistive devices have been developed to help the aging client maintain hygiene routines. Tub seats that fit over the tub with handles to grasp make it easier to get in and out of the tub. Handles can be installed in showers to grasp while bathing. Rubber mats prevent skidding or slipping and are essential for clients of any age.

Many aging clients find the toilet seat too low. With reduced muscular strength, it is difficult enough to descend to the level of the average toilet, but even more difficult to pull oneself off. The client can be advised that there are seats that fit over the toilet and raise the level. To ascertain the difficulty clients may have in this area, the nurse can note the type of chair they choose to sit in and the difficulty they have pushing themselves out of the chair.

Fire Hazards. Overloading of old circuitry, especially with additional heating appliances, can be dangerous in older buildings and homes. At times one finds an array of wires, resembling spaghetti, plugged into the same outlet. Again, the client's diminished visual acuity may fail to discern frayed electrical cords on lamps or appliances. The residence should be checked for smoke alarms. In many cities the fire code has made this device mandatory in apartments. For the elderly in any setting, it is essential. Clients should also be warned about the hazards of extra heating devices, kerosene stoves, gas heaters, electric heaters and about exposed steam pipes.

Intruders. Today one of the major considerations for the elderly is safety from intruders. As a precaution, many have extra locks on doors, alarm systems, and gates on the windows. The nurse should ascertain how gates on windows are opened; those requiring keys are not only illegal but extremely hazardous in the event of fire.

When the Client Lives Alone. If the client lives alone, the nurse should find out who checks on him or her each day. In some cities, the mailman informs the building superintendent if the mail is not picked up on a daily basis. More often it is a relative or next door neighbor who provides surveillance. One elderly woman with a hearing impairment had a neighbor who checked on her twice a day. He had synchronized a light to flash when the doorbell rang as an alternative cue for this woman's hearing deficit. The elderly are usually very adaptive and even inventive in the arrangements they make.

Recently the telephone company in some areas of the country has promoted the Vial-of-Life, a small plastic container which encloses a brief health history of the client, including diagnosis, medications, name of physician, and person to call in emergency. The vial is stored in the top right shelf of the refrigerator and a Vial-of-Life sticker is posted on the refrigerator door. Should the client be unable to give information to the rescue squad, vital information might be stored in the refrigerator. The idea seems to be taking hold and could be lifesaving to an aging client.

Nutrition. One of the major assessments that must be made on the home visit is the nutritional status of the client. This is discussed in Chapter 10. However, a 24-hour recall in the home setting can be helpful in a number of ways. It may give an accurate picture of the client's nutrition. Granted that clients sometimes relate what they think the nurse wants to hear, the information still allows the nurse to assess the client's level of knowledge about nutrition. If the nurse follows up by asking to see if food storage facilities are adequate, this provides an opportunity to confirm whether the food supplies match the stated diet.

Medications. The client's home is also the best place to determine what medication regimen has been prescribed and the manner in which the schedule is being followed. The nurse should ask clients to bring out their medications and show what they are taking and how they are taking them. One client, in recent memory, appeared with a soup tureen filled to the brim with prescription medications, not too many of which had ever been taken. She dutifully had the prescriptions filled, for fear perhaps of offending her physician. It is important to know if the client has a rationale for each drug being taken. Frequently the physician will say "these are water pills or pills for blood pressure or arthritis" but the client has little or no understanding about the manner in which the drug works or what side effects to expect. It is best not to overdramatize side effects, since it provides the client with a rationale for not taking the medications at all. Clients do need to know what side effects are potentially dangerous and thus need to be reported and which can be expected and, usually, tolerated. Another aspect of

medication is the need to ascertain how the client is taking the prescription. One client who had faith in folk remedies ignored the physician's prescription while her blood pressure soared! She, in turn, faithfully adhered to a schedule of chestnut pills and other home remedies that may have buoyed her morale but did nothing for the adaptation at hand.

Activities of Daily Living. The client's ability for self-care as well as care of the home, cooking, cleaning, and shopping activities are more easily assessed in the home than anywhere else. It is a good idea to ask what kinds of activities are presenting the most difficulty. Are there problems in any of these areas? Is outside assistance needed? If so, to what extent?

Socialization. Social contacts provide critical information about elderly clients' functioning. How many times do they go out to visit friends during the week? How often are they able to entertain friends at home? How often do they call friends on the phone? To whom do they turn when assistance is needed? What social and recreational activities do they find enjoyable? Is there a library near where they live?

Although data collection can be done in any situation, assessment in the home setting is one of the best ways of securing comprehensive data. It is here that the data are most readily observable and available. The home is also the least intimidating setting for a client interview. Since clients feel in control, they can afford to relax and share information more freely. More sensitive areas, like sexuality and financial status, are more likely to be discussed in this atmosphere.

SUMMARY

Assessment techniques for the healthy elderly client were presented in this chapter. The nursing history, physical assessment, interpretation of laboratory data, and psychosocial assessment were discussed.

Nurses who work with elderly clients in clinics or community settings often spend more time than other health professionals with these clients. The nurse is in a favored position to identify subtle changes in the client's physical status. These may be normal concomitants of the aging process or indicators of early signs of pathology. The nurse is also in a position to identify changes in mental, functional, and social status. The onset of confusion or a disorder of mood or behavior is very often the first sign of physical illness in the elderly client (Caird and Judge, 1974). A changing mental status may also signal an untoward reaction to drugs the client is receiving.

The psychosocial assessment should be comprehensive. Only in this way can the nurse uncover the stresses, whether social or economic, that are affecting health and mental status. Stresses that lead to depression and anxiety are often clearly identifiable if the data base is complete, enabling the nurse to offer effective counseling. By making a comprehensive base line health assessment of the client, the nurse can monitor changes as they occur and make necessary referrals for further evaluation.

REFERENCES

Agate J: Common symptoms and complaints, in Rossman I (ed), Clinical Geriatrics, 2nd ed. Philadelphia, Lippincott, 1979

Anand MP: Accidents in the home, in Anderson WF, Isaacs B (eds), Current Achievement in Geriatrics. London, Cassel, 1964

Anderson F: Preventive medicine in old age, in Brocklehurst JC (ed), Textbook of Geriatric Medicine and Gerontology, 2nd ed. London, Churchill Livingstone, 1978

Anderson F: Practical Management of the Elderly, 3rd ed. London, Blackwell, 1976

Babu TN, Nazir F, Rao DB, Luisada AA: What is "normal" blood pressure in the aged? Geriatrics 32(1):73, 1977

Balazs EA: Intercellular matrix of connective tissue, in Finch C, Hayflick L (eds), Handbook of the Biology of Aging. New York, Van Nostrand Reinhold, 1977

Baserga RL: Aging and the cell, in Finch C, Hayflick L (eds), Handbook of the Biology of Aging. New York, Van Nostrand Reinhold, 1977

Bates B: A Guide to Physical Examination, 2nd ed. Philadelphia, Lippincott, 1979

Beck AT, Ward CH, et al: An inventory for measuring depression. Archives of General Psychiatry 4:561, 1961

Blazer D: Life events, mental health functioning and the use of health care services by the elderly. American Journal of Public Health 70(11):1174, 1980

Botwinick J: Aging and Behavior: A Comprehensive Integration of Research Findings, 2nd ed. New York, Springer, 1978

Brocklehurst JC: The urinary tract, in Rossman I (ed), Clinical Geriatrics, 2nd ed. Philadelphia, Lippincott, 1979

Brody H, Vijayashanker N: Anatomical changes in the nervous system, in Finch C, Hayflick L (eds), Handbook of the Biology of Aging. New York, Van Nostrand Reinhold, 1977

Brown DG: Gynaecological disorders in the elderly, in Brocklehurst JC (ed), Textbook of Geriatric Medicine and Gerontology, 2nd ed. London, Churchill Livingstone, 1978

Burch GE: The special problems of heart disease in old people. Geriatrics 32(2):51, 1977

Burnside IM: Nursing and the Aged, 2nd ed. New York, McGraw-Hill, 1981

Busech SA: Visual status of the elderly. Journal of Gerontological Nursing 2(5):34, 1976

Butler RN, Lewis MI: Love and Sex After Sixty. New York, Harper & Row, 1977

Caird FI: Clinical examination and investigation of the heart, in Caird FI, Dall FLC, Kennedy RD (eds), Cardiology in Old Age. New York, Plenum, 1976

Caird FI, Dall FLC: The cardiovascular system, in Brocklehurst JC (ed), Textbook of Geriatric Medicine and Gerontology, 2nd ed. London, Churchill Livingstone, 1978

Caird FI, Judge TG: Assessment of mental state, in Assessment of the Elderly Patient. Marshfield, Mass, Pitman Medical, 1974

Calloway NO, Foley CF, Lagebloom P: Uncertainties in geriatric data. II. Organ size. Journal of American Geriatrics Society 13(1):20, 1965

Carotenuto R, Bullock J: Physical Assessment of the Gerontologic Client. Philadelphia, Davis, 1981

Carpenter RR: Maintaining the general health of aging women. Clinical Obstetrics and Gynecology 20(1):215, 1977

Carter AB: The neurologic aspects of aging, in Rossman I (ed), Clinical Geriatrics, 2nd ed. Philadelphia, Lippincott, 1979

Clifford GO, Bewtra AK: Hematologic problems in the elderly, in Rossman I (ed), Clinical Geriatrics, 2nd ed. Philadelphia, Lippincott, 1979

Cohen S, Harris E: Programmed instruction: Mental status assessment. American Journal of Nursing 81(8):1493, 1981

Comfort A: Non-threatening mental testing of the elderly. Journal of American Geriatrics Society 28:261, 1978

Comfort A: Sexuality in later life, in Birren J, Sloane R (eds), Handbook of Mental Health and Aging. Englewood Cliffs, NJ, Prentice-Hall, 1980

Conrad AH Jr: Dermatologic disorders, in Steinberg FU (ed), Cowdry's The Care of the Geriatric Patient, 5th ed. St. Louis, Mosby, 1974

Conrad D: Foot education and screening programs for the elderly. Journal of Gerontological Nursing 3(6):11, 1977

Corso JF: Sensory processes and age effects in normal adults. Journal of Gerontology 26(1):90, 1971

Cutler RP, Kurland HD: Clinical quantification of depressive reactions. Archives of General Psychiatry 5:280, 1961

Dales LG, Friedman GD, Collen MF: Evaluation of a periodic multiphasic health checkup. Methods of Information in Medicine 13(3):140, 1974

DeGowen EL, DeGowen RL: Bedside Diagnostic Examination, 2nd ed. New York, MacMillan, 1970

Duke-OARS: Multidimensional Functional Assessment: The OARS Methodology, 2nd ed. Durham, NC, Duke University Center for the Study of Aging and Human Development, 1978

Elkowitz EB: Geriatric Medicine for the Primary Care Practitioner. New York, Springer, 1981

Exton-Smith AN, Overstall PW: Guidelines in Medicine. Volume 1: Geriatrics. Baltimore, University Park Press, 1979

Feinstein EI, Friedman EA: Renal disease in the elderly, in Rossman I (ed), Clinical Geriatrics, 2nd ed. Philadelphia, Lippincott, 1979

Foley W, Schneider D: A comparison of the level of care predictions of six long-term care patient assessment systems. American Journal of Public Health 70(11):1152, 1980

Frank-Stromborg M, Stromborg P: Primary Care Assessment and Management Skills for Nurses: A Self-Assessment Manual. Philadelphia, Lippincott, 1979

Gerstenblith G, Frederiksen J, et al: Echocardiographic assessment of a normal adult aging population. Circulation 56(2):273, 1977

Glover BH: Sex counseling of the elderly. Hospital Practice 11(6):101, 1977

Goldfarb AI: The evaluation of geriatric patients following treatment, in Hoch PH, Zubin J (eds), Evaluation of Psychiatric Treatment. New York, Grune & Stratton, 1964

Goldfarb AF: Geriatric gynecology, in Rossman I (ed), Clinical Geriatrics, 2nd ed. Philadelphia, Lippincott, 1979

Goldman R: Speculations of vascular changes with age. Journal of American Geriatrics Society XVIII (9):765, 1970

Goldman R: Decline in organ function with aging, in Rossman I (ed), Clinical Geriatrics, 2nd ed. Philadelphia, Lippincott, 1979

Goodhill V: Deafness, tinnitus and dizziness in the aged, in Rossman I (ed), Clinical Geriatrics, 2nd ed. Philadelphia, Lippincott, 1979

Gordon D: Eye problems of the aged, in Chinn A (ed), Working with Older People. Vol. 4. Clinical Aspects of Aging. DHEW, Rockville, MD, 1971

Gray MJ: Ambulatory gynecologic services: Special needs and perspectives of the aging patient. Clinical Obstetrics and Gynecology 20(1):183, 1977

Grob D: Common disorders of muscles in the aged, in Reichel W (ed), Clinical Aspects of Aging. Baltimore, Williams and Wilkins, 1978

Gurland B: The assessment of the mental health status of older adults, in Birren J, Sloane R (eds), Handbook of Mental Health and Aging. Englewood Cliffs, NJ, Prentice-Hall, 1980

Gurland B, Copeland J, Sharpe L, Kelleher M: The geriatric mental status interview (GMS). International Journal of Aging and Human Development 7:303, 1976

Gutman E: Muscle, in Finch C, Hayflick L (eds), Handbook of the Biology of Aging. New York, Van Nostrand Reinhold, 1977

Habermann ET: Orthopaedic aspects of the lower extremities, in Rossman I (ed), Clinical Geriatrics, 2nd ed. Philadelphia, Lippincott, 1979

Habot B, Libow B: The interrelationships of mental and physical status and its assessment in the older client: Mind–body interaction, in Birren J, and Sloane R (eds), Handbook of Mental Health and Aging. Englewood Cliffs, NJ, Prentice-Hall, 1980

Hamilton M: A rating scale for depression. Journal of Neurology, Neurosurgery and Psychiatry 23:56, 1960

Harnes JR: Normal values with increasing age. Journal of Chronic Diseases 33(10):593, 1980

Harris R: Cardiac arrhythmias in the aged, in Caird FI, Dall JLC, Kennedy RD (eds), Cardiology in Old Age. New York, Plenum, 1976

Harris R: Special problems of geriatric patients with heart disease, in Reichel W (ed), Clinical Aspects of Aging. Baltimore, Williams and Wilkins, 1978

Harris R: Cardiopathy of aging: Are the changes related to congestive heart failure? Geriatrics 32(2):42, 1977

Harvey AM, Johns RS, et al (eds): The Principles and Practices of Medicine, 20th ed. New York, Appleton-Century-Crofts, 1980

Hatton J: Aging and the glare problem. Journal of Gerontological Nursing 3(5):38, 1977

Hesch RD, Gatz J, et al: Total and free triiodothyronine and thyroid-binding globulin concentration in elderly human persons. European Journal of Clinical Investigation. 6(2):139, 1976

Horney K: The Neurotic Personality of Our Time. New York, Norton, 1957

Howell TH: Senile deterioration of the central nervous system. British Medical Journal I:56, 1949

Hughes G: Changes in taste sensitivity with advancing age. Gerontologica Clinica 11(4):224, 1969

Hyams DE: The blood, in Brocklehurst JC (ed), Textbook of Geriatric Medicine and Gerontology, 2nd ed. New York, Churchill Livingstone, 1978

Jahss MH: Geriatric aspects of the foot and ankle, in Rossman I (ed), Clinical Geriatrics, 2nd ed. Philadelphia, Lippincott, 1979

Kahn RL, Goldfarb AI, Pollack M, Peck A: Brief objective measure for the determination of mental status in the aged. American Journal of Psychiatry 117:326, 1960

Kannel WB, Gordon T, Schwartz MJ: Systolic versus diastolic blood pressure and risk of coronary heart disease. The Framingham Study. American Journal of Cardiology 27:335, 1971

Keating FR, Jones JD, Elvebach LR, Randall RV: The relation of age and sex to distribution of values in healthy adults of serum calcium, inorganic phosphorus, magnesium, alkaline phosphatase, total proteins, albumin and blood urea. Journal of Laboratory and Clinical Medicine 73(5):825, 1969

Keim R: How aging affects the ear. Geriatrics 32(6):97, 1977

King PA: Foot assessment of the elderly. Journal of Gerontological Nursing 4(6):47, 1978

Klocke RA: Influence of aging on the aging lung, in Finch C, Hayflick L (eds), Handbook of the Biology of Aging. New York, Van Nostrand Reinhold, 1977

Knoop AA, Hoitink AWJK, vanden Bos GC: Cardiovascular effects in aging. Bibliotheca Cardiologia XXI:7, 1968

Koepke JA: Guide to Clinical Laboratory Diagnosis. New York, Appleton-Century-Crofts, 1979

Kohn RR: Heart and cardiovascular system, in Finch C, Hayflick L (eds), Handbook of the Biology of Aging. New York, Van Nostrand Reinhold, 1977

Kornzweig AL: The eye in old age, in Rossman I (ed), Clinical Geriatrics, 2nd ed. Philadelphia, Lippincott, 1979

Langer A: Oral signs of aging and their clinical significance. Geriatrics 31(12):63, 1976

Lawson JS, Rodenburg M, Dykes J: A dementia rating scale for use with psychogeriatric patients. Journal of Gerontology 32:153, 1977

Lewis HP: The History and Physical Examination. New York, Appleton-Century-Crofts, 1979

Libow PC: Senile dementia and pseudosenility: Clinical diagnosis, in Eisdorfer C and Friedel RO (eds), Cognitive and Emotional Disturbance in the Elderly. Chicago, Yearbook, 1977

Lombardo PC: Dermatologic disorders in the elderly, in Rossman I (ed), Clinical Geriatrics, 2nd ed. Philadelphia, Lippincott, 1979

Lubowe II: Treatment of the aging skin by dermatologic methods. Journal of the American Geriatrics Society XXIV(1):25, 1976

Luisada AA: Using noninvasive methods to study the aging heart. Geriatrics 32(2):58, 1977

MacKinney AA Jr: Effect of aging on the peripheral blood lymphocyte count. Journal of Gerontology 33(2):213, 1978

Maekawa T: Hematologic disease, in Steinberg FU (ed), Cowdry's The Care of the Geriatric Patient, 5th ed. St. Louis, Mosby, 1976

Mahoney EA, Verdisco L, Shortridge L: How to Collect and Record a Health History. Philadelphia, Lippincott, 1976

Malasanos L, Bar Kauska V, et al: Health Assessment. St. Louis, Mosby, 1977

Matteson MA: A report of sensory assessment at a senior citizens' center. Journal of Gerontological Nursing 5(1):39, 1979

Mayfield P: Physical assessment of the older adult, in Hogstel MO (ed), Nursing Care of the Older Adult. New York, Wiley, 1981

McCormick D: The normal range for serum creatine phosphokinase. Irish Journal of Medical Science 145(3):86, 1976

Mezey MD, Rauckhorst LH, Stokes SA: Health Assessment of the Older Individual. New York, Springer, 1980

Mezey M, Rauckhorst LM, Stokes SA: The health history of the aged person. Journal of Gerontological Nursing III(3):47, 1977

Neugarten BL: Adaptation of the life cycle. Journal of Geriatric Psychology 4:71, 1970

O'Kell RT, Elliott JR: Development of normal values for use in multitest biochemical screening of sera. Clinical Chemistry 16(3):161, 1970

Pathy MS: Acute cardiac problems, in Coakley D (ed), Acute Geriatric Medicine. Littleton, MA, PSG, 1981

Pathy MS: Clinical presentation and management of neurological disorders in old age, in Brocklehurst JC (ed), Geriatric Medicine and Gerontology, 2nd ed. London, Churchill Livingston, 1978

Patient assessment: Examination of the male genitalia. Programmed instruction. American Journal of Nursing 79(4):689, 1979

Pearson LJ, Kotthoff ME: Geriatric Clinical Protocols. New York, Lippincott, 1979

Perez GL, Jacob M, et al: Incidence of murmurs in the aging heart. Journal of the American Geriatrics Society XXIV(1):29, 1976

Pfeiffer E: A short portable mental status questionnaire for the assessment of organic brain deficit in elderly patients. Journal of the American Geriatrics Society 23:433, 1975

Pfeiffer E: Ways of combining functional assessment data, in Duke-OARS, Multidimensional Functional Assessment: The OARS Methodology, 2nd ed. Durham, NC, Duke University Center for the Study of Aging and Human Development, 1975, chap 8

Prior JA, Silberstein JS: Physical Diagnosis. The History and Examination of the Patient. St. Louis, Mosby, 1973

Rakoff A, Nowroozi K: The female characteristic, in Greenblatt RB (ed), Aging. Volume 5. Geriatric Endocrinology. New York, Raven, 1978

Reed AH, Cannon DC, et al: Estimation of normal ranges from a controlled sample survey. 1. Sex- and age-related influence on the SMA 12/60 screening group of tests. Clinical Chemistry 18(1):57, 1972

Remnet V: The home assessment. A therapeutic tool to assess the needs of the elderly, in Burnside IM (ed), Nursing and the Aged. New York, McGraw-Hill, 1976

Richardson JL: Colorectal cancer: A mass screening and education program. Geriatrics 32(2):123, 1977

Rodstein M: Heart disease in the aged, in Rossman I (ed), Clinical Geriatrics, 2nd ed. Philadelphia, Lippincott, 1979

Rodstein M: The ECG in old age: Implications for diagnosis, therapy and prognosis. Geriatrics 32(2):76, 1977

Rodstein M, Zemen FD: Arcus senilis and arteriosclerosis in the aged. American Journal of Medical Science 245(1):70, 1963

Rossman I: Anatomic and body composition changes with aging, in Finch C, Háyflick L (eds), Handbook of the Biology of Aging. New York, Van Nostrand Reinhold, 1977

Rossman I: Mortality and morbidity overview, in Rossman I (ed), Clincial Geriatrics, 2nd ed. Philadelphia, Lippincott, 1979a

Rossman I: The anatomy of aging, in Rossman I (ed), Clinical Geriatrics, 2nd ed. Philadelphia, Lippincott, 1979b

Rowe JW: Clinical research on aging: Strategies and directions. New England Journal of Medicine 297(24):1332, 1977

Sana JM, Judge RP: Physical Appraisal Methods in Nursing Practice. Boston, Little, Brown, 1975

Schouten J: Important factors in the examination and care of old patients. Journal of the American Geriatrics Society XXIII(4):180, 1975

Selmanowitz VJ, Rizer RL, Orentreich N: Aging of the skin and its appendage, in Finch C, Hayflick L (eds), Handbook of the Biology of Aging. New York, Van Nostrand Reinhold, 1977

Selye H (ed): The Stress of Life. New York, McGraw-Hill, 1956

Shafer WG, Hine MK, Levy BM, A Textbook of Oral Pathology, 3rd ed. Philadelphia, Saunders, 1974

Shanas E, Townsend B, Wedderburn D: The psychology of health, in Neugarten BL (ed), Middle Age and Aging. Chicago, University of Chicago Press, 1968

Shanas E: Self-assessment of physical function: White and black elderly in the United States, in Hayne SG, Feinleib M (eds), Proceedings of the Second Conference on the Epidemiology of Aging. Washington, D.C., U.S. Department of Health and Human Services, NIH Publication No. 80-969, July, 1980

Shank MJ, Conrad D: A survey of the well-elderly: Their foot problems, practices and needs. Journal of Gerontological Nursing 3(6):10, 1977

Shapleigh JB, Mayes S, Moore CV: Hematologic values in the aged. Journal of Gerontology 7(2):207, 1952

Shock NW: System integration, in Finch C, Hayflick L, Handbook of the Biology of Aging. New York, Van Nostrand Reinhold, 1977

Sherman JL, Fields SK: Guide to Patient Evaluation, 2nd ed. Flushing, NY, Medical Examination Publishing, 1976

Sjögren AL: Left ventricular wall thickness determined by ultrasound in 100 subjects with heart disease. Chest 60(4):341, 1971

Steffl B: Sexuality and aging: Implications for nurses and other helping professionals, in Solnick R (ed), Sexuality and Aging. Ethel Percy Andrus Gerontology Center, University of Southern California Press, 1978

Stern TN: Clinical Examination: A Textbook of Physical Diagnosis. Chicago, Year Book, 1964

Straus B: Disorders of the digestive system, in Rossman I (ed), Clinical Geriatrics, 2nd ed. Philadelphia, Lippincott, 1979

Sweeten JC, Thomson WHS: Revised normal ranges for six serum enzymes: Further statistical analysis and the effects of different treatments of blood specimens. Clinica Chemica Acta 48:49, 1973

Syzek BJ: Cardiovascular changes in aging: Implications for nursing. Journal of Gerontological Nursing 2(1):28, 1976

Tichy AM, Malasanos LJ: Physiological parameters of aging. Journal of Gerontological Nursing 5(1):42, 1979

U.S. Department of Commerce, Bureau of the Census. Current Population Reports: Social and Economic Characteristics of the Metropolitan and Nonmetropolitan Population, 1974 and 1970. Washington, D.C., U.S. Government Printing Office, 1975, Series P/23, No. 55

Vaidya PN, Bhosley PN, Rao DB, Luisada AA: Tachyarrhythmias in old age. Journal of American Geriatrics Society XXIV(9):412, 1976

Vaillant G: Theoretical hierarchy of adaptive ego mechanisms. Archives of General Psychiatry 24(2):107, 1971

Villaverde MM, MacMillan CW: Ailments of Aging. New York, Van Nostrand Reinhold, 1980

Wilding P, Rollason JG, Robinson D: Patterns of change for various biochemical constituents detected in well population screening. Clinica Chemica Acta 41:375, 1972

Williamson J, Lowther CP, Gray S: The use of health visitors in preventive geriatrics. Gerontologica Clinica 8(6):362, 1966

Wilson A: Nursing and eye problems of the aged. The Sight Saving Review 41(4):171, 1971–1972

Wilson L, Grant K, Witney P, Kerridge D: Mental status of elderly hospital patients related to occupational therapist's assessment of activities of daily living. Gerontologia Clinica 15:197, 1973

Wynne JW: Pulmonary disease in the elderly, in Rossman I (ed), Clinical Geriatrics, 2nd ed. Philadelphia, Lippincott, 1979

Zach L: The oral cavity, in Rossman I (ed), Clinical Geriatrics, 2nd ed. Philadelphia, Lippincott, 1979

Zung WK: A self-rating depression scale. Archives of General Psychiatry 12:63, 1965

Zung WK: A rating instrument for anxiety disorders. Psychosomatics 12:371, 1971

8

Preparing the Client for Healthy Aging

Preparation for aging should begin in the first decade of life. That we age as we live is a truism. Patterns that affect physical and psychosocial development and health are established early in life. However, since the human organism is continuously changing, new, healthier patterns can be developed at any point in the life cycle. Primary prevention techniques are used by the nurse to assist the middle aged and the "young-old" to develop and consolidate behaviors that will improve the quality of their lives in old age. Central to primary prevention in the old age group is assisting clients to assume a personal accountability for their own health status. Clients can engage in many self-care activities that promote health. Nurses must support these activities. The old model of passive patients relieved of responsibility and with the care-provider in control must be discarded. A model that is based on client–provider partnership and that encourages an active, independent role for clients in their own health care will be more effective. This is particularly true for elderly clients who may be experiencing stresses that undermine independence. Being responsible and accountable for their own health is one way the elderly can maintain independence and control over their lives well into advanced old age.

NURSE–CLIENT RELATIONSHIP

Establishing an effective relationship with the aging client is basic to the counseling and guidance techniques used in prevention of illness and promotion of health. First, the relationship must be based on trust. Trusting relationships are arrived at over time if the nurse allows the expression of positive feelings and anger or other negative feelings by the client without withdrawing or retaliating. The nurse should avoid false reassurances, probing, minimizing complaints, interrupting, making quick judgments or being inconsistent. The nurse should be open, frank, available, and supportive (Longo and Williams, 1978; Hames and Joseph, 1980). In working with elderly clients the nurse should be alert to the possibility of being placed in a surrogate role (daughter, son, nephew, niece) by the client. Clear and correct use of language is important. Expanded or slow speech, clearly pronounced, may improve communication. Modern slang should be avoided since it may not be understood or may be offensive to the client. Immigrant clients may never have learned English and a translator may be required. Nonverbal behavior should also be slowed down. Walking, gesturing, assisting, and moving need to be done at the client's pace. This may require great patience on the part of the nurse (Stone, 1969).

Touching may communicate understanding and support or a willingness to listen and be a confidant of the client. The nurse should be alert to the client's response to touch. Client preference must be respected. Use of space is also important. Older people may prefer more distance between themselves and others. Decreasing eye contact or sitting beside or at right angles to the client may decrease personal space intrusion (Gioiella, 1980).

ANTICIPATORY GUIDANCE

In order to prepare for healthy aging clients need to understand what changes should be expected as a result of normal aging. This information can be presented by the nurse in structured teaching sessions or in more informal encounters. Individual clients may need guidance in modifying behavior to cope with anticipated changes more effectively. Guidance implies a degree of directiveness by the nurse. Counseling, a less directive technique, is also useful, especially when change in behavior leads to anxiety for the client. Counseling is discussed in more detail later in this chapter.

First, clients must understand that changes of normal aging cannot be prevented. However, the degree to which these changes impair the quality of life can be influenced by a variety of actions on the part of the client. Individual genetic history is important and cannot be changed. Knowing one's family history for certain diseases such as diabetes, heart disease, and cancer enables the client to exert vigilance in prevention and early detection of these problems.

Some changes in each of the senses are common in later life. Decreased vision due to presbyopia can be treated and corrected. Regular examination by the ophthalmologist should be a routine part of health care. Intensity of lighting may have to be increased for reading. Larger print in books and newspapers may also improve reading capacity. Color discrimination by the aging eye is less accurate. If color coding is used on medications or other items the older client should verify capacity

to distinguish the colors. Black ink is easier to read than blue or green. Obtaining advice when buying clothes or makeup can be useful in coping with this change in vision. Changes in hearing occur gradually and may not be noticeable to the client until they are well advanced. High-frequency sounds disappear first. Increasing the volume will only partially compensate for the hearing loss. Attention to nonverbal cues may expand comprehension. Artificial aids should be explored if indicated. Periodic examination for cerumen buildup and removal when necessary will eliminate this impediment to hearing. Having audiometry testing in early aging (before age 60) will provide baseline data before presbycusis begins. The senses of taste and smell also decrease with aging. Use of new spices should be tried to enhance the pleasure of eating. Care should be taken to avoid excessive use of salt or sugar.

Dryness of the skin may be a problem for some elderly clients. Use of lubricants and moisturizers on clean skin will help prevent cracking and peeling. Mild soaps may be used sparingly. Frequency of bathing may need to be decreased. Skin should be dried through blotting rather than rubbing. Heavily perfumed cosmetics should be avoided. Gloves should be worn for housework. Older skin tans more easily; a good sun screen should be used to prevent drying. The development of age spots and some wrinkling cannot be prevented but can be slowed by avoiding overexposure to the sun. Particular attention should be given to the feet. Trimming of nails and calluses should be done with extreme care or by a podiatrist. Careful drying between the toes and prevention of blisters is important as decreased healing capacity may turn minor sores into major problems in older clients. This is discussed further in the section on Safety.

Many elderly clients may require dentures in late life. Dentures should be removed for 6 to 8 hours each day. They should be brushed and stored in cool water or denture-cleansing solution.

Changes in digestion and elimination require careful attention to diet in the aging client. Fluid intake must be maintained to prevent constipation or dehydration. Elderly clients experiencing some problems with stress incontinence or frequency may try to avoid accidents by decreasing fluids. This should be discouraged. Planning to ensure regular access to toilet facilities or even the use of protective clothing are more effective ways of dealing with bladder problems. Some bladder problems may be corrected by surgery or other interventions. Physical examination will indicate if treatment is possible. Adequate intake of roughage, fresh fruits, and vegetables and regular exercise will also assist digestion and elimination. Mild laxatives may be needed occasionally but regular use of enemas or other electrolyte and energy-depleting remedies should be avoided. In general, elderly people require fewer calories but the same daily intake of nutrients, vitamins, and minerals as younger adults. Maintaining correct weight and nutritional status will be discussed in detail in Chapter 10.

Elderly clients are frequently aware of diminished muscle strength and tone and feelings of stiffness. Difficulty in locomotion, bending, grasping, and other movements may develop. Slowing of response in the central nervous system is a normal part of aging, as is loss of muscle tissue, increased fatty deposits, and some arthritic changes in joints. However, a regular exercise regimen will markedly reduce the debilitating effects of the aging process. Lack of exercise can lead to premature aging (Birren and Sloane, 1980). Beginning an exercise program at any age may improve functioning, body image, and cardiovascular and pulmonary capacities. Clients who have exercised regularly throughout life may find that they need to decrease the intensity of their exercises as they get older. People new to exercise should obtain medical clearance before beginning a high-intensity program (jogging, swimming, tennis). An exercise program should involve stretching, bending, and moving all joints at least three times a week. Walking and exercise that involves the cardiovascular system should be included as tolerated. Exercise may prevent many of the problems that accompany decreased mobility. People feel better, look better, and function better with regular exercise. One recent study showed that anxiety decreased in elderly subjects who exercised (Wiswell, 1980). Yoga and other relaxation exercises have been used to lower blood pressure and relieve tension. Participating in a regular exercise program may be the most important thing the elderly client can do to prepare for healthy aging. The nurse may need to assist the client in developing a program. Few in this generation of older clients had

physical education in school. Also, many exaggerate the risk involved and underrate their own capacities. A basic exercise program for the reasonably healthy should begin with a warmup of jogging and walking. Someone new to exercise should jog a short distance, then walk an equal distance, then jog, and then walk approximately 1 mile a day. The heart rate should be increased 40 percent over its resting rate for 20 minutes at least three times a week. This warmup should be followed by mild calisthenics aimed at moving all joints and strengthening large muscles. A cooling down period of stretches such as those used in yoga exercises completes the program. Isometric or static contraction of muscles is less desirable, as they stimulate the vasovagal response and raise the blood pressure. If jogging is ruled out for orthopedic or other reasons, swimming may be substituted as a cardiovascular conditioning and warmup exercise. A similar program has been used with a group of elderly subjects over a 6-month period. Significant improvement in cardiac and pulmonary functioning and in fitness was achieved by the study group (deVries, 1980).

Decrease in energy and strength may be lessened through exercise and diet. However, changes in capacity to work, travel, and participate in activities should be anticipated. Obtaining assistance in the home, traveling at off-peak hours, planning to cut down on the amount of work done in a given time period, allowing time to rest between activities, and using energy-saving devices will help the client to cope with this part of aging. The client may blame the decrease in energy on lack of sleep. Sleep patterns do change with age. Sleep periods are shorter and shallower. Waking up at night is common, as is napping during the day. Acceptance of these changes and a degree of insomnia is important to healthy aging. Sedatives should be avoided unless the insomnia is undermining health. Avoiding caffeine and doing relaxation exercises in the evening may decrease the insomnia.

Two other physical changes occurring in old age for which the client should be prepared are decrease in height and in immune system functioning. Changes in height are of minor importance unless severe kyphosis develops. Attention to good posture and exercise is useful in minimizing change. Changes in the immune system are more significant.

The elderly are more susceptible to severe adaptations to common pathogens. Yearly immunization against influenza and pneumonia is recommended. Early diagnosis and treatment of upper respiratory infection is essential. Antibiotics have greatly reduced mortality in the elderly; however, the incidence of infection that can lead to complications is still high. Good hygiene, maintaining good nutrition, and avoidance of undue stress, fatigue, and crowded places during influenza season are important measures aimed at decreasing susceptibility to infection.

A few changes in psychosocial functioning should be anticipated as part of the normal aging process. Some clients will begin to experience difficulties with memory, especially for recent events. Writing notes to oneself, preparing reminder cards to be placed on the refrigerator or near the bedside lamp or clock, using an appointment book, and making lists may all serve to aid in declining memory.

Clients may also find that they become more focused on their own thoughts and more involved in activities that do not require interaction with others. Cautiousness, especially in new situations, may increase. Care should be exercised by the aging individual to be sure these changes do not become exaggerated and develop into social isolation.

The nurse's role in helping the client to cope with changes that affect mental health is discussed further in the Counseling section of this chapter.

SAFETY

Falls

Preparing to meet the safety needs that develop as a client ages requires careful consideration. All too often it is only after an accident that could have been prevented occurs that proper precautions are instituted. Falls cause the highest number of accidents in the elderly, and people over 75 have the highest accidental death rate of any age group (Hogue, 1980). This may be related to problems of vision, balance, or slowed reaction time. Clients should change position slowly to avoid orthostatic hypotension, stay off of ladders and stepstools, and have handrails and nonskid tracks put on bathtubs. Loose rugs should be secured or removed, and electric cords, small pieces of furniture, and other po-

tential obstacles should be removed from the environment. Stairs may be a place of particular danger to the elderly. Treads should be marked with a painted strip to increase visibility. Handrails should be present and secure. Uneven surfaces and cracks should be repaired. Shoes should provide adequate support and have nonslip heels. Extra caution is required in rainy, windy, or snowy weather.

Research on falls in a nursing home indicates that use of tranquilizers and unfamiliarity with the setting may increase the number of falls (Feist, 1978). These variables may apply to the elderly in the community as well. When traveling and staying in strange surroundings extra caution should be taken.

Hazards Related to Poor Vision

With age, peripheral vision is reduced, that is, the visual field is reduced. Clients with reduced peripheral vision are at risk for safety hazards. They may not be aware of moving objects at their side and out of their direct line of vision. They may report that they frequently bump into things. Decreased peripheral vision, if combined with an unsteady gait, can limit ambulation. Teaching such clients to scan their environments is helpful. Lens opacities also occur as a *normal* consequence of aging, causing light to scatter and increasing sensitivity to glare. As a result, the aging client is at risk for stresses affecting safety. Failure to see a street curb because it is in shadow may lead to a fall. To maximize vision and prevent accidents, the environment should not include dimly lit areas.

Care should be taken to ensure that there are no great lighting differences in the visual field, as between a hallway and a stairwell. Providing walls and furnishings with a matte finish will diffuse light and reduce glare. Uncontrolled natural light, such as that from a large picture window, should be replaced by subtle shading of large windows. Exposed light bulbs and single, intense lamps should not be used. Instead, fluorescent or frosted bulbs or several smaller lamps will provide adequate light but without glare. When in the sun, a brimmed hat helps to reduce glare. Glare may make driving hazardous. The aging client should be told never to look at oncoming headlights.

Aging persons also experience a decrease in *dark adaptation* and a greater proportional loss of visual acuity in dim illumination. The aging should be instructed to allow enough time to make visual adaptations when turning on a light in a dark room. Night-lights should be installed in the home. The aging often get up at night, and moving about in the dark can be hazardous. The night-light should be soft, indirect lighting. It may be left on all night or attached to a switch that can be easily reached from the bed. Phosphorescent tape on switches makes them more visible.

As the lens yellows with age, older people also experience a diminution of color discrimination, particularly of low-tone colors, such as violets, blues, and greens. Reds and yellows tend to be seen best. If not recognized, difficulty distinguishing between blues and greens can create special problems. If the client has been prescribed several types of pills in blue and green colors, the client must have some other basis for distinguishing between them. To assist the aging in locating doors, reading signs, and finding other important elements in the environment, strong color contrasts should be used in decorating (Andreasen, 1980).

Traffic Hazards

Traffic accidents are the second leading cause of accidental death in the elderly (Cooper, 1981). Driving difficulties probably result from decreased reaction time and vision problems. Changes in depth and color perceptions and sensitivity to glare put elderly drivers at risk for accidents. The American Association of Retired Persons sponsors a course "55 Alive/Mature Driving" in many states. This course assists elderly drivers in detecting changes in themselves that may impair their driving abilities. Elderly pedestrians also need to take special precautions. Crossing streets requires careful attention to the traffic lights, checking for cars turning into the street, and ensuring that there is sufficient time to cross before the light changes. Crossing streets at night is the most dangerous since the elderly person may neither see nor hear a car and the driver may not see the pedestrian.

Burns

Decrease in the sense of smell may hamper the detection of smoke or gas. Smoke detectors can be installed. Great caution should be used in the kitchen, with clear reminders to turn off the stove or oven.

Loose, flowing clothes should not be worn when cooking. An elderly client should not smoke in bed or if sedated. Decrease in sensitivity to temperature and pain requires careful monitoring of water temperature. Heating pads, electric blankets, and hot water bottles should be well covered and used cautiously.

Hazards Related to Climate

Since temperature regulation is more precarious at this age extremes in temperature should be avoided if possible. Heat exhaustion and freezing have been regular causes of death in the elderly. The elderly client should be alert to heat-related illnesses whenever the temperature is close to body temperature and the humidity is high. Wearing light, loose-fitting clothing, using shades to insulate the home from excessive heat, maintaining ventilation, cooking only early in the morning or late evening, avoiding exertion, and maintaining hydration are all measures that can be used to prevent heat exhaustion. If temperature elevates or nausea, weakness, and disorientation occur during very hot periods, medical assistance should be sought.

Dressing warmly in cold weather to prevent frostbite is important. Layers of clothing provide more warmth than one heavy garment. All surfaces, including the face, should be covered in very cold weather. Home temperature should be maintained around 68°F. Taping windows, hanging heavy curtains, and closing off extra rooms may conserve heat. Extra blankets, quilts, thermal underwear, heavy sweaters, socks, and the like are also useful for maintaining warmth in cold climates.

Foot Problems

Poor circulation and decreased healing capacity necessitate quick attention to small cuts and abrasions, avoidance of constricting clothing or rough materials, and good hygiene, especially foot care. Foot care is important to prevent infection and ulcers. Foot disabilities in the elderly may compromise mobility and independence and should be prevented or minimized. Attention should be given to shoe fit, and care of calluses, corns, and nails. Using foot lotion to treat dry skin, soaking nails before cutting, cutting nails straight across, filing rough edges with an emory board, and padding calluses with moleskin or sponge rubber may prevent disability. A podiatrist should be consulted for removal of corns, painful calluses, and ingrown nails (Rossman, 1979).

Emergencies

A decreased gag reflex can lead to choking and suffocation. Food should be well chewed and eaten slowly. All elderly clients should have a telephone that is easily accessible and emergency numbers should be in plain sight. All medications should be clearly labeled. Using different textured materials on tops may be helpful to those whose color discrimination is impaired. Old medication should be discarded. Immediate assistance should be sought if the wrong medication is taken. Early-alert services exist in some communities. These services will call an elderly client on a regular basis to be sure the client is well. They will notify someone designated by the client if they get no answer on the telephone.

Fear of crime is common in the elderly. They feel less safe than their younger neighbors (Conklin, 1976). Actually, the elderly are less likely to be victims of crime than other age groups. However, the elderly are more frequently the victims of some types of crime. Robbery with injury, and crime in the dwelling rather than on the street are the most common. Safety devices and practices such as chain locks, peepholes in doors, not entering apartment house elevators with strangers, and careful securing of windows and doors can offer some protection. Advice from local police can be sought regarding security measures.

PREPARATION FOR RETIREMENT

One of the most important events in the life process of older clients is retirement. Planning for post-retirement years is an essential part of preparation for healthy aging. This topic is also discussed in Chapter 11 as a stress that may put the client at risk. Proper planning will help to prevent adaptations that decrease the level of health.

Provision for adequate income is an essential aspect of preretirement planning. Social security benefits provide minimal support. Clients should be encouraged to provide other pension, annuity, in-

vestment, or savings income for themselves after regular salary ceases. Income can be supplemented by part-time work, food stamps, and other benefits if necessary. Consultation with retirement counselors in local agencies or other experts should be considered by the client. Financing adequate health care is discussed later in this chapter.

Living arrangements after retirement need to be considered. The pros and cons of giving up large country homes for urban apartments or retirement communities require discussion and investigation. Ease of maintenance, accessibility of health care, transportation and services, cost, and giving up ties to neighbors and friends are issues that need to be examined. Family participation in decision making is preferable if the client intends to maintain family ties after retirement. Realistic planning is important; however, it must be understood that reality includes emotional investment in home and community. Moving to new housing, unless it involves improvement in living conditions, has little impact on morale (Birren and Sloane, 1980). It may require finding new friends and facilities. Moving to age-segregated housing does increase the potential for finding age-appropriate social contacts and new friends.

Relocation of the elderly has been the subject of many studies in gerontology. Early work demonstrated that mortality rates increased following institutionalization (Lieberman, 1961). However, no control for health of the subject was employed. Subsequent studies have demonstrated that many factors play a role in determining the effects of relocation. Wolanin (1978) has reported that if relocation is planned, gradual, and accompanied by orientation to the new facility no ill effects ensue. Another large study by Borup (1979) confirmed these results. At this time it appears that relocation of the healthy young-old to a retirement community will be handled successfully by most individuals. Relocation to a nursing home frequently involves the frail or ill old-old, making outcomes less certain. If well planned, relocation from facility to facility is not apt to have ill effects.

Use of leisure time should be of primary concern in preretirement planning. This period can become a time to do many of the things put aside in younger years due to lack of time. Travel, reading, crafts, political activity, volunteering, music, games, and new learning are just some of the leisure activities available. Attendance at university programs for senior citizens is a popular way to spend time and continue to stimulate the intellect. A variety of activities are sponsored by religious institutions and senior citizen centers. Again, realistic planning is important. Some activities are expensive, and many require mobility and energy. In general, the broader the activity range developed in younger years the more varied one's interests and possibilities in retirement. Planning at least some regular meaningful activity outside the home is important to maintaining social interaction and self-esteem.

Role changes should also be anticipated after retirement. For some, leaving the worker role is a traumatic experience. If this role has been the major or exclusive source of satisfaction and energy expenditure for many years, then giving it up will constitute a significant loss and require great effort to work through. Anticipating this loss by developing new roles in the last few working years can ease the transition when retirement occurs. Tapering off at work and building participation in other organizations is a healthy way to prepare for role change.

Role changes within the family will also occur. Wives should prepare to have their husbands more involved in domestic activities. This requires adjustment of territory and authority within the marital dyad. The wife may feel threatened by this shift of interest by her husband. Ability to deal with these changes will be enhanced if they are discussed openly between the couple before retirement as well as during the adjustment period after retirement. The single person upon retirement will not have to work out changed marital relationships; however, loss of social contacts related to work may lead to loneliness for the single person who has been totally involved in the work role. Again, anticipating this possibility by seeking new contacts before retirement is important.

COUNSELING

Some of the changes associated with the aging process may affect the mental health of the client. A long-term counseling approach to preparing for these changes can prevent problems associated with decreased morale. Anticipating such changes as decreased secondary memory, increased introversion and personal space needs, and heightened cautiousness in trying new things or making decisions is important, as is developing potential strategies to cope with these changes. These strategies may include reviewing one's life, reminiscing about past achievements, planning legacies for the future, increasing self-awareness to improve relationships with family and friends, stimulating one's intellect, exercising, and meditation.

Another essential strategy that may be difficult for some is building a support network. This may include repairing family relationships, making new friends, joining support groups, and making an effort to keep in touch with relatives and old friends. Bitterness, anger, and constant complaining will hamper these efforts. Counseling can assist clients to avoid being their own worst enemy by modifying these behaviors if they are dominant coping mechanisms used by them. Acquiring a pet or plants may be a good strategy to help offset the loneliness associated with the inevitable loss of family and friends due to death. Social networks engender a sense of belonging. Disappearance of regular contacts leads to a constricting of life space, decrease in self-esteem, apathy, and withdrawal. To avoid this, one's social network should be wide enough to spread the demand for support in a crisis and to provide regular positive feedback. Different people have different network styles. Four basic styles have been identified. The kinship style implies a network primarily built on relatives. The friendship style involves friends rather than family. The associate style refers to networks largely related to groups, including those associated with work. The restricted style is one in which the network is limited or nonexistent (Longo and Williams, 1978). Clients whose styles have been associate or restricted may need to be encouraged to expand their styles. However, it is very important to keep in mind that patterns of successful aging are very individual. There is no strategy appropriate to all.

Sexuality is affected by aging but less so than many people believed. Discussing sexual behavior is not something many clients are used to doing. However, frank discussion in a counseling session of changes to be expected and ways to continue sexual satisfaction into late life is an important part of preparing for healthy aging. Aging clients need to know that regular stimulation via intercourse or through masturbation helps to maintain strength of response and lubrication. Female orgasm is not diminished by age. Male orgasm may be less strong. Both the male and female may also find arousal requires longer preparation. The male may find that erection is less firm and diminishes faster after ejaculation but may last longer than in younger years (Corby and Solnick, 1970). Consistency of activity and pattern may improve performance. Oral and digital manipulation also help to strengthen response. Women may need to use a lubricant to prevent irritation of dry tissues. If vaginal tissue becomes fragile an estrogen cream may return tissues to a healthy state. Aging clients should be cautioned that certain drugs and alcohol will decrease response. Also if the client tires late in the day then sex may be more pleasurable in the morning. Most important, clients should be comfortable with their sexuality. Achieving a degree of acceptance of sexual feelings and modes of expression is difficult for some clients at any age. For aging clients it may be more difficult since their previous experiences and attitudes may have inhibited sexual activity. Counseling can assist these clients to grow, even in later life.

FINANCING HEALTH CARE

Medical care expenses are the single largest cause of personal bankruptcy in the United States (Harris, 1975). Elderly clients need to know what sources of funds are available to cover the high cost of health care in their post retirement years. Most important, there is no such thing as total coverage for medical care and almost no coverage for health maintenance and promotion. About half of total costs for health care for people over 65 are paid by Medicare. Approximately 50 percent of the population over 65 carry private insurance in addition to Medicare. However, this extra coverage pays only a small portion of the expenses uncovered by Medicare. Some out-of-pocket expenditures are required for most elderly people every year (Krizay and Wilson, 1974).

In 1965 the Social Security Act was amended to provide health insurance for the elderly. Medicare, as the amendment is called, became effective in 1966. It has two components. Part A is a hospital insurance plan that covers most in-hospital costs. It also covers expenses of home visits or costs of a skilled nursing care facility. All reimbursements under Part A are regulated by "benefit periods." A benefit period begins when a client is hospitalized and ends when the client has been out of the hospital for 60 consecutive days. During the benefit period, 90 days of in-hospital care, 100 days of skilled facility care, and 100 home visits are covered. There is no limit to the number of benefit periods. There is also a lifetime reserve of 60 additional hospital days if a client must go over the 90 days allowed in a single period. During each benefit period the client pays a deductible, or fixed fee, before benefits begin. The client also pays a portion of the cost in a hospital after 60 days and in a skilled care facility after 20 days.

Part B of Medicare is a voluntary medical insurance plan. Monthly premiums are deducted from social security payments. An annual deductible must be paid. Then the plan pays 80 percent of charges for medical and surgical services and additional home health care if needed. There are a variety of services not covered by Medicare, such as routine eye examination and foot care. Also there are several stipulations that govern whether home care or skilled nursing facility costs will be covered, such as, a physician must order these services. For details regarding regulations and services covered information can be obtained from the local Social Security Office. Pamphlets explaining coverage are available from them.

Medicaid is a medical assistance program for certain low-income groups, including the elderly poor. It is also a part of the 1965 social security amendments. Designed in part to cover expenses not covered by Medicare in the over-65 age group, eligibility varies from state to state. Most elderly clients are eligible only after they have expended all their savings and resources. About 15 percent of the elderly are covered by Medicaid (Krizay and Wilson, 1974).

In general, the elderly client should be prepared to pay for most of the cost of preventative services and some of the cost of acute and long-term illnesses from income and savings. For information about programs that may offer additional or related services at reduced rates for the elderly, local groups such as Council on Aging or Area Agencies on Aging should be consulted.

SUMMARY

Clients should be encouraged to look forward to old age. Preparation can facilitate adjustment to changes of normal aging and contribute to satisfaction in advanced life. Opportunities in later life include decreased obligations, increased leisure time, and increased freedom from social constraints. It can be a time to continue to grow, to try new things, and to help others. Morale in the elderly is generally high. The stereotype of loneliness and negativism is not supported by current research (Birren and Sloane, 1980). Most elderly people do not experience major changes in personality or life-style as they age. Behavior is an outgrowth of earlier behavior. The nurse and other health care professionals through guidance and counseling can assist the aging client to accept responsibility for healthy aging (Gioiella, 1983).

REFERENCES

Andreasen ME: Color vision defects in the elderly. Journal of Gerontological Nursing 6(7):383, 1980

Birren J, Sloan R (eds): Handbook of Mental Health and Aging. Englewood Cliffs, NJ, Prentice-Hall, 1980

Borup J, Gallego D, Heffernan P: Relocation and its effects on mortality. Gerontologist 19:135, 1979

Brill EL, Kitts DK: Foundations for Nursing. New York, Appleton-Century-Crofts, 1980

Burnside I: Nursing and the Aged. New York, McGraw-Hill, 1976

Comfort A: Sexuality in later life, in Birren J, Sloane RB (eds), Handbook of Mental Health and Aging. Englewood Cliffs, NJ, Prentice-Hall, 1980

Conklin J: Robbery, the elderly and fear: An urban problem in search of a solution, in Goldsmith J, and Goldsmith SS (eds), Crime and the Elderly. Lexington, MA, Lexington Books, 1976

Cooper S: Accidents and older adults. Geriatric Nursing 2(4):287, 1981

Corby N, Solnick R: Psychosocial and physiological influences on sexuality in the older adult, in Birren J, Sloane RB (eds), Handbook of Mental Health and Aging. Englewood Cliffs, NJ, Prentice-Hall, 1980

deVries H: Physiology of exercise and aging, in Lesnoff-Caravaglia G (ed), Health Care of the Elderly. New York, Human Sciences Press, 1980

Diekelmann N: Pre-retirement counseling. American Journal of Nursing 78(8):1337, 1978

Feist RR: A survey of accidental falls in a small home for the aged. Journal of Gerontological Nursing 4:1, 1978

Field M: Aging with Honor and Dignity. Springfield, IL, Charles C. Thomas, 1968

Gioiella E: Give the older person space. American Journal of Nursing 80(5):888, 1980

Gioiella E: Healthy aging through knowledge and self-care, in Simsons, et al (eds), Aging and Prevention. New York, Haworth, 1983

Griggs W: Sex and the elderly. American Journal of Nursing 78(8):1352, 1978

Hames CC, Joseph DH: Basic Concepts of Helping. New York, Appleton-Century-Crofts, 1980

Harris S: The Economics of Health Care. Berkeley, CA, McCutchan, 1975

Hess P, Day C: Understanding the Aging Patient. New York, Robert J. Brady, 1977

Hogue CC: Epidemiology of injury in older age, in Epidemiology of Aging. NIH Publication No, 80-969, July 1980

Kart G, Metress E, Metress J: Aging and Health. Menlo Park, CA, Addison-Wesley, 1978

King PA: Foot problems and assessment. Geriatric Nursing 1(3):182, 1980

Knopf O: Successful Aging. Boston, G.K. Hall, 1975

Krizay J, Wilson A: The Patient as Consumer. Lexington, MA, Lexington Books, 1974

Lesnoff-Caravaglia G: Health Care of the Elderly. New York, Human Sciences Press, 1980

Lieberman M: Relationship of mortality rates to entrance to a home for the aged. Geriatrics 16:515, 1961

Litwack L, Litwack J, Ballou M: Health Counseling. New York, Appleton-Century-Crofts, 1980

Longo D, Williams R: Clinical Practice in Psychosocial Nursing: Assessment and Intervention. New York, Appleton-Century-Crofts, 1978

Rossman I (ed): Clinical Geriatrics, 2nd ed. Philadelphia, Lippincott, 1979

Shindell S, Salloway J, Obevembt C: A Coursebook in Health Care Delivery. New York, Appleton-Century-Crofts, 1976

Stone V: Give the older person time. American Journal of Nursing 69(10):2124, 1969

Wiswell R: Relaxation, exercise, and aging, in Birren J, Sloane RB (eds), Handbook of Mental Health and Aging. Englewood Cliffs, NJ, Prentice-Hall, 1980

Witle N: Why the elderly fall. American Journal of Nursing 79(11):1950, 1979

Wolanin MO: Relocation of the elderly. Journal of Gerontological Nursing 4:47, 1978

Woods NF: Human Sexuality in Health and Illness, 2nd ed. St. Louis, Mosby, 1979

Yurick A, Robb SS, et al: The Aged Person and the Nursing Process. New York, Appleton-Century-Crofts, 1980

9

Developing Resources
for the Aged

The aging process is inextricably connected to the stress of change and loss. Most elderly clients need assistance in achieving healthy adaptations to these stresses. The nurse should be aware of the resources available to the elderly to provide this assistance. Knowledge of gaps in resources or barriers to utilization of resources is also essential. Most important, the professional nurse should be able to develop new resources and improve existing services in the community.

COMMUNITY RESOURCES

There is no coherent comprehensive program of resources and services for the aged in the United States. The social security programs that include Medicare and Medicaid have the largest impact on the elderly. Most elderly citizens receive retirement income and health care benefits. However, the retirement income from social security is minimal and the health care portions of this program are acute-illness oriented. Support for long-term care is still fragmentary and inadequate. Details of individual benefits available under Medicare are discussed in Chapter 8. Fewer elderly are affected by other government or voluntary agency programs. Despite the relatively few affected a substantial investment has been made by the government in helping aging citizens. It has been estimated that if the majority of elderly eligible took advantage of services such as home health care, the cost would overwhelm the economy. In general, attitudes toward the aged determine services available. A society that values its

elderly will provide comprehensive, universal services to those in need. The United States is slowly developing more positive attitudes toward its aged. This has led to growth of resources under the aegis of multiple laws and agencies. The result is a confusing array of programs that meets some of the needs of some of the elderly. At least three types of agencies are involved in planning services for the elderly. Health Systems Agencies (HSAs), Area Agencies on Aging (AAAs) and Community Mental Health Agencies (CMHAs) all have some legislative authority for planning. The number of agencies involved in delivery of services is vast. When policy-making bodies and interest groups are added the array of groups involved in care for the aged is staggering. The following list is a partial representation of these groups:

- The President's Task Force on Aging
- Senate Special Committee on Aging
- Senate Subcommittee on Aging
- Nursing Homes
- Hospitals
- Community Nursing Services
- Veterans Administration
- National Institute on Aging
- Nutrition Centers
- Day Care Centers for the Elderly
- National Council on Aging
- National Council of Senior Citizens
- Society Security Administration
- State Committees on Aging
- Area Agencies on Aging

• Health Systems Agencies
• Community Mental Health Centers

The array of services may change drastically in the near future as federal support for health care and other social services is withdrawn.

UTILIZATION OF RESOURCES

Resources and services are utilized by some and not by others. Determining patterns and degree of utilization is often the first step in a comprehensive assessment of the resources in a community. This involves data such as number of client visits, types of services offered, time of day and day of week when services are utilized, and who uses which services when. Unfortunately few guidelines exist for the evaluation of resources for the elderly. Health Systems Agencies that have some responsibility for determining what resources should be available lack criteria on which to base decisions (Raffel, 1980). A complete assessment that will be of value to the nurse will go well beyond utilization and will focus on the expressed needs of the community. Criteria for evaluation should include:

1. Utilization
2. Availability
3. Accessibility
4. Acceptability
5. Gaps in service
6. Quality

Barriers to utilization will emerge from the analysis of this data.

AVAILABILITY

Determining the availability of resources involves finding out what services exist in a community. The nurse must first decide the boundaries of the community to be assessed. A city, region, town, or neighborhood may be the most appropriate locality to meet the needs of the clients with whom the nurse is concerned. Once the community has been defined, the agencies that service the elderly must be identified. Some communities have an information

and coordinating council that will list the agencies. In some areas the Department of Health may provide information about health and social agencies. Local senior citizens' councils may act as clearing houses for agencies dealing with the aging. If no central listing of resources and their functions exists, the nurse may need to develop one. This is time consuming but an invaluable asset in referring clients appropriately.

ACCESSIBILITY

Once the various resources have been identified the nurse must evaluate their accessibility. Are the hours convenient? Is transportation readily available? Are the personnel interested? What are the fees? Are waiting times too long? Is the language congruent with the population's language?

ACCEPTABILITY

Some agencies are available and accessible to elderly clients but remain underutilized. This may be due to barriers that make the agency unacceptable to the potential clients. Agencies that do not consider the mores and norms of the client's culture, the socioeconomic status of the client, the age range of the client, the religious beliefs of the client, or do not meet the perceived needs of the community may be unacceptable to potential clients. The presence of local people on the advisory board of an agency in an active capacity is often a positive signal that the agency is interested in being acceptable to its clients.

Once data on utilization, availability, accessibility, and acceptability are obtained, further investigation will determine the state of the resources for the aged in a community. To identify gaps in resources the nurse must categorize the resources into types of services.

GAPS IN SERVICE

Most communities need a variety of resources for their elderly citizens. The nurse should be aware of the sources of assistance in several categories.

Mental Health Services

These may be provided through community mental health centers, voluntary agencies, private counselors, physicians, nurses, and social workers. This is an area where resources are often scarce. There is little belief by mental health workers that the elderly can be effectively helped to deal with emotional problems (Kobata et al., 1980). Services should include counseling, group work, protective services for the psychotic and incompetent, crisis intervention, rehabilitation including long-term psychotherapy, day care, foster care, and suicide prevention.

Home-Based Health Care

Home-based health care is aimed at assisting the elderly to remain in their own homes at maximum levels of independence. Effective home health care decreases the total cost of care for the elderly by decreasing the number of elderly in institutions. It also meets the needs of those wishing to remain independent and safe at home. Home health care programs also assist families in maintaining elderly relatives in the community. A complete home-based health care program involves nurses, physicians, social workers, and other therapists as needed. It may be connected with a hospital or independent. Necessary elements of a home-based program include nursing, medical, social, physical therapy, speech therapy, nutrition, homemaking, and laboratory services. Transporation to clinics or other facilities should also be provided. Comprehensive programs will provide a full range of these services through a single coordinated effort. If no comprehensive program exists then the nurse may need to coordinate several agencies to provide the necessary services for the client. Some funding has been available for this type of program through Title XX of the Social Security Act and through Title III of the Older Americans Act.

Long-Term Care

Long-term care is usually provided in institutional settings. Care may range from custodial to skilled nursing care 24 hours a day. Standards and terminology for institutions offering long-term care to elderly clients vary from state to state. In general, a skilled nursing care facility offers care under the supervision of a licensed nurse 24 hours a day. An intermediate care facility will have less nursing care available. An extended care facility is meant for short-term post-hospital discharge clients only (Raffel, 1980). Further discussion of institutions for the elderly is provided in Chapter 16.

Adult Day Care

These programs, first developed in Europe in the 1940s, are health oriented. Some emphasize health services, others the social program. Preventive services aimed at assisting the aging to maintain function are the core of most programs. Assistance with some activities of daily living is provided. These programs aim to help the frail elderly who need less than 24-hour supervision or assistance. Keeping the elderly in their own homes or with family as long as possible is the goal. Recreation programs, some meals, education and referral services may be offered (Kart, 1978).

Senior Citizen Centers

A familiar resource in most communities, these centers may focus on recreation and meals or may offer a wide range of services for the healthy aged. A comprehensive center might include a friendly visiting program and telephone reassurance link for homebound clients, escort service for visits to clinics or shopping, legal assistance and advice relating to wills, benefits, and rent laws, education programs, crafts, trips, health clinics, counseling, physical fitness programs, social services, and information services.

Outreach Programs

These services are designed to identify elderly clients in need of care who are unable to seek out assistance themselves. The frail, impaired, or isolated elderly, often in substandard housing and living in poverty, need these programs. Home visits and clinics in hotels or other areas where these clients live are essential to outreach programs. Outreach programs are also discussed in Chapter 12.

Other Services

Transportation for the elderly is an important service. It has an impact on many of the services already discussed. Lack of transportation may be a barrier to utilization of many agencies. Automobile ownership declines with age. Public transportation, convenient, easy to use, and low cost, is necesssary to most aged. Communication services are also important. How the elderly find out information about resources, health, nutrition, medications, and so on should be a planned effort. Television programs, local newspapers, special leaflets, and radio are all important media for transmitting information to this population. Legal services were mentioned under senior citizen centers.   If this service is not available through a local center then it should be available from some other agency. Legal assistance to the homebound of limited means should also be provided. Nutrition services including counseling, education, and meals at centers and at home are essential programs. Quality of meal programs is discussed further in Chapter 10. The elderly are important consumers of educational and recreational resources. Programs for the elderly are becoming big business in many parts of the country. The decrease in college-age population has stimulated many institutions to develop adult education programs for the retired. Providing some access to these facilities for the low-income elderly is an important consideration for those involved in caring for the aged. Housing is often a problem for the elderly. Tenants' associations may offer some assistance to their elderly members. Assistance with investigation of rent laws, exemption, subsidies, and public housing should be provided by some agency in the community. A volunteer repair squad is a useful service for the aged. Counseling and assistance in exploring options for sharing residences, foster homes, and life-care communities is an important service. Finally, no discussion of resources for the elderly would be complete without citing the importance of religious establishments in offering programs for the aging. The nurse should be aware of the client's religious affiliation and the sources of support this may provide for the client.

Once the nurse has determined which of these services do not exist in the community, gaps in service can be identified. The nurse now combines information about utilization, availability, accessibility, acceptability, and gaps in service with data from the next category (quality) for a complete evaluation of services for the elderly.

QUALITY OF RESOURCES

Information related to types, availability, accessibility, and acceptability of resources and data that show degree and patterns of utilization together provide the base for a comprehensive analysis of services in any given community. This analysis is crucial to the nurse in the role of coordinator and change agent. However, it does not provide information that will describe the quality of service being provided by any agency. Few attempts have been made to assess quality. Few standards have been developed against which to measure the service (Lowy, 1980). The nurse usually learns by word of mouth from clients or other health professionals that an agency is providing effective service in the eyes of the person expressing the opinion. Some attempts have been made to determine factors that affect client satisfaction with a service. Studies have found that waiting time has the most impact on satisfaction in agencies offering direct client assistance (Aday et al., 1980). Distance from home of major services has been identified as an important factor in measuring residents' satisfaction with housing for the elderly (Hamovitch and Peterson, 1969). Given the decreased mobility and stamina of the aging these findings are not surprising. Quality can also be measured by assessing the number and qualifications of personnel, continuity of care provided, cost effectiveness of care, and outcome of care provided. This type of assessment requires specific objectives and criteria against which the care can be measured. Research to identify the long-term impact of services on the quality of life of the elderly still needs to be undertaken.

THE FAMILY AS RESOURCE

Contrary to popular myth, families continue to be a strong support system for most elderly. They may provide stability, affection, emergency care, economic supports and social interaction. The family is a resource for the aged and as such must be assessed by the nurse. Although most elderly prefer to live in separate households, many more over the age of 75 live with children than are in institutions (National Nursing Home Survey, 1979). The three-generation extended family living in one home is no longer common. This type of living arrangement, an economic necessity in the past, has given way to four- and five-generation families living in separate, often distant homes but tied together by affection and complex patterns for exchange of services.

Family structure has changed in the past few decades. The number of widows is increasing. Smaller families have resulted in fewer children to share the responsibility for elderly parents and fewer young people in general to provide the economic base for assistance to the aging. Divorce. has affected family structure. Complex groupings of relatives from second marriages often develop. Change in roles for women has led to more middle-aged daughters being involved in careers and having less time for aging parents. Change in life expectancy has led to families where young-old children (55–65) may be caring for old-old parents (75 +).

A family assessment to determine the capacity of the family to act as a resource for the elderly client is a complex process requiring skill in interviewing, observing, and analyzing. Developing the family as a resource demands sensitive negotiation by the nurse. It is essential to focus on the whole family as a client rather than just a provider of care for an elderly member. Eighty percent of care for the frail elderly is provided by families (Dunlop, 1980). Assistance for the family may be important in keeping the burden of care manageable and thus preserving the family as a resource. Careful assessment allows the nurse to determine what assistance is necessary. A family assessment includes a family history. How have functions been fulfilled over the years? Are communications open, clear, supportive, direct? Who assumes which role? Who makes the decisions? Is this a flexible arrangement? Is each member's role equally important? Are family conflicts confined to single generations? If not, is fighting done through parents or children? Are there unresolved tensions between daughter or son and in-laws that are projected on parents or grandchildren? Are there old conflicts that are reemerging now that parents are becoming dependent on the children? Does the family have strong ties to external social networks? Is the family afraid to care for an ill member? Can the family cope with changes

in mental status of an elderly parent? Does the family respect and value its elderly members? These are some of the important questions to be asked by the nurse. Each generation is a system within the larger system of the extended family. In open systems, interactions are continuous. The nurse can help the family with intergenerational negotiations, especially in dealing with conflict related to autonomy versus dependence. The presence of a frail elderly parent or relative in the family requires new adjustments related to the independence–dependence continuum by all family members. Just as continuous adaptation is required of families as children grow up, continuous change is also required as elderly parents become more dependent and move toward death.

Very little is known about patterns of sibling relations among older men and women but there are indications that sibling rivalries and support systems continue into old age. Therefore assessment of these relationships is also important. Finally, inflation has increased the financial burden to families of caring for aging members. It is not only conflict, but also increased life expectancy, changing roles, smaller families, and divorce that have made outside support essential in helping families serve as a resource. Economic realities often mean that caring for a frail elderly member may tax the family beyond its resources.

Total responsibility for care of the elderly has gradually been shifting from the family. Society now supplements the family as a resource. Homemakers, home health services, day care, counseling, and self-help groups are some of the services that supplement family care. Relatively few people at this time benefit from these services. Also there are no data yet available to document that these services decrease the number of impaired elderly who are placed in institutions or that family stress is decreased. Research is needed to determine if increasing services to supplement family care really does assist the family significantly (Dunlop, 1980). Even when supplementary services are used families continue to assist the frail elderly with appearance, roles, transportation, emotional support, and monitoring changes. Mental health, especially self-esteem, has been linked to family feedback. How important this is for the elderly is not clear. Family support may not be essential to high morale in all elderly people (Bengston and Treas, 1980). Even with supplemental support some families will not and should not care for elderly members. Some clients do not wish to be involved with their families. The nurse must respect this situation when it occurs and assist the client to find resources elsewhere.

THE CARETAKER

Family members who care for the chronically ill elderly at home may face role conflict or role fatigue. If caretakers are younger family members they may have many other responsibilities and roles. Becoming caretakers may result in role conflict for them. If the caretaker is an older family member who has fewer obligations, conflict is less apt to develop. However, older caretakers tend to have less physical and emotional energy to expend in this role. All other activities may need to be subordinated to the caretaker role. This may lead to role fatigue. In either situation the level of dependence and disability of the ill client and the level of health of the caretaker as well as degree of other assistance available will affect the development of role conflict or fatigue. The nurse must assist the caretaker in developing strategies to cope with role conflict or fatigue if they develop. Involving additional caretakers, using visiting nurse services, and seeking relief through hobbies and friends are potential mechanisms for relieving this problem (Goldstein et al., 1981).

THE DATA BASE FOR PLANNED CHANGE

Developing new resources and improving the quality of care provided by existing services are ways the professional nurse functions as a leader in health care delivery. The health care system today is still geared to acute illness. The elderly, many of whom are chronically ill, require a broader range of services and services that focus on health maintenance rather than cure. Maintaining maximum independence and limiting disability should be the goals of

programs that serve this population. This does not mean refusing to meet real dependency needs but rather supplying the aid necessary to foster independence. Human services organizations are big business. Few professional managers work in these agencies. The services often compete rather than cooperate, they are usually reactive rather than proactive, and they rarely wield influence to improve services in their community. The nurse can play a significant role in influencing goals and attitudes of individuals, groups, and organizations in the community. Successfully wielding this influence requires leadership skills and understanding of the community itself.

The first step in understanding a community, as previously mentioned, is to define the boundaries. The nurse must determine whether a neighborhood, health district, health system agency area, town, or county is the most logical community to study in depth and which of these levels of system has the most impact on the clients with whom the nurse is concerned. Once the system to be studied is established data that describe the system and its subsystems must be gathered. This data gathering should be goal-directed. Why is the nurse studying the community? The purpose discussed in this chapter is to develop new services and improve the quality of service available for the elderly. Data relevant to this purpose should be sought.

A recent study of health care in the United States, funded by Robert Woods Johnson, demonstrated that education, income, and insurance coverage had an important impact on utilization of health resources (Aday et al., 1980). Data related to three variables would therefore be important. Data related to other demographic variables such as age, race, ethnicity, sex, marital status, and religion would be helpful. Information about housing, transportation, media, facilities for shopping, recreation, sanitation, and safety as they apply to the elderly should be obtained. Census data, observation, and interviewing are the best sources for these data. Information about the health status of the residents of the community is useful. Mortality and morbidity statistics are available from local health departments. More detailed data related to health status can be obtained through more time consuming and costly investigation, including the use of questionnaires. Agencies who service the elderly can be surveyed. Elderly people themselves can be questioned about their health status. The nurse also needs information about the services available for the elderly. Assessing these services has been discussed in the previous sections of this chapter. Information obtained through analysis of utilization, availability, accessibility, acceptability, and quality can now be added to demographic data to form a more complete base for formulating plans for initiating change. Two additional types of information are essential to planning for change. Informal and formal associations, including religious, political, social, and educational groups, may be significant forces in a community. The nurse needs to identify them and the role they play in the community under study. The last type of information needed relates to opinion leaders and power in the community.

Opinion leaders may be part of the formal leadership structure of the community or an informal or grass roots structure. Informal opinion leaders are individuals who, through a network of personal contacts, eventually influence large groups. These networks include family structures, small social or ethnic clubs, and even gangs. Formal leaders are more likely to be from the ethnic majority and the upper-middle class. Informal leaders are often from minority groups, including women, and may be economically disadvantaged.

To identify these leaders the nurse must find out who the local elected officials are. Visiting local organizations, churches, schools and businesses, and reading the local newspapers will assist the nurse to develop knowledge of the formal opinion leaders. Identifying informal leaders requires becoming known and trusted in a community. The nurse who is trusted will meet and identify the informal leaders through personal contact with community residents. The nurse may establish these contacts through clients, joining local groups, volunteering in a community project, or through planned house-to-house surveys. Once the leaders are identified the nurse must assess the relative power of each in practice situations under study.

Power is an important concept for nurses to understand. Power is an interaction of energy, strength, and action. When used, power results in control, or at least influence, over people and events.

The energy component is the energy of an individual or a group that is available to be expended in a particular situation. The strength component refers to the capacity of the individual to reward or punish. This may be done through legal sanctions, or through giving or withholding of money, titles, publicity, jobs, or other rewards. The action component of power is the degree to which the individual or group translates the energy and strength into real deeds. Therefore, to assess the power of an individual opinion leader the nurse must gather data related to:

1. the enthusiasm of the individual for or against a project;
2. the amount of time the individual has available;
3. the ways in which the individual can reward or punish members of the community;
4. the willingness of the person to use the rewards or punishments; and
5. the ways to carry out the rewards or punishments already in existence.

Once gathered, these data are evaluated to yield a picture of the degree of power held by the leader.

Power in a community resides not only in individual leaders but also in various groups. Governmental groups like the local board of education, political groups such as a local party organization, businesses, for example, a large industrial plant, social groups like a church fellowship, special interest groups such as a chapter of the Gray Panthers, and many others may all be sources of power in a community.

The same technique for identifying opinion leaders should also be used by the nurse to identify sources of power in the community.

The data base the nurse needs to influence resources for the elderly can be summarized as follows:

1. Community boundaries
2. Demographic data
3. Services
4. Groups
5. Power and leadership

Analysis of this information will identify needs and size and scope of unmet needs of the elderly. It will also provide information about ways and means to activate the change process.

THE NURSE AS AGENT OF CHANGE

To be an effective agent of change the nurse uses knowledge of the change process and the leadership process as a base for action. The change process involves a change agent, a target system, planning, initiating, reducing barriers, overcoming resistance, and consolidating gains. The leadership process as defined by Yura et al. (1976) involves deciding, relating, influencing, and facilitating. In the context of improving services to the elderly, the first step, deciding, relies on the data base discussed in the previous section. Once the problems are identified and the target groups selected, a plan for change can be developed. This plan should include goals, objectives, strategies, resources needed, timetable, alternatives, and evaluation. At times, it may be wiser to focus on a problem such as transportation rather than the age group. This may attract wider community interest and support.

The second step, relating, requires multiple actions on the part of the nurse. Becoming known in the community, establishing a network of contacts, developing expertise, developing trust, cooperating, collaborating, and helping are all behaviors used in this phase. It is important to communicate to the community respect for diverse values and various points of view while supporting and explaining the changes felt to be important.

Influencing may require a series of efforts by the nurse. Raising the level of awareness of the problem by the community is necessary. Both mass media and interpersonal contact should be used. The message should be explicit, emphatic, and frequently repeated. Involving others, especially the opinion leaders, is crucial. A movement that will stimulate enough agitation to overcome inertia and resistance must be created. This requires innovators and followers working together (Quesada, 1980). It is important to include the local Health Systems Agency (HSA) since planning for health services is their legal responsibility and this group is potentially a powerful ally.

The final step in the leadership process is fa-

cilitating. Building an organization to support and explain proposals for change is one method of facilitating. Negotiating between different groups to achieve consensus may facilitate change. Proposal and grant writing to obtain new funds or establish a demonstration project is one way the professional nurse can help bring about change. Encouraging the community to be realistic in its goals, to begin with small projects such as establishing an escort service, is a part of facilitating. An effective change agent is also a risk taker. All steps in the leadership process require some willingness to risk reputation, privacy, and wasting time. Professionalism demands concern for the quality of care available to clients. Achievement of quality through change can occur when a knowledgeable, skillful, courageous nurse assumes the change agent role.

The nurse can also act as a change agent through political action. Health policy is developed on the national, state, and local level. Influencing this development is the goal of the politically active nurse and is an important part of good citizenship (Cowert, 1981). There are many actions the nurse can take to become politically active. Voting in all elections is of course the easiest action. Writing to legislators and telephoning and visiting them are other common means of exerting political power. The individual nurse may have little impact through this type of activity; however, groups of nurses can exert greater power acting together as a bloc.

The nurse may form a coalition of peers to lobby on a particular issue. A coalition of nurses and consumers is also a powerful alliance for lobbying. It is important to present facts clearly and concisely and have available supporting data to use in letters, calls, or visits. Communication with legislators and their aides before a bill is introduced or while it is being marked up may assist the coalition in influencing its content. Continued contact after a bill is introduced may assist in its passage or defeat. Coalitions should become aware of which local, state, and national legislators have a particular interest in the health and welfare of the aged and establish contact with them.

The next step in political involvement can take several forms. Joining N-CAP, the political action arm of the American Nurses' Association assists the nurse to influence the election of individuals.

N-CAP endorses and contributes to the campaigns of candidates running for Congress who are health-care oriented. State nurses' associations also have political action committees (PACs) that perform the same functions at a state level. State and district nurses' associations may also have legislative committees that monitor current legislation. Involvement with these committees allows the nurse to lobby for particular legislation; joining a political action committee is a way of influencing elections.

Nurses can also increase their political involvement by joining local groups. A party organization, a political club, or the campaign staff of a particular candidate are all examples of political groups. For information on becoming involved at this level the pamphlet "Getting Involved in Politics, a How-to-Do-it Guide" published by N-CAP, the Nurses' Coalition for Action in Politics, can be obtained by writing to:

N-CAP
Suite 408
1030 15th Street N.W.
Washington, D.C. 20005

THE ELDERLY AS A RESOURCE

The elderly themselves are emerging as a political force capable of stimulating change on their own behalf. In the past, elderly citizens were often led to believe they were powerless in a youth-oriented society. This is less true today. Growing numbers, increased economic status, increased voting power, and social guilt have combined to undermine ageism in the United States. Many elderly refuse to accept the stereotyped role of dependent, passive, and powerless citizen. Many have become politicized, seeking new routes to power in order to effect change. The National Council of Senior Citizens, the Gray Panthers, and the American Association of Retired Persons are some of the better known national organizations for the elderly that engage in political activity. New groups are being formed, such as the Older Women's League, which hopes to be a national organization, based in Washington, that would deal strictly with the concerns of older women. The professional nurse working with the aged should become familiar with the work of these groups and

actively seek their support for improving the quality of services for the elderly.

OTHER HEALTH CARE PROVIDERS

The nurse is, of course, only one of many professionals and technicians who provide care for the elderly. The physician, social worker, nutritionist, psychologist, physiotherapist, podiatrist, home health aide, and a host of others are involved in delivery of care. These individuals form a complex network of resources for care for each individual client. Coordinating the efforts of this network to achieve a team approach to care is frequently the role of the nurse. A team approach requires the maintenance of harmonious relationships among the disparate members of the network even in the face of occasional professional disagreement regarding care. The nurse must be able to negotiate and conciliate as well as advocate to achieve this end. The valuable contribution of all professionals will be facilitated by a coordinator who respects the contributions of each and recognizes areas of expertise overlap. Most important to the client is a clear, consistent, mutually agreed-upon plan for health care.

Other health care professionals also represent logical collaborators in developing and improving resources for the aged. Initiating collaborative efforts or participating in those begun by others is an expected behavior of any nurse working in gerontology. Multidisciplinary efforts are characteristic of this field and participation by nursing is essential.

REFERENCES

Aday L, Anderson R, Fleming G: Health Care in the U.S. Beverly Hills, CA, Sage Publications, 1980

Bengtson V, Treas J: The changing family context of mental health and aging, in Birren J, Sloane R (eds), Handbook of Mental Health and Aging. Englewood Cliffs, NJ, Prentice-Hall, 1980

Bevil C, Gioiella E: The Community Assessment. New York, The School of Nursing of the City College of CUNY, 1980

Bott E: Family and Social Network, 2nd ed. London, Tavistock, 1971

Brickner P: Home Health Care for the Aged. New York, Appleton-Century-Crofts, 1978

Brody E: A Socialwork Guide for Long-term Care Facilities. Rockville, MD, NIMH, 1974

Brody S, Poulshock S, Masciocchi C: The family caring unit: A major consideration in the long-term care support system. Gerontologist 18(6):556, 1978

Brody S, Masciocchi C: Data for long-term care planning by Health Systems Agencies. American Journal of Public Health 70(11):1194, 1980

Burnett I, Walsh G: Caring for single room occupancy tenants. American Journal of Nursing 73(12):1752, 1973

Butler R: Why Survive? Being Old in America. New York, Harper and Row, 1975

Cowert ME: Implementing Health Policy in Baccalaureate Curricula. New York, NLN Publication No. 15-1844, 1981

Damone H, Harashbarger D: A Handbook of Service Organizations. New York, Behavioral Publications, 1974

Donley R Sr: An Inside View of the Washington Health Scene. American Journal of Nursing 79:1946, 1979

Dowd J: Aging as exchange: A preface to the theory. Journal of Gerontology 30:585, 1975

Dunlop B: Expanded home based care for the impaired elderly, solution or pipedream? American Journal of Public Health 70(5):514, 1980

Duvall E: Marriage and Family Development, 5th ed. Philadelphia, Lippincott, 1977

Field M: The Aged, the Family and the Community. New York, Columbia University Press, 1972

Friedman M: Family Nursing. Theory and Assessment. New York, Appleton-Century-Crofts, 1981

Goldstein V, Regnery G, Wellin E: Caretaker role fatigue. Nursing Outlook 29(1):24, 1981

Hamovitch M, Peterson J: Housing needs and satisfactions of the elderly. Gerontologist 9:30, 1969

Hanchett E: Community Health Assessment. New York, Wiley, 1979

Horn M: Hospital-based home care. American Journal of Nursing 75(10):1811, 1975

Jarvis L (ed): Community Health Nursing: Keeping the Public Healthy. Philadelphia, Davis, 1981

Karl S, Rosenfield S: The residential environment and its impact on the mental health of the aged, in Birren J, Sloane R (eds), Handbook of Mental Health and Aging. Englewood Cliffs, NJ, Prentice-Hall, 1980

Kart C, Metress E, Metress J: Aging and Health: Biological and Social Perspectives. Menlo Park, CA, Addison-Wesley, 1978

Kobata F, Lockey S, Moriwaki S: Minority issues in mental health and aging, in Birren J, Sloane R (eds), Handbook of Mental Health and Aging. Englewood Cliffs, NJ, Prentice-Hall, 1980

Laslett P: Societal development and aging, in Binstock R, Shanas E (eds), Handbook of Aging and the Social Sciences. New York, Van Nostrand Reinhold, 1976

Lawton MP, Brody E, Turner-Massey P: The relationships of environmental factors to changes in well-being. Gerontologist 18:133, 1978

Lesnoff-Caravaglia G: Health Care of the Elderly. New York, Human Services Press, 1980

Lowy L: Mental health services in the community, in Birren J, Sloane R (eds), Handbook of Mental Health and Aging. Englewood Cliffs, NJ, Prentice-Hall, 1980

National Nursing Home Survey. National Center for Health Statistics, 1979, PHS Publication No. 79-1794

Neugarten G, Havighurst R (eds): Social Policy, Social Ethics and the Aging Society. Washington, D.C., National Science Foundation, 1976

Newgarten B, Maddox G: Our Future Selves: A Research Plan Towards Understanding Aging. Washington, D.C., NIH, 1978

Padilla A, Ruiz R, Alverez R: Delivery of community mental-health services to the Spanish-speaking/surnamed population. American Psychologist 30:892, 1975

Patterson R: Services for the aged in community mental health centers. American Journal of Psychiatry 133(3):271, 1976

Quesada G: Campaigning for health programs. American Journal of Nursing 80(5):952, 1980

Raffel M: The U.S. Health System: Origins and Functions. New York, Wiley, 1980

Schwartz A, Mensh I (eds): Professional Obligations and Approaches to the Aged. Springfield, IL, Charles C. Thomas, 1974

Shanas E: The family as a social support system in old age. Gerontologist 19(2):169, 1979

Shanas E, Hauser P: Zero population growth and the family of older people. Journal of Social Issues 30:492, 1974

Shindell S, Salloway J, Oberembt C: A Coursebook in Health Care Delivery. New York, Appleton-Century-Crofts, 1976

Taber M, et al: Handbook for Community Professionals. Springfield, IL, Charles C. Thomas, 1972

Weiter P, Rathbone-McCuan E: Adult Day Care. New York, Springer, 1978

Yura H, Ozimeck D, Walsh M: Nursing Leadership. New York, Appleton-Century-Crofts, 1976

Yurick A, Robb S, Spier B, Ebert N: The Aged Person and the Nursing Process. New York, Appleton-Century-Crofts, 1980

10

Nutrition Counseling

DIET MODIFICATIONS IN NORMAL AGING

Nutritional practices may be the most important variable affecting health status that the nurse can influence. The aging client should be aware of the elements of a normal diet for older adults and should be assisted by the nurse to modify eating patterns to maintain good nutritional status.

Changes associated with the normal aging process influence dietary requirements and preferences. Decrease in basal metabolic rate with age occurs slowly. Stare (1977) has suggested that most individuals should decrease their calorie consumption between the ages of 25 and 70 by 24 percent. Decrease in mobility may also decrease calorie requirements in many elderly. The average male (5'9") requires 2400 kcal per day, the average female (5'5") only 1800 kcal per day (Table 1). The client should take into consideration that older adults may expend more energy doing the same activities as a younger adult. Therefore, if activity level is high then calorie requirements may exceed those recommended. National Institute on Aging studies (1979) of longevity indicate that *mild* obesity accompanies a longer life span.

Changes in bone density in the elderly predispose to tooth loss, which may affect nutritional status. Several nutrition surveys done in the United States in recent years—the Health and Nutrition Examination Survey in 1974, 1975, and 1978, the Ten-State Nutrition Survey in 1972, and The Household Consumption Survey in 1972—have revealed that calcium requirements are often not met in the elderly. (Halpern, 1979) This lack of calcium may compound the problem of bone and tooth loss.

Decrease in the secretion of saliva and changes in taste and smell may affect nutritional status. Decreased numbers of functional papillae in the tongue reduce the ability to distinguish sweet, sour, bitter, and salty flavors. The elderly client may compromise good nutrition by overusing salt and sugar to compensate for this decrease in taste acuity. Swallowing difficulties may inhibit the client from eating all but soft or liquid foods for fear of choking.

Changes in the gastrointestinal tract occur with aging. Decreased secretions may be associated with some food intolerances. No evidence of a direct effect on vitamin or mineral deficiencies has been found. Decreased motility of the tract may contribute to constipation, a common complaint of the elderly. Overuse of laxatives may lead to vitamin or other deficiencies, most notably vitamin A deficiency if mineral oil is used. Increasing roughage and fluid intake is the preferred method of handling this problem.

Decrease in insulin production in many aging individuals leads to a decrease in glucose tolerance. Adult-onset diabetes is a common adaptation in later life. Limited use of sugar and other concentrated sweets should be encouraged even before changes in glucose tolerance are noted.

Other deficiencies found frequently in the elderly include inadequate intake of vitamin C, riboflavin, niacin, and iron. These deficiencies are not related to changes due to aging but are more often associated with poor diet.

For the normal, healthy aging client the only change in recommended dietary allowances from young adult levels is a decrease in calories. Protein intake should remain at 0.8 mg per kilogram of body weight. Iron allowances for men and women are equal (10 mg) once menopause has occurred. A slight reduction in niacin and riboflavin is suggested since energy requirements are lower. Six to eight glasses of fluid should be included, along with high intake of fiber to maintain adequate elimination.

STRATEGIES FOR THE PROMOTION OF OPTIMAL NUTRITION

Assessment

A comprehensive assessment of nutritional status involves obtaining a dietary history and a physical examination that includes anthropometry and laboratory data. Because nutritional status is also determined in part by heredity, past exposure to environmental hazards, disease, treatment regime, eating habits, mental status, income, kitchen facilities, and transportation to shopping areas, the nutritional assessment should initially be part of a complete health appraisal of the client.

The dietary history is often the most difficult to obtain accurately. If the nurse relies on recall from elderly clients during an examination or interview for the past 24 hours' intake, an incomplete picture of the diet may result. Asking the client to keep a 3-day (with one of the days a weekend day) diary of food and fluid intake may result in a better data base. Quantities should be recorded using

household measures. Discussion of this diary with the client that includes questions referring to the basic four food groups, patterns of eating, cooking and storage facilities, shopping habits, difficulties in eating, and the meaning of food to the client will elicit a full dietary history. The interview will require considerable time and should be open-ended in format. If the nurse suspects that a full and accurate picture has still not been obtained and a nutritional problem is indicated by other data then a home visit may clarify the situation. Visiting clients' kitchens and interviewing at the time of the midday meal often reveals foods eaten but not recorded or the absence of foods clients claim to eat regularly.

Physical examination data should include height, weight, mobility status, and neurological status, especially taste, smell and swallowing. Mouth examination, including the teeth, and appraisal of skin, hair and nails are important. Anthropometry, measurement of skinfold thickness, is used to determine if the client is obese. The skinfold (subcutaneous tissue not muscle) over the triceps is the site most frequently used for this test. The examiner gently pinches the skinfold over the triceps until the skin surfaces are parallel. The calipers are then applied next to the fingers to measure the thickness of the fold. A minimum skinfold thickness of 23 mm in men and 30 mm in women is used to define obesity. Some researchers have found that in the elderly abdominal circumference is a better indicator of body weight in men (Vir and Love, 1980).

Laboratory data should minimally include hemoglobin, blood sugar, urinalysis, and feces (color, texture, and guaiac for occult blood). A more complete workup is indicated if health appraisal indicates an unidentified or unconfirmed problem.

Nutrition Teaching and Counseling

Analysis of the data obtained from the assessment described above may reveal a client in good nutritional status or the presence of inadequate nutrition. In either instance the nurse should follow through with some information related to the basic food groups (Table 2). For the healthy client a quick review and positive reinforcement may be all that is necessary. For others a much more elaborate plan of care may be required.

Planning daily menus for a 2-week period with a client is one teaching technique that is useful for

TABLE 1. RECOMMENDED DIETARY ALLOWANCES AGE 51 AND OVER

	Female	Male
Calories (kcal)	1800	2400
Protein (g)	44	56
Vitamin A (μRE)	800	1000
Vitamin E (mg)	8	10
Vitamin C (mg)	60	60
Niacin (mg)	13	16
Riboflavin (mg)	1.2	1.4
Thiamine (mg)	1.0	1.2
Calcium (mg)	800	800
Iron (mg)	10	10

From Recommended Dietary Allowances, 9th ed. Washington, D.C., National Academy of Sciences, 1980.

TABLE 2. BASIC FOOD GROUPS

Food Group	Servings per Day
Fruits and vegetables	4
Bread and cereal	4
Meat and legumes	2–3
Milk and milk products	2

demonstrating the use of the basic food groups. In general, increasing intake of complex carbohydrates such as pasta, potatoes, breads, and legumes and decreasing sugars, fats, and sodium will improve nutrition. Foods dense in nutritional value should be emphasized to keep calories down without sacrificing nutrients. Small, frequent meals are often better for the elderly. Use of condiments to enhance flavor should be suggested (lemon, pepper, spices). Including ethnic foods and occasional "splurges" as well as some alcohol if desired is critical to making the diet acceptable. The use of low-fat milk and cheeses helps reduce fat and caloric intake and provides needed calcium. Casseroles and puddings can be fortified with dry skim milk if necessary to increase protein and calcium.

Foods that are difficult to chew may be cut into small pieces for soups and stews. Using moist foods, sips of water with foods, and careful attention to positioning when eating helps clients with swallowing difficulties. Encouraging clients to chew food thoroughly, avoid high-fat foods, keep regular meal times, and increase fiber and fluids will assist them in avoiding problems of digestion and elimination.

Clients should be instructed that different foods from each of the food groups should be included in any given week to assure that vitamin and mineral intake is adequate. A typical serving of fruit or vegetables is $1/2$ cup; of meat, 3 ounces; of bread and cereal, 1 slice or $2/3$ to 1 cup; and of milk, 8 ounces or $1 1/2$ cups cottage cheese or 2 ounces of hard cheese (Table 3).

To be appetizing, meals should have variety, be attractive, have texture and flavor, provide enough fat and protein for satiety, and be eaten slowly in pleasant surroundings. Encouraging clients who eat alone to cook full meals and make mealtimes a relaxed, comfortable experience is important. Food

should not be overcooked, especially vegetables, if vitamins are to be retained.

Shopping, storage, and cooking may each present a problem for the elderly client. If income is adequate, then purchasing frozen main dishes, small cans, fresh fruits, and vegetables in small quantities and having food delivered may be strategies for coping with problems involving mobility and facilities. However, for the elderly client with limited income other strategies may be needed.

Searching for supermarket bargains, buying generic rather than name-brand products, limiting meat, skipping garnishes, and avoiding convenience foods may be necessary. Obtaining assistance with shopping, "Meals on Wheels," or going to a center for lunch may be the best way for some elderly clients to maintain adequate nutrition. In general the elderly client should read labels carefully, be aware that "health foods" may not be any more nutritious than other foods, select a market for quality and price, and avoid impulsive buying (never shop when hungry).

Teaching elderly clients requires that the nurse

TABLE 3. SERVING SIZE AND NUTRIENT SOURCE

Food Group	Serving Size	Nutrients
Fruits and vegetables	$1/2$ cup	Vitamin C (juicy fruits, dark green vegetables) Vitamin A (dark green leafy, yellow vegetables)
Bread and cereal	1 slice $2/3$–1 cup	B vitamins Iron
Meat and legumes	3 ounces	Protein, iron, vitamin B_{12}
Milk and milk products	8 ounces $1 1/2$ cups cottage cheese, 2 ounces hard cheese	Protein Calcium Vitamins A and D

use basic principles of learning and teaching modified for older adult learners. Readiness to learn is a crucial factor in successful learning. Older adults are motivated to learn if the material is relevant and specific to an immediate need. The client must recognize that changing dietary patterns is important to alleviating a complaint or to feeling better in the near future.

The nurse must also keep in mind that the client is an adult learner with a wealth of past experience, self-directed, oriented to learning in the context of performing a social role, and interested in solving a problem rather than obtaining general knowledge. The nurse should relate the material to past experience. Participatory learning strategies that allow self-direction are useful. The proposed change must be highly valued by the client.

Barriers to teaching and learning in the elderly include short attention span, decreased hearing and eyesight, anxiety, slowing of response, lack of trust in the nurse and denial. Building a relationship is the first step in overcoming these barriers. Anxiety can be decreased by proceeding slowly, using patience, respecting old habits, and creating a pleasant atmosphere. Illustrations using colored charts and large print are useful aids. Tape recording information for the client to play at home and providing written information allows for repetition at the client's own pace. If the client is using denial as a defense mechanism, trying to teach the client a new diet that relates to the illness being denied will only trigger the denial mechanism. In this instance, the client is not ready to learn. Many nurses have found that teaching the client at home is more effective. In this setting the nurse is able to demonstrate cooking techniques, prepare menus and shopping lists, color code boxes, jars and cans, put up charts in the kitchen, and find energy-saving ways for the elderly client to prepare meals.

If the changes in dietary habits required to improve the level of adaptation are major, then counseling as well as teaching will be necessary. The nurse must carefully explore with the client the significance of the changes required, the meaning of the changes to the client, and the ramifications for the client's life-style and family. Long-term support during the change process may be required. Referral for more intensive treatment (psychotherapy, hypnotism, behavior modification) should be considered for clients experiencing difficulty developing new dietary habits. The nurse should never decide that a client is too old to change or learn new habits. Evidence indicates that the aging learn where motivated just as younger individuals do. However, motivation in the elderly often requires a clear, immediate need to solve a problem, such as eliminating a chief complaint.

NUTRITION FOR GROUPS OF ELDERLY CLIENTS

Congregate feeding of elderly clients has been funded since 1973 by the US Congress under the Older Americans Act. Meals are provided for individuals over 60 and their spouses (no age limitation) at sites approved for this purpose. Meals are also provided for the homebound elderly in some areas in their homes. "Meals on Wheels" programs are also run by private, voluntary groups. To be eligible for meals at home the client must be over 60, unable to either cook or shop, and have no one else to do it for them. Transportation to and from the eating site is provided by some centers. Meals are planned to provide one-third of the recommended daily allowances. Therefore, the clients using this service must also prepare some meals for themselves in order to maintain adequate nutrition.

A recent evaluation of these programs in the Boston area found that they provided one good meal per day, increased socialization, and provided indirect financial benefits. No evidence of improved nutrition was found; however, a significant improvement in quality of life was cited by the participants since scarce funds could be used for things other than food (Posner, 1979).

Services often provided with the meal programs include nutrition education sessions. A nurse working in such a setting or in the local community might become involved in conducting the education sessions. The principles of teaching the elderly discussed early in this chapter should be implemented. The following points can serve as a guide:

1. Keep the group small
2. Keep participation voluntary
3. Encourage discussion

4. Start with expressed concerns
5. Keep it practical
6. Use visual aids
7. Keep sessions short
8. Include cultural, emotional aspects
9. Relate to exercise, medications, cost
10. Stress benefits ("feeling good")
11. Be positive
12. Go slowly
13. Aim for improvement rather than dramatic changes

The nurse whose client is eating daily in a congregate setting or is receiving meals at home from an agency should stay alert to the possibility that the client may not eat the meal provided. Also the client may not prepare any meals in addition to the ones provided. Encouraging clients to supplement the meals provided with appropriate food and to eat the meals provided may be essential, especially for the elderly living alone who may neglect their nutritional health due to loneliness, grief, depression, lack of energy, decreased mobility, or inadequate income.

FOOD SERVICE IN NURSING HOMES

Elderly clients in nursing homes have almost no control over their own meals. Malnutrition can become a problem in these settings, even in relatively healthy individuals, unless care is taken to provide acceptable food service. Consideration should be given to ethnic, religious, and other personal beliefs about certain foods. A variety of types of food should be offered. Food should be attractively served in pleasant surroundings. Clients should be fed in group settings as much as possible. Less able clients can be fed by their more independent peers.

Attention to preparation, storage, quality, and seasoning is important to avoid food-borne diseases and to make the meals palatable. Families and friends should be encouraged to supplement institutional food with favorite snacks allowed by the dietary regimen. Clients should use the toilet before meals; meals should be paced slowly. More information related to diet therapies is provided in Chapter 16.

IDENTIFYING THE HIGH-RISK CLIENT

The decrease in lean body mass that occurs with aging puts elderly clients experiencing increased stress at risk for developing nutritional problems. Protein depletion occurs rapidly in the elderly, compromising the immune response and wound healing. Electrolyte imbalance occurs readily in older clients also.

The following stresses are frequently associated with poor nutrition in aging clients:

1. Obesity
2. Loneliness
3. Grief
4. Depression
5. Impaired mental status
6. Chronic illness
7. Drug interactions
8. Radiation or other therapies
9. Decreased mobility
10. Inadequate income

The nurse should be especially alert to the possibility that poor nutrition may lead to learning difficulties, confusion, and depression, as well as vice versa. Drug interactions are also an important source of malnutrition. Aspirin blocks vitamin C absorption; many drugs affect the utilization of the B vitamins. The nurse should carefully check the pharmacology of any drug the client is taking for nutritional consequences.

THE INFLUENCE OF MISINFORMATION ON NUTRITION

Food has been associated with health and disease since primitive times. The medicine man, witch doctor, priest, and early physician often prescribed certain foods as cures and prohibited the use of others in order to prevent disease. Despite the growth of nutrition as a science many beliefs about food that are untrue are a part of folklore.

Fallacies (false beliefs), fads (current fashions), and quackery (false claims) can lead to economic waste, malnutrition, and poor health. Older people are particularly susceptible to promises of health and vitality. Over one-half billion dollars a year is spent in the United States as a result of food quackery (Weg, 1978). So-called health foods and organic foods may be as much as twice as expensive as other equally nutritious food (Robinson, 1978).

The nurse should determine if the client subscribes to nutrition fallacies, fads, or quackery. If so, the impact of these beliefs must be assessed. Many people hold some false beliefs that have minor effects on their eating habits. The nurse should not be overly concerned about these beliefs. However, the nurse must intervene if the misinformation is causing the client to:

1. Spend scarce resources unnecessarily
2. Refuse to seek appropriate medical care
3. Refuse to follow a treatment regimen
4. Become malnourished
5. Develop a toxicity

The most common problems the nurse will encounter in the elderly related to nutrition misinformation involve fallacies, fads, and quackery. The elderly client may believe that honey will cure arthritis or garlic lower blood pressure. Despite the lack of scientific evidence the client may believe that vitamin E promotes long life and that vitamin C cures a variety of diseases. The elderly client may shop in health food stores, believing the current fad that organically grown foods or certain other foods such as brown sugar are more nutritious. The elderly client may believe that large dosages of vitamins are necessary for health or may follow a diet deficient in essential nutrients on the advice of a "quack."

The nurse must be able to explain to clients why their beliefs have no scientific validity and what potential or actual harm they may be doing themselves. Obtaining pamphlets for the client from the American Dietetic Association, 430 North Michigan Avenue, Chicago, IL 60611, may help reinforce the right information. Care should be taken not to ridicule the client who holds false beliefs about food; nevertheless, the nurse is accountable

for presenting correct scientific information to the client.

REFERENCES

Albanese AA: Nutrition for the Elderly. New York, Alan R. Liss, 1980

Barckley V: How to eat on $1.18 per day. Geriatric Nursing 1(1):50, 1980

Bille DA: Educational strategies for teaching the elderly patient. Nursing and Health Care 1(5):256, 1980

Bozian A: Nutrition for the aged or aged nutrition. Nursing Clinics of North America 11(1):169, 1976

Ebert NJ: Nutrition and elimination in the aging and the aging process, in Yurick A et al (eds), The Aged Person and the Nursing Process. New York, Appleton-Century-Crofts, 1980

Gillis D: Seniors: A target for nutrition education. Canadian Nurse 76:28, 1980

Halpern SL: Quick References to Clinical Nutrition. Philadelphia, Lippincott, 1979

Lewis C: Nutritional Considerations for the Elderly. Philadelphia, Davis, 1978

Moehrlin BA, Wolanin MO, Burnside IM: Nutrition and the elderly, in Burnside I (ed), Nursing and the Aged, 2nd ed. New York, McGraw-Hill, 1981

National Institute on Aging. Special Report on Aging: 1979. Bethesda, MD, The Institute, NIH Publication No. 79-1907, 1979

Posner BM: Nutrition and the Elderly. Lexington, MA, Lexington Books, 1979

Robinson CH: Fundamentals of Normal Nutrition. New York, Macmillan, 1978

Stare FJ: Three score and ten plus more. Journal of the American Geriatrics Society 25:529, 1977

Steffee WP: Nutritional intervention in hospitalized geriatric patients. Bulletin of the NY Academy of Medicine 56:6564, 1980

Townsend CE: Nutrition and Diet Modifications, 3rd ed. Albany, NY, Delmar, 1980

Vir SC, Love AAG: Anthropometric measurements in the elderly. Gerontology 26(1):1, 1980

Weg RB: Nutrition and the Later Years. Los Angeles, University of Southern California Press, 1978

Winick M (ed): Nutrition and Aging. New York, Wiley, 1976

Yen PK: What is an adequate diet for the older adult? Geriatric Nursing 1(1):64, 1980

III

Level Two Adaptation: The Aging Client at Risk

11

Stresses that Place
the Aging Client at Risk

A variety of events such as retirement and widowhood occur in the lives of many healthy aging. Also, several conditions such as powerlessness may develop with age. These events and conditions constitute stresses that put the elderly client at risk for a change in health status. The nurse should be aware of the most common of these stresses to assure that in screening clients the implications of these stresses will be fully evaluated.

RETIREMENT

Retirement is a significant life event for most men and an increasing number of women in Western society. Research has demonstrated that health status and attitudes about retirement are the best predictors of satisfaction following retirement. The individual in poor health who has a negative attitude toward retirement will be less satisfied with life after retirement (Kimmel et al., 1978). If the individual retires voluntarily greater ease of adjustment may be expected. However, if retirement is forced on the client by ill health or mandatory retirement laws then more difficulty adjusting and less satisfaction with the retired state may be anticipated. In either event there is no evidence to indicate that retirement itself causes a major change in health status for the majority (Haynes et al., 1978). Instead the adaptation seen in most retirees is a gradual adjustment to a new life-style.

Preparation for this change may enhance adjustment. Anxiety about retirement peaks before the event and involves uncertainties such as loss of income and friends associated with work. Planning for adequate retirement income and a realistic life-style after retirement is important. Also anticipating loss of friends at work by early involvement in groups not associated with work may decrease this worry. Where possible, slowly disengaging oneself from the job is another useful strategy. This will allow time and energy to develop concrete plans for use of leisure time. Long vacations and shorter days during the final working years may stimulate the individual to try new types of relaxation activities and new patterns for the use of time. Further, it offers the opportunity for a married couple to spend extended time together. The increased time available for a couple to spend together after retirement may be a burden to either spouse if it increases the intensity of the relationship or changes the role each plays. Loss of structure of one's day may be anxiety producing for highly structured individuals. Developing alternate daily routines is an important part of planning and eventual adjustment. Awareness of the phases of adjustment to retirement that will occur may also ease the transition. These phases include the retirement event, such as luncheon or party, often coupled with exhilaration followed by a let down. This is followed by the "honeymoon" phase when many new things are tried in an attempt to develop a new life-style. A period of disenchantment may come next until a satisfying routine is developed. Finally a new pattern emerges and develops into a routine, leading to satisfaction.

Unfortunately, for some individuals retirement constitutes a crisis. Suicide rates among men between 65 and 69 are five times that of women and two and one-half times that of the general population. Those who view retirement as a loss of power, who derive their sense of self-esteem mainly from their success at work, who use busy work schedules to avoid dealing with other conflicts, or who see themselves becoming a burden to others due to loss of income are especially vulnerable to unhealthy adaptations to retirement. Careful history taking by the nurse may identify this stress underlying many physical or psychosocial adaptations in the recently retired.

DECREASED MOBILITY

Other factors in addition to retirement may precipitate change in life-style in later life. Decrease in mobility due to normal aging or arthritis or osteoporosis often hampers the aging person in a variety of activities. Very active sports may become too taxing. Use of public transportation, especially during crowded rush hours, may be difficult. Routine housework that involves climbing stairs, bending, and carrying may need to be curtailed. Activities requiring fine coordination may be impaired. Changing activities is one possible adaptation to the stress of a decrease in mobility. Another adaptation is obtaining assistance to accomplish some goals. Seeking and accepting assistance may be difficult for the elderly client. Giving up certain sports, allowing more time to go places, and planning appointments to avoid traveling with crowds implies acceptance of aging and a life-style alteration that may constitute a threat to independence. A change in health status may occur if the elderly client adapts to this stress by becoming too sedentary, afraid of going out, or too dependent. Some life-style change will be required by most older clients to adjust to the decrease in mobility. Radical change is rarely necessary and may constitute an additional stress if it does occur.

BODY IMAGE

Changes in physical appearance and function related to normal aging may affect an individual's body image and possibly life-style. Body image is a part of one's self-concept. It is the mental image one has of one's body's appearance and function. The importance of body image to self-concept varies from person to person. It is affected by external stimuli such as skin condition, muscle tone, and hair color and by internal stimuli such as strength, energy, digestion, bladder capacity, and sexual stamina. Body image is dynamic; it may fluctuate over short time periods depending to some degree on feedback from social interaction or feelings of poor health and physical inadequacy. Differences between ideal and real body image perceived by an individual may lead to changes in health status. Aging clients whose ideal body image is one of youthful vigor and appearance and whose self-concept is strongly related to this ideal body image may become anxious when they find themselves faced with changes in appearance and physical capacity. Gradual modifying of life-style to deemphasize the physical norms and expectations of youth is the adaptation that is seen in most aging clients. However, for those unable to modify their life-style due to the anxiety generated by the conflict between ideal conditions and reality, then a change in health status may occur. Lying about one's age, dressing in styles designed for youth, and frantic attempts at keeping up with activities associated with the young are adaptations that may lead to disappointment. This disappointment may in turn lead to hypochondria, alcohol abuse, and depression.

LOSS

Although retirement, decreased mobility, and body image changes may result in a sense of loss for the aging client, the most profound loss asssociated with aging is the death of significant others. Research has shown that this type of loss is a stress that for many results in a decrease in level of wellness. Different adaptations occur in each phase of the grieving process (Murray et al., 1980). Physical symptoms associated with anxiety such as weakness, tremors, shortness of breath, hyperventilation, and anorexia, along with feelings of disbelief, helplessness, and confusion, mark the *shock* phase, which may last from minutes to several days. The second phase, *defensive retreat,* may last from hours to days. During this period clients withdraw, isolating themselves from emotion. Varying degrees of denial may be used to cope with anxiety. Helplessness and confusion may persist.

The third phase begins with *acknowledgment* of the loss. Fluctuations of denial and acknowledgment may occur at first. Anger is common during this period. Gradually the mourner becomes preoccupied with the loss. Physical symptoms involving many systems may develop, including some similar to those experienced by the deceased. This unconscious physical identification process is related to guilt feelings for previous angry feelings toward the deceased. Depression and self-hate may be experienced during this phase. If guilt is not resolved, preoccupation with the loss, self-hate, and depression may continue. *Idealization* and *identification* are the next phase of grieving. Conscious adoption of some of the characteristics of the deceased may occur. As identification occurs, normal behavior patterns return and *resolution,* the last phase of grieving takes place.

The length of time needed to accomplish the grieving process, its intensity, and its outcome are related to the individual. Previous experiences with loss, degree of dependency on the deceased, number of other recent losses, present health status, and feelings of anger and guilt toward the deceased will all affect the process. If a long illness preceded the death some anticipatory grieving may have been done. Also, during a long illness the healthy client may have been occupied with activities of caring. After the death lack of these activities may be disabling until new activities are found.

If the loss is not effectively resolved change in level of wellness may become severe. Mortality rates are higher in those recently bereaved. The anniversary syndrome may occur, in which the survivor becomes ill or dies on the same day as the spouse. Depression may become acute, leading to suicide. The socially isolated client has a more difficult time adjusting to loss. The nurse's role in assisting aging clients through this process is discussed in detail in Chapter 22. The goal of nursing intervention is to assist the client to develop a satisfactory single-person image and to function independently.

ISOLATION

Social and/or emotional isolation are stresses common to aging clients that may affect health status. Social isolation results from a lack of network of involvements with peers. It is associated with feelings of loneliness, boredom, and marginality. Emotional isolation is the result of lack of intimate ties to significant others and is accompanied by feelings of anxiety and emptiness (Weiss, 1973). The aged may experience both types of isolation as a result of retirement, decreased mobility, loss of friends and relatives, and roles associated with younger life-styles. Reaction to isolation-producing stresses is individual. Some elderly clients experience little discomfort with isolation. These are frequently lifelong isolates, the result of personality traits. Other clients experience distress when isolation develops in old age due to situations beyond their control. In these clients depression, low morale, or various somatic adaptations occur. Anger and hostility may develop leading to reciprocal withdrawal (Weiss, 1973).

Isolation, if severe, may lead to a decrease in self-esteem and to sensory deprivation. Decreased self-esteem may precipitate further isolation, interfere with ability to find new social contacts or seek appropriate health and social assistance. Sensory deprivation has been linked with changes in cognitive functioning (Brownfield, 1972). Varied stimuli are necessary for complex behavior. Monotony tends to free the unconscious and undermine defenses long used to cope with conflict. For some this may be a destructive experience.

Women are at greater risk for the stress of isolation. One-half the women over sixty in the United States are widows. Eighty-five percent are widows by the time they reach their eighties. Women in the present generation of elderly have frequently had little life outside their home or families. Developing an independent life-style as a single person may therefore be especially difficult. Socialized to marry young to older men they may have few skills useful in developing ties to a largely female peer society. Widowers are encouraged to seek out younger women companions. Societal norms do not sanction this behavior in older women. To avoid isolation widows may consider living with their children. If this involves a move to another locality it may further disrupt peer relationships among neighborhood friends. Living with a son or daughter may constitute a stress for the family. Such arrangements should be carefully thought through by parent and child. Some researchers have found that widows prefer to live alone, maintaining emotional ties at a distance (Weiss, 1973).

POVERTY

For many, old age holds few rewards. One out of every four Americans 65 or older lives below the poverty line. Despair, deprivation, and desolation characterize their lives. This poverty may be the result of a lifetime of being poor or may be due to inflation's effect on retirement income or an inability to build sufficient savings during a lifetime that included the Great Depression of the 1930s, and several inflation/recession periods following World War II. Many elderly find their savings wiped out by a catastrophe such as illness, fire, or job loss late in life. Elderly women suffer from poverty more than men. They have frequently earned lower salaries, have fewer benefits, or receive less income from their husbands' retirement pensions.

Poverty constitutes a stress for millions of the elderly. One adaptation to poverty that negatively affects health status is living in substandard housing. One-third of the aged live in deteriorating urban areas. Potential hazards created by this type of housing include fire, lack of heat, lack of refrigeration, unsafe stairs or elevators, and higher crime rates. Another adaptation is poor nutrition. Many elderly are unable to buy sufficient quantities of reasonably nourishing food to maintain health. Poverty may limit an individual's ability to obtain adequate health care. If inexpensive transportation and activities for the elderly are not accessible then the elderly poor may be forced to become social isolates. Social programs available to assist with some of the adaptations to poverty are discussed in Chapter 9. The nurse can serve as a major advocate for elderly clients in obtaining services available and in stimulating society to increase its responsiveness to this stress.

POWERLESSNESS

Ageism is a term coined in 1968 by the noted psychiatrist Robert Butler to describe prejudice against the elderly in Western society (Butler, 1975). Negative views of aging and disparaging attitudes toward the elderly are common. Society often rejects and neglects its elderly members, characterizing them as senile, crotchety, and the like. Acceptance of this stereotype by aged people themselves is pervasive. Ageism contributes to feelings of power-lessness in many elderly people. Social exchange theory postulates that since the elderly have few resources and have less value to the society they have less power in the eyes of society. Thus powerlessness may be the result of both prejudice and lack of resources. Powerlessness is a stress that puts aging clients at risk. Low self-esteem and a sense of powerlessness are closely linked. Lack of power undermines self-esteem, compounding problems the elderly have in coping with living in a complex society. Aging clients may experience a sense of inability to maintain control over their own lives. They may feel they have no voice in matters which concern them. Adaptations that decrease health status that may result from powerlessness include withdrawal, dependency, constriction of life-style, hostility, and depression.

One way in which powerlessness most adversely impacts the elderly is by making them vulnerable to many kinds of crime. The degree to which elderly citizens are the victims of crime is not known. Many elderly victims do not report crime and often the age of victims who do report is not recorded. Despite the lack of exact data reading the daily newspaper verifies that crimes of all types are a serious problem for this age group. Decreased strength and mobility and residence in poor neighborhoods with high crime rates increase the vulnerability of the aging to robbery and assault. Loneliness, lack of education in early life, and illness increase the vulnerability to fraud. Living in institutions or the homes of others increases the vulnerability to abuse. Avoiding victimization is an important factor in limiting the risks of powerlessness.

No discussion of powerlessness would be complete without drawing attention to the problems of aging in minority populations. Minority populations suffer from dual prejudices. Life expectancy among minorities is lower than in white populations. Income levels are lower and services are often inadequate in minority neighborhoods. Lifelong experience with discrimination may lead to increased bitterness and submissiveness. Powerlessness in these groups has been a continuous experience now exaggerated by old age. Recent studies have indicated some changes in patterns associated with aging in minority groups. Among blacks, life expectancy is improving and the income gap is slowly closing. However, the extended family pattern, in which elderly women provided day care, foster care, and adoption for children, is being eroded under pressures from inflation and middle class values (Hill, 1978). Despite the double jeopardy experienced by minority elderly studies show that differences between ethnic and racial groups, especially in measures of life satisfaction, decrease as age increases (Dowd and Bengtson, 1978). The role that expectation of happiness plays in these findings is unknown.

PREVIOUS LIFE PATTERNS

Research in the field of preventive health has revealed that many lifelong patterns of behavior contribute significantly to pathological changes that complicate the normal aging process and put the older person at risk. Poor nutritional habits may lead to obesity or low-level anemias. Obesity adds an additional work load to the cardiovascular system, produces poorly oxygenated tissue, and limits mobility. It is associated with diabetes mellitus and hypertension. Chronic low-level anemia leads to chronic fatigue and may affect the work load of the cardiovascular system. In both situations limited mobility may lead to muscle wastage and many other changes associated with a decrease in mobility (see Chapter 19). Poor eating habits are difficult to change for the older client. Long-term dependence on food to cope with unconscious conflicts requires carefully planned supportive assistance from the nurse to overcome.

Cigarette smoking and alcohol abuse are also patterns that lead to pathological changes. Cigarette smoking causes paralysis and eventual destruction of the cilia, thus undermining the body's natural defenses. Decrease in elasticity of lung tissue and destruction of alveoli occur and may result in emphysema. Cancer of the lung, the third most common cancer in humans, is associated with heavy smoking. Cardiovascular disease is also linked with smoking. Alcohol abuse, which is characterized by an excessive consumption of alcohol over a prolonged period, is associated with degenerative changes in many organ systems. Cirrhosis, pancreatitis, gastric distress, cardiomyopathy, encephalopathy related to thiamine deficiency, and degeneration of the thalamus may occur. Many of these changes are associated with chronic alcoholism. However, varying degrees of degeneration may oc-

cur merely with prolonged overuse. Changes in both of these patterns are again difficult for the aging person to undertake. Group support has been shown effective with many clients.

Two additional lifetime patterns may have major significance for developing pathology in later life. One is the "type A" personality pattern. First described by Dr. Meyer Friedman, this type of behavior is characterized by a hard-driving, intense life-style. Type A individuals are success oriented, likely to be involved in more than one task at a time, and do not know how to relax. This behavior pattern is associated with early coronary disease and may be a pattern evolved to cope with anxiety associated with a variety of conflicts.

Another lifelong pattern related to activity regulation that undermines health is the sedentary lifestyle. Clients who have never exercised, never walk when they can ride, and avoid work through the use of labor-saving devices may approach old age with limited mobility and little cardiac or respiratory reserve. Lack of exercise may be the most important stress, leading to pathology that complicates the aging process. Planned concerted efforts on the part of clients to change either of these activity patterns may decrease risk of major illness.

Clients suffering from chronic illness are not ordinarily considered healthy. However, if managed carefully, some illnesses have little effect on health status except over a long period. One such condition is hypertension. Lifelong hypertension is associated with coronary artery atherosclerosis, myocardial changes, and changes in the kidney. These changes can eventually cause severe illness from renal failure or cardiac failure. Vascular damage may also occur in the brain, leading to cerebral vascular accidents. Early diagnosis and conscientious management often keep hypertension well controlled and significantly decrease the risk of early severe complications occurring. Controlled hypertension can therefore be considered a lifelong pattern that puts an essentially healthy aging client at risk.

SUMMARY

Stresses that put the elderly client at risk for adaptations that decrease the level of functioning need to be identified by the nurse. Relationships between adaptations such as depression and a precipitating stress such as powerlessness should be recognized. Techniques used to identify clients at risk and appropriate nursing interventions are discussed in following chapters.

REFERENCES

Antunes G, Cook FL, et al: Patterns of personal crimes against the elderly. The Gerontologist 17:321, 1977

Baker J, Kelley L: Loss: Some origins and nursing implications, in Longo D, Williams R (eds), Clinical Practice in Psychosocial Nursing: Assessment and Intervention. New York, Appleton-Century-Crofts, 1978

Binstock R, Shanas E (eds): Handbook of Aging and the Social Sciences. New York, Van Nostrand Reinhold, 1976

Birren J, Schaie KW (eds): Handbook of the Psychology of Aging. New York, Van Nostrand Reinhold, 1977

Bloom K: Age and the self-concept. American Journal of Psychiatry 118:534, 1961

Brownfield C: The Brain Benders. New York, Exposition, 1972

Busse E, Pfeiffer E: Behavior and Adaptation in Late Life. Boston, Brown, 1977.

Butler R: Why Survive? Being Old in America. New York, Harper and Row, 1975

Cull J, Hardy R: The Neglected Older American. Springfield, IL, Charles C. Thomas, 1973

Diekelmann N: Pre-retirement counseling. American Journal of Nursing 78:1337, 1978

Dowd J, Bengtson V: Aging in minority populations. Journal of Gerontology 33:427, 1978

Esberger K: Body image. Journal of Gerontological Nursing 4:35, 1978

Gore J: Death, Grief, and Mourning. Garden City, Anchor, 1967

Haynes S, McMichael A, Troyler H: Survival after early and normal retirement. Journal of Gerontology 33:269, 1978

Hill R: A demographic profile of the black elderly. Aging 278:2, 1978

Kellett A: Update on aging: Its problems, its promises. Image 7:20, 1975

Kimmel D, Price K, Walker J: Retirement choice and retirement satisfaction. Journal of Gerontology 33:575, 1978

Kleemier R (ed): Aging and Leisure. Oxford, Oxford University Press, 1961

Knoph O: Successful Aging. Boston, G.K. Hall, 1975

Murray R, Huelskoetter M, O'Driscoll D: The Nursing Process in Later Maturity. Englewood Cliffs, NJ, Prentice-Hall, 1980

Rasmussen J (ed): Man in Isolation and Confinement. Chicago, Aldine, 1973

Robb S: The nurse's role in retirement preparation. Journal of Gerontological Nursing 4:25, 1978

Schoenberg B, Carr A, Peretz D, Kutscher A (eds): Loss and Grief: Psychological Management in Medical Practice. New York, Columbia University Press, 1970

Weiss R: Loneliness: The Experience of Emotional and Social Isolation. Cambridge, MA, M.I.T. Press, 1973

12

Identifying the Client at Risk

Identifying the healthy aging client at risk for a change in level of adaptation is a complex and costly process. The interaction of the changes due to normal aging and changes related to pathology need to be determined and evaluated. Too frequently decline in function is attributed to aging alone, rather than more appropriately to pathology plus aging. If the pathology is identified early enough, decline in function may be modified. Determining the changes related to pathology plus aging is difficult. Adaptations to disease may vary greatly in different age groups. Hyperthyroidism and diabetes in the aged are almost totally different diseases than in the young (Bierman and Brody, 1978). Also, norms for some parameters such as glucose tolerance, blood pressure, and pulmonary function are different in the elderly (see Chapter 5). Some tests have no clearcut standards for the aged. Despite the difficulties involved in identifying clients at risk programs can be and have been established for this purpose.

SCREENING, CASE-FINDING, OUTREACH

Screening programs are established to separate the well from the at-risk or apparently not well. The techniques used are not necessarily aimed at a definite diagnosis. Once the apparently not well client is identified a thorough diagnostic workup can be initiated. When a client at risk is identified interventions aimed at limiting the risk can be instituted, following careful exploration of the stresses involved. Screening programs are usually designed to examine large numbers of people in a short period

of time at minimal cost. The better organized the program the more cost-effective it will be.

Hypertension screening is an example of this type of program. The goal of the program would be to identify all the individuals in a given area who are hypertensive and then to refer these individuals for treatment. Multiple sites for the testing such as churches, supermarkets, health stations, and mobile units might be used. At the initial contact the blood pressure would be taken in the arm with the client sitting down. Clients who have abnormal readings are asked to return for a second testing. At this visit the blood pressure is measured sitting, standing, and lying down. If results continued to be abnormal the client is referred for further testing.

This type of screening program can be combined with other testing such as vision, urinalysis, weight, and hematology to identify additional health problems. When several tests are done together the program is known as a multiphasic screening program. The more comprehensive the program the more costly it will be to establish and maintain. However, if stresses that put elderly clients at risk are to be identified, only a comprehensive, multiphasic program will be sophisticated enough to assess the changes related to age–pathology interaction.

A good screening program for the elderly would include periodic multiphasic testing and a health appraisal. The health appraisal would include a health history and physical examination as well as several other tests to identify the common stresses discussed in Chapter 11. Details of such a program are discussed later in this chapter.

Case-finding or identification of clients at risk

is a result of a screening program. However, not all potential clients will come to the screening sites. The elderly may not know that the services are available. They may be reluctant to be examined for fear of being given "bad news." They may be feeling well and not see the need to be screened. Transportation difficulties may keep some from reaching the sites. Cost of screening may be an inhibiting factor. Language or culture may constitute barriers to attending screening clinics. To maximize case-finding among the elderly a program of outreach activities should be added to the screening process.

Outreach implies going out to the elderly in their homes. In rural areas this may include setting up a mobile screening unit and calling house to house. In urban areas transporting elderly residents of apartment houses or hotels to clinics for screening or setting up screening sites in hotels or housing for the elderly is an option. Outreach programs include establishing networks for referral. The police, fire department, church personnel, block associations, community center workers, and landlords can all be involved in identifying elderly clients for screening programs. An escort service to assist the elderly reluctant to travel on their own and personnel capable of explaining the need for screening to individuals and groups can improve the level of case-finding.

Another factor crucial to effective case-finding is a positive, helpful attitude on the part of the health care team. Society, including health care personnel and the elderly themselves, often expects older people to be sick. Aging itself is viewed as illness by many. This view may influence care-providers to think there is little they or their clients can do to improve their health status. This negative attitude may set up a self-fulfilling prophecy, where decline in functioning is expected, and thus accepted, thereby undermining motivation to seek care. Conversely, some health care workers view elderly clients as too demanding, or being frequent complainers. Aging clients who may be experiencing the beginning stages of multiple chronic diseases should be expected to have numerous adaptations to these stresses. Careful evaluation of these changes requires detailed reporting by the client. Unfortunately, health care terminology, which emphasizes health *problems* and chief *complaints*, focuses on the client in

a negative manner, making the projection of a positive attitude more difficult. Further, negative attitudes related to unconscious conflicts involving aging or parents as discussed in Chapter 3 may be communicated by health care providers to their clients, thus decreasing their motivation. Decreased self-esteem is a stress for many elderly. Nurses and their health care colleagues should be alert to any action that may signal lack of respect or caring if screening, case-finding, and outreach are to be successful and if an attitude of personal accountability for health is to be fostered in elderly clients.

IDENTIFYING ADAPTATIONS TO COMMON STRESSES

A periodic health appraisal, with history and physical examination, should include collection of data relating to the stresses identified in the preceding chapter. To obtain accurate information the nurse must be careful to observe three important aspects of communicating with the elderly. First, the history must be a *life* history, not just a recent history. This means a single visit may not be enough to establish baseline data for accurate assessment. Second, the nurse must pace the interview and examination slowly enough to cope with the aging client's slowing of response. Third, the nurse should respond frankly to all questions; evasion or platitudes are demeaning to any client, but especially undermining to aged clients with lowered self-esteem. Fear of being considered too demanding may influence the elderly to underreport significant adaptations, especially if clients feel they are taking too much time from an obviously busy nurse.

Assessing Adaptations to Retirement
Assessing the adaptations to retirement requires detailed questioning. The following areas should be covered:

1. Attitudes toward retirement
2. Major changes in life-style after retirement
3. Feelings about present life-style
4. Financial status
5. Attitude of spouse
6. Changes in friendships
7. Present use of time

Assessing Activity Level

In obtaining information about use of time an activity inventory can be a useful tool. Asking the client to fill in a weekly schedule may suggest new options to the client as well as provide data for the nurse. A simple activity inventory is provided in Table 1.

Assessing Mobility

Evaluating changes in mobility will involve determining range of motion, strength of muscles, gait, assessment of pain, and ability to perform usual tasks. Questions regarding walking capacity, ability to do work in the home, participation in sports, exercises, dancing, and coping with public transportation should be asked. Degree of independence and amount of assistance required should be determined.

Assessing Body Image

Assessing body image involves obtaining information about clients' perceptions of their bodies' appearance and functioning in the past and the present. The nurse should be alert to subtle cues to conflict between real and ideal body image. Reluctance to discuss feelings, bitterness about loss of youth, and anger at changes in sexual stamina may be significant signals. The physical appearance of the client, including grooming, posture, makeup, and dress, is important. Dental disease often affects appearance. Dental history and examination should be included in the periodic appraisal.

Assessing Adaptations to Loss

Assessing adaptations to loss involves collecting data about the client's significant relationships. If a recent loss has been experienced the nurse should determine what stage in the grieving process the client has reached and if physical symptoms are related to that process. Exploring feelings about the loss may not be possible in a screening visit but need for a follow-up visit may be determined at this time. The nurse should be alert to signs of depression or impending crisis. Crisis intervention is discussed in Chapter 13.

TABLE 1.   WEEKLY ACTIVITY RECORD

Each day fill in number of times you participated in any of the activities listed. Total at the end of the week.

	M	T	W	T	F	S	S	Total
1. Visiting others								
2. Watching television								
3. Listening to radio or phonograph								
4. Reading								
5. Going to place of worship								
6. Meeting attendance								
7. Social gathering								
8. Going to movies								
9. Playing games								
10. Shopping trips								
11. Meals with others								
12. Attending class								
13. Exercising								
14. Volunteer work								
15. Concerts/plays								
16. Telephoning								
17. Writing letters								
18. Other								

Grand Total

Assessing Social Interactions

In evaluating effects of retirement an activity inventory was suggested. This will also provide some data regarding the degree of social interaction the client is maintaining. Further information related to social isolation can be determined through the use of the "isolation index" shown in Table 2, which focuses on roles rather than activities. Various forms of this instrument, developed by Tec and Granick, have been used to study social isolation in the elderly in a number of studies (Bennett, 1973; Hoch and Zubin, 1961). To determine if the client is a new isolate or a lifelong isolate, a history of inter-

action patterns 5, 10, or 20 years ago must also be obtained. One weakness of this method is that it does not address quality of interaction.

Assessing Living Conditions

Assessment of socioeconomic status is discussed in Chapter 7. If data obtained indicate that the client has limited or inadequate resources the nurse should explore the impact of this stress on the client's standard of living. Housing, nutrition, access to health care, and social activities should be evaluated.

The home visit has been advocated by Anderson (1978) as an essential component of health ser-

TABLE 2.   PAST MONTH ISOLATION INDEX

Category	Role Contacts	Score
1. Organizations	A. Individual did not report attendance at any organization, such as place of worship, social club, or political club, during the past month.	0
	B. Individual reported attendance at one organization during the past month.	1
	C. Individual reported attendance at two or more organizations in the past month.	2
2. Children	A. Individual did not report any contact with children during the past month.	0
	B. Individual reported contact with one child during the past month.	1
	C. Individual reported contact with two or more children.	2
3. Neighbors	A. Individual did not report any contact with neighbors during the past month.	0
	B. Individual reported contact with one neighbor during the past month.	1
	C. Individual reported contact with two or more neighbors.	2
4. Friends	A. Individual did not report any contact with friends during the past month.	0
	B. Individual reported contact with one friend during the past month.	1
	C. Individual reported contact with two or more friends.	2
5. Relatives	A. Individual did not report contact with any relatives other than children in the past month.	0
	B. Individual reported contact with one such relative during the past month.	1
	C. Individual reported contact with two or more relatives.	2
6. Marriage	A. Individual was not married during past month.	0
	B. Individual's spouse is living but separated from subject.	1
	C. Individual lives with spouse.	2

vices for the aging. It provides a way of contacting that portion of the aging population that is isolated or homebound. It allows for an assessment of the aging person's day-to-day environment and living conditions, where a few basic modifications may improve its safety and prolong the client's ability to live independently.

Assessing Powerlessness

Determining if feelings of powerlessness are a stress can be accomplished through discussion with clients of how much control they feel they have over their lives. Questions relating to victimization should be indirect. The elderly client who has been a victim of fraud or abuse or who is currently being victimized may be afraid or ashamed to discuss it. Careful observation of the client's manner and physical condition may produce clues of abuse. Exploration of the client's living conditions and relationships may lead the nurse to suspicion of fraud. Follow up to obtain more data is essential in either case.

Assessing Self-Esteem

All of the stresses discussed so far can lead to the adaptation of low self-esteem. To assess this adaptation the nurse may evaluate information ob-

tained through interviewing that indicates how clients see themselves. If a more formal assessment, which may be more reliable, is preferred the following simple test can be administered. Label several small disks as illustrated in Figure 1. Put them in a container, mix them up, and dump them out in front of the client. Ask the client to put them in order of importance from left to right in a line. The further to the left the client places the disk labeled "myself" the higher the client's self-esteem. This test was devised by Ziller (1964) and correlated well with other tests of self-esteem.

Assessing Stresses Related to Previous Life-Style

Data needed to determine stresses related to previous life-style will emerge from the history and physical. Nutrition assessment is discussed in Chapter 10. Cigarette smoking is determined by simple questions regarding the daily intake and type of cigarettes smoked now and in the past. Use of alcohol may be more difficult to evaluate. Quantity of alcohol consumed may not give an accurate assessment. Different individuals tolerate greater or lesser amounts of alcohol with little effect. To determine whether the elderly client is abusing alcohol, behavior related to drinking needs to be de-

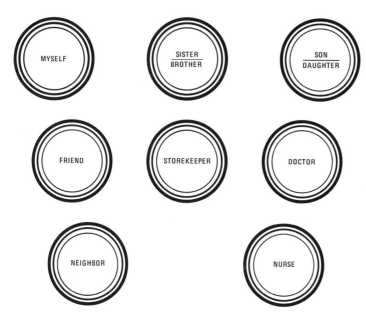

Figure 1. To test self-esteem, simple disks, such as the ones depicted here, can be mixed up and placed in front of the client. Ask the client to place them in a line from left to right, in order of importance. Placing the disk labeled "myself" to the left indicates high self-esteem.

termined. The following points should be covered by the nurse:

1. Frequency of drinking
2. Time of day drinking begins
3. Control of behavior, i.e., falls, aggressive behavior
4. Blackouts
5. Past drinking habits

If the nurse ascertains that the client drinks early in the day and then continues at frequent intervals, has periods of uncontrolled behavior, has blackouts, has increased drinking significantly in recent months, or any combination of these then a drinking problem should be suspected. Validating behavior with family or friends may be useful since denial is a common defense in alcohol abusers.

Identifying the type A individual requires data related to the use of time. Clients who seek a high-stimulus environment and plan multiple commitments and tight schedules, and who hate waiting or unfilled time may have this personality type. Techniques useful in changing this life-style include yoga, meditation, and biofeedback-relaxation exercises.

A few well chosen questions about physical activity will identify the chronically sedentary individual. Before an exercise program is planned a "stress" test may be useful. This provides information about the client's response to exercise and usually involves a treadmill that can be adjusted so that the subject walks or runs at varying speeds on the level or up a gradient. During the test, blood pressure and ECG responses are measured. Oxygen uptake can also be measured. The subject's verbal reports of pain, fatigue, or dizziness are also assessed. In the elderly, the test can establish tolerance for exercise and may establish the presence of asymptomatic coronary heart disease.

Exercise capacity is governed by heart rate and stroke volume. Heart rate and systolic blood pressure increase during exercise. When maximal heart rate and systolic blood pressure are reached, physical exhaustion forces the subject to stop exercising. Maximal heart rate and systolic blood pressure vary with age, physical conditioning, and cardiovascular disease. In healthy male adults aged 55 and over maximal heart rate ranges from 180 to 170 beats per minute. Maximum systolic blood pressure may

be as high as 240 mm Hg. Women have lower exercise capacities. The physically trained will have higher exercise capacities. Cardiovascular disease will lower capacity (Sivarajan and Halpenny, 1979).

An exercise test may have a single stage or multiple stages. Work load is held constant in a single-stage test and increased at intervals in a multistage test. Duration of the test varies with the procedure used at each institution. Any test is terminated if severe symptoms occur. Monitoring occurs at rest before the test, during the test, and during the recovery period. Informed consent is required. Persons qualified to administer the tests are certified by the American College of Sports Medicine. The nurse should prepare clients for the test. This involves finding out the exact procedure used in the local institution. Clients should be advised to get adequate rest the night before the test, to eat a light meal 2 hours before the test, omitting coffee, tea, or alcohol, and to wear loose-fitting clothes (not nylon) and comfortable rubber soled shoes. A warm, not hot, shower may be taken no less than 1 hour after the test. Results of the test are used to plan a safe exercise program for the client.

PERIODIC HEALTH APPRAISAL

It is advisable for older people to undergo health assessments more frequently than young adults. All individuals over age 45 should have an annual health assessment (Anderson, 1978; Villaverde and MacMillan, 1980). It is generally agreed that the health assessment of the aging person must include a comprehensive health history and physical examination. The guaiac test for detecting occult blood in the stool should also be part of the annual assessment for all persons over age 35. This test is easy to perform, low in cost, and highly effective in detecting carcinoma and other stresses of the colon and rectum (Carpenter, 1977; Dales et al., 1974). Other tests recommended for the aging on an annual basis are electrocardiogram (ECG), urine testing for sugar and acetone, complete blood count (CBC), coagulation time, and blood chemistry (Villaverde and MacMillan, 1980; Anderson, 1978). Testing for visual acuity and tonometry should also be performed annually (Kornzweig, 1979). Regular dental examinations are suggested to detect dental disease as well as cancer of the mouth. Frequency depends on condition of the teeth and gums.

The merits of performing other screening techniques as part of the health assessment have been debated. However, the efficacy of performing specific screening techniques with the aging has not been studied sufficiently. Researchers at Kaiser-Permanente undertook a 7-year study of the outcomes of health screening regimens. They followed 10,000 men and women ages 35 to 54, but their results were inconclusive. For example, they found that annual mammography was not a necessary part of the health assessment for women under 54, but suggested that it may be beneficial for selected groups, such as the aging (Dales et al., 1974).

Annual rectal examinations for the aging have also been urged (Anderson, 1978). The incidence of colon and rectal cancer increases with age. Straus (1979) believes the rectal examination is useful in the detection of colorectal cancer, since 35 to 50 percent of colonic cancers are apparent during rectal examination. In addition rectal examination provides essential information about the status of male and female reproductive organs. On the other hand, Richardson found that the rectal examination provided little useful information about the presence of colorectal cancers because most cancerous lesions are located too high in the colon (Richardson, 1977).

There are also differences of opinion about the frequency at which Papanicolaou smears should be taken in aging women. Practitioners have urged that cervical cytological examinations be performed as often as every year (Mezey et al., 1980) and as infrequently as every 2 to 4 years (Carpenter, 1977; Burnside, 1981; Strauss, 1979). According to Goldfarb (1979) the need for an annual Papanicolaou smear in women over 65 without abnormal gynecological adaptations is debatable. Because the yield on routine Papanicolaou smears is fairly low, there is a question about whether or not the procedure is cost-effective.

The value of an annual chest x-ray has also been discussed (Anderson, 1978; Dales et al., 1974). In general, chest x-ray and other radiographical studies, such as those of the sinuses and mastoids, should be performed only if indicated by the client's adaptations (Villaverde and MacMillan, 1980).

Clients should be carefully prepared for any tests done. If waiting periods are required, explanations should include this information. If fluids are being restricted or forced, careful attention to dehydration or diminished bladder capacity is required. Intolerance to various dyes is also more common in the elderly. Assistance with moving and undressing and reassurance during such procedures is essential to motivate elderly clients to participate voluntarily in these procedures. It cannot be emphasized enough that a patient, caring attitude is crucial to good client care.

Assessing Mental Status

Finally, the nurse should routinely screen the elderly client for changes in mental status. This assessment is discussed in Chapter 7. Particular attention should be paid to the development of depression, a common adaptation to many stresses in the aging. Scales for rating depression can be used to augment data obtained through interviewing. A self-rating depression scale that is self-administered, brief, and state rather than trait related is the Zung Self-Rating Depression Scale (Zung, 1965). A comprehensive discussion of other scales is presented by Gorland in *The Assessment of the Mental Status of Older Adults* (Birren and Sloane, 1980). Depression as a health problem and its nursing management in the aged are discussed in Chapter 16.

REFERENCES

Anderson F: Preventive medicine in old age, in Brocklehurst JC (ed), Textbook of Geriatric Medicine and Gerontology, 2nd ed. London, Churchill Livingstone, 1978

Bennett R: Social isolation and isolation reducing programs. Bulletin of the NY Academy of Medicine 49:1143, 1973

Bierman E, Brody H: Our Future Selves: A Report of the Panel on Biomedical Research. Washington, NIH Publication, 1978

Birren J, Sloane R (eds): Handbook of Mental Health and Aging. Englewood Cliffs, NJ, Prentice-Hall, 1980

Brickner P, Bolger AG, et al: Outreach to welfare hotels, the home bound, the frail. American Journal of Nursing 76:762, 1976

Burnside, I: Nursing and the Aged, 2nd ed. New York, McGraw-Hill, 1981

Carnavali D, Patrick M (eds): Nursing Management for the Elderly. Philadelphia, Lippincott, 1979

Carpenter RR: Maintaining the general health of aging women. Clinical Obstetrics and Gynecology 20(1):215, 1977

Dales LG, Friedman DG, Collen MF: Evaluation of a periodic multiphasic health checkup. Methods of Information in Medicine 13(3):140, 1974

Goldfarb FF: Geriatric gynecology, in Rossman I (ed), Clinical Geriatrics, 2nd ed. Philadelphia, Lippincott, 1979

Hoch P, Zubin J (eds): Psychopathology of Aging. New York, Grune and Stratton, 1961

Kornzweig AL: The eye in old age, in Rossmann I (ed), Clinical Geriatrics, 2nd ed. Philadelphia, Lippincott, 1979

Lee G: A rural hypertension control program. American Journal of Nursing 74:1451, 1974

Mezey MD, Rauckhorst LH, Stokes SA: Health Assessment of the Older Individual. New York, Springer, 1980

O'Flynn-Comisky A: The type A individual. American Journal of Nursing 79:1956, 1979

Reichel W (ed): The Geriatric Patient. New York, H.P. Publishing, 1978

Richardson JL: Colorectal cancer: A mass screening and education program. Geriatrics 32(2):123, 1977

Shindell S, Salloway J, Oberembt C: A Coursebook in Health Care Delivery. New York, Appleton-Century-Crofts, 1976

Sivarajan E, Halpenny C: Exercise testing. American Journal of Nursing 79(12):2163, 1979

Straus B: Disorders of the digestive system, in Rossman I (ed), Clinical Geriatrics, 2nd ed. Philadelphia, Lippincott, 1979

Villaverde MM, MacMillan CW: Ailments of Aging. New York, Van Nostrand Reinhold, 1980

Ziller R: Self social constructs of normals and acute neuropsychotic patients. Journal of Consulting Psychology 24:59, 1964

Zung W: A self-rating depression scale. Archives of General Psychiatry 12:63, 1965

13

Management of Risk Factors

Old age, like adolescence, is a prolonged period of susceptibility to crisis. Personal losses head the list of the myriad stresses encountered during this period. The loss of a spouse or of relatives and friends—as well as the personal threat of a deteriorating body image—makes death a reality as never before. Other stresses impact on the elderly: the economic and social losses so often associated with retirement, social losses that occur through relocation, the loneliness occasioned by these losses, and the isolation brought about by reduced levels of activity. Add to this the wear and tear of a style of living that may have included such things as smoking, overeating, and lack of exercise and it is no wonder that the elderly experience reduced self-esteem.

With so many risk factors at hand there is always the potential for erupting crisis. Crisis situations can magnify out of proportion if accustomed coping mechanisms have been eroded by the aging process. For example, it is not unusual for people facing crisis to increase their activity level as a way of coping. For the elderly person, decreased mobility brought on by cardiac problems or arthritis may eliminate this long-standing coping behavior. Or consider the person who customarily talks a crisis out. In the absence of a partner to use as a sounding board, a crisis situation may escalate. In cases such as these, not only is the aging person at risk for more losses, but the aging process itself may necessitate a change in coping behaviors normally used to deal with those losses.

Knowing that losses will accrue to the aging, the nurse can help the person through discussion and guidance to anticipate stresses and develop new coping skills or strengthen old behaviors in order

to meet these eventualities. Such guidance can be viewed as primary prevention. Historically, the concept of prevention has held little interest for our society, since it has always been difficult to prove that prevention results in a reduced incidence of illness or a better quality of life. Despite this lack of interest by the health field generally, nursing has long focused on preventive teaching, especially in the area of child care and prenatal counseling. Today there is a need to expand this focus to include the aging population in our society.

There are a number of interventions the nurse can undertake for the elderly client at risk. Providing a vehicle for discussion, cognitive learning, and problem solving through the medium of group work is one; enlarging the support system or encouraging networking via religious groups and community supports is another. Finally, when crises erupt, as inevitably they will, the nurse can engage in crisis intervention and attempt to restore the client to a pre-crisis level of functioning. Since working with the client at risk is not a solitary task, the nurse must frequently call upon other members of the health care team for consultation, support, and, at times, direct intervention.

GROUP WORK FOR THE CLIENT AT RISK

Although little research exists to prove the value of therapeutic groups for the elderly, there is much clinical agreement that such groups serve an important function in the care of the elderly. Richardson and Lowman (1980), in their fine historical perspective on group work for the elderly, suggest that the group is a particularly effective therapeutic modality for meeting the developmental, social, and psychological needs of older adults and for enhancing their sense of well-being. In addition to meeting the need for socialization and affiliation, the group can be a vehicle for developing new coping behaviors, enhancing self-esteem through creative problem solving, and increasing both cognitive awareness of health and conformity to acceptable health behaviors through peer pressure.

The group is also a medium for providing the elderly with a social support system, and an intact social support system is positively correlated with mental health (Evans, 1979). Evans suggests that the nurse might offer aging clients an opportunity to meet regularly in small discussion groups at neighborhood health centers or senior centers, where the group itself has the potential for becoming a continuing support system for its members. An example of this type of group support was experienced by an aging member of a church senior citizen center that offered a regular luncheon program. Larry, separated from his wife and children and experiencing severe bouts of loneliness, began to drink excessively and was finally evicted from his apartment for not paying his rent. Although the social agency helped him relocate, it was a member of the group who tuned in on his loneliness and regularly invited him to visit her in her apartment. Group activities and shared meals had contributed to a degree of cohesiveness within the group that eventually provided Larry with a support system.

Brower (1981) points out that the group can serve many purposes, ranging from the emotional education that comes from involvement in the group process to the enhancement of self-esteem that results from the attention and support of a peer group. Since health can encompass all problems of life and living, the group may range from a highly structured discussion of hypertension to an informal discussion of a topic chosen by the group.

Richardson and Lowman (1980) note that the group is an especially acceptable medium for today's cohort of elderly who were raised to rely heavily on themselves. Despite their vulnerability to mental distress because of losses and diminished resources for coping, few older persons seek assis-

tance from mental health professionals (Kramer et al., 1973). Having grown up in a society that paid little attention to mental health, they lack sophistication in this area. Moreover, they prize their independence and view seeking help as a form of weakness. In a group setting they can help others while working out solutions to their own problems. The activity involved in group problem solving is much preferred to the passivity of being treated by a mental health professional.

Group work is also a more efficient modality for the professional's time, since it enables the leader to work with as many as eight clients at a time. There is also evidence to support the effectiveness of group work. Peer pressure is the strongest force mobilizing us toward conformity, a critical factor in compliance with health teaching. Finally, people in a group are more likely to accept new ideas and adopt new attitudes and values when they see themselves as members of a group dedicated to those principles (Lewin, 1943). Given the fact that the group is more acceptable to the elderly client, that it makes more efficient use of the professional's time, and that it provides a more effective way of meeting a variety of goals—not the least of which is meeting an individual's dependency needs without fostering dependence—the group is one of the best modalities for the nurse interested in helping aging clients.

Yalom (1977) identified twelve curative factors that operate within a group setting. Although these have not yet been researched with regard to the elderly, Burnside (1978) sees the application of a number of these curative factors:

1. *Group cohesiveness, or solidarity:* This is a measure of the attractiveness of the group and how well it confers the feeling that one is accepted. Hartford (1972) finds evidence of cohesiveness when members refer to themselves as "we."

2. *Universality:* Universality is the feeling that, whatever problem is being experienced, members are not alone. By listening to others coping with problems, one is able to make a better adjustment.

3. *Interpersonal learning:* As members receive feedback (input) from the group, they learn about their ability to communicate. They also improve

their skills in getting along with others (output) and begin to feel more trusting as they learn how they relate to other members.

4. *Catharsis:* Members have an opportunity through catharsis to express both positive and negative feelings toward other members or the group leader. They are able to say what is bothering them without holding it in.

5. *Identification:* Members find someone in the group to pattern themselves after, leading to an increase in self-esteem. They may, for example, begin to imitate a member who is better adjusted.

6. *Instillation of hope:* Members may learn that others have been able to solve problems with the help of the group.

To these might be added:

7. *Altruism:* Helping others increases one's self-respect; being important to others enhances one's self-esteem.

8. *Family reenactment:* Members may have the same characteristics, foibles, and strengths that significant others have. Understanding current relationships facilitates learning about past relationships.

While Yalom's curative factors address the value of the group as a medium for problem solving and change, they touch only marginally on the other major focuses of group work for the elderly in community settings today. Traditionally, group activities filled leisure hours for the elderly. During the seventies a tremendous growth in the use of group treatment approaches occurred, including the introduction of behavior modification, problem-solving, and actualization groups designed to prevent mental health problems (Lieberman and Gourash, 1979; Brown, 1977). The elderly were no longer considered patients in need of amusement, but citizens who could develop new and caring relationships and exert control over their lives by confronting the problems of living, thereby enhancing their self-esteem.

Purposes of Groups

Today both directive and nondirective groups are offered to the elderly in community settings to meet their wide range of needs. Generally speaking, a directive format is utilized for traditional didactic groups where the main focus is on teaching, or for lecture–discussion groups which focus on special health problems. A nondirective format is utilized when the needs of the group are first identified by problem solving and the findings are translated into group goals.

Miller and Solomon (1980) suggest that the purposes for groups fall into four categories:

1. *Formal and informal educational groups,* which may include anything from cooking to poetry discussion to health.

2. *Life task,* the purpose of which is to overcome feelings of loneliness, helplessness, and hopelessness. Members may include recent retirees, the recently bereaved, the disabled, and those contemplating a move from independent to institutional living. Life task groups may be further subdivided into anticipatory guidance, crisis groups, and tertiary prevention or postcrisis groups.

3. *Self-government groups* are generally for people at senior citizen centers or for the institutionalized who are trying to maintain control over their lives by influencing administrative policy.

4. *Social action groups* provide opportunities for people to exert control over their lives by affecting political and social issues of concern to older people. Advocacy groups like the Gray Panthers are a good example.

Miller and Solomon note that each of these groups makes different demands of group members; specifically, each demands a different degree of mutual aid and interdependence. In formal and educational groups these demands may be rather low, while in life task or problem-solving groups they may be very high. While groups are more acceptable to many people than one-to-one interactions, not all members are ready for high level input. For example, Miller and Solomon describe a group formed in an institutional setting to improve aspects of daily life. This was a high demand group with an expectation of mutual participation and interaction. The group members, however, knew each other only casually and had developed little trust. It was only by forming low-demand activity oriented groups that members came to know and trust each other. They then regrouped to accomplish their original purpose.

Guidelines for Group Formation

In selecting members for the group it is wise to consider the need for common interests. Ethnicity and socioeconomic class should be viewed as factors that influence the way group members feel about certain subjects. For example, while working with a predominantly black group, a student leader focused on the subject of "soul foods" remembered from childhood. This triggered a discussion of childhood memories of the South and produced a cohesiveness that normally was not seen in the group. Brower (1981) notes that sexuality may be more explicitly and comfortably discussed by the affluent elderly than by a group of inner city, poor elderly. Although a similar level of mental alertness is required for any active problem solving group, life experience can often compensate for educational differences.

Ground Rules

Yalom (1977) points out that a large part of the group leader's task in group maintenance is performed before the first meeting. One important task for the leader is to develop a group culture through the establishment of group norms. Some of the guidelines for participation might include one person speaking at a time, respectful listening, and active participation by all members. The group leader may need to set limits on digression and restore focus when the group strays from the topic.

Conducting the Group

Miller and Solomon (1980) suggest that the group begins by focusing on group purpose and how it is to be accomplished. This lends structure and safeguards members from unnecessary intrusion. The initial gathering should include a statement from the leader as to why the group is offered and a period to allow for feedback from members.

All groups struggle with basic issues of dependence versus independence (Yalom, 1977), but for groups of older people who have accepted the societal view that young people know what is best for the elderly, the resolution of these issues requires more time. The elderly have a tendency to acquiesce to the leader's perception of the group

purpose. Acquiescence, however, need not mean acceptance or mutuality. Miller and Solomon warn that if difficulty arises in getting members to focus on the purpose or attendance falls off, it may signal the need for further discussion on the purpose of the group. Research has shown that the elderly find it extremely difficult to confront each other or express negatives, so it behooves the leader to provoke this discussion (Lakin et al., 1977). Another aspect of the dependence versus independence issue arises when members expect the leader to assume complete responsibility for following through on group decisions, especially when they involve contact with external systems. Fearful that this will only enhance group feelings of powerlessness and helplessness, the nurse leader may be reluctant to take on this responsibility. Miller and Solomon suggest that it may be necessary initially to assume this responsibility as a demonstration of respect and caring. Once needed support is given, dependency needs are likely to decrease.

Ongoing Phase. During the ongoing phase the group is actively involved in the problem-solving process. The leader can often facilitate this process by breaking down larger problems into more manageable ones. By providing technical help and expressing faith in the group's ability, the nurse leader can lend sufficient support while still allowing the group to arrive at its own solution.

The issue of scapegoating often surfaces during this phase as members berate or belittle the authoritarian or acting-out group member. The nurse leader must be on guard against moving too quickly to protect the scapegoated member, thereby driving the conflict underground.

Termination. Endings are always difficult because they reawaken past separations, many of which have not been resolved. For the nurse leader who sees termination as yet another loss inflicted on the elderly, it is well to keep in mind that the elderly are experienced survivors of loss. It does little good to avoid the issue, as some do, by offering the group a farewell party which permits only positive sentiments to be expressed. Termination is a process which must be started early enough to allow for avoidance, anger, acceptance, and final farewells to take place. Moreover, it should be a reciprocal process wherein the nurse leader can share personal insights and feelings about the group. It is important to summarize group achievements and the growth that has occurred.

Frequently the question of gifts surfaces at the end of a group. While professionals disagree on the appropriateness of accepting gifts, if the gift is viewed by the nurse leader as an expression of thanks it may be an important way for the group member to equalize the relationship. If the gift is refused the group member may feel rejected along with the gift.

Meeting Developmental Tasks through Group Work

Groups are especially effective in assisting older people to accomplish developmental tasks (Richardson and Lowman, 1980). Erikson (1963) defined the main developmental task of the aging period as integration, by which he meant that people must become reconciled with their lives and recognize that the past cannot be changed; life must be realistically accepted and positively evaluated. Butler (1963) proposed the purposefulness of the Life Review (reminiscing, dreaming, and reflecting on the past) in order to reexamine both its successes and failures as a way of gaining perspective. Butler proposed that the garrulousness and "living in the past" attitude that often characterize the elderly are actually attempts to resolve lifetime conflicts in preparation for death. Terming it the "Life Review," Butler considered it an adaptive process, but warned that certain individuals, particularly those who had injured others, who were arrogant, and who tended to live in the future rather than the present, might be subject to anxiety and depression in the process. He recommended a trained participant/observer to facilitate the Life Review process.

Reminiscence, the act of recalling and narrating past experiences, can help the elderly order the events of their life and rework aspects of the past to make them more acceptable. To remember coming to America alone at seventeen for political or economic freedom and struggling to survive, raise children, and achieve success, is to remember one's contribution to the present.

Although everyone reminisces almost on a daily basis, until recently the process was considered pathognomonic of old age. Today the recall of positive aspects of life as it was prior to dependence and

disability is considered both necessary and therapeutic. Hala (1975) describes an experiment in reminiscence therapy with a group of older clients who had lost self-esteem as they lost some of their self-sufficiency. She concluded that the experiment fostered socialization by allowing common areas of interest and feelings to be explored. Socialization and reminiscing continued outside the group. Moreover, as participants developed more self-confidence, they showed less automatic compliance to the staff.

Ebersole (1976) cautions the group leader not to seek to be entertained. Knowing that there will be many colorful characters with rich backgrounds in the group, the nurse leader may become angry or frustrated when group members fail to participate at an expected level. Miller and Solomon (1980) note that constant repetition of themes may reflect unresolved conflicts. Probing the situation may bring to light stresses that were life threatening or guilt about acts committed or omitted that can be resolved. To achieve an ongoing cohesive reminiscence group, Ebersole suggests that members be chosen carefully and with some commonalities in mind. The group should be closed, with new members admitted only with the group's approval.

DEVELOPING COPING SKILLS

The group can be used to enhance mental health by aiding in the development of new coping skills. Many older persons lack assertive skills because of their cultural upbringing. Zarit (1980) points out that most elderly have been raised to respect the authority and judgment of the physician without question. Yet they often feel frustrated and powerless when the doctor does not listen or fails to answer questions. Many elderly consider it impolite to be direct with others in expressing their feelings, preferences, and needs. Most were raised to anticipate the needs of their parents; when their own children fail to act in a like manner, the elderly parent is often unable to make a direct request.

The nurse can play a major role in helping clients understand that assertiveness is not used to manipulate others but to make one more effective in recognizing and stating one's own preferences. Assertiveness training has two aspects—learning assertive beliefs that facilitate assertiveness, and practicing assertive behaviors. Through role playing in a group situation elderly clients can learn ways of asking questions and persisting until an answer is forthcoming. They can also learn to express feelings and preferences so that anger and resentment do not have an opportunity to build. Although there is no specific guide to assertiveness training for the elderly, several excellent books can be adapted for that purpose (Clark, 1978; Phelps and Austin, 1975).

Another important coping behavior with wide application for the elderly is *relaxation*. Relaxation techniques can be beneficial in the treatment of insomnia, hypertension, and other psychosomatic disorders, or as an adjunct to other treatments. Studies are underway at Columbia Presbyterian Medical Center in New York City to explore the value of relaxation in hypertensive disease. Both biofeedback and consistent relaxation techniques have been found to lower the medication requirement. Relaxation can also be used as an adjunct to assertiveness training or in any situation that induces anxiety. Using relaxation techniques the nurse can teach elderly clients to monitor their own tensions more accurately. Clients learn deep muscle relaxation by tensing various muscle groups for ten seconds, then relaxing them for fifteen seconds. By learning to distinguish between the two feelings, clients are able to locate the source of tension, whether in the back, neck, arm, or thighs. They can then focus on the part of the body where tension is lodged.

Exercise is another coping behavior that appears to have a beneficial effect on the individual's ability to cope with stress, particularly when used in conjunction with other stress reduction techniques such as biofeedback or relaxation. Exercise is rather like a two-edged sword. Not only does it relieve tension, it also promotes a general sense of well-being. From a physical standpoint, some researchers believe that exercise decreases the risk of degenerative states such as osteoporosis, muscle atrophy, and even bladder and bowel dysfunction. In 1975, during an international track meet in Toronto that attracted participants from 30 to 90, two researchers had an unusual opportunity to study the relationship between continued exercise and aging (Fixx, 1977). After examining 128 male and 7 female participants, the researchers concluded that the oxygen processing ability of the aging athlete declines more slowly than it does in the general population, and that heart abnormalities among these individuals are rare.

Exercise for the elderly can take many forms. Some elderly who are deemed fit by a physician may gradually begin an aerobic exercise program like jogging. For the sedentary, simple stretching exercises and isometric exercises are a possibility (Table 1). Despite the minimal muscle fiber shortening involved, isometric exercises do improve muscle tone. Caution must be taken not to elevate blood pressure in the hypertensive. For those at an intermediate level of fitness, Yoga, T'ai Chi, or creative movement might be a more acceptable alternative.

Boots and Hogan (1981) report that dance exercise increases sensory stimulation, provides greater range of motion for general health maintenance, and even helps develop one's nonverbal communication skills. Creative movement begins with a process called "centering," which is essentially derived from relaxation techniques. Muscles are tensed on inspiration and relaxed on expiration, the process moving sequentially from the feet to the legs, thighs, buttocks, and so on. The technique can be done in a sitting position, making it easy for older clients.

Nurses need not be professional dancers to incorporate principles of dance into their practice. Nor do older clients need to be agile and flexible. The important concept is to increase the activity level of the client, since inactivity breeds depression, discouragement, and apathy. In her work with the emotionally disturbed, Harris (1975) found that while behavioral disturbances can lead to a deterioration in physical fitness, the reverse is also true. An absence of physical fitness can result in further emotional disturbance. In the interests of better mental and physical health, the nurse should engage older clients in an exercise program. Since most people find it difficult to move from sedentary status to an active exercise program, group support can be an important mobilizing force.

ANTICIPATORY GUIDANCE

Usually people are formally and systematically trained to deal with the next stage of their development. Until recently, however, little attention was paid to

TABLE 1. SEDENTARY EXERCISES

Isometric Exercises

The following exercises are done to the count of four, working from toes to the nose.
1. Sit up straight in a chair, touching both feet to the ground.
2. Press toes into the ground.
3. Press heels into the ground.
4. Press both feet together at toes.
5. Press both feet together at heels.
6. Cross feet and press feet together, knees apart.
7. Cross feet opposite direction, feet together, knees apart.
8. Place right hand on right knee, press hand down as you push knee up.
9. Place left hand on left knee, press hand down as you push knee up.
10. Place hands inside knees, push knees in as you push hands out.
11. Place hands outside knees, push knees out as you push hands in.
12. Place hands on waist, press in while inhaling deeply.
13. Make a fist with right hand and place left hand over it. Push up as left hand pushes fist down. Push fist into center as left hand pushes out. Push fist down as left hand pushes up, and push fist out as left hand pushes in.
14. Make a fist with left hand and place right hand over it. Push fist up as right hand pushes fist down. Push fist into center as right hand pushes out. Push fist down as right hand pushes up, and push fist out as right hand pushes in.
15. Make a fist with right hand. Cover fist with left hand and squeeze.
16. Make a fist with left hand. Cover fist with right hand and squeeze.
17. Press fingers of right hand into left palm one at a time to the count of two.
18. Press fingers of left hand into right palm one at a time to the count of two.
19. Press hands together at the chest, elbows out. Press hands together at forehead. Press hands together over head.
20. Catch fingers together at chest and pull, elbows out. Catch fingers together over head and pull.
21. Place hand under chin, press chin down, and push hand up. Place hand on right side of face, push face toward right as hand pushes left. Place hand on left side of face, push face toward left as hand pushes to right.
22. Place both hands on forehead, push head forward as hands pull head back. Place both hands on back of head, push head backward as hands pull forward.

Stretching Exercises

The following exercises can be done while sitting in a chair, to the count of four.
1. Stretch both legs out in front. Do not point toes.
2. Turn feet to one side, then straight, then to other side, then straight, etc.
3. Lift right leg and make four circles, lift left leg and make four circles.
4. Hands on waist, bend to right, bend to front, bend to left.
5. Hold both arms out to the side and make 8 small circles; rest arms and then make 8 medium circles; rest arms and then make 8 big circles. Shake out arms.
6. Hold arms straight over head and bob arms to the count of eight; rest arms.
7. Hold arms over head and try to reach as high as possible, first right, then left.
8. Sit up straight, try to touch right ear to right shoulder, left ear to left shoulder, etc.
9. Try to bring shoulders up to ears. Do this quickly to count of eight.
10. Circle head to right trying to keep as close to shoulders as possible. Do this slowly.
11. Turn head to right and try to look back as far as possible. Repeat, turning head to the left.
12. Holding the head steady, look from right to left and left to right to the count of eight. Look up and down to the count of eight.
13. Tighten face, close eyes, purse lips, then open eyes wide, mouth wide, and relax face.

one of the most stressful stages—retirement. Despite the loss of important social roles critical to one's self-concept and self-esteem, the older person was expected to handle the crisis alone. Rosow (1973) points out that the elderly, although subject to the same pressures and role losses as other people, seldom muster a peer support system in the way adolescents, for example, do to confront these stresses. A gold watch, a farewell dinner, and a handshake often become the only rites of passage into the retirement period.

Kimmel (1979) points out that one of the leading implications of recent retirement studies is the importance of anticipatory socialization for the new set of roles that the retired person will occupy. These studies also suggest that preretirement counseling should focus particular emphasis on health maintenance and attitudes about retirement. Kimmel concludes that planning for a reliable source of income, anticipating the different kinds of roles and activities desirable and available to the retiree, as well as developing a few interests that may deepen into leisure activities involving new friends, would all be helpful in the preretirement phase.

Today many firms offer preretirement counseling to employees. Estes (1978) describes a course format developed by the Omaha Gerontology Program at the University of Nebraska. In seven two-hour sessions the topics of mental health, the process of aging, leisure, estate planning, finance, and every day law for the senior citizen are covered. Prior to and following the series preretirees are given the Nathan Kogan Attitude Scale, which determines both negative and positive attitudes toward aging. The program also provides very practical information about the nature of maturing sexuality and the individual differences seen in physical aging. Preretirees are encouraged to pursue their fantasies of a future life and focus on their options and life potentials. They are encouraged to practice communication skills, reflect on available support systems in the event of illness or death, and familiarize themselves with community organizations and activities as they evaluate their own needs for leisure, volunteer, and work activities. They are even encouraged to reminisce on past experiences of youth. From reminiscing to projecting and planning for a future, the program anticipates and deals with, at

some level, most of the crises that are likely to erupt in the retirement period.

The role for nurses in anticipatory guidance to preretirees is a large one. Whether functioning at the worksite or in a community-based setting, nurses are in a favored position, by virtue of education and experience, to conduct groups for preretirees. With the exception of financial and legal matters they are prepared to deal with all of the topics suggested for a preretiree course. Not only can they teach vital aspects of health maintenance, they can also discuss changing physiology and alterations in sexual functioning that occur during this period. Being knowledgeable about the community, they can also help the preretiree seek new roles in the community. Their knowledge of established groups and organizations would be useful in providing the preretiree with a broader based support system. Given adequate time the nurse can also teach new coping skills, while the group itself might become the nucleus for new relationships during the postretirement period.

Setting

For the occupational health nurse the worksite is the logical setting for a preretirement group. For the community nurse reaching preretirees with counseling sessions is more difficult because of the lack of a central location. Clients are not likely to be found at senior centers or mental health centers while they are still pursuing an active work role. One frequently overlooked setting is the place of worship. For many elderly people, the religious gathering place remains a social setting of great influence. Among blacks, for example, the church has traditionally been a source of renewal. The counseling sessions might also be conducted as part of the outreach program of a local community mental health center.

Community Resources

The nurse conducting preretirement counseling can explore both continuing education and service opportunities with clients. Elderhostel (Nemy, 1981) has been one of the most remarkable success stories in the area of higher education for older adults. The program, which started in 1975 with only a handful of institutions in New Hampshire, now offers programs in fifty states and on four hundred campuses to more than 21,000 seniors. The program itself consists of one-week sessions in which participants live on campus in student housing, take their meals in dining halls, attend up to three special noncredit classes, and take part in a variety of field trips and cultural activities. Previous college experience is not required and many participants have not graduated from high school. Best of all, the cost is reasonable. A catalogue of programs is available free-of-charge by writing to Elderhostel at 100 Boylston Street, Suite 200 T, Boston, MA 02116.

Second Careers Volunteer Program offers an opportunity to former business executives, teachers, principals, and administrators to serve as volunteers in agencies and organizations where their help is sorely needed. Some of these volunteers are using skills they perfected during years of gainful employment; others are enjoying the opportunity to develop new talents or employ talents they never had a chance to use in their previous careers. For more information, write to the Second Careers Volunteer Program care of ACTION, 806 Connecticut Avenue NW, Washington D.C. 20525.

Foster Grandparenting offers still another opportunity for the elderly to feel both useful and loved. Started by the Administration on Aging and the Office of Economic Opportunity in 1965, this program is also under the aegis of ACTION. It offers older men and women a chance to give love and attention to institutionalized and handicapped children, receiving in return a small stipend and the great satisfaction of being needed and loved. The usual work period is 20 hours a week and the pay is set at the minimum wage.

A more complete listing of opportunities and services for older Americans can be found in Department of Health and Human Services Bulletin (OHD) 75-20807.

SELF-HELP GROUPS

Although self-help groups are usually spontaneously organized and consumer initiated, nurses have an opportunity to promote, organize, and introduce the self-help approach in outpatient settings. Clients with chronic illnesses, such as hypertension,

diabetes, arthritis, and cerebrovascular and cardiovascular disease, often feel inferior and consider themselves helpless victims of a disease process beyond their control (Strauss, 1975). Too often they isolate themselves from social support systems and fail to follow prescribed regimens. Acute illnesses can follow. Cole et al. (1979) believe that noncompliance is a visible manifestation of the dysfunctional relationship between client and health professional, with the client seeking advice from friends or relatives that is based on experience rather than professional knowledge.

Since the establishment of Alcoholics Anonymous in the mid-thirties, self-help groups have provided an important source of social support and an opportunity for group members to change their lives. The self-help principle focuses on commonality of experience and in many instances on the perception of being deviant and stigmatized by the larger society. Self-help groups act as a reference group for persons with the same condition. Not only do these groups provide emotional support, they also encourage members to assume greater responsibility for their own lives. As members seek strategies that enable them to cope more effectively, they become convinced of the value of such change.

Self-help groups are especially effective as tertiary prevention. Groups organized for specific chronic conditions, such as stroke, diabetes, arthritis, and hypertension, have provided a sense of belonging and, with it, the encouragement to change life-styles in compliance with the illness. By contrast, people who are socially isolated with minimal primary group or work-related social ties have a heightened vulnerability to chronic disease (Rabkin and Struening, 1976).

In addition to organizing self-help groups for the elderly, the nurse can play a major role in referral. For example, new groups have been surfacing in recent years to help champion the cause of older women. Recognizing their longer life expectancy and greater economic privation, these groups are trying to help older women cope with feelings of powerlessness and low self-esteem in positive, action-oriented ways.

Economic inequities are reflected in a startling statistic from 1977 that reveals that the median income for men 65 and over was $5526; for women of the same age, it was only $3088 (Carlson, 1980). Moreover, an estimated 72 percent of the elderly poor are unmarried women. And the lot of the married woman is not always any better. Many married women have not worked enough years to be eligible for a pension or have worked in service areas where pensions were either nonexistent or small. Adding insult to injury, a 1974 law permits a husband to collect a larger pension by foregoing the survivor's benefit—without consulting his wife. If he dies before she does, she loses all her pension rights.

Some of the advocacy groups that have begun to redress both economic and political inequities through research, education, and distribution of information are listed below:

- *The Older Women's League Educational Fund* investigates issues of concern to older women and publishes reports on how women can help themselves. Contact Tish Sommers or Laurie Shields. Address: 3800 Harrison St., Oakland, CA 94611.
- *The National Action Forum for Older Women* provides information on problems affecting elderly women and suggests steps women can take to improve their condition. Address: School of Allied Health Professions, the State University of New York, Stony Brook, NY 11794.
- *The Older Women's Committee of the National Organization for Women* promotes political action to reform institutions that discriminate against older women. Address: 425 13th St. NW, Washington, D.C. 20004.
- *The Displaced Homemaker Network* acts as referral service for women seeking help and provides technical aid. Contact Sandra Burton, executive director. Address: 755 H. St. NW, Washington, D.C. 20001.
- *The Older Americans Program of the American Association of Community and Junior Colleges* provides education, job training, and improved access to employment opportunities for older persons. Address: One Dupont Circle NW, Suite 410, Washington, D.C. 20036.
- *The Women's Division of the National Retired Teachers Association/American Association of Retired Persons* serves as a clearinghouse for all national women's organizations in coordinating programs for older women. Address: 1909 K St. NW, Washington, D.C. 20049.

- *The Older Women's Caucus of the National Women's Political Caucus* deals with issues in Congress and state legislatures to promote women's rights. Address: 53 Monte Vista, Novato, CA 94947.
- *The Women's Equity Action League* lobbies for legislation to reform Social Security and improve retirement income of older women. Address: 805 15th St. NW, Washington, D.C. 20005.

CRISIS INTERVENTION

When losses occur to the elderly through death, retirement, relocation, disability, or criminal victimization such as assault, it is not unusual for normal coping mechanisms to fail. It is equally true, however, that the older person's ability to handle losses continues to reflect a lifelong pattern of dealing with loss. As in so many aspects of the elderly, the spectrum ranges from those who function effectively with a variety of adaptive skills to those who function ineffectively with chronic deficits and maladaptive skills.

For example, one young-elderly client comes into a senior center on a regular basis with a crisis situation. Her level of anxiety is always high and utterly contagious. One month an important document substantiating her need for assistance has been lost; the following month food stamps have been cut off; another visit is filled with psychosomatic symptoms but no access to a health care facility; yet another month goes by and the landlord is threatening to raise the rent. This client reflects a lifelong pattern of maladaptive skills. Any precipitant can be magnified to crisis proportions.

Far more typical is the octogenarian who appeared recently asking to have her blood pressure monitored. When a comment was made about the swelling in her face and the ecchymotic area under her eye, she claimed to have been mugged. In discussing the mugging further she admitted that the assault had been made by her 82-year-old husband who came home drunk and abused her. Her first response was that she "didn't understand what had gotten into him," but later, as her trust in the interviewer began to grow, she admitted that the husband had beaten her on many occasions during their marriage and that he was now threatening to take the money from their joint account and return alone to Europe. She had learned to cope with the beatings over the years, but the threat of losing her life savings, which would have made her helpless and totally dependent, had caused a crisis that overwhelmed her usual coping skills. In this instance a referral was made to a social service agency serving the elderly. A case worker accompanied her to the bank, where the manager made joint signatures mandatory for any future withdrawals from the account.

The word "crisis" comes from the Greek work "krinein", which means "to decide". It is the need for decision and the reluctance or perhaps inability to make that decision that so often produces a crisis. Interestingly, the Chinese character for the word "crisis" is a combination of characters meaning "danger" and "opportunity". Crisis is thus the turning point which offers both danger and opportunity to the individual. Any change, regardless of its source and desirability, is likely to precipitate a crisis. Silverman (1977) states that crisis is a result of the interaction of a stressful event and the perceived lack of resources either to overcome it or accommodate to it. Perlman (1975) believes that coping mechanisms are put into play on one of three levels: defense mechanisms are used at the unconscious level; preconscious mechanisms produce an automatic response but are easily brought to awareness; and conscious coping behaviors are those which are used selectively as the result of a decision-making process.

Crisis intervention has evolved over the past forty years into a growing body of theory and techniques. The literature reflects much general agreement about both the causes and stages of crisis development and the process of intervention. It is interesting to note that long before the theory emerged nurses were in the forefront of crisis intervention as they dealt with crisis situations in the home and hospital on a daily basis.

Baldwin (1978) has outlined the typical phases of a crisis situation:

1. *Onset:* An emotionally hazardous situation occurs, producing an uncomfortable affect. Previously learned coping behaviors are brought into play to minimize the discomfort.

2. *The Emotional Crisis:* When coping behaviors fail to work, discomfort intensifies along with cognitive disorganization. This failure calls forth an attempt at new coping behaviors and problem-solving techniques. During this phase the individual usually seeks out a support system.

3. *Crisis Resolution:* With assistance the problem is defined, feelings are dealt with, and decisions are made or new problem-solving methods are learned to cope with the crisis. Underlying conflicts that are frequently reactivated by crisis events are identified and at least partially resolved. At this point the individual is restored to a pre-crisis level of functioning. In the event that the person fails to seek or find adequate help, deal with feelings, or initiate effective coping behaviors or sources of support, the uncomfortable affect may be reduced but the individual will return to a less adaptive level of functioning.

4. *Post-crisis Adaptation:* As a result of the successful resolution the individual is less vulnerable when confronted with similar or new problem situations. Underlying conflicts have been resolved, new and more adaptive coping or problem-solving skills have been learned, and overall improved levels of functioning and personal growth have occurred. In the event that the crisis is not appropriately resolved, the person becomes much more vulnerable to future crises because self-esteem has been further eroded.

Baldwin recapitulates a number of well-established corollaries that flow from crisis theory:

• Crises are not restricted to the emotionally fragile; they can happen to anyone.

• Crises are self-limiting, lasting no more than six weeks. During this period crisis resolution, whether adaptive or maladaptive, will take place.

• During a crisis psychological defenses are weakened or absent and the individual is more susceptible to external intervention.

• Help should be made available within the first two weeks of the crisis. Even a small external influence during a crisis can produce a disproportionate result within a short period of time.

• Every emotional crisis reflects an actual or anticipated loss that must be resolved as part of the crisis solution.

• Effective resolutions prevent future crises by removing vulnerabilities from the past and increasing available coping skills.

Types of Crises

Although the literature describes as many as six types of crises (Baldwin, 1978), three major classifications would seem to cover most crises. *Developmental*, or maturational, crises occur when the person is unable to make role changes appropriate to his or her new level of maturity. As Rosow (1973) points out, role losses may be institutionalized and inevitable for the aging person, but socialization to those losses is not. Since there is no clear definition of the role, people must adapt in the best way they can. Berezin (1963) speaks of aging as a crisis of slow-motion. It is punctuated by critical events such as widowhood or retirement and results in losses that are cumulative and, in many ways, irreversible.

Situational crises represent yet another type. They can result from an external event—one not necessarily part of normal living, often sudden and unexpected—that looms larger than the person's immediate resources or ability to cope. Illness, relocation, and the threat of reduced finances all represent situational crises.

Adventitious crises are those involving groups of people and usually involve disaster situations like floods, earthquakes, tornadoes, or fires.

Bereavement as a Crisis

One of the developmental tasks of aging is to adjust to the loss of one's spouse (Duvall, 1967). Typically it is the widow who survives her husband by eight years (Fell, 1977). Normally a grief reaction undergoes three stages and is successfully resolved by the individual without lasting impairment (Engel, 1964). The first stage is one of shock and disbelief that can last from minutes up to days. The second stage is initiated when the bereaved begins to face the reality of the loss with crying, anger, or even sudden attack upon relatives or the health care providers. The third stage, the actual grief work or restitution phase, lasts up to a year, during which the survivor must deal with the painful void through reminiscence, idealization, and finally realistic appraisal of both good and bad qualities of the deceased.

Heyman and Gianturco (1973) conducted a pilot study on the activities, attitudes, and mental and physical health of the elderly prior to and subsequent to widowhood. Their data indicate that older people adapt reasonably well to the loss of a spouse when supported by deep religious faith and a stable social network of family and friends. This is especially true if other life changes are held to a minimum. Jeffers (1961) also found that religion provided the elderly with a source of comfort in dealing with their feelings toward death.

Identifying Clients at Risk for Abnormal Grief Reactions. Some elderly clients are more prone to abnormal grief reactions than others. Certainly underlying personality structure and dependency needs are factors placing an individual at risk for an abnormal bereavement. One of the first clues to the "at risk" client is the frequency of clinic or office visits for psychosomatic symptoms. Parkes (1964) found that older widows showed a significant increase in the number of consultations for physical ailments such as headache, blurred vision, indigestion, weight loss, fatigue, palpitations, chest pains, and osteoarthritic and rheumatic symptoms. In some instances the symptoms replicate those of the deceased spouse. Contrary to the generally held belief that a long drawn-out illness better prepares the survivor to cope with the death of a spouse are the findings of Schwab et al. (1975) and Gerber et al. (1975). They found that an extended death watch of more than six months created greater psychological and physical health problems in the surviving spouse than in those whose mate died suddenly. Another danger signal is the bereaved who seeks isolation and pushes friends and loved ones away. Still another predictor of abnormal bereavement is the individual who shows intense grief, anger, and self-reproach during the first six weeks of bereavement. In summary, the "at risk" group consists of those who have had to care for an ill or dying spouse longer than six months; who have no prior experience with bereavement; who either have no available support system or have isolated themselves from such supports; who are depressed, conscience stricken or angry two months following the death of the spouse; or who make multiple visits to the doctor for psychosomatic type symptoms.

It is worth noting that a prolonged death watch has implications for primary prevention. The community nurse who makes home visits and the gerontological specialist in the nursing home would do well to assist the spouse with anticipatory grief work, encouraging discussion of feelings and even resentments associated with the dying process. Evans (1979) points out that we need to know how those who adapt to loss are able to resolve the problem. When losses occur, do they perceive a need for continued social interaction? If so, how do they increase their opportunities for social interaction? She concluded that nursing research on the elderly who adapt to loss might hold clues for our interventions with those who experience a crisis.

Secondary prevention involves early detection and treatment of abnormal grief reactions. The nurse's assessment includes the determination of the following: 1. the meaning of the death of the spouse; 2. whether the loss is perceived realistically or not; 3. whether the client has coped with grief before; 4. whether this current experience has awakened unresolved grief episodes from the past; and 5. the kind of support system in operation. A mental status assessment is always included, along with assessment of suicidal ideation.

Mr. M, a 72-year-old divorced male with a grown son, had been living with a woman friend who was being seen by the community nurse. The woman had been diagnosed at a major medical center as having a benign brain tumor without any suggestion of surgical intervention. Despite her deteriorating condition, the woman elected to return to her native country. Mr. M helped her make all the arrangements. Within two months of her return, and before Mr. M could join her for a visit, she died in her native country. Mr. M began to experience intermittent chest pain and shortness of breath, symptoms he had not complained of before. He accused the doctors and faulted himself for not having demanded surgical intervention. Lemasters (1978) points out that the guilt which attends bereavement is often related to the survivor's wish to have acted differently during a terminal illness. Along with the self-recrimination for negligence, Mr. M began to fault himself for his divorce that had occurred more than thirty years before.

In all intervention the initial goal is to help the client gain insight into the cause–effect relationship of crisis and stress. Mr. M understood this relationship all too clearly. The client was encouraged to express feelings about the loss and to verbalize any associated anxiety and tension. Mr. M was both highly verbal and sensitive, and able to verbalize his sentiments freely. Lindemann (1966) cautions

that widowers often need more support in order to ventilate, based on the cultural dictum that "grown men don't cry." Unfortunately, religious support was unavailable to Mr. M since he held a long-standing resentment to the "church," no matter what denomination, based on his belief that it had a markedly suppressive influence, especially on the young. Other supports, his brother and son, were available by phone but not easily accessible.

In working with Mr. M the nurse tried to propose a more realistic view, namely that he was blaming himself for a decision the experts had misjudged. The nurse also allowed time for reminiscence about life with his friend. He shared many tender moments of the relationship along with taped recordings of her voice and youthful photos from an earlier, happier time. Mr. M also began to talk about his feelings of guilt surrounding the divorce; the loss had reawakened memories of having "let down" still another person in his life.

Finally Mr. M was encouraged to join a senior luncheon program where he met another gentleman with similar interests in art, literature, politics, and culture. They were able to share these interests during and following their luncheon meetings. He was also encouraged to volunteer in a nursery school program because of his expressed interest in children.

At termination the nurse reviews the problem, the agreed upon plan, and the solution, emphasizing the client's present level of functioning, new coping skills, and the backdrop of community supports currently available.

Providing Support Groups. One additional strategy which might often prove helpful is referral of the client to a group of peers who have also suffered loss. Silverman (1969) found that widows and widowers who reached out to the recently bereaved for support found them more helpful than professionals. They reported that professionals and friends tended to push them into new relationships while those who had undergone a grief reaction merely offered support.

Support groups for the normal grieving process can now be found throughout the country. One hundred and one Widowed Person Service (WPS) groups are scattered across the nation, serving more than 5,000 persons a year. The purpose of the program is to help widowed persons recognize that they are still whole people in spite of their loss. Further information can be obtained by writing to WPS, care of the American Association for Retired Persons, 11909 K Street, N.W. Washington, D.C. 20049.

THE FAMILY AS A SUPPORT SYSTEM

The value of groups in the community has already been discussed in light of the support rendered before, during, and following crisis periods that face the elderly. One neglected area of support has been the family. Part of this stems from the misconception that adult children in American society are incapable of providing parents with adequate care (Silverman and Brahce, 1979). Shanas' (1979) report of her 25 years of research indicates that the elderly who have children not only live close to at least one of these children but also see their children often. There is also full recognition by the children that elderly parents need more support from their families.

The problem is not that family members are unwilling to give support so much as they lack the know-how and skills required (Kahn and Silverman, 1976). Many are under the misconception that they must act alone in providing assistance to aged parents. They also find themselves in the position of caring for aging parents and providing for children who have extended their dependency beyond adolescence, while at the same time, trying to meet personal needs, including adjustment to their own aging process (Strieb and Thompson, 1960; Brody, 1966).

Providing Support Before a Crisis
Gerontologists like Robert C. Benedict (1978) believe it is highly desirable to strengthen the family's role in supporting elderly persons, especially those who continue to live in the community. To this end Silverman and Brahce (1979) organized a group program for adult children. They blended didactic and therapeutic approaches, with the intent of increasing knowledge about the aging process, increasing understanding of the emotional reactions

of older people, providing access to community supports, and facilitating a support system within the group itself. During problem-solving sessions it became evident that children often increase the dependency of aging parents by their overconcern and overprotection. Grief, anger, role loss, and issues of dependence and role reversal were frequently discussed by the adult children who felt overburdened by parental needs. As a result of these sessions many group members were able to communicate more openly with their parents, especially when alternative care situations were discussed. They also realized that community services were open to all, not just the destitute.

Working with the Family in a Crisis Situation
In working with the elderly the nurse will often be called upon to confer with an extended support system representing children or even grandchildren of an aging client. Once it is ascertained that the crisis is one affecting the whole family and not just the individual, some assessment of the support system should be made. A number of researchers have developed family assessment tools (Lowe and Freeman, 1981; Pless and Satterwhite, 1973; Smilkstein, 1978), but the tools have been geared toward families with young children or adolescents. It is difficult to find a tool that assesses structure and relationships in a family with an elderly member. Several major aspects of functioning can provide helpful guidelines. These are described in Table 2.

Counseling the Family
Herr and Weakland (1978), in discussing the role of counseling with the elderly and their families, call attention to a major problem—the general reluctance to share feelings. In their experience they found that it helps to approach the family as though they are doing the counselor a favor. They suggest reframing the approach with questions like "I wonder if you could help me understand this situation better?" To find out exactly what the family is trying to achieve it becomes important to clarify goals. As the problem emerges, reflective techniques like "I think I hear you saying that . . ." or "Am I hearing you correctly? . . ." should be used to encourage the correction of inaccurate perceptions.

Determining how the family has been trying

TABLE 2. FAMILY INVENTORY

Structure

1. How many members are in the family? What are their ages and health statuses? Are there coalitions within the family? Factions are an important consideration, since one faction may subvert plans made by another.
2. How physically and emotionally close are the members? How often do they come together for reunions? Families can be physically close and emotionally distant, or emotionally close though separated by great distances.
3. What kind of living arrangements are available? Housing conditions or sheer lack of space may preclude having an older person join the family.
4. What is the financial situation of the family members? Does the family lack the resources to care for an aging parent? In some situations the older person's social security check may be the only reason that person is welcome in the household.
5. What community resources are available to assist the family in the care of an aging member? A check with the local social services office or one of the religious charitable organizations can provide specific referral information.

Function

1. Is one family member the gatekeeper, who permits or withholds access to the other members?
2. Is decision making shared or is one member vested with the power of decision?
3. What is the mood—warm, affectionate, and optimistic, or cool, distant, and pessimistic?
4. What is the level of trust between family members? Is there internal scapegoating of a member?
5. What is the level of trust between this family and the outside community? Is there scapegoating of the community?
6. Are there any family rules, that is, any unspoken agreements among family members about the conduct of the family (for example, to act logically and unemotionally)?
7. What is the communication pattern?
   a. Is communication clear or clouded?
   b. Can members express deep emotion, including angry feelings?
   c. Can members negotiate with each other without rancor?
   d. Are ego boundaries clear or are members invasive? For example, does one member speak for another?
   e. Are members able to respect each other's differences?
8. Are members goal-directed and able to deal with the task at hand?
9. Are members able to share responsibility?
10. What is the level of somatic complaints? Somatizing may reflect a level of depression and dependence that does not permit family members to reach out and help a parent.
11. What is the relationship of married children to their spouses?
    a. Are there strong emotional ties?
    b. Is the spouse supportive of the elderly member?
12. What is the relationship of children to the elderly family member?
    a. Does the older member have a role in the family?
    b. Is the older person given opportunities to exhibit control and competence?
    c. Is the older member overprotected to the extent that challenges are denied, leading to a decreased sense of competence?
    d. Is the older member physically or emotionally neglected by the family?
    e. Is the older member subjected to physical abuse?
    f. Does the family allow the older person to engage in activities of daily living without criticism, even when the results are less than perfect?
    g. Does the family reward the older person for independent functioning or do they tend to reinforce helplessness?
13. What is the family's cultural and socioeconomic status?
    a. What role does culture play in the intensity level of family relationships with an older member?
    b. How does the family's religious tradition influence values and beliefs about acceptance of an older member?
    c. How does the family's socioeconomic status influence their ability to provide both physical and emotional support to an older member?

to solve the problem is another useful technique. Herr and Weakland advise giving the family credit for intelligence by eliciting both the effective and ineffective strategies that have been called into play. This will eliminate solutions that have already been tried and failed and at the same time give the family credit for the active attempt at solving their own problems. In presenting alternative solutions to the family, beware of the "Yes, but . . ." response. Any solution involving an older member that is unacceptable to the family is a nonsolution. Wherever possible, offer alternatives and step aside, allowing the family to work out a solution. The nurse's role is that of a facilitator, guiding the family around roadblocks and to a solution.

Postcrisis Intervention

The nurse's role following a crisis is to facilitate linkage with existing support systems in the community. Referral may be made to a senior citizen group, a special widows' bereavement group, or a self-help group for the client with a chronic illness. When additional social services are required the nurse can refer the family to a community social service agency. One frequently overlooked support system is the client's place of worship. In addition to providing a spiritual support system, such meeting places frequently offer recreational activities and social services, and are organized to offer supportive services to senior members in the form of transportation, shopping assistance, luncheons, and telephone reassurance.

THE HEALTH CARE TEAM

It goes without saying that the nurse cannot support an aging client through crisis situations without assistance. Loneliness, financial distress, illness, and loss of independence and self-esteem cannot be resolved by any one person. A supportive health care team should be in operation.

In the past decade millions of dollars have been spent to investigate ways in which health care teams can facilitate the delivery of care to clients. While heralded as the answer to health care delivery to the elderly, the team concept is not without its flaws in practice. Although Great Britain has been in the forefront of the team concept, professionals are still uncertain about their colleagues' roles. A study done at the University of Aberdeen in Scotland in 1978 (Milne, 1980) demonstrated that students of nursing, medicine, and social work have rather stereotypic views of each others' functions. All three groups viewed visiting nurses as giving bedside care; public health nurses as looking after children; social workers as providing access to services for clients; and physicians as diagnosing and medicating. They also viewed many of the shared psychosocial functions as exclusively the purview of one discipline or another.

Similar reports can be found on the American scene (Balassone, 1981). The question of territoriality is without a doubt a major unresolved problem. The questions who does what, and why?, have not yet been successfully answered. Role definition still tends to follow stereotypes or lack precision. Interdisciplinary education has been suggested as part of the solution to this problem. The experience of working together while learning could develop a mutual appreciation for the true extent of each discipline's professional role.

A second problem is that of leadership. Bottom (1980) points out that the team approach automatically challenges the age-old concept that the doctor should be captain of the health care team. Clients have needs that go beyond medical management, making a type of rotating leadership within the health care team a more responsive approach to client management.

The geriatric team should consist of a full spectrum of members—general practitioner, nurse, social worker, occupational therapist, physical therapist, psychologist, dietician, dentist, optometrist, and minister. Such teams could be based both in hospital settings and in the community. This chapter has already discussed the multifaceted role that the nurse can play on such a team. In addition to expertise as teacher, care-giver, counselor, and crisis interventionist, the nurse is often in the most favored position to coordinate client care. The nurse generally has the most abiding contact with the client and, in essence, becomes the go-between, monitoring the client, alerting other members when special help is needed, and interpreting the nature of this help to the client.

Finally, as in all endeavors, communication between and among team members is a critical aspect of survival of the team concept. Members must be able to communicate their needs, expectations, and differences openly and honestly. Bottom (1980) believes that most of the impediments to team operation can be overcome by regular team sessions where members reaffirm their goals and reexamine their roles in an open and honest atmosphere.

REFERENCES

Aguilera D, Messick J: Crisis Intervention Theory and Methodology, 4th ed. St. Louis, Mosby, 1982

Balassone P: Territorial issues in an interdisciplinary experience. Nursing Outlook 29(4): 229, 1981

Baldwin BA: A paradigm for the classification of emotional crises: Implications for crisis intervention. American Journal of Orthopsychiatry 48: 538, 1978

Bankoff E: Support from Family and Friends, What Helps the Widow? Committee on Human Development, University of Chicago, Chicago, 1980

Benedict R: The future of aging: An interview with the commissioner. Aging, Dept. of Health, Education and Welfare pub. no. 279-280, 1978

Berezin M: Some intrapsychic aspects of aging, in Zinbert N, Kaufman I (eds.), Normal Psychology of the Aging Process. New York, International Universities Press, 1963

Bininger C, Kiesel M: Assessment of perceived role losses in the gerian. Journal of Gerontological Nursing 4(5): 24, 1978

Blackman JC: Group work in the community: Experiences with reminiscence, in Burnside IM (ed), Psychosocial Nursing Care of the Aged, 2nd ed. New York, McGraw-Hill, 1980

Boots S, Hogan C: Creative movement and health. Topics in Clinical Nursing 3(2): 23, 1981

Bottom W: Teaming up for geriatrics. Geriatrics 35(10): 106, 1980

Brewer G: Promoting healthful aging through strengthening family ties. Topics in Clinical Nursing 3(1): 45, 1981

Brody EM: The aging family. Gerontologist 6(4): 201, 1966

Brower HT: Groups and student teaching: Putting health education into practice. Journal of Gerontological Nursing 7(8): 483, 1981

Brown BR: The effects of three group dynamics treatments on nursing home residents. Long Term Care and Health Services Administration Quarterly 1: 226, 1977

Burgess AE, Baldwin BA: Crisis Intervention Theory and Practice: A Clinical Handbook. Englewood Cliffs, NJ, Prentice-Hall, 1981

Burnside IM: Principles from Yalom, in Burnside IM (ed.), Working with the Elderly: Group Process and Techniques. North Scituate, MA, Duxbury Press, 1978

Butler RN: The life review: An interpretation of reminiscence in the aged. Psychiatry 26(1): 65, 1963

Carlson, E: Older women—the problem and the promise. Modern Maturity Oct–Nov: 28, 1980

Clark CC: Assertive Skills for Nurses. Wakefield, MA, Contemporary Publishing, 1978

Cobb S: Social support as a moderator of life stress. Psychosomatic Medicine 38(5): 300, 1976

Cole S, O'Connor S, Bennett L: Self-help groups for clinic patients with chronic illness. Primary Care 6(2): 325, 1979

Dennis H: Remotivation therapy for the elderly: A surprising outcome. Journal of Gerontological Nursing 2(6): 28, 1976

Duvall E: Family Development. New York, Lippincott, 1967

Ebersole P: Problems of group reminiscing with the institutionalized aged. Journal of Gerontological Nursing 2(6): 23, 1976

Engel G: Grief and grieving. American Journal of Nursing 64(9): 93, 1964

Erikson E: Childhood and Society. New York, Norton & Co., 1963

Estes D: Pre-retirement series for hospital personnel. Journal of Gerontological Nursing 4(1): 15, 1978

Evans L: Maintaining social interaction as health promotion in the elderly. Journal of Gerontological Nursing 5(2): 19, 1979

Fell J: Grief reactions in the elderly following death of a spouse: The role of crisis intervention and nursing. Journal of Gerontological Nursing 3(6): 17, 1977

Fixx J: The Complete Book of Running. New York, Random House, 1977

Gerber I, Rusalem R, Hannon N, et al: Anticipatory grief and aged widows and widowers. Journal of Gerontology 30(2): 225, 1975

Gershowitz S: Adding life to years: Remotivating elderly people in institutions. Nursing and Health Care 3(3): 141, 1982

Hala M: Reminiscence group therapy project. Journal of Gerontological Nursing 1(3): 34, 1975

Halfman M, Jojnacki L: Exercise and the maintenance of health. Topics in Clinical Nursing 3(2): 1, 1981

Harris MR, Kalis BL, Freeman EH: Precipitating stress: An approach to brief therapy. American Journal of Psychotherapy 17: 465, 1963

Harris R: Physical activity and mental health in the aged. RN 38(8): 130, 1975

Hartford M: Groups in Social Work. New York, Columbia University Press, 1972

Herr J, Weakland J: The family as a group, in Burnside I (ed.) Working with the Elderly: Group Process and Techniques. North Scituate, MA, Duxbury Press, 1978 chap 20

Heyman D, Gianturco DT: Long term adaptation by the elderly to bereavement. Journal of Gerontology 28(3): 359, 1973

Ingersoll B, Goodman L: History comes alive: Facilitating reminiscence in a group of institutionalized elderly. Journal of Gerontological Social Work 2(4): 305, 1980

Jeffers FC: Attitudes of older persons toward death. Journal of Gerontology 16: 53, 1961

Kahn BH, Silverman AG: An unmet need: The other generation gap. Family service highlights. Family Service Association of America 2(5):4, 1976

Kimmel DC: Adulthood and Aging: An Interdisciplinary Developmental View, 2nd ed. New York, Wiley, 1979

Kramer M, Taube CA, Redick RW: Patterns of use of psychiatric facilities by the aged: Past, present and future, in Eisdorfer C, Lawton MP (eds.), The Psychology of Adult Development and Aging. Washington, DC, American Psychological Assn, 1973

Lakin M, Mooney KS, Havasy S: Interactions among the aged and group therapy intervention. Gerontologist 17(5)(part II):85, 1977

Lebowitz B: Old age and family functioning. Journal of Gerontological Social Work 1(2): 111, 1978

Lemasters G: The effects of bereavement on the elderly and the nursing implications. Journal of Gerontological Nursing 4(6): 22, 1978

Lewin K: Forces behind food habits and methods of change. Bulletin of Natural Resources Council 108: 35, 1943

Lieberman MA, Gourash N: Evaluating the effects of change groups on the elderly. International Journal of Group Psychotherapy 29: 283, 1979

Lindemann E: The meaning of crisis in individual and family living. Teachers College Review 57: 310, 1966

Lowe M, Freeman R: Appendix A: A family coping index. Freeman R, Heinrich J: Community Health Nursing Practice. Philadelphia, Saunders, 1981

Maney J, Edinberg M: Social competency groups: A training and treatment modality for the gerontological nurse practitioner. Journal of Gerontological Nursing 2(6): 31, 1976

McMahon AW, Rhudick PJ: Reminiscing: Adaptational significance in the aged. Archives of General Psychiatry 10(3): 292, 1964

Miller I, Solomon R: The development of group services for the elderly. Journal of Gerontological Social Work 2(3): 241, 1980

Milne MA: Training for team care. Journal of Advanced Nursing 5: 579, 1980

Nemy E: College vacations for the over 60's. New York Times, July 9, 1981

Parkes MC: Effects of bereavement on physical and mental health—A study of the medical records of widows. British Medical Journal 2: 274, 1964

Parsons T: The Social System. New York, The Free Press, 1951

Perlman HH: In quest of coping. Social Casework 56: 213, 1975

Phelps S, Austin N: The assertive woman. Fredericksburg, Virginia, Impact, 1975

Pless I, Satterwhite B: A measure of family functioning and its application. Social Science and Medicine 7: 613, 1973

Rabkin JG, Struening E: Life events, stress and illness. Science 194: 1013, 1976

Rauseo L: Separation of generations—Who benefits? Journal of Gerontological Nursing 3(1): 40, 1977

Richardson K, Lowman R: Group intervention strategy with the aged. Paper presented at the American Gerontological Society Convention, San Diego, California, Nov 25, 1980

Robb S: The nurse's role in retirement preparation. Journal of Gerontological Nursing 4(1): 25, 1978

Rosow I: The social context of the aging self. Gerontologist 13(1) 82, 1973

Ryden M: Nursing intervention in support of reminiscence. Journal of Gerontological Nursing 7(8): 461, 1981

Schwab JJ, Chalmers JM, Conroy SJ, et al: Studies in grief: A preliminary report, in Schoenberg B, Gerber I, Wiener A, et al (eds.), Psychosocial Aspects of Bereavement. New York, Columbia University Press, 1975

Shanas E: Social myth as hypothesis: The case of the family relations of old people. Gerontologist 19(1): 3, 1979

Silverman A, Brahce C: 'As Parents Grow Older': An intervention model. Journal of Gerontological Social Work 2(1): 77, 1979

Silverman P. The Widow to Widow program: An experiment in preventive intervention. Mental Hygiene 53: 333, 1969

Silverman WH: Planning for crisis intervention with community mental health concepts. Psychotherapy: Theory, Research and Practice 14: 293, 1977

Smilkstein G: The Family APGAR: A proposal for a family function test and its use by physicians. The Journal of Family Practice 6(6): 1231, 1978

Strauss A: Chronic Illness and the Quality of Life. St. Louis, Mosby, 1975

Streib G, Thompson W: The older person in a family context, in Tibbitts C (ed.), Handbook of Social Gerontology. Chicago, University of Chicago Press, 1960

Yalom I: The Theory and Practice of Group Psychotherapy, 3rd ed. New York, Basic Books, 1977

Zarit H: Aging and Mental Disorders: Psychological Approaches to Assessment and Treatment. New York, Free Press, 1980

IV

Level Three Adaptation: The Aging Client with a Chronic Health Problem

14

Nursing the Client Experiencing Oxygen Deprivation

A wide range of stresses that affect the aging heart, lungs, and vasculature may cause oxygen deprivation. The resulting adaptations may be either local or systemic. In both cases, the adaptations result in progressive, chronic disability that restricts the older person's quality of life. Older clients with chronic oxygen deprivation cannot expect marked improvement in their level of adaptation. Often they must modify their plans for an active, rewarding retirement period and their activities of daily living. They must learn to manage a variety of complex and time-consuming treatment regimens, including diet modifications, exercise regimens, medications and new equipment. In most cases, clients must live with the knowledge that because their stresses cannot be eliminated, they must learn to live with disabling adaptations that increase in number as their condition worsens. The nurse plays an important role in helping clients set realistic goals, utilize their strengths, and modify their life-style so that they can maintain a maximum level of independence while implementing a complex treatment plan.

SIGNIFICANT PROBLEMS

Angina Pectoris

Angina is an adaptation to myocardial ischemia. Many stresses precipitate myocardial ischemia, but the most important one in the elderly is coronary artery disease. The two processes involved in the development of coronary artery disease are arteriosclerosis and atherosclerosis.

Arteriosclerosis is a normal consequence of aging. Gradually, arterial walls thicken and the number of arterial muscle fibers declines. As a result, the arteries become rigid tubes that no longer expand and contract. Their ability to adapt to changing oxygen needs is reduced. Hypertension is known to accelerate this process. Because the arterial changes are gradual, adaptations may not develop for years (Dobrowolski, 1979).

Atherosclerosis is a pathological complication of arteriosclerosis and not a normal aging process. Changes in the arterial intima allow the entry of harmful lipids, especially cholesterol, into the intimal layer. The trapping of lipids and other harmful matter elicits a low-grade inflammatory reaction in the vessels (Kohn, 1977). As lipids collect, occlusion of the vessel lumen results. The wear and tear of hemodynamic forces operating over a period of years and genetic factors also play a role in the development of atherosclerotic lesions (Harris, 1978).

Because arteriosclerosis and atherosclerosis develop slowly, adaptations may not be exhibited until advanced age. Lesions may occur anywhere in the arterial tree, including the cerebral arteries, coronary arteries, or the terminal aorta and peripheral arteries. Adaptations vary according to the location of the lesion. For example, lesions of the cerebral artery may produce confusion, behavior changes (see Chapter 16), or strokes (see Chapter 18). Lesions of the terminal aorta or peripheral arteries result in intermittent claudication, discussed later in this chapter. When lesions affect the coronary vasculature, the term "ischemic heart disease" is used. Lesions develop in the main branches of the coronary arteries, constricting the lumen of the vessel, reducing coronary arterial blood flow, and producing ischemia. Adaptations to ischemia range from arrhythmias and myocardial infarction (see Chapter 18) to angina pectoris.

Angina may precede or follow myocardial infarction. It is a common adaptation in the elderly, but its frequency declines after age 80 (Caird et al., 1976). Angina indicates myocardial ischemia resulting from an intermittent disruption of the balance between oxygen demand and oxygen supply. The resting myocardium extracts almost 75 percent of the oxygen that flows through the coronary vessels. When myocardial oxygen demand increases, the heart cannot significantly increase its oxygen extraction rate, therefore increased oxygen must come from increased perfusion. Healthy coronary arteries can dilate in response to myocardial hypoxia and increase perfusion by 500 percent. If stresses such as arteriosclerosis and atherosclerosis are present, the coronary artery is unable to increase perfusion and temporary myocardial ischemia results. Over time, angina becomes a stress that results in fibrosis of the myocardium, cardiac enlargement, and heart failure (Harris, 1978).

In people with coronary artery disease, angina is usually precipitated by one or more stresses that increase the oxygen need of the myocardium. Normal exertion, such as climbing stairs or rapid walking, may provoke an attack. Other stresses include eating a meal, any form of physical exercise, cold, frosty, windy weather, weather changes from cold and dry to hot and humid, emotional stress, and nightmares (Harris, 1978; Kleiger, 1976; Pathy, 1976). Other stresses exacerbate angina. For example, if anemia develops in a person with coronary artery disease, the angina may be so severe that it results in congestive heart failure (Wedgewood, 1976). Other stresses that exacerbate angina include hyperthyroidism, obesity, hypotension, tachyarrhythmias, and hypoglycemia (Caird et al., 1976). The elderly who are medicated for diabetes, hypertension and hypothyroidism are at high risk should they develop toxic effects to these medications.

About 10 percent of those with angina have normal coronary arteries. Stresses that precipitate angina in this group include aortic valve disease, syphilitic aortitis, hypertension, and severe anemia.

Peripheral Vascular Disease

The term peripheral vascular disease is used to describe a variety of conditions affecting the arteries, veins, and lymphatic vessels of the extremities. Important stresses in its development are obstruction and abnormal vasodilation or vasoconstriction. Adaptations are a result of ischemia to the area served by the vessel. Because of their distal and dependent position, the legs are most likely to exhibit adaptations. In the elderly, conditions associated with the artery include arteriosclerosis obliterans (ASO), thromboangiitis obliterans (TAO or Buerger's disease), Raynaud's disease, erythromelalgia, and many others. Arteriosclerosis obliterans is the most frequently encountered arterial condition in older people. Varicosities, venous thrombosis, and chronic venous insufficiency are the most frequently encountered venous conditions in the elderly.

Arteries.   Arteriosclerosis of the branch arteries, which compromises their lumen and results in reduced peripheral blood flow or occlusion, is most often involved in the development of ASO. As blood flow is progressively reduced, there is a concomitant development of collateral circulation. This condition occurs most often in men aged 50 to 70 (Haimovici, 1979; Elkowitz, 1981). The specific process by which ASO develops is not known. In part, the process involves deposition of calcium in arteries, thickening of the arterial lining, and atrophy of muscle fiber, all of which make the arteries more rigid (Dobrowolski, 1979). Stresses associated with its development include hypercholesteremia, disturbed lipid metabolism, diabetes mellitus, smoking, obesity, lack of physical exercise, nervous tension, and mechanical stresses. In particular, diabetes speeds up the process by which ASO develops. ASO progresses at rates and in locations that vary widely from one individual to another. In the elderly the femoral, popliteal, and tibial arteries are most frequently involved. The process may also involve the aortoiliac arteries. When it does, this is called Leriche syndrome. Occlusion is usually bilateral, affecting buttocks, thighs, and calves.

Veins.   With age, veins become dilated and stretched. Venous muscle tone and efficiency of venous valves decrease. Consequently, blood is returned less efficiently to the heart, increasing the congestion of veins. Age-related changes are responsible in part for an increase in the incidence of varicose veins, thrombophlebitis, and venous insufficiency in the elderly.

Varicose veins usually affect the superficial veins, particularly the greater saphenous vein and less often the lesser saphenous vein. They are believed to be due to structural changes in the vein walls and valves that make the veins sensitive to hydrostatic pressure (Herndon, 1976). Consequently, blood pools, edema develops, and the veins become tortuous and serpentine and increasingly dilated. Varicose veins have a strong hereditary tendency and usually affect females.

The aging client with varicose veins is at high risk to develop venous thrombosis. However, age alone is an important risk factor in the development of venous thrombosis. The increased incidence among the elderly seems to be directly related to the progressive enlargement of the intramuscular calf veins that occurs with advancing years. Any stress that injures the intima of vessels, alters the blood's coagulability, increases venous stasis, or results in an accumulation of tissue breakdown products may precipitate venous thrombosis. Stresses include prolonged sitting or bed rest, surgery, fractures of the lower limbs, obesity, debilitating conditions such as congestive heart failure, neoplasms, infections or stroke, or medications such as hormones. The older client who is healthy may develop venous thrombosis after a long trip in a car or airplane. The elderly client who is hospitalized may develop it in the postoperative period following an exploratory laparotomy. Clients with a history of this condition are at high risk for recurrences. Venous thrombosis is called phlebothrombosis when thrombosis in the vein is a primary phenomenon and inflammation of the venous wall is secondary to it. The term thrombophlebitis indicates that the inflammatory reaction of the vessel wall is primary and thrombosis is secondary.

There are two types of venous thrombosis: deep and superficial. Deep thrombosis involves the deep veins of the calf, including the peroneal and posterior tibial veins. The client with deep vein thrombosis is at high risk to develop pulmonary emboli. Superficial venous thrombosis, which usually involves the greater or lesser saphenous veins, is less likely to produce dangerous adaptations. Occasion-

ally, the thrombosis extends toward the groin and affects communicating veins linking the superficial to the deep venous system. This condition places the client at high risk for thromboembolism and requires surgical ligation.

A potential stress associated with venous thrombosis is chronic venous insufficiency. It may also result from leg injury. The venous valves are damaged, collateral circulation develops, and the veins become incompetent.

Chronic Obstructive Pulmonary Disease

Chronic airway obstruction is the major reason for pulmonary disability in the elderly. Chronic bronchitis, chronic emphysema, and asthma are the conditions most often associated with airway obstruction in the elderly. The terms Chronic Obstructive Pulmonary Disease (COPD) and Chronic Obstructive Lung Disease (COLD) are used to describe all of these conditions. It is rare for an older client with airway obstruction to exhibit only one disorder. In fact elements of all three conditions may be present.

Although each condition is precipitated by a unique pattern of stresses, all have at least some adaptations in common. Since interventions are aimed largely at helping clients modify or cope with ineffective adaptations, the principles for managing all forms of COPD are similar.

Chronic Bronchitis. Chronic bronchitis is defined according to the adaptation most often exhibited by clients as the presence of a productive cough at least 3 months out of the year for 2 or more consecutive years. Smoking is the most important stress associated with its development. Mortality due to bronchitis is 20 times higher among persons who smoke at least 25 cigarettes a day than among nonsmokers (Lowe, 1969). Smoking also triggers a chain of adaptations in the airways that are similar to those seen in chronic bronchitis. Other pollutants, such as those found in urban areas and industries, also precipitate chronic bronchitis.

The onset of chronic bronchitis usually occurs by age 50, well before old age. However, adaptations that threaten the client's level of adaptation may not be apparent until old age. The prevalence of established cases continues to rise throughout the life span (Exton-Smith and Overstall, 1979). Chronic bronchitis is much more common in men than in women, presumably because men are more likely to smoke and to hold jobs involving exposure to industrial pollutants.

Airway obstruction associated with chronic bronchitis develops very gradually. Smoking and other pollutants stimulate a hypersecretion of mucus. At the same time, these irritants paralyze the cilia, inhibiting their ability to sweep mucus and foreign substances up and out of the airways. Consequently, a buildup of mucus, bacteria, and other foreign materials occurs in the airways. Other changes also occur, including hyperplasia and hypertrophy of the mucous glands in the submucosa of large airways, chronic inflammation, edema, and hyperplasia of smooth muscle and goblet cells in small airways, and bronchospasm. The increased volume of sputum coupled with the structural damage to the walls of these airways contributes to obstruction.

In bronchitis, the obstruction of the airways causes alveolar hypoventilation and a serious ventilation-perfusion mismatch. Although ventilation is reduced in those alveoli beyond the mucus plugs, the underlying pulmonary capillary bed is well preserved. Shunting of blood through these areas results in hypoxemia and carbon dioxide retention. As carbon dioxide increases, the respiratory drive diminishes. The increase in mucus production, the airway plugging, the mucosal hypertrophy, and the loss of support for the walls of airways all increase the resistance to airflow, particularly during expiration. To overcome the resistance to airflow, the client must work harder to breathe. Accessory muscles are brought into play, further increasing the work of breathing. Both the work of breathing and the relative lack of hypoxic drive in the client with bronchitis contribute to hypoxemia (Fig. 1).

Emphysema. Emphysema is defined by its morphological characteristics, not by its adaptations, as the distention of air spaces distal to the terminal bronchioles with destruction of alveolar walls. There are two types of emphysema: centrilobular and panlobular. In centrilobular emphysema, the process of alveolar destruction begins in the center of the lobule, and moves to the periphery, often leaving alveoli at the lobule edges intact. It is found more often in upper than in lower portions of the lungs

and is frequently seen in combination with bronchitis. Panlobular emphysema is characterized by diffuse enlargement and destruction of the alveoli in the lobe and tends to occur in dependent regions of the lungs.

The stresses that contribute to the development of emphysema are not completely known. Hereditary factors play a role in the development of some cases of panlobular emphysema. The stress is an inherited deficiency of α_1 antitrypsin, a protein that inhibits trypsin, an enzyme released from white blood cells to fight infection. When trypsin is uninhibited, it destroys lung tissue. This form of emphysema occurs in nonsmokers, usually between ages 30 and 45. The emphysema most often seen in older people is centrilobular. It is believed to be due to prolonged exposure to toxic substances such as cigarette smoking, environmental pollutants, and other irritants. By age 90, the lungs of nearly everyone exhibit some emphysematous changes (Pathy, 1976).

The process by which emphysema develops is not completely understood. Apparently, two mechanisms are involved: dynamic airway collapse and loss of lung elastic recoil, both of which decrease airflow and account for the adaptations seen in the client. Emphysematous lungs have fewer elastic fibers and a lower elastin-to-collagen ratio than do normal lungs (Motomiya et al., 1979). The elastic recoil of the lung decreases with loss of alveolar septa, presumably because the reduced alveolar surface area exerts a lower surface tension. Because of lost elastic recoil, the bronchioles are poorly supported and tend to collapse on expiration when compressed by surrounding alveoli (COPD Manual Committee, 1973). Air is trapped, alveoli are distended, residual volume is increased, and the lungs are hyperinflated. The hyperinflated lungs flatten the diaphragm, reduce its effectiveness, and necessitate the use of accessory muscles to move air in and out of the lungs. The reduced alveolar surface area also results in a loss of diffusing capacity and impaired gas transport. However, because the client hyperventilates and because there is minimal left-to-right shunting, the balance of ventilation and perfusion is fairly well maintained. Therefore, blood gases are maintained near normal limits and the hypoxic drive is preserved if the client remains in the compensated state. When emphysema is in an advanced stage or when infection or other compli-

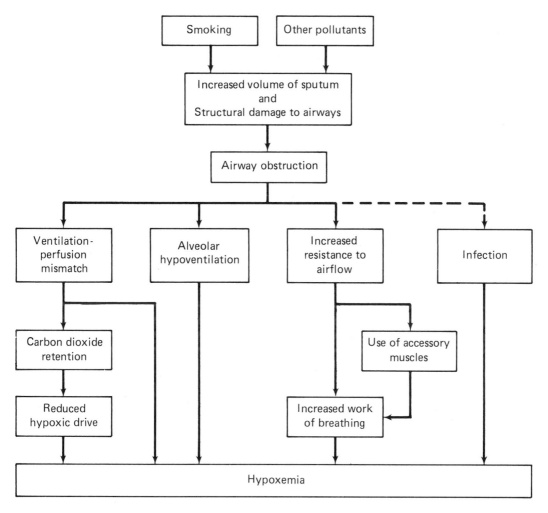

Figure 1. Steps in the development of chronic bronchitis.

cations develop, additional demands are placed on the lungs, and hypoxemia and carbon dioxide retention develop. With emphysema, cyanosis is usually a late development and reflects central anoxia and polycythemia.

Asthma. In contrast to other types of COPD, airway obstruction associated with asthma is reversible. Asthma has been classified as extrinsic (allergic) or intrinsic (nonallergic) (Table 1). An important difference between the two types involves the nature of the stresses that precipitate each.

When exposed to antigens, individuals with allergic asthma have been found to produce excessive amounts of the antibody IgE, which attaches to mast cells. If the individual is reexposed to the antigen, the mast cells release a number of chemical mediators which contract bronchial smooth muscle, alter vascular permeability, stimulate mucus secretion, and attract eosinophilic cells to the airway. In asthmatic individuals, the release of these mediators appears to be related to intracellular levels of cyclic guanosine monophosphate (GMP). In normal persons, cyclic GMP, which causes bronchoconstriction, is increased by stimulation of vagus-mediated

TABLE 1.   DIFFERENCES AMONG ADAPTATIONS TO EXTRINSIC AND INTRINSIC ASTHMA

Adaptation	Extrinsic Type	Intrinsic Type
History		
Age of onset	Before age 30	After age 40
Allergic history	Has had other allergic disorders: eczema, hay fever, rhinitis	Unremarkable
Family history	Strong family history of allergic disorders or asthma	Family history of allergic disorders
Precipitating stress	Allergens	Infection, especially viral. Unknown.
Skin test	Positive: wheal and flare reactions to small doses of allergens	Positive: to large doses of nonspecific agents
Respiratory changes	Little or no wheezing between attacks Prognosis good	Continuous wheezing May be severely disabling

cholinergic reflexes, and cyclic adenosine mono-phosphate (AMP), which causes bronchodilation, is increased by β-adrenergic stimulation. Persons with allergic asthma have been found to have a decreased responsiveness to β-adrenergic stimulation and a heightened sensitivity to cholinergic reflexes. Persons with allergic asthma usually experience its onset before age 30. Exposure to allergens precipitates attacks and seasonal variations are frequent.

Intrinsic (nonallergic) asthma is the type most often seen in the elderly. The onset usually occurs after age 40. Stresses that precipitate intrinsic asthma are poorly understood. Exposure to dust, cigarette smoke, air pollution, a change of temperature, and infections, especially viral infections, may precipitate or worsen adaptations. In these clients, serum IgE levels are normal. In the elderly, this type of asthma is more likely to become disabling.

Many elderly persons with asthma experience characteristics of both intrinsic and extrinsic types. This is termed "mixed asthma."

Asthma is characterized by increased responsiveness of both the trachea and the bronchi to various stimuli, manifested by a general narrowing of airways. Bronchospasm, bronchial wall edema, and hypersecretion of mucous glands all contribute to airway narrowing and airway obstruction. In asthma, airway narrowing is dynamic and the degree of nar-

rowing changes frequently. In some persons, airway resistance is increased during an asthmatic attack but may be close to normal during remission. Airway resistance is increased permanently in elderly persons with long-standing asthma.

Histological changes of asthma include an increase in the size and number of goblet cells and mucous glands, thickening of the bronchial basement membrane and smooth muscle, submucosal infiltration of mononuclear inflammatory cells, and blockage of airways by eosinophils and mucus plugs. Pulmonary perfusion patterns are usually preserved until the late stages of the disease; therefore, blood gases are often maintained within normal limits except during an exacerbation (Davies, 1981).

Potential Stresses.   Chronic airway obstruction and the hypoxemia that accompanies it are stresses that place the client at risk for polycythemia, right ventricular hypertrophy and failure, arrhythmias, acute respiratory failure, and numerous other disorders. The nurse needs to be aware of these when assessing the client with COPD and planning care.

Polycythemia.   Chronic arterial hypoxemia increases the production of erythropoietin, resulting in bone marrow stimulation and erythrocytosis. If the erythrocytosis is accompanied by higher hemo-globin levels and increased oxygen-carrying capacity, this adaptation is favorable. However, the increased blood volume may strain a weak heart. The increased blood viscosity increases resistance to blood flow through the lungs and coronary vessels, further taxing the myocardium. Continuous oxygen therapy to correct hypoxemia removes the stress that stimulates erythropoiesis and gradually relieves the polycythemia. Clients with chronic bronchitis, which is characterized by ventilation-perfusion defects, are at high risk of developing hypoxemia and secondary erythrocytosis. This process accounts for the cyanotic appearance of many clients with chronic bronchitis.

Cor Pulmonale. Two stresses that underlie the process by which cor pulmonale develop are arterial hypoxemia and respiratory acidosis. These factors exert a strong vasoconstrictor effect on pulmonary vessels, leading to increased pulmonary vascular resistance, pulmonary arterial hypertension, and increased right ventricular systolic pressure. Eventually, right ventricular hypertrophy and failure result. In emphysema without bronchitis, right ventricular hypertrophy and failure usually develop later than in bronchitis. Adaptations to right ventricular failure include increased end-diastolic pressure and dilation of the right ventricle, visible on x-ray. Distended neck veins, hepatomegaly, and peripheral edema also develop, due to impaired salt and water clearance. Since the process involves reversible pulmonary vasoconstriction and not permanent loss of pulmonary capillaries, cor pulmonale can be prevented if hypoxemia and acidosis are corrected.

Spontaneous Pneumothorax. The rupture of pulmonary blebs, usually in the apex of the lung, may occur spontaneously or as a consequence of chest trauma. Lung collapse is accompanied by an alarming increase in dyspnea that can be fatal. Because breath sounds and chest expansion are already reduced in the client with COPD, assessment of a pneumothorax is difficult. Intrapleural suction is the usual treatment for pneumothorax.

Arrhythmias. Clients with severe COPD are at risk of developing life-threatening cardiac arrhythmias. Hypoxemia, hypercapnea, and acidosis, often ac-

centuated by hypokalemia, adrenergic drugs, and digitalis, are the stresses that precipitate arrhythmias. Prevention involves correcting the underlying alveolar hypoventilation by giving oxygen and improving ventilation.

Peptic Ulcer. Approximately 25 percent of clients with COPD will have a peptic ulcer at some time. Increased gastric acidity, carbon dioxide retention, decreased arterial oxygen saturation, and emotional stresses are believed to contribute to the development of ulcers. Clients treated with corticosteroids are at high risk for the development of peptic ulcer.

Pulmonary Thromboembolism. Pulmonary thromboembolism is common in clients with COPD. Adaptations include a worsening of dyspnea, tachycardia, arrhythmias, wheezing, and congestive heart failure.

Acute Respiratory Failure. Acute respiratory failure is a life-threatening adaptation that develops abruptly when alveolar ventilation is inadequate for the body's needs. A sudden rise in P_{CO_2} above 50 mm Hg, with a fall in pH below 7.3, are hallmarks of acute respiratory failure. Arterial hypoxemia precedes carbon dioxide retention. An acute bronchopulmonary infection most often precipitates acute respiratory failure in clients with COPD. Hypoxia and acidosis damage the central nervous system and myocardium, accounting for many of the adaptations the client exhibits. Early adaptations include anxiety, restlessness, dyspnea, and headache. Later, drowsiness, mental confusion, diminished tendon reflexes, papilledema, asterixis, and coma may develop. The client is cyanotic, with rapid, shallow respirations, and an ineffective cough. Sinus tachycardia and other arrhythmias, hypotension, and congestive heart failure signal myocardial involvement. Treatment is aimed at correcting the hypoxemia and acidosis by providing oxygen and restoring adequate alveolar ventilation. Studies indicate that older clients can be treated successfully for respiratory failure. Over 50 percent of clients over age 70 who require mechanical ventilation recover and leave the hospital. In the elderly, it is especially important to maintain adequate nutrition and muscle tone during the acute phase of illness (Petty, 1976).

ASSESSING THE CLIENT'S ADAPTATIONS

Angina Pectoris

The assessment of anginal pain is more difficult in the elderly than in younger people. Older clients with memory deficits or a diminished appreciation of pain may not be able to give a reliable history. The incidence of diseases with adaptations similar to angina increases in the aged and may be mistaken for angina. These include diseases of the chest wall or lungs, hiatal hernia, ulcers, gallbladder disease, and esophagitis. Finally, the perception of anginal pain varies widely among the aged. Pain, if present, is usually much less severe than in middle-aged clients. It may vary from substernal oppression to a severe, dull, constant gripping or choking pain behind the sternum. Pain may extend across the chest, up the neck and jaw, or radiate down the left arm or both arms. Occasionally, pain is experienced only in the wrists. With pain, the client experiences an overwhelming need to stop whatever activity brought on the pain. If the client rests, the pain lasts only a short time, anywhere from a few minutes to an hour. In the elderly, the intensity of the pain may be overshadowed by the simultaneous development of mental confusion, presumably due to a reduction of cardiac output and cerebral perfusion. Other neurological adaptations and gastrointestinal adaptations may develop as well. Anginal pain may be accompanied by lightheadedness or followed by syncope, possibly due to a simultaneous transient arrhythmia.

In the elderly, angina may not present as pain but as dyspnea or weakness on effort, syncope with exertion, sudden cough with emotional stress, or palpitation and sweating with exercise. These unusual adaptations are attributed to transient cardiac failure, ischemic arrhythmias, or a sudden reduction in cardiac output. In short, angina is characterized by a pattern of provoking stress, pain, or other adaptation and relief with rest or medication.

Stable angina is characterized by a predictable pattern of adaptations provoked by predictable stresses. Unstable angina, or crescendo angina, is a more serious form of angina and indicates that the client is at high risk for myocardial infarction and death. Unstable angina is characterized by a changing pattern of adaptations that occurs with increasing frequency and severity.

Blood pressure changes and an increased pulse rate reflecting hemodynamic changes may accompany angina. Usually, there are no distinctive auscultatory changes during an anginal episode. A systolic murmur may be auscultated during an anginal attack if the ischemia is severe enough to cause dysfunction of papillary muscles. Electrocardiographic changes occur during, but not after, angina pain and indicate ischemia. They are apparent in the leads that reflect the distribution of the involved coronary artery. The ST segment and T wave that reflect repolarization of the ventricles are most often affected. ST depression and inversion of the T wave are frequent changes.

Assessment must include identification of those stresses that provoke an anginal episode. The client should be examined for the presence of anemia, hyperthyroidism, and other conditions that might worsen an anginal episode. The client's coronary risk profile, including family history, smoking habits, blood sugar, blood pressure, and serum cholesterol, triglycerides, and lipoproteins, should also be obtained. In the elderly, the prognostic significance of coronary risk factors differs in some respects from that found in the young. Nevertheless, when these factors exist in an aging client, they should be identified and controlled.

Peripheral Vascular Disease

Arteries. Because adaptations to peripheral vascular disease are progressive, a thorough assessment is necessary to collect baseline data and pinpoint alterations over time. Adaptations to arteriosclerosis obliterans depend on the rapidity of onset, the site and extent of arterial occlusion and insufficiency and the extent of collateral circulation. Usually, collateral circulation is adequate to keep tissues viable but inadequate to meet the needs of a working muscle. The most common adaptation is intermittent claudication, which is pain during exercise caused by an inadequate supply of blood to the contracting muscles. Arterial blood flow cannot be increased to meet tissue demands. Most often, the pain occurs in the calf, causing clients to limp and forcing them to stop exercising. It develops more quickly if clients walk rapidly or uphill. The pain is relieved by rest. Early in the process, intermittent claudication may be the only adaptation.

As the condition advances and collateral vessels become occluded, other adaptations may develop, including resting pain, trophic skin changes, color changes of the skin, sensations of coldness, paresthesias, numbness, ischemic ulcers, ischemic neuropathy, disuse atrophy, and diminished or absent arterial pulses. The resting pain associated with arteriosclerosis obliterans is aggravated by raising the leg and relieved by lowering the leg to a dependent position, which promotes arterial blood flow. Integumentary changes include cool, thin, shiny taut skin, thickened opaque nails, and scanty or absent hair. Since hair growth declines with age, this adaptation alone is not indicative of arteriosclerosis obliterans. A sharp difference in skin temperature between proximal and distal areas indicates recent arterial occlusion. If color changes are present, these indicate the condition is advanced. When the leg is elevated high above the head, marked blanching of the toes and foot occurs, and when the leg is returned to the dependent position, hyperemia and rubor develop. Ischemic neuropathy is a late adaptation characterized by severe, paroxysmal burning or a shooting pain that begins in the foot and radiates up the leg. Feet and toes must be carefully assessed for ischemic ulcers, particularly between the toes. In contrast to diabetic ulcers, those associated with ASO are painful. Examination of the arteries should include palpation and auscultation of femoral, popliteal, posterior tibial, and dorsalis pedis pulses. Pulses proximal to the diminished or absent pulses should be assessed to pinpoint the level of arterial occlusion. Absent pulsations are often accompanied by gangrene. A bruit may be heard in the femoral artery if it is more than 50 percent obstructed. Three classifications of arteriosclerosis obliterans have been identified, depending upon the adaptation:

- Stage I—intermittent claudication
- Stage II—rest pain without lesions
- Stage III—ischemic lesions (ulcers and gangrene)

Clients with aortoiliac occlusion (Leriche syndrome) may not exhibit adaptations to ischemia for years because of well-developed collateral circulation. Eventually clients may experience fatigue or weakness of the legs. Later, rest pain, impotence, and gangrene may occur.

There are a number of well-established diagnostic tests to provide an objective assessment of vascular insufficiency. These measure the arterial pressure at various levels of the extremities and provide flow measurements. They include the Pulse Volume Recorder, Doppler Ultrasonic Velocity Detector, and radioisotopes. If corrective surgery is being contemplated, arteriography will be used.

Veins. Varicose veins are visible under the skin as dilated, tortuous, elongated veins best seen when the client is standing. The nurse should note their size and distribution. Some varicosities, called cords, are palpable veins with the consistency of rubber tubing. The client may complain of cramping pain, paresthesia, or a dull, aching heaviness and feelings of fatigue brought on by periods of standing. Nonpitting ankle edema, which is worse at the end of the day, may also occur. When circulation has been impaired for a long time, venous stasis occurs and can result in stasis dermatitis, with thinning and brown pigmentation of the skin above the ankles, itching, eczematous changes, and ulcers in the area of the medial malleolus.

Early adaptations associated with deep thrombosis of the calf vary widely. These include a sensation of heaviness, a dull ache, frank pain or cramps in the leg, and pain in the foot or along the length of the involved vein. The pain increases when the limb is in a dependent position or during walking. The client often feels anxious or restless. The ankles and calves should be measured to determine the presence of edema. If it is present, it is usually mild or moderate. Pain and spasm of the calf muscles produced by dorsiflexion of the foot (Homan's sign) is present in only a small percentage of cases (Haimovici, 1979). Warmth of the affected leg, low-grade fever, tachycardia, and tenderness, induration, and cyanosis of the involved limb may also occur. Sensory and motor functions are intact, and arterial pulsations should be present.

If the iliofemoral segment is involved, the swelling may involve the entire lower extremity, including the thigh. Other adaptations include a general aching of the involved extremity, cyanosis, tenderness of the upper thigh over the femoral vein, and engorgement of superficial veins.

Thrombosis of superficial veins is characterized by spontaneous onset of pain, particularly when adjacent muscles are used or when pressure is applied. The area over the affected vein may be warm and red; when palpated, the involved vein feels like a thickened cord. The client may have a low-grade temperature, but never a significant elevation or chill.

Chronic venous insufficiency is characterized by ankle edema, which progresses to edema of the leg. Itching and dull discomfort occur and are made worse by periods of standing. The skin is thin, shiny, atrophic, and cyanotic. Eventually, brownish pigmented areas develop. Eczema and superficial areas of weeping dermatitis may occur in the lower one-third of the leg. Subcutaneous tissues become thick and fibrous and are subject to recurrent ulceration. When ulcers occur, they are most often located on the malleolus, and they are extremely painful.

Chronic Obstructive Pulmonary Disease

Bronchitis and Emphysema. The relationship between bronchitis and emphysema is such that most older clients with chronic airway obstruction exhibit elements of both conditions. Most elderly clients are in the advanced stage of disease. Because adaptations develop slowly and insidiously, some older clients may attribute their declining exercise tolerance and breathlessness to old age or heart disease and delay seeking health care until disability is advanced or until a complication develops.

Clients with emphysema and bronchitis are usually males with a long history of cigarette smoking. When talking with the nurse they may sit leaning forward with their weight on their forearms to facilitate breathing. Depending on the severity of the obstruction, clients complain of breathlessness on exertion, shortness of breath, or dyspnea at rest.

Dyspnea is the foremost adaptation to airway obstruction. In clients with COPD, it may vary from day to day, depending upon the degree of bronchial edema and the amount and character of sputum. It may be worse in the morning until sputum is coughed

up, in high humidity or high altitudes, or after eating a heavy meal. The feeling of dyspnea is related in part to the increased work of breathing. With emphysema, the respiratory drive may be preserved until a late stage and the client may complain of profound dyspnea.

The following classification of dyspnea is useful:

Grade I.   Can keep pace when walking on the level with a healthy person of same age and build, but unable to do so on stairs and hills.

Grade II.   Can walk one mile at own pace without dyspnea, but cannot keep pace with a healthy person when walking on the level.

Grade III.   Becomes breathless after walking 100 yards or a few minutes on the level.

Grade IV.   Becomes breathless when dressing or talking.

In addition, the client often complains of fatigue due to the increased work of breathing, repeated coughing, and inability to sleep at night.

The term "pink puffer" has been used when emphysema predominates, since arterial oxygen is maintained close to normal limits. The client is unusually thin, undernourished, and debilitated. Skin turgor is poor. Weight loss and poor nutrition are common for many reasons. Clients are anorexic; aerophagia and gastric distention cause early satiety; chewing contributes to breathlessness; and large meals interfere with breathing. At the same time there is an increased energy expenditure associated with the increased work of breathing. Clients with bronchitis have been described as "blue bloaters"—overweight, edematous, and drowsy due to hypoxia, carbon dioxide retention, polycythemia and pulmonary hypertension. Most clients seen by the nurse fall somewhere in between these two extremes.

Many physical signs reflect both emphysema and bronchitis. The anteroposterior diameter of the chest is increased, producing a barrel-shaped inspiratory condition. Respiratory movements depend upon the use of accessory muscles. Breathing is labored and hyperpnea is evident. The diaphragm, which is low and flat, is almost immobile during respiration. In advanced cases, the abdominal muscles contract on inspiration. On palpation, respiratory movements are decreased. In advanced cases, the liver is displaced downward due to the fixed inspiratory position of the chest.

When auscultated, inspiratory sounds are prolonged and breath sounds are more distant due to hyperinflation. Wheezing due to airway collapse may be heard. With bronchitis, scattered rhonchi, due to mucus in the airways, are present. With emphysema, the intensity of breath sounds is decreased due to hyperinflation and alveolar damage.

During the physical assessment, clients should be asked to exhale rapidly through the open mouth, after fully inflating the lungs and until no further air can be expelled. Prolongation of forced expiration beyond 4 to 5 seconds indicates airway obstruction.

Clients with emphysema and bronchitis usually have a chronic cough, productive of whitish sputum. With emphysema, efforts to cough are usually out of proportion to the amount of sputum produced and may be exhausting.

Heart sounds may be decreased at the base due to hyperinflation of the lungs. In severe cases, heart sounds may be inaudible except at the xiphoid area. The area of cardiac dullness is decreased. Tachycardia is present with slight or moderate exertion.

The electrocardiogram (ECG) is usually normal in mild or moderate COPD. In more severe stages, particularly with emphysema, characteristic changes develop in the P wave and QRS complexes. The ECG is affected by the positional and rotational changes of the heart associated with several factors, including increased lung volume, depression of the diaphragm, and vascular changes. A frequent change is the shift of the P-wave axis toward the right. In leads II, III, and VF, P waves are peaked. There is a negative deflection of the P wave in lead AV_L. The QRS complex often shows low voltage in the limb and precordial leads.

The chest roentgenogram does not show significant changes in mild or moderate COPD. However, it is used to rule out the presence of other stresses, such as tuberculosis or tumors, which also compromise the client's respiratory function. In well-established bronchitis, the chest roentgenogram shows hyperinflation and increased lung markings. In moderate and severe emphysema the chest roentgenogram shows clear hyperradiolucent, overinflated lungs, bullous areas, and loss of peripheral

vascular markings. The domes of the diaphragm are flattened, the rib spaces are widened and the retrosternal space is increased in depth. If a right ventricular enlargement is present, there are changes in the cardiac contours and pulmonary artery. An increased prominence of basal vascular markings and a widened transverse diameter of the heart indicate combined right and left ventricular failure.

Pulmonary function studies are of particular significance when performed in the early stages of chronic obstruction because changes and findings can be useful in monitoring the client's status. These studies should not be done during an acute exacerbation. They are performed with and without a bronchodilator in order to determine its potential effectiveness. There are few differences in the changes in lung volumes and flow rates exhibited with emphysema and bronchitis (Table 2). One of the most characteristic findings associated with COPD is the reduction in the ratio of forced expiratory volume at 1 second (FEV_1) to forced vital capacity (FVC). This is particularly useful in differentiating between obstructive impairment and restrictive impairments, such as fibrosis, lung resection or congestive heart failure. When the FEV_1 drops to 1.5 to 2 liters, mild dyspnea is usually present. As the FEV_1 continues to drop, dyspnea worsens. An FEV_1 below 1.00 liter is usually associated with severe dyspnea and disability and a poor prognosis. If the test results do not improve after inhalation of a nebulized bronchodilator, emphysema is indicated. If bronchitis is present, inhalation of a bronchodilator usually results in slight improvement.

Diffusion capacity is a measure of the health of the alveolar–capillary surface area. Diffusion is usually significantly decreased in emphysema, but it may be normal or only slightly altered in chronic bronchitis.

Hematological and arterial blood gas studies also exhibit changes with COPD. Chronic hypoxia stimulates the production of red blood cells. Therefore, the hematocrit, mean corpuscular volume, and mean corpuscular hemoglobin are elevated. Concomitantly, hemoglobin values remain within a normal range. Hemoglobin values rarely go above 18 g/dl (Exton-Smith and Overstall, 1979). The mean corpuscular hemoglobin concentration is reduced.

Changes in arterial blood gas values vary widely from one client to another. When considered with

TABLE 2. CHANGES IN PULMONARY VOLUMES AND FLOW RATES WITH EMPHYSEMA AND BRONCHITIS

Parameter	Definition	Change with Normal Aging	Change with COPD	Remarks
Lung Volumes				
Vital capacity (VC)	Maximal volume expelled by complete expiration after a maximal inspiration.	Reduced	Variable: low, normal, or high	This measurement is of little value by itself.
Forced vital capacity (FVC)	Vital capacity performed with expiration as rapid and forceful as possible.	Reduced	Reduced	Reduction due to air trapping. Significant standard measurement.
Functional residual capacity (FRC)	Volume of gas in lungs at resting expiratory level.	Increased	Increased, especially in emphysema	An early change.
Residual volume (RV)	Volume of gas in lungs after maximal expiration.	Increased	Increased	Due to air trapping and alveolar impairment. An early change.
Total lung capacity (TLC)	Volume of gas in lungs after maximal inspiration (VC + RV).	Unchanged	Increased (or normal in chronic bronchitis)	Due to loss of elasticity.
Flow Rates				
Forced expiratory volume in 1 second (FEV_1)	Volume of gas exhaled in 1 second when performing forced vital capacity.	Reduced	Significant reduction	Important indicator of severity of airway obstruction due to airway collapse.
FEV_1/FVC ratio	Relationship of time to volume. Ratio of forced expiratory volume in 1 second to forced vital capacity.	Reduced somewhat	Reduced	Indicates airway obstruction due to airway collapse and loss of elastic recoil.
Forced expiratory flow (FEF 200–1200) (or MEFR—maximum expiratory flow rate)	Average rate of flow for a specified portion of the FEV, usually between 200 and 1200 ml.	Reduced	Reduced, especially in bronchitis	Reflects changes in large airways. Values change with client effort.

TABLE 2. (CONTINUED)

Parameter	Definition	Change with Normal Aging	Change with COPD	Remarks
Forced midexpiratory flow (FEF 25–75%) (or maximum midexpiratory flow rate)	Average rate of flow during the middle half of the FEV.	Reduced	Reduced, especially in emphysema	Reflects obstruction in smaller airways. Cannot be improved by client effort.
Maximal voluntary ventilation (MVV) (or maximum breathing capacity)	Volume of air that a subject can breath with voluntary maximal effort for a given time.	Reduced	Reduced	Correlates with complaint of dyspnea. Airway obstruction, air trapping, reduced lung recoil, fatigue, pain, and weakness influence this measurement.

other assessment data, they are an indication of the severity of airway obstruction and the adequacy of alveolar ventilation. Increased ventilatory efforts help to maintain values within a normal range when disturbances of ventilation, perfusion and diffusion are not severe. Then, as obstruction progresses, arterial Po_2 is maintained at rest, but not with exercise. In severe, chronic COPD, Po_2 is low and Pco_2 is elevated. Because COPD is usually well established in the elderly, clients usually exhibit hypoxemia and some degree of CO_2 retention. The pH is maintained near the normal range due to compensatory increases in serum bicarbonate. If blood gas changes develop gradually, clients tolerate an arterial Po_2 of 35 to 40 mm Hg and a Pco_2 of 80 mm Hg. When caring for the elderly client, the nurse should bear in mind that a Po_2 of 70 to 85 mm Hg is considered normal. It is helpful to know baseline blood gas and pH values for clients with COPD for use in monitoring changes in the severity of the client's condition or the onset of respiratory failure.

With deteriorating blood gas exchange, gradual impairments of mental acuity, memory, and judgment, irascibility, headache, and insomnia may occur. If changes in Po_2 and Pco_2 are gradual the central nervous system is able to adapt. If abrupt changes in blood gases or pH occur signs of central nervous system depression may result. These in-

clude drowsiness, mental confusion, disorientation, asterixis, coma, and death.

Asthma. In the elderly, asthma is likely to be a long-standing disorder. Unlike younger clients, the elderly seldom experience severe asthmatic attacks punctuated with periods of normal airway resistance. Instead, the elderly usually exhibit continuous wheezing, dyspnea, and coughing. The degree of wheezing does not always correlate with the degree of respiratory impairment. The dyspnea is often most severe at night and the cough is characterized by difficulty expectorating the thick, tenacious sputum. These adaptations may gradually worsen if the client develops a respiratory infection or comes in contact with a respiratory irritant. The fatigue associated with these worsening adaptations is often the reason why the older asthmatic seeks health care. The client who is exhausted by dyspnea and coughing lies passively in bed, the chin sags, and respiratory movements are confined to the upper chest.

Because asthma is usually long-standing, the elderly client often exhibits signs of airway resistance even between exacerbations of the condition. In particular, the FEV and FEV_1 are likely to be reduced. An exacerbation further reduces these volumes as a consequence of airway obstruction. An

TABLE 3.   PATTERNS OF BLOOD GAS CHANGES IN ASTHMA

Severity	pH	Pco$_2$ (mm Hg)	Po$_2$ (mm Hg)
Mild	Normal	Normal or low (35–44)	Moderate reduction (60–70)
Moderate	Normal or alkaline	Low (30–35)	Moderate to severe reduction (50–60)
Severe	Normal or acid	Normal or moderate elevation (40–50)	Severe reduction (40–50)

Source: From Davies BH, 1981, with permission.

important difference between asthma and other types of COPD is that the FEV$_1$ usually improves by more than 20 percent when bronchodilators are given to the asthmatic. Frequent flow measurements should be taken because they are a reliable indicator of the degree of respiratory impairment.

Accurate assessment of the client is difficult because adaptations exhibited by the older asthmatic closely resemble other health problems seen in the elderly, including congestive heart failure and bronchitis. A careful health history to identify the age of onset of adaptations and any family or personal history of allergy or asthma is important. Sputum and blood tests should indicate eosinophilia. Allergy testing may be helpful in determining the presence of allergic asthma. The roentgenogram usually indicates hyperinflation. Some segmental or lobar collapse due to plugging may also be visible. Arterial blood gas studies are helpful in pinpointing the severity of the asthma (Table 3). Because the asthmatic tends to hyperventilate, blood gas values may be nearly normal until later stages. Carbon dioxide retention usually does not occur except during a severe asthmatic attack. When it does, it indicates a poor prognosis. If the client is having a severe asthmatic attack, tachycardia and pulsus paradoxus are present. Central cyanosis is usually not apparent in the elderly client except during a severe asthmatic attack.

NURSING INTERVENTIONS

Realistic Goal Setting

Setting realistic goals with the aged chronically ill is a challenging task that faces every health care provider who works with the aged. Doing so is a crucial step in helping the aged chronically ill to slow the processes of deterioration and maintain the highest possible level of adaptation. Realistic goals depend upon a comprehensive assessment of the client's physical and psychosocial adaptations. Because of the wide range of stresses and adaptations exhibited by the elderly, the nurse may collaborate with several other members of the health team in the goal-setting process. Clients and family must also be involved in this process if their preferences and needs are to be considered. Group conferences in which client and family discuss the client's condition and their feelings and desires with the health team can be helpful. Clients should be asked what they view as their most troubling problem. Priorities should be established. They should be asked what they would like to be doing a year from now. Finally, they should identify what they would like to accomplish in 1 month, 2 months, 6 months, and so on. Identifying realistic short-term achievements along the road to a long-term goal allows the client to experience successes along the way and improves motivation.

Setting realistic goals is a difficult accomplishment for some clients. Many older people have anticipated retirement as an opportunity to do all those things they never had the time to do. However, plans to travel are abandoned when the client's efforts to walk even a few blocks are interrupted by intermittent claudication. Dreams of growing prize-winning roses are modified when digging in the garden produces angina. Even plans to sit in a rocker and enjoy doing absolutely nothing cannot be realized when every breath is a struggle. Many elderly clients who are chronically ill need help in revising their goals. Denial is a normal part of the grief process and some clients may be unable to admit a need to revise goals until they have worked through their loss. An open, honest nurse–client relationship in which the client is free to express feelings can assist the work of grieving. Some clients may be so discouraged by what they view as a relentless process of increasing disability that they are reluctant to make the necessary efforts involved in setting and meeting revised goals. It is a challenge to create meaningful goals for improved well-being of the aged who have been "given up" by themselves or society. These clients must be helped to see that modifying only a few adaptations is often enough to compensate for a serious disability. Even the partial restoration of function can make the difference between a useful and a useless life.

Setting realistic goals can also be difficult for nurses. The aging process is inevitable and brings with it decline in physical abilities. Chronic illness usually implies a continuous process of deterioration, punctuated by plateaus of varying lengths. Dramatic improvement cannot be expected. Damage done by lifelong stresses cannot be completely erased, whether it is the buildup of atherosclerotic plaques or the destruction of alveolar membranes and airway walls. Goals must be aimed at compensating for irrevocable losses and slowing the process of additional disability. Setting realistic goals for the aged chronically ill does not always mean setting higher goals. It may mean aiming for modest gains, maintaining the status quo, or even adjusting goals downward. Doing so can be difficult for anyone oriented to "cure" rather than "care."

A belief in the inherent value of human life is fundamental to setting and meeting realistic goals for the aged chronically ill. For every elderly person, aging marks the culmination of the life process. It is a time to review what went before and to prepare for what lies ahead. In this context, improving the quality of any aged person's life, however small that improvement, is a viable goal in itself.

Therapeutic regimens may require several hours of the client's day, every day. Realistic goals allow clients to experience small gains and help them to maintain their involvement in the plan of care. If goals are overly optimistic, clients may become discouraged by their seeming lack of progress, lose

confidence, become depressed, and abandon the plan of care. Failure to set realistic goals also has consequences for nurses who may attribute the client's inability to improve to a lack of their own professional expertise. In one study of nurses caring for elderly stroke victims, less than 40 percent of nurses set short-term goals and less than 70 percent set long-term goals. Their failure to do so may have led to a variety of negative feelings they expressed, such as frustration, depression, and a lack of enthusiasm about working with these clients (Bevil, 1978).

Goals should be set down in writing and shared with the client, the client's family, and other health care providers working with the client. If goals are to remain appropriate, they must be evaluated and revised. Because change is a constant element in caring for the elderly, evaluation of goals must be a constant process.

Angina Pectoris

The goal of treatment is to modify the client's adaptations by reducing the myocardial demand for oxygen. Treatment involves medication therapy and changes in life patterns, such as activity patterns, that are related to the onset of anginal episodes.

The medications most often prescribed for the client are short-acting and long-acting nitrates, β-adrenergic blocking agents, and sedatives or tranquilizers. Because all of these medications have potentially dangerous side effects or toxic effects, the nurse must assure that the client is knowledgeable about their use.

Nitrates reduce the cardiac oxygen demand by reducing blood pressure, reducing venous return and heart size, and shortening the systolic ejection period. They reduce blood pressure by decreasing arterial resistance and reducing venous tone. Nitrates may also aid by dilating collateral circulation. Some of their benefit is reduced due to a reflex increase in heart rate and contractility.

Sublingual nitroglycerin in small doses (0.5 mg or less) is prescribed for the prevention and treatment of angina. The client should be taught that this medication should be taken prophylactically prior to performing those activities that are known to produce anginal pain. If anginal pain develops, the medication is most effective if it is taken promptly before the pain becomes severe. If pain is not relieved after three tablets in about 15 to 20 minutes, the client should be advised to call the physician. Some clients may need reassurance that nitroglycerin is not a dangerous substance. Because nitroglycerin is unstable, clients should be instructed in proper storage procedures. They should keep the medication tightly capped in the original container, but without cotton. Extra supplies should be refrigerated and the prescription should be refilled regularly. The client should be aware that nitroglycerin which is still potent will produce a slight burning or tingling sensation under the tongue. If it does not do so, the medication may have lost its potency and the pills should be replaced. Some clients may avoid taking nitroglycerin when angina occurs because it produces a feeling of fullness in the head or a headache; they should be told that if the medication is taken regularly, in time these unpleasant sensations will abate.

The use of long-acting nitrates is somewhat controversial. All forms are poorly absorbed and, in some clients, they may be ineffective. The elderly are especially sensitive to the hypotensive effects of nitrates and may faint or fall as a consequence. Clients who are given these medications should be warned about their side effects and advised to use caution when moving about or changing position. Since the long-acting nitrates tend to raise intraocular pressure, they should be avoided in the aged client with glaucoma. Sublingual isosorbide dinitrate (5 mg four times daily) has been an effective long-acting agent for some elderly clients.

β-Adrenergic blocking agents, such as propranolol (10 to 20 mg four times daily), decrease myocardial oxygen demands by reducing blood pressure, slowing the heart rate and reducing cardiac contractility. On the other hand, they increase ventricular size and prolong the duration of systolic ejection. Thus propranolol and nitroglycerin have synergistic effects.

If angina is provoked by anxiety or other emotional stress, the physician may prescribe mild sedatives or tranquilizers for the client.

Nursing interventions are aimed at helping the client modify activity and other patterns of behavior related to the angina. Clients should be advised to slow the pace of activity and curtail those activities that provoke anginal episodes. They should exercise up to, but not beyond, the limits of their tolerance. Clients should be urged to engage in whatever exercise they most enjoy—walking, dancing, golfing, and so on. The nurse can help the client work out a regular exercise plan and evaluate the client's tolerance to it. Stresses that provoke anginal pain should also be controlled. This may entail assisting clients to modify their meal patterns from a few large meals to several small ones, discussing ways to modify sexual activities so these are less taxing, or helping the client deal with emotional stresses. The nurse may also need to help the client modify those stresses that exacerbate anginal pain. This might mean helping the client who is obese, diabetic, or anemic to plan appropriate meals. Risk factors should also be controlled. These include the avoidance of caffeine, excessive alcohol, and smoking, and the monitoring of blood pressure.

If medication and modification of activity are ineffective, or if the client has unstable angina or disabling angina, surgery may be indicated. Vein grafts, using saphenous veins or internal mammary arteries, are inserted into the lumen of narrowed arteries. Age is not a risk factor in this surgery, although congestive heart failure, left ventricular impairment, and cardiomegaly are. In 90 percent of cases, revascularization relieves angina and increases exercise capacity even in the aged. Preliminary data indicate this procedure also improves survival (Lawson and Starr, 1976).

Another surgical procedure with limited use in disabling angina refractory to medical regimens is carotid nerve stimulator insertion. This allows the client to stimulate the carotid nerve by activating a small battery-operated transmitter. Stimulation reduced blood pressure, heart rate, cardiac contractility, and venous return and shortens the ejection period.

Fostering Sexual Adjustment

Masters and Johnson (1968) identified six physical and psychosocial factors that alter sexual responsiveness in the aged.

1. Monotony in sexual relationships, leading to loss of interest and boredom.
2. Male preoccupation with economic pursuits and financial security.

3. Mental and physical fatigue.
4. Overindulgence in food and alcohol, resulting in secondary impotence.
5. Fear of failure.
6. Physical and mental infirmity.

Acute and chronic health conditions are especially important factors after age 60. Even when stabilized, chronic illness can interfere directly or indirectly with sexual ability or impair sexual drive. Medications prescribed for these health conditions may also alter sexual responsiveness. Very few research studies have focused on the sexual adjustment of the chronically ill and disabled, especially among persons over age 60. Even less work has been done with female subjects than with males. Sadoughi et al. (1971) studied 55 clinically ill persons whose median age was 50 and found a decline in frequency of sexual activity as well as a decline in interest in sex and satisfaction during sexual activities. The lowest levels of frequency, interest, and satisfaction were reported by the older subjects. In this study and in another by Tuttle et al. (1964), a majority of subjects reported that they had received only vague, nonspecific information or no information at all about sexual activity. Many subjects felt they would have benefited from advice.

Some health problems, such as diabetes, radical surgery, or renal failure, affect sexual performance directly. For example, new male diabetics or those who are poorly controlled have transient incidences of impotence, which cease once the diabetes is controlled. In chronic male diabetics, neuropathy of the autonomic nervous system results in retrograde ejaculation or impotence. By age 60, almost one-half of male diabetics are impotent and they are at greater risk to become impotent the longer they have the disease, no matter how well controlled. Women diabetics may be unable to achieve orgasm due to a variety of factors, including neuropathy, changes in the microvasculature and vaginal lubrication, and the presence of vaginal infections (Belt, 1973).

The permanent change associated with prostatectomy is another instance when physical factors are directly responsible for changes in sexual function. Impotence occurs when the nerves that control penile erection are cut. This may occur during rad-

ical perineal prostatectomies, but rarely with transurethral and suprapubic procedures (Finkle and Prian, 1966). A more frequent consequence of prostatectomy, especially transurethral procedures, is retrograde ejaculation (Bowarsky, 1976). This may result from any type of radical abdominal surgery such as colon resection and is due to interference with the autonomic nervous system. Sexual dysfunction has also been related to chronic renal failure and hemodialysis, which results in reduced plasma testosterone levels and spermatogenesis, anemia, and neuropathy.

In most instances, chronic illnesses do not affect potency directly but stimulate a network of physical and psychosocial responses that influence sexual abilities and activities. Illness that affects the cardiovascular and respiratory systems results in a slow but progressive reduction of physical ability. Although this decline limits all physical activity, the client often cuts back the frequency or intensity of sexual activity first. The continuous pain and fatigue that accompany many chronic health problems, such as arthritis and osteoporosis, reduce the client's desire for sexual activity. In addition, when mobility in the hips and legs or other areas is reduced, the ability to have intercourse may also be impaired. Some clients may experience adaptations during intercourse that cause them to cut back on sexual activity. This may be the case with older women who have untreated senile vaginitis, cystocele, or rectocele, for whom intercourse is an uncomfortable or painful experience. Clients with coronary artery disease who experience angina, palpitations, or breathlessness during intercourse reduce the frequency of sexual activity more than those who do not experience adaptations (Hellerstein and Friedman, 1970).

Medications alter sexual activity through a variety of chemical mechanisms. Some act on the brain, altering the function of sexual centers and diminishing or enhancing libido. Others alter the response of genital blood vessels. Others influence the peripheral nerves of the autonomic nervous system that regulate the function of the sex organs. Drugs that block sympathetic impulses affect ejaculatory function and those that interfere with parasympathetic stimulation affect penile erection (Woods, 1979). The effects of drugs on males is better understood than females, partly because a male's response is more visible and quantifiable. Not all persons who take medications affecting sexual response experience alterations in sexual function. The reasons for the variable responses are unclear. Drugs that may affect sexual activity are listed in Table 4.

Elderly clients who have been prescribed medications that may alter sexual functioning have a right to know about the possible side effects. This discussion must be undertaken with great care because fear of becoming impotent is a powerful stress that may become a self-fulfilling prophecy. Some physicians believe it inadvisable to tell clients beforehand about this potential side effect. Once clients have begun taking the medications, they must be assessed regularly for any changes in their sexual life-style. If this is not done, clients may attribute new difficulties in sexual functioning to aging or other factors. They may avoid sexual encounters, believing their problems to be permanent. Older clients should also be aware that some medications that affect sexual ability can be bought over the counter. If a drug is found to affect potency, reducing the dosage or withdrawing it altogether, if possible, usually alleviates the problem.

Psychosocial adaptations to chronic illness are more likely than the illness itself to result in sexual dysfunction. Sexual performance is an expression of a healthy, well-adjusted individual. It reflects the person's self-image and the quality of the person's interpersonal relationships. Psychosocial adaptations to chronic illness vary widely, depending upon the symbolic significance of the illness to the client. Grief, loss of ego strength, changes in body image, negative self-concept, depression, anxiety, and dependence are frequently experienced. For the elderly, the many losses associated with chronic illness merely compound the losses that accompany the aging process. These may challenge the client's self-esteem and feelings of masculinity or femininity and alter sexual functioning. For example, while there is no evidence that hysterectomy reduces sexual desire, performance, or response, many women report feelings of weakness and emptiness, depression of desire, or inability to reach climax. In many women, the uterus is a sexual organ and a source of youth and feminine attractiveness and they experience complex psychological responses to its removal (Weg, 1978; Steffl, 1978). Myocardial infarctions and prostatectomies are viewed by many men as a threat to their manhood. Some men may give up having sex altogether. Others may overcompensate, generating a cycle of anxiety and sexual dysfunction. For the older client as well as the young, some radical surgical procedures, such as mastectomy or colostomy, may lead to concern about sexual attractiveness and deter the sexual expression or reduce the sexual desire of the client or the spouse.

Fear of death is another factor that affects the sexual activity of many chronically ill older clients or their partners. Fear is most often associated with clients who have coronary artery disease or strokes. The level of fear regarding sudden death during coitus is out of proportion to its occurrence. Less than 1 percent of all coronary deaths occur as a consequence of sexual intercourse. In men over age 60, the incidence of coital death is even lower, due in part to the decreased physical demands of sexual activity with aging. Sudden death is a possibility only if the older client already has an underlying cardiovascular or cerebrovascular disease process (Massie et al., 1969). Acute coronary insufficiency, cerebral hemorrhage, and pulmonary embolus are the most common reasons for sudden death during intercourse (Trimbel, 1970). As sexuality is inhibited, anxiety, depression, and hostility can accompany these fears (Butler and Lewis, 1977).

The presence of a willing partner is often the determining factor in whether or not the older chronically ill client remains sexually active (Finkle and Prian, 1966; Finkle et al., 1959). For the elderly, many of whom have lost their sexual partner of many years, this is an especially significant factor. For some chronically ill clients, particularly those with coronary artery disease, it is not usually advisable to seek out a new partner. The heightened anxiety and excitement may increase the client's energy expenditure during sexual activity, making it dangerous.

The long-term goal for the chronically ill client—to lead as normal a life as possible—includes sexuality. Neither chronological age nor chronic illness removes sexual interest or drive. Clients need help to make sexual adjustments at new adaptive levels, commensurate with their age, abilities and preferences. A realistic goal is to help clients resume sexual patterns similar to the ones they enjoyed

TABLE 4. DRUGS THAT ALTER SEXUAL FUNCTIONING

Category	Examples	Mechanism of Action	Adaptations
Antihypertensives	Reserpine (Serpasil) Guanethidine (Ismelin) Mecamylamine (Inversine) Trimethaphan (Arfonad) Methyldopa (Aldomet) Pentolineum (Ansolysen)	Sympathetic blocking agents	Reduced sexual desire in women Reduced erectile ability or impotence Possible altered ejaculation
Diuretics	Spironolactone (Aldactone)	Interfere with normal resorption of sodium ions	Impotence Gynecomastia
Antispasmodics	Methantheline (Banthine)	Ganglionic blocking agent	Impotence
Antihistamines	Diphenhydramine (Benadryl) Chlorpheniramine (Chlor-Trimeton)	Block parasympathetic nerve impulse to sex organs	Impaired erection Reduced sexual desire in women
Estrogens	Diethylstilbestrol (Stilbestrol)	Antagonize male sex hormones	Reduced desire and potency in men
Antidepressants			
Tricyclic compounds	Imipramine (Tofranil) Amitriptyline (Elavil)	Have peripheral anticholinergic effects	Impotence
MAO inhibitors	Phenilzine sulfate (Nardil) Tranylcypromine sulfate (Parnate)	Block peripheral ganglionic nerve	Inhibited erection; impotence
Narcotics	Morphine sulfate Heroin	Depress central nervous system	Depressed sexual performance and ability
Barbiturates	Amobarbital (Amytal) Pentobarbital (Nembutal) Secobarbital (Seconal)	Depress central nervous system	Depressed sexual performance and ability
Major tranquilizers	Phenothiazines: Chlorpromazine (Thorazine) Prochlorperazine (Compazine) Thiodazine (Mellaril)	Modify sensory input to reticular formation in brainstem May block adrenergic impulses and cholinergic synapses	Reduced libido Ejaculatory disorders; impotence
Minor tranquilizers	Chlordiazepoxide (Librium) Diazepam (Valium) Meprobamate (Equanil)	Affect cholinergic and adrenergic aspects of central nervous system	Reduced libido Inhibited erection Altered ejaculation
Alcohol		Depress central nervous system	Depressed sexual performance and ability
Antiparkinsonism agents	Levodopa (L-dopa)	Mechanism uncertain. May be secondary to increased feelings of well-being	Increased libido and penile erection

before they became ill. Not all older clients wish to continue to be sexually active. Some may have found sex a burden and cooperated with a sexual partner out of a sense of duty. If older clients wish to use chronic illness as a reason for avoiding sex, their wishes should be respected.

Nursing responsibilities include assessing the client's past, present, and potential levels of sexual adjustment and planning and implementing appropriate care. The nurse is in a strategic position to educate and counsel clients and their partners regarding stresses that interfere with sexual function and ways to adapt to those stresses. When the client's sexual problems require intervention beyond the scope of nursing, the nurse makes referrals to appropriate resources.

Assessment.   Information about sexual activity is a routine part of every health history. By inquiring about sexual activity, the nurse lets clients understand that sexual behavior is a normal and important part of life and invites them to discuss problems they are having in this area. As older clients become more aware of their sexuality, they will expect sexual health care from nurses and other professionals. If sexual interest and activity are introduced as a routine part of the health history and discussed in an objective, professional manner, most older clients do not react with anxiety or evasion (Pfeiffer, 1979). If discussion of sexual topics was not acceptable during most of their lifetime, elderly clients may be hesitant to introduce this topic themselves and reluctant to admit the existence of any problems. These older clients may be more willing to discuss sexuality if the nurse explains the reasons for doing so. Clients may be relieved that the nurse has taken the initiative and asked pertinent questions.

The sexual assessment need not be lengthy and should focus on the *client's perception* of the problem. Questions should be asked to obtain the following data:

- Self-concept and level of self-esteem.
- Nature and quality of interpersonal relationships.
- Ability to fulfill role expectations.
- Current ability to function sexually.
- Changes in ability to function sexually.

- Reasons for any change in ability to function sexually.
- Satisfaction with current sexual activities.
- Expectations and goals for future sexual functioning.

This information is integrated with other data about the client's physical and psychosocial adaptations and medication history and used to identify stresses in the area of sexual functioning. The sexual history provides a data base for the client's current level of sexual behavior for later comparison. It is also used to identify areas where sex education or counseling are needed.

Education and Counseling.   Misinformation is a major reason for sexual dysfunction in chronically ill elderly clients (Tuttle et al., 1964). Because many of the current population of older people did not have access to sex education, they may lack accurate, basic information about sexual behavior. Consequently, when confronted with a health problem, they make decisions about their sexual abilities and activities based on incorrect information, superstitions, or fears. The nurse may need to initiate client education or supplement what is already known. The chronically ill aged often need reassurance that sexual activity is not the reason for the illness and will not worsen their condition. In fact, because sexual activity is a way to relieve tensions and a form of physical activity, it can relieve emotional distress and contribute to an overall sense of well-being. Most chronically ill clients need information about what types of sexual activities are safe, when they can be resumed, and how often they can be undertaken. They need specific information about how to modify previous sexual patterns to accommodate chronic stresses, and they need to know what to do if adverse adaptations develop during or after sexual activity.

Most clients need help to cope with the fatigue, pain, and impaired mobility that usually accompany chronic illness and prevent a fulfilling sexual relationship. If it is acceptable to the client and partner, they may be taught new positions, with the ill person assuming a more passive role. The client may sit in a low chair or assume the on-bottom position, or both partners may assume side-lying positions. These positions reduce energy expenditure and would be appropriate for clients with reduced cardiovascular or respiratory functioning, for those who are too weak to assume the on-top position, such as the stroke client, or for those with painful conditions such as arthritis or osteoporosis.

To prevent fatigue, clients should be advised to nap before sexual activity or to plan sexual intercourse in the morning after a good night's sleep. In addition, clients should avoid other strenuous activities soon after intercourse. If the client is overweight, losing weight reduces the energy cost of sexual activity. Clients should also be advised to avoid sex up to 3 hours after a large meal, after drinking alcoholic beverages, when the temperature is extremely hot or cold, or when experiencing any negative emotions, such as anxiety or anger. Sexual encounters that are illicit, involve a new partner, or are undertaken in unfamiliar surroundings with a time limit also increase the energy cost and contribute to fatigue. Sexual activity that is relaxed, unhurried, and shared with a familiar, compatible partner requires the lowest energy cost.

To reduce pain, taking a warm bath and any prescribed pain medications shortly before sexual activity may be helpful: Clients with pain often need to experiment to find the most comfortable position for sexual intercourse. Because the activity associated with intercourse stimulates the production of cortisone by the adrenal glands, it may reduce pain and improve the status of clients with arthritis.

Before clients undergo surgical procedures that have long-term implications for sexual functioning, they need information about how the procedure will influence sexual abilities and when they can expect the return of sexual function. For example, men who are undergoing prostatectomies need to know how the procedure will affect their potency and ability to have children. If sterility is a prospect, older men married to younger women may wish to place sperm in a sperm bank. Clients must be prepared for the dressing, tubes, and bloody urine that characterize the immediate postoperative period. Otherwise, they may misinterpret these things and believe that complications have occurred. Clients should also be warned if retrograde ejaculation is likely to occur. Although this does not interfere with the sensation of orgasm, there is no sensation of emission. Many clients who are about to undergo radical procedures, and their partners, need extensive counseling to help them deal with their fears that such procedures will alter sexual desire, attractiveness, or ability.

The nurse also counsels clients for whom chronic illness makes sexual intercourse dangerous or impossible. Sexual needs persist, including the need for warmth, closeness, and being valued as a person. The nurse should encourage other activities such as touching, stroking, kissing, and embracing. If the client's condition can tolerate them and if the client is willing, masturbation and oral sex should be encouraged.

The presence of a willing partner has been cited as the determining factor in sexual adjustment of many older chronically ill clients (Finkle et al., 1959; Finkle and Prian, 1966). For this reason, the nurse includes the client's partner when planning and implementing care aimed at sexual adjustment. The partner's needs for teaching and counseling must be met as well. The nurse should encourage the client and partner to keep communication about sexual activities open. One way to do so is to conduct mutual teaching sessions in which both partners participate.

Referral. When the client's sexual dysfunction is severe or due to psychosocial factors, the nurse should determine whether the client wishes a referral to a sex therapist or other qualified professional. Some clients have physical conditions that can be corrected and should be referred to a physician. A vaginal pessary or surgery may benefit women with a prolapsed uterus or cystocele. Penile implants may restore some function to the client who has had a radical prostatectomy (Escamilla, 1975). Diabetics who are poorly controlled, women with senile vaginitis, and clients the nurse suspects of having adverse side effects to medication should also be referred to a physician.

Promoting Sexual Function in Clients with Coronary Artery Disease. The sexual needs of older clients who have angina or who have had a myocardial infarction typify those of many of the chronically ill aged. The cardiac condition is a source of concern to the client and partner and provokes many questions about sexual activity. The nurse can assure the couple that sex is another form of exercise. Like other activities, clients can resume sexual activities in a careful, graded manner, while monitoring their responses to it. The nurse helps the client modify sexual activity when necessary for optimal cardiac function. Those clients who wish to do so can maintain a satisfactory sex life.

The level of sexual activity the client maintains depends upon several factors:

1. Sex drive, performance, and patterns before the onset of illness.
2. Age-related changes in sexual function.
3. Partner's health, attitudes, and decisions.
4. Emotional response to coronary artery disease.
5. Extent of myocardial damage and level of cardiovascular functioning.
6. Responses to drugs, progressive exercise regimens and other treatments (Hellerstein and Friedman, 1970).

Clients with coronary artery disease who do not receive sexual education and counseling most often experience sexual dysfunction as a consequence of their emotional responses. Following myocardial infarction, 66 percent of clients permanently cut back their sexual activity and 10 percent became impotent. Their sexual patterns were based on misinformation and fear (Tuttle et al., 1964). Without appropriate information, most clients and their spouses believe that sexual intercourse will precipitate sudden death or another heart attack (Sheingold and Wagner, 1974).

Clients who have had a myocardial infarction or an anginal attack need specific directions about how soon they can engage in sexual activities, what kinds are safe, and under what circumstances. Following an uncomplicated myocardial infarction, the absence of adaptations and the results of exercise tests are used to determine the resumption of activity. On average, older clients burn 6 to 8 calories per minute when walking vigorously or climbing two flights of stairs. The older client who has sexual intercourse with a familiar partner expends only 6 calories per minute for less than 30 seconds at orgasm and only 4.5 calories per minute before and after orgasm. Therefore, if clients can perform stair climbing or vigorous walking without experiencing

angina, palpitations, or other difficulty, they should be told that sexual activities are also safe (Hellerstein and Friedman, 1970). Clients should know that those who are physically reconditioned have the best chance of resuming normal sexual activities. Therefore, they should be encouraged to maintain a regular exercise program (Naughton, 1975).

Clients should be counseled about ways to resume normal sexual relationships without promoting anxieties about performance. In most cases, the couple can be encouraged to give sensate pleasure to nongenital areas within 1 or 2 months after myocardial infarction. The couple should be encouraged to focus on reexperiencing and enjoying one another, rather than on male performance. If it is acceptable to them, clients can be encouraged to masturbate 2 months after myocardial infarction. Masturbation requires a lower energy expenditure than intercourse and is one way for clients to find out if they are still able to have an erection and orgasm. This can eliminate much of the anxiety when intercourse is resumed, usually within 12 to 14 weeks following infarction (Woods and Herbert, 1979; Naughton, 1975).

Clients should be informed about positions that reduce the energy cost during intercourse. They should be advised to avoid the on-top position, which involves isometric contractions of small muscle groups, elevates central aortic pressure, and may produce angina or arrhythmias (Scheingold and Wagner, 1974). The client should also be advised about other circumstances, discussed earlier in this chapter, that increase the energy costs of intercourse.

The nurse should advise clients about what to do if breathlessness, dyspnea, or angina occur during sexual activity. Clients who experience angina should be advised to take nitroglycerin prophylactically (Hellerstein and Friedman, 1970). Usually difficulties will occur in the resolution phase of intercourse so no action is needed. If they occur prior to that, clients should be advised to slow down or stop intercourse. Signs of overexertion include palpitations for 15 minutes or more during or after intercourse, sleeplessness, or fatigue the day after intercourse. If any adaptations occur either during or after intercourse, clients should be instructed to contact their physician.

The client's partner must be an integral part

of the teaching and counseling. The nurse should encourage partners to express their fears openly. They need to be reassured that sexual activity will not worsen the heart condition. The emotional security and physical activity that accompany a good sexual relationship can reduce the level of tension, help clients face other stresses with more confidence, and promote physical and mental well-being. Partners usually need facts about sexuality and the physiological responses during sexual activity. They need to understand that the energy costs associated with sexual intercourse are minimal. Together, the nurse, client, and partner can help devise ways to further reduce energy costs during sexual activity. With ongoing support from the nurse, the partner can be a source of support as the client resumes sexual activity.

Peripheral Vascular Disease

Arteriosclerosis Obliterans. The most effective treatment for intermittent claudication is a progressive walking program. Clients should be advised to walk slowly, to take short steps, to avoid stairs and hills as much as possible, and to stop frequently. Clients should exercise every 4 to 5 hours throughout the day, stopping when the pain starts. They should gradually increase the distance walked until they are able to cover a couple of miles every day. Exercise develops collateral circulation. The success of the program can be measured by evaluating how much further the client is able to walk before the pain develops. Many clients with arteriosclerosis obliterans also have angina. For these people, a less vigorous program of exercise is needed in order to prevent anginal pain. Clients should be taught that when resting, the best position to promote circulation is the reverse Trendelenberg. If the client exhibits any of the risk factors associated with ASO, such as obesity, smoking, diabetes, or hypercholesteremia, the nurse should work with the client to control these. The client with intermittent claudication usually does not benefit from medication. Analgesics are not necessary since the pain lasts only for a few seconds. Vasodilator drugs do not appear to affect the involved areas and anticoagulants are of little value.

Clients with advanced ASO should be referred to a physician for a complete examination and treatment. Clients with Stage II or III ASO require analgesics or narcotics for pain relief during the day and at night. In clients with intractable rest pain and ischemic lesions, surgical intervention may be the only way to save the limb. Procedures such as thromboendarterectomy, arterial grafts, lumbar sympathectomy, or a combination of these are used with excellent results in the elderly. If ischemic gangrene develops, an amputation may be the only recourse.

Foot Care. In all clients with arteriosclerosis obliterans, assuring that the client carries out meticulous daily foot care is an essential part of the plan of care. The goals are to prevent ischemic ulcers and infection. Clients should be taught to inspect the feet systematically for signs of trauma or skin breakdown. In addition, clients should be taught the following procedures for foot care:

CLEANSING. The feet should be washed daily in tepid water with a mild soap. Water should be tested first to prevent burning of the foot. The client should pat, not rub, the feet dry, especially between the toes. After drying, a bland lubricating cream should be massaged into the feet, with special attention to calluses, the base of the toenails, and the heels. Excess cream should be wiped off and foot powder applied, especially between the toes.

NAIL CARE. The nails should be cut after bathing when they are soft. They should be cut straight across and never shorter than the end of the toe, Sharp nail edges can be filed gently with an emory board. The podiatrist should cut nails if the client has limited vision or mobility.

FOOTWEAR. Lamb's wool should be used to separate toes that overlap. The client must not go barefoot or wear slippers during the day. Clean dry stockings or socks should be worn. Socks that have holes or have been mended should not be worn, since these areas may cause friction. Before being worn, shoes should be inspected for foreign objects or nails projecting through the sole and for worn or wrinkled linings that might cause friction. Shoes must have sturdy toes to prevent injury. Open-toed and open-heeled shoes are not advisable, nor are shoes with rubber soles. Shoes should be alternated daily to allow them to air out between wearings and to prevent pressure areas. New shoes should be broken in gradually.

SAFETY. Extremes of heat and cold must be avoided. Heating pads, hot water bottles, and hot soaks must never be used, since these may result in burns, infection, and eventually gangrene, necessitating amputation. If the client is cold at night, thick cotton or wool socks can be worn to bed. The client should avoid sitting too close to fireplaces and stoves. Socks and boots should be worn outside in cold weather; when possible, however, going out in the cold should be avoided.

CIRCULATION. Constricting garments such as girdles, garters, tight hose, or shoes should be avoided, as should sitting with knees crossed, which causes constriction. Tobacco should be avoided. A progressive walking program should be started and Buerger-Allen exercises performed regularly to develop collateral circulation.

SPECIAL PROBLEMS. A podiatrist should be visited regularly (every 4 to 6 weeks) for special attention to nails, corns, calluses, and for injury. Corns and calluses should not be cut, nor should over-the-counter medications be used to remove corns and calluses since these may cause chemical burns.

If the client develops ischemic foot lesions, the goals of care include avoidance of trauma, control of infection, relief of pain, and preservation of muscle strength and joint range of motion. The physician usually drains purulent material from beneath eschars and debrides scabs. Wet dressings with normal saline, antibiotics, or potassium permanganate soaks (1:10,000 solution) are often ordered.

Varicose Veins. The client with varicosities should be taught several measures to reduce uncomfortable adaptations and prevent complications. Elastic protective stockings should be used from the proximal foot to just below the knee when sitting or standing. These compress dilated superficial veins, preventing edema and aiding the muscular pumping action essential for good venous return. Legs should be elevated periodically during the day for a total of 1 or 2 hours. Clients should exercise, by walking, on a regular basis to prevent venous stasis and should know how to recognize thrombophlebitis and stasis ulcers, two common complications of varicosities. If varicose veins are severe the client should be referred to a physician for medical or surgical treatment. This includes the injection of sclerosing solutions such as sodium tetradecyl sulfate, administration of small doses of heparin to prevent venous thrombosis, or surgical ligation and stripping of involved veins.

Venous Thrombosis. Because adaptations to venous thrombosis vary widely or may be absent altogether, the nurse may be uncertain about whether or not a problem exists. Whenever venous thrombosis is suspected, the client should be referred promptly to a physician. A number of diagnostic tests, including contrast venography, ultrasonic techniques using the Doppler method, radioactive-labeled fibrinogen, impedence plethysmography, and phleborheography are used to confirm the diagnosis.

Intervention varies widely depending on whether the thrombosis involves a deep vein or a superficial one. If a superficial vein is involved and if edema and pain are absent, bed rest and elevation of the limb may not be prescribed. The limb is wrapped with an elastic stocking or Ace bandage to promote venous return and the client is given antiinflammatory agents such as Butazolidin or Tandearil. Resolution of the local process takes from 2 days to 2 weeks. If the superficial thrombosis extends above the knee, bed rest, elevation of the limb, moist heat, anticoagulants, and possibly surgery are prescribed.

The goal of treatment for deep vein thrombosis is to prevent the formation of emboli or thrombi. Usually, absolute bed rest for 5 to 10 days is prescribed. The Trendelenberg position to elevate the legs above the level of the heart promotes venous return, prevents venous stasis, and reduces edema and pain. This position can be accomplished by placing the bed on blocks or using a hospital bed. The use of pillows to elevate the legs may interfere with venous drainage and should be avoided. The client's head should not be elevated when the legs are elevated because venous stasis and thrombosis may develop in the iliac area, a dependent part of the body. If the older client cannot tolerate the head down position, the head should be elevated and the legs placed in a horizontal position. Elastic stockings may be used while the client is in bed and should always be used when the client is out of bed. Moist heat is usually applied to the full length of the involved extremity. The nurse should assure that the client is well hydrated to prevent hemoconcentration, which predisposes to thrombosis of the veins.

During the acute phase, the client should not breathe deeply or strain at stool. Once the danger of emboli is passed, bed exercises should be encouraged. When the client is permitted out of bed, the nurse should encourage walking and discourage sitting or standing since these positions increase hydrostatic pressure and predispose to peripheral edema.

Anticoagulation therapy is generally prescribed for clients with venous thrombosis. Usually, the treatment involves the administration of heparin followed later by warfarin sodium (Coumadin). Oral therapy may be continued for 3 to 6 months. Fibrinolysins and low-molecular-weight dextran are given to some clients. Their value has not been definitively established. In the elderly, dextran must be given with caution to prevent circulatory overload.

Interventions for chronic venous insufficiency are aimed at preventing potential stresses, such as emboli and stasis ulcers. Clients should be instructed to elevate their legs at night and intermittently during the day. They should avoid long periods of standing and use well-fitting elastic stockings from mid-foot to just below the knees. Clients should also be instructed in proper foot hygiene to prevent infection.

Treatment of stasis ulcers differs in several ways from that of ischemic ulcers. If clients develop venous ulcers, their legs are elevated and warm packs are applied to reduce inflammation and pain. Once edema has been reduced, applications such as Unna's paste boots may be made to promote healing. In some cases, surgical grafting may be required for complete healing.

Chronic Obstructive Pulmonary Disease

When planning a therapeutic regimen for the client with COPD, it is important to individualize each treatment according to the client's needs and wishes. Usually, the therapeutic regimen involves numerous medications and pieces of equipment and a series of structured exercises and activities that consume many hours of every day. A successful treatment plan requires the client's complete cooperation and involvement. Clients must have realistic expectations about what treatment can achieve. Otherwise, they may become discouraged and cease to participate in their plan of care. Because chronic airway obstruction cannot be cured, marked or permanent

improvement of pulmonary function should not be expected. The therapeutic regimen is aimed at controlling adaptations, thus preventing exacerbation and complications that necessitate hospitalization and improving the client's mobility, independence, and quality of life.

The elements of a comprehensive regimen for COPD include

- Client education
- Medication management
- Bronchial hygiene
- Oxygen therapy
- Nutrition
- Progressive exercise
- Modification of life-style
- Coping with psychosocial stresses.

Client Education. The first step toward obtaining the client's cooperation in the plan of care is education. Because chronic airway obstruction requires continuing care, the client needs ongoing education. Clients need information about the anatomy of the respiratory system, the disease process, and their prognosis. They need to be informed about every aspect of their treatment plan, including the reasons for each therapeutic measure and instructions on how to carry the measures out. Famiy members need to be included in the educational process in order to appreciate the importance of a regular treatment regimen. They need to understand the physical and psychosocial problems with which the client has to deal. Often, the spouse is involved in the treatment plan, preparing appropriate meals, assisting with pulmonary physical therapy, assisting with the maintenance of nebulizers and other equipment and in many other ways. It is important for the spouse to know which adaptations signal the onset of an exacerbation, an infection, or respiratory failure. Often, a worsening of the client's condition is accompanied by changes in mentation and judgment and it is the spouse who must take the responsibility for obtaining the appropriate medical care. Many pamphlets and booklets about COPD written for laymen are available and are excellent supplements to the teaching provided by the nurse. The American Lung Association is an excellent resource and might be the first place to contact regarding educational material for clients.

Medication Management. Most clients with COPD have been prescribed a large number of medications, including bronchodilators, antibiotics, and steroids (Table 5). These medications help to control adaptations but do not halt the disease process. These drugs have numerous side effects, some of which are particularly dangerous in the elderly. If clients with COPD are to manage their medication regimen safely and effectively, they must be knowledgeable about each medication.

Mucolytic agents and *expectorants* have been used to thin and liquify mucus. Acetylcysteine (Mucomyst) is one of the most widely used agents, but because it is a hypertonic solution, it may induce bronchospasm unless administered with a bronchodilator. Saline solutions have been found to be just as effective as Mucomyst in treating clients with chronic bronchitis (Freeman, 1978; Wynne, 1979). Both mucolytic agents and expectorants are believed by many to be of questionable value in helping clients loosen and expectorate mucus.

Some medications have been contraindicated for use with the client with respiratory obstruction. Although *anticholinergic* and *antihistamine* drugs do have bronchodilating effects, these are not recommended, because of their drying effects on bronchial secretions. Clients should be warned that many over-the-counter drugs, including some sedatives, contain antihistamines.

Mild sedatives such as chlorodiazepoxide (Librium) and diazepam (Valium) and mood elevators may be prescribed for some clients if their condition warrants it. Any client taking sedatives or tranquilizers should be assessed for lethargy, depression, and other adaptations that may contribute to underventilation. Because narcotics and barbiturates depress respiration, these medications should not be used with clients with COPD.

Bronchial Hygiene. Bronchial hygiene includes all measures to improve airway clearance and prevent bronchial irritation.

Minimizing Airway Irritants. Every client with COPD must be urged to discontinue smoking, the single most important source of respiratory irritation. Cigarette smoking not only aggravates bronchitis and emphysema but involves the inhalation of carbon monoxide, which interferes with red cell oxygen transport. Pointing out what clients have to gain by conquering this habit may help them to do so. Clients should be told that if smoking is discontinued, cough will improve, sputum volume will decrease, and further deterioration of lung function is less likely.

The nurse must encourage and support older clients, many of whom must give up a lifelong habit and feel they "can't quit." Helping clients examine the reasons why they smoke may help them to give up the habit. Smoking cigars and pipes, provided they are not inhaled, or switching to low tar and nicotine, filtered cigarettes, while reducing the number smoked, are better practices than not quitting at all.

Other respiratory irritants should be identified and avoided. These may vary widely from one client to another. The nurse can help the client examine "bad days" for factors that may have worsened adaptations. Avoidance of irritants may involve staying indoors during periods of high environmental pollution or cold weather, using air conditioners and air purifiers, and using humidifiers in winter to counteract the hot, dry air provided by many heating units.

Preventing Infection. For clients with COPD, infection is the most common reason for increased sputum production, exacerbation of the condition, and respiratory failure. Simple preventive measures include seasonal influenza vaccination and avoidance of people with respiratory infections and crowded and closed areas in winter months. Some physicians prescribe antibiotics to prevent infections in susceptible individuals. Clients must be well informed about the symptoms that signal infection. These include increased cough or sputum, changes in the color or viscosity of sputum, increased shortness of breath, tightness in the chest, fever, or chills. Clients must understand what they are to do if they suspect an infection. This may include promptly instituting antibiotic therapy and contacting the physician. Sputum cultures are taken in an acute exacerbation, but they have limited diagnostic value. Antibiotic therapy is instituted before the sputum culture reports are available, since the flora of clients with COPD is usually predictable. Later, if needed, the specific antibiotic can be changed.

TABLE 5. MEDICATIONS COMMONLY USED IN COPD

Drug Group	Actions and Indications	Nursing Implications with the Elderly	Commonly Used Drugs
β-Adrenergic stimulators	Stimulate β_2 receptors, relaxing smooth muscle of bronchi and skeletal muscles, thus relieving swelling, edema, and spasm, improving movement of mucus, and causing bronchodilation. Also cause β_1 stimulation, resulting in inotropic and chronotropic effects on the heart. Especially useful with asthma. Sometimes useful with clients who wheeze or have bronchitis.	Many side effects, including nervousness, tachycardia and other arrhythmias, anorexia, nausea, vomiting, sleeplessness, weakness, and drowsiness. Should be used with caution in elderly since they stimulate the cardiovascular system and may aggravate hypertension. Contraindicated in clients with angina or arrhythmias. May stimulate urinary retention in men with prostatic obstruction. If possible, suggest clients take medications in morning to prevent sleeplessness. Caution clients that overuse of these agents tends to produce tolerance. Since oral forms are poorly absorbed, aerosols have become popular.	Bronkosol (isoetharine) Isuprel (isoproterenol) Vaponefrin (racemic epinephrine) Phenylephrine Ephedrine Newer drugs include: Alupent (meta-proterenol sulfate) Brethine (terbutaline sulfate) Salbutamol—observe for tremors as a side effect These newer drugs have proportionately less β_1 effects. Therefore, they are more satisfactory for use in the elderly.
Methylxanthines	Cause brochodilation by inhibiting the action of phospho-diesterase, which catalyzes the breakdown of cyclic AMP. Especially useful with asthma. Sometimes useful with clients who wheeze or have bronchitis.	Side effects include supraventricular tachycardia, seizures, nausea, vomiting, anorexia, headache, sleeplessness, nervousness. Use with caution in clients with liver dysfunction and congestive heart failure. Because	Aminophylline (Elixophylline): With repeated doses, toxic effects such as nausea and vomiting may become troublesome. Theophylline: has a very narrow therapeutic range between an ineffective dose and

(continued)

TABLE 5.   (CONTINUED)

Drug Group	Actions and Indications	Nursing Implications with the Elderly	Commonly Used Drugs
Methylxanthines (continued)	These agents are often combined with β-adrenergic stimulators.	these clients metabolize xanthines more slowly, they are at high risk for toxicity. Caution clients that overuse of these agents tends to produce tolerance.	onset of side effects. Combination drugs include: Tedral (theophylline, epinephrine, phenobarbital) Bronkotabs (quaifenesin, theophylline, phenobarbital) These combination drugs often produce an effect superior to that produced by either drug alone.
Corticosteroids	Antiinflammatory agents that relax bronchial muscles by preventing antigen–antibody reactions, increasing cellular concentrations of cyclic AMP and inhibiting other cellular mechanisms associated with bronchoconstriction. Especially effective with asthma.	Elderly are at higher risk than the young for side effects including bleeding, skin fragility, and fractures of the ribs or vertebrae. Teach client to monitor for common side effects. To lessen side effects, give every other day or for three consecutive days each week. To minimize inhibition of endogenous cortisol production, give in morning. Encourage use of antacids to prevent gastrointestinal bleeding. If therapy is prolonged, clients with positive tuberculin tests may require Isoniazid prophylactically.	Oral: Hydrocortisone Prednisone Inhaled: Vanceril (beclomethasone diproprionate) Inhaled agents are especially valuable in the elderly, since systemic side effects are minimal.
Antibiotics	Used during exacerbations due to infection against the bacteria most often responsible: *Hemophilus influenza* and	Ensure client understands correct principles and procedures for taking antibotics. Ensure client understands	Preferred: Tetracycline Ampicillin Others: Doxycycline Chloramphenicol Erythromycin

(continued)

TABLE 5. (CONTINUED)

Drug Group	Actions and Indications	Nursing Implications with the Elderly	Commonly Used Drugs
Antibiotics (continued)	*Diplococcus pneumoniae* Used prophylactically; especially effective for clients with a history of respiratory infections.	importance of calling physician or nurse at first sign of infection. May be given prophylactically throughout the year or winter months daily, on one week–off one week, or on three weeks–off one week. Clients often given a supply of antibiotic and instructed to begin a 7- to 10- day course of treatment at the first sign of respiratory infection.	Cephalosporin Sulfamethoxazol

Hydration. The most effective way to liquefy bronchial secretions is through systemic hydration. Elderly clients without heart disease benefit from drinking 2 to 3 liters of fluid daily. The nurse should work with the client to develop a satisfactory plan of fluid intake. Many elderly clients must consume the bulk of the fluid well before bedtime to avoid interrupting their sleep. Keeping a written record of fluid intake may help clients with memory lapses to maintain the needed intake.

Water may also be added to the airways locally. Some clients may benefit from long hot showers in the morning to moisten and raise secretions although others may find this suffocating. Humidifiers, vaporizers, and nebulizers are some of the devices used for this purpose, but they may not be needed unless airways are unusually dry. Humidifiers may be costly and nebulizers may be a source of infection if not kept scrupulously clean. Certainly, the simple habit of drinking water is more effective and less costly in lessening mucus viscosity and aiding expectoration. The goal is to develop a plan that is effective and that the client is willing to follow.

Pulmonary Physical Therapy. Breathing exercises, controlled expulsive coughing, postural drainage, percussion, and vibration are measures that help to mobilize secretions and improve alveolar ventilation. The nurse may be involved in teaching these techniques to clients, helping them devise a regular schedule for therapy, and modifying particular techniques to meet the needs and limitations of the elderly. Difficult, complicated maneuvers to drain lung segments are deleterious to any client, particularly an elderly one. After assessing the client's musculoskeletal status, the nurse can help the client find a comfortable position that places the tracheal–bronchial tree in a downward tilt. This might be accomplished with several pillows or tightly rolled blankets, a simple knee–chest position, or the use of an exercise board. Percussion and vibration techniques must be performed gently in the elderly and may not be tolerated at all. If percussion is done improperly, ribs and vertebrae can be fractured.

Equipment. Bulb nebulizers, power nebulizers, and intermittent positive pressure machines are some of the devices used by the client with COPD to deliver aerosols to the airway. Elderly clients who are given a handheld bulb nebulizer must be carefully evaluated to ensure they can use it effectively. Taking a deep breath while simultaneously squeezing the bulb requires muscle strength and coordination. This may be difficult to impossible to learn if the older client has diminished coordination or strength. For weak or poorly coordinated clients, power driven devices may be preferable. Intermittent positive pressure machines (IPPB) are used to reduce airway obstruction and remove secretions when all other methods have failed. Because the benefits of IPPB in clients with COPD have not been clearly demonstrated and because the machines are expensive, IPPB is not recommended for routine use by clients living at home.

Because any reusable equipment is a potential source of infection, it must be cleaned thoroughly and regularly. Whenever equipment is part of the therapeutic regimen, the client must have written instructions for its use, cleaning, and maintenance.

Oxygen.   In recent years, oxygen therapy for clients living at home has become a widely accepted practice. Portable liquid oxygen systems have made continuous oxygen therapy available and convenient, even for mobile clients. Oxygen therapy forestalls the development of potential stresses, such as cor pulmonale, polycythemia, and cardiac failure. Although oxygen therapy does not alter the natural course of severe COPD or improve pulmonary function, it can improve exercise tolerance and stamina in activities of daily living and reduce the number of days spent in the hospital (Wynne, 1979). Although oxygen therapy is expensive, its cost is offset by the reduced costs of hospitalization.

When the arterial PO_2 drops below 50 mm Hg at rest, the physician may prescribe oxygen, designating a specific flow rate. Usually this is 2 to 3 liters if nasal prongs are used or 24 percent if the Venturi mask is used. Oxygen may be prescribed continuously or periodically, such as at night. The nurse is often involved in teaching clients and family members how to use oxygen safely and correctly and in monitoring their ability to use the oxygen system.

Nutrition.   The emaciation that often accompanies advanced airway obstruction makes the nurse's role of maintaining good nutrition a challenge. Some clients, particularly bronchitics, are overweight, which increases dyspnea by decreasing respiratory excursion. These clients need assistance in losing weight (see Chapter 16). Clients with COPD should endeavor to stay at or below their desired weight. The effort of chewing and the breath-holding required when swallowing make eating a fatiguing experience. Clients often swallow air when eating, which distends the abdomen and gives a feeling of fullness. The large amounts of fluid needed to hydrate clients may make them feel too full to eat. Even moderate-sized meals impede the movement of the diaphragm, increasing dyspnea. Many of the aerosol drugs used by the client leave a foul taste in the mouth, compounding the client's anorexia. Many clients are encouragd to eat high-protein, high-calorie meals simply to maintain their weight. Vitamin and mineral supplements are helpful. The nurse needs to work with the client to find innovative ways to maintain nutrition. Eating four or five small feedings daily is one way. The client should be discouraged from drinking fluids with meals, since this contributes to an early feeling of satiety. Performing pulmonary physical therapy techniques before meals may reduce breathlessness. Frequent oral hygiene, particularly before meals, may improve the appetite. Careful diet planning to avoid any foods that may cause gastric distress or gas is also a valuable practice.

Exercise.   Progressive exercise programs for clients with COPD improve their sense of well-being and short-term exercise tolerance. The improvement is thought to be due to improved muscle function rather than altered lung function (Freeman, 1978). Walking, the regular performance of household duties, socializing, and even stair climbing should be encouraged within the limits of fatigue and dyspnea. The client should not attempt activities that result in dyspnea. Any exercise program must be carefully planned and graded and closely supervised. Clients are more likely to continue regular exercise if there is close follow up. The nurse is in an excellent position to provide needed support while evaluating the client's responses to exercise. The nurse can also help the client learn new habits that increase exercise tolerance. These include walking at a slower pace, controlled breathing during exercise, abdominal breathing, and resting before fatigue or dyspnea become severe.

Modification of Life-Style. The progressive nature of COPD requires that the client and the family make extensive adjustments in their habits of daily living. Simply performing activities of daily living such as bathing, dressing, and eating, and implementing the treatment regimen may consume larger and larger portions of every day. The nurse needs to assess clients' usual patterns of daily activities and work with them to develop a schedule that includes their preferences and encompasses the treatment regimen. Most clients find the morning hours to be particularly difficult. Dyspnea can be extreme until the client has raised secretions that pooled at night. Clients need ample time in the morning if they are to be ready for clinic appointments or social events later in the day. Frequent rest periods must be scheduled, particularly before major activities, to prevent debilitating fatigue or dyspnea. Organizing the household to conserve energy expenditure may also be necessary. Placing a commode by the bed or moving the client's bedroom to the first floor to minimize stair climbing may be helpful. Nighttime can be a real source of concern for clients. Some may fear choking to death in their sleep; others need to use their machines or cough frequently at night and may worry about disturbing their spouse. Depression or dyspnea may make sleep impossible.

Some clients may consider moving to a warmer, drier climate, hoping it will improve their condition. Clients with severe COPD may not tolerate altitudes above 4000 feet. For some clients with allergies or frequent respiratory infections, moving may result in some improvement. However, changing one's place of residence is always a stress and may be particularly so if it involves leaving behind a life-long home, cherished possessions, loved ones, and support systems. The nurse should help the client considering such a decision to explore the consequences and alternatives carefully. Before making a final decision, the client should make an extended visit of at least 3 months to the proposed area.

Coping with Psychosocial Stress. Progressive disability often necessitates early retirement and other role changes and losses. Plans and dreams of a vigorous retirement must be abandoned or modified. As a consequence, clients with COPD, like all clients who are chronically ill, undergo a grieving process. Disability brings fears about being a burden and results in a loss of self-esteem. Breathlessness and dyspnea limit the ability to participate in social events. Even quiet conversation can become fatiguing. These changes promote social isolation. The diagnosis of COPD is accompanied by a specific pattern of psychosocial adaptations. Depression, somatic concern, and conversion tendencies have been identified in hospitalized clients (Kimbel et al., 1971).

The nurse should encourage clients to verbalize their feelings in order to work through the grieving process and come to terms with their altered lifestyle. Joining an "emphysema club" or a similar group gives the client an opportunity to share feelings and problems. Encouraging the client to participate in exercise, recreational activities and hobbies where achievements can be realized helps to improve self-esteem.

As elderly clients with COPD become more disabled, they are forced to relinquish their role functions to other family members. In the aging family unit this is usually the spouse. The elderly client may have been forced to take an early retirement and may no longer be able to keep up the tasks previously performed in the household. As the client gives up these tasks, someone, usually the aging spouse, must fill the gap. Clients may also relinquish or modify other roles, such as companion and sex partner. Concomitantly, the spouse is expected to participate in the planning and implementation of the client's treatment regimen. These changes may cause conflict in family members, resulting in resentment, frustration, depression, or guilt.

The nurse should assess the past and present coping behaviors of the aging spouse and identify the willingness and ability to participate in the client's plan of care. Whenever possible, the spouse should be encouraged to be involved in the client's care but to avoid encouraging dependency in the client. The nurse plays a critical role in teaching and counseling the spouse about all aspects of the client's condition and treatment. If the spouse has a willing listener, subtle problems can be identified and dealt with before they compromise the spouse's level of adaptation.

Home Care

Because the elderly comprise a heterogeneous group, a variety of alternative resources must be available if their needs and preferences for long-term care are to be met. Institutional facilities, such as homes for the aged and nursing homes, are an important mechanism for the provision of long-term care (see Chapter 18). However, this mechanism does not meet the needs of all older people, many of whom would prefer to stay in their own homes as long as possible. Home health care is not intended to replace the hospital or the long-term care institution but rather to provide an alternative mechanism for delivering care and allowing older people who want to remain in the community to do so.

Home care consists of supportive health and social services provided in the home. These services encourage independence through preventive, supportive, and therapeutic interventions. Historically, nurses have been leaders in the delivery of home care to clients of all ages. Visiting nurses, public health nurses, and independent practitioners have been caring for clients in their homes since the advent of the first settlement house. The growth of home care programs in the United States was slow until the passage of Medicare, which provided some impetus for their development. Home care programs utilize family, community, and interdisciplinary professional resources, coordinating all of these to meet the client's unique needs. Nurses have assumed a major responsibility for the implementation of these services, administering programs, supervising personnel, coordinating services, and delivering direct care (Kahana and Kahana, 1976).

There is no single form of organization necessary to the establishment of an effective home care agency. Home care programs are organized under a variety of auspices: voluntary and public hospitals, visiting nurse associations, local health departments, rehabilitation centers, prepaid group practices, or a combination of these. Most are administered by health departments and visiting nurse associations (Kahana and Kahana, 1976). Proprietary home health agencies have also been formed in many cities.

Services offered may include provision of basic nursing and medical care, social services, physical therapy, occupational therapy, nutrition counseling, portable meals, supplies, equipment, transportation, homemakers, home health aides, drugs, and laboratory services. In reality, few home care services have full-time physicians on their health teams. This weakness is a major difficulty for such programs (Rossman, 1979). Perhaps nurse practitioners could fill this gap. In fact, nearly half of home care programs provide nursing and just one other service (Kahana and Kahana, 1976). The services may be provided by the administering agency itself or by an outside cooperating agency. Services vary widely from one program to another. They may be comprehensive, specialized, or limited, continuous or intermittent. This variation can be advantageous because the elderly vary widely in their needs.

In recent years, home care programs have expanded the types of services they deliver. Elderly clients who were previously excluded from home care programs because of the special nature of their problems are now being cared for. These include clients with terminal illnesses and cancer and those with illnesses such as emphysema and rheumatoid arthritis that require highly specialized treatments.

Nurses provide a range of services essential to the successful implementation of home care programs. Their first responsibility is a comprehensive assessment of the client and the home environment. These data are critical to determining whether or not home care is the best way to meet the client's needs. Some important questions are:

- How much assistance, if any, does the client need to perform activities of daily living? Personal care? Household activities? Marketing?
- How much nursing care does the client need? What level? How often?
- Does the client require medical visits? Special procedures? Specialized monitoring? How often?
- Are the home conditions appropriate for home care?
- What support systems are already available to the client? Family? Friends? Neighbors?
- What are the client's preferences?

The assessment data are used to identify what kinds of services the client needs. When planning a home care program, the nurse must be clear about the objectives of the program: prevention, maintenance of the status quo, support through decline or death, or rehabilitation. The decision to provide home care depends upon whether or not the kinds of services clients need are available. The elderly who might benefit from home care are a diverse group. Ideally, home care should provide services that are appropriate to the client's level of adaptation. The following types of services are important:

Preventive services for the elderly serve those who are functioning well in the community but who are at high risk to develop a problem. Early interventions that foster independence can help this group utilize and retain their capacities and may forestall institutionalization. The emphasis of preventive care should be on self-help. Some of the services that should be made available to clients include health assessment, care on an outpatient basis, dental services, health education, home safety, legal protection services, socialization, recreation, part-time employment, volunteer work, and educational opportunities.

Supportive services are aimed at helping the client with chronic, disabling physical and psychosocial adaptations to remain at home. Many of the clients in this group have multiple disabilities, are homebound, and could no longer remain at home without service. This group might need many of the following services: nursing care, homemaker, nutrition, transportation, handyman, legal, financial, religious, friendly visiting, telephone reassurance, recreation, information, and referral.

Rehabilitative services are aimed at the more acutely ill elderly, with or without chronic impairments. Services enable hospitalized older persons to shorten their hospital stays and avoid placement in long-term care institutions. Services also enable acutely ill elderly persons to remain in their homes and avoid hospitalization. Elderly clients in this group need many of the supportive services listed above. They might also need physical, occupational or other therapies, a home health aid, pharmaceutical and laboratory services, night sitters, and respite care.

Elderly clients require different levels of home care at different times. In addition, not all require lifetime or even lengthy care. In a year-long study of 420 home care recipients, the average length of stay was less than 2 months (Widmer et al., 1978).

Many elderly clients need only transitional services until they or their families learn how to perform care themselves. Still others require lengthy ongoing maintenance care.

Essential nursing responsibilities are setting goals, planning treatment, and evaluating care. The nurse also provides a range of direct services for the home care client, including ongoing assessment, health education, providing medically indicated treatments, and performing personal care.

When the older client lives with family members the home care program must consider their needs as well. The nurse assesses the family's capabilities and willingness to participate in home care. Family members who feel hesitant or anxious about caring for a loved one may appear indifferent or unwilling to do so. The nurse can help family members resolve these feelings by providing them with the teaching and support they need to feel confident about their role in the client's care.

Families may be able to provide limited care for the older client, but find 24-hour-a-day, 7-day-a-week care a burden. This is especially true with the trend toward both partners working. Although home care may be the treatment of choice for some older persons, it can be burdensome to family members who live with them, compromising the family's adaptation. Respite services are intended to provide support for these family members. They are important if the family is to remain involved in a client's care. Using day or night sitters is one way to provide relief for the family. Night sitters may be especially helpful when the client needs attention at night, as they allow family members an opportunity to rest. Another solution is to refer the client to a day care program for treatment or custodial care, with the client returning home at night. This service is extremely beneficial for working families or for families where caretakers need a brief respite. In some communities, arrangements can be made to have the older person check into a nursing home for weekends, holidays, or vacations to give the family a chance to rest.

Provision of home care involves a team of people who provide a network of needed services. Coordination and management of care is essential to the success of a home care program. Most often, the nurse serves as the coordinator of care (Widmer et al., 1978; Butler and Lewis, 1977). Another essential nursing role is supervision. Utilization patterns in home care programs indicate that most services are provided by paraprofessional workers, such as home health aides and homemakers. The nurse meets regularly with paraprofessional workers, particularly home health aides, to obtain data about the client and discuss the client's care. Since most paraprofessionals receive very brief training programs prior to their employment, the nurse provides ongoing education and careful supervision of workers to assure high quality of care.

Benefits of Home Care. Home care benefits not only the elderly, but families and communities as well. Most home care for older people is provided by their families. Although most families are willing to help an older member, they may seek institutionalization for the older client when the situation becomes too burdensome. If supports are available to help the family care for the client at home and to provide the family with opportunities for respite, families may be more willing to care for an older member at home.

National health care costs have continued to rise throughout the last two decades. Medicare provided an impetus for institutional care and these costs have comprised a major component of all health care costs. Home care is an effective way of reducing the costs of hospitalization by reducing hospital stays. Typically, the length of stay of a post-surgical client can be reduced by 30 to 50 percent. Home care programs can offer added benefits to homebound clients who have been discharged from the hospital by providing borrowed equipment and therapy that help the client maintain or improve skills learned in the hospital (Rossman, 1979). Nielson et al. (1972) found that when home health aid services were provided to the elderly after discharge from a rehabilitation facility, the need for rehospitalization significantly declined. Studies have indicated that the costs of home care also compare favorably with those of skilled nursing facilities and health-related facilities and that home care is at least as effective in meeting the client's needs (Colt et al., 1977; Peabody, 1977; Widmer et al., 1978).

Cost effectiveness is an argument frequently used to point out the desirability and feasibility of home care as an alternative form of long-term care,

but it should not divert attention from an important issue—some clients prefer it. This is a nation of homeowners, and the concept of home is deeply engrained in its older citizens. Sixty-seven percent of older people own their own homes and 85 percent, if given a choice, would prefer to spend their remaining years at home (Hennessey and Gorenberg, 1980). Estimates vary but the need for home care for the elderly is considerable. About 14 percent of Americans over age 65 and living at home are bedfast, homebound, or limited in mobility and require some form of help at home (Morris, 1974; Shanas et al., 1968). One study indicated that one out of every six older persons not in institutions needed some type of home care. In addition, about 25 percent of the elderly now in nursing homes might be able to manage in the community if sufficient support services were available to them (Pepper, 1976). These people are in institutions because the resources to maintain them at home were not available and not because they had major medical or nursing problems.

Limitations of Home Care Although home care might be a preferred alternative to institutionalization, a number of problems limit its effectiveness. First, home care is not available to all those who need it. The development of home care services has been slow and many smaller towns do not have home care programs of any kind. In those communities where home care programs do exist, development has been sporadic and has been guided more often by the goals of the sponsoring agencies or the perceptions of community leaders than by the results of a comprehensive needs assessment. Proprietary health agencies have been cited as a particular problem, often duplicating existing services in areas where they were available (Peabody, 1977). It is estimated that only 10 percent of the elderly who could benefit from home care services actually receive them (Kahana and Kahana, 1976). For a number of reasons, the elderly often do not qualify for home care programs. Reimbursement mechanisms are often so restrictive that the elderly who wish to take advantage of the services do not qualify for reimbursement and cannot afford to pay for the care out of their own pockets. In some instances, home care is reimbursed only if *skilled* nursing or medical care is required, only following a hospitalization, only when services rendered are physician supervised, or only for a prescribed number of visits. Some private insurance companies still do not reimburse for home care. In one study, where 80 percent of clients had Medicare coverage and 96 percent had some kind of third party coverage, only 25 percent of home care costs were covered by Medicare. In addition, one-third of all home care costs in this study were not reimbursed by any third-party payer (Widmer et al., 1978).

Another problem is that home care programs that emphasize preventive care for the well or nearly well elderly rarely exist. Those that do exist do not qualify for reimbursement by third-party payers. Eligibility requirements set by the programs themselves may further restrict their use. For example, many programs insist that the elderly client be living with a relative who is willing to assist with care.

Policies and practices of the federal government have limited the scope of home health care programs. After committing funds to home care following the passage of Medicare, the government made serious cutbacks in home care funding in the 1970s. In addition, the focus of Medicare is on coverage for short-term, acute conditions rather than for the more chronic conditions of the elderly. By 1984, the government still had not made a clear commitment to home care as an alternative form of long-term care for the elderly.

Finally, home care programs do not seek out those who might benefit from their services, but depend upon a referral system. This practice severely limits the possibility that these programs will reach those most in need. The homebound aged, who constitute at least 5 percent of those over age 65, are abandoned, ignored, hidden, and unable to call attention to themselves (Brickner, 1979).

SUMMARY

Elderly clients adapting at Level Three must learn to cope with lifelong stresses that precipitate long-term, progressively worsening adaptations. Three health problems—angina pectoris, peripheral vascular disease, and chronic obstructive pulmonary disease—that affect large numbers of elderly people were discussed. All are stresses that precipitate chronic oxygen deprivation. With appropriate in-tervention, clients with these health problems can learn to cope with or modify their adaptations and maintain an independent life-style.

The nurse plays an important role in helping older clients with chronic oxygen problems to set realistic goals, modify old patterns and practices, and accommodate new behaviors that promote optimal functioning in spite of oxygen deprivation. The nurse may teach clients to manage new medication and diet regimens, modify exercise patterns and sexual activities and use specialized equipment. Most older clients with chronic oxygen deprivation can manage successfully in the community, provided they want to do so and receive appropriate, supportive health and social services in the home. The nurse can expect that clients with chronic oxygen deprivation will experience exacerbations or complications that temporarily move them to lower levels of adaptation. For example, clients with chronic obstructive lung disease who develop infections, arrhythmias, peptic ulcers, and other stresses are no longer able to adapt successfully. They require temporary hospitalization and bedside nursing care to meet basic needs until the additional stresses have been resolved. Older clients with chronic oxygen deprivation usually cannot expect marked improvement in their level of adaptation, but, with appropriate support, they can maintain independence and quality of life.

REFERENCES

Akhtar AJ: Recent advances in respiratory diseases, in Anderson WF, Judge TG (eds), Geriatric Medicine. New York, Academic, 1974

Belt BG: Some organic causes of impotence. Medical Aspects of Human Sexuality 7(1):152, 1973

Bevil CA: Professional Nurse Behaviors Exhibited in Selected Aspects of Care of the Patient with a Cerebrovascular Accident. EdD dissertation, Teachers College, Columbia University, 1978

Bowarsky RE: Sexuality, in Steinberg U (ed), Cowdry's The Care of the Geriatric Patient, 5th ed. St. Louis, Mosby, 1976

Bowers LM, Cross RR, Lloyd FA: Sexual function and urologic disease in the elderly male. Journal of American Geriatrics Society XI(7):647, 1963

Brickner PW: Home Health Care for the Aged. New York, Appleton-Century-Crofts, 1979

Burnside IM: Sexuality and the older adult: Implications for nursing, in Burnside IM (ed), Sexuality and Aging. Ethel Percy Andrus Gerontology Center, University of Southern California, 1975

Burnside IM, Moehrlin BA: Health care in the confused elderly at home. Nursing Clinics of North America 15(2):391, 1980

Butler RN, Lewis MI: Aging and Mental Health, 2nd ed. St. Louis, Mosby, 1977

Caird FI, Dall JLC: The cardiovascular system, in Brocklehurst JC (ed), Textbook of Geriatric Medicine and Gerontology, 2nd ed. Edinburgh, Churchill Livingstone, 1978

Caird FI, Dall JLC, Kennedy RD: Cardiology in Old Age. New York, Plenum, 1976

Coakley D: Acute Geriatric Medicine. Littleton, MA, PSG Publishing, 1981

Coe RM: The geriatric patient in the community, in Steinberg FU (ed), Cowdry's The Care of the Geriatric Patient, 5th ed. St. Louis, Mosby, 1976

Colt AM, Anderson N, Scott HD, Zimmerman H: Home health care is good economics. Nursing Outlook 25(10):632, 1977

COPD Manual Committee of the Oregon Thoracic Society. Chronic Obstructive Pulmonary Disease: A Manual for Physicians. American Lung Association, 1973

Davies BH: Acute respiratory disease in the elderly, in Coakley D (ed), Acute Geriatric Medicine. Littleton, MA, PSG Publishing, 1981

Dobrowolski LA: Arteriosclerosis and atherosclerosis, in Orimo H, Shimada K, et al. (eds), Recent Advances in Gerontology. Amsterdam, Excerpta Medica, 1979

Elkowitz EB: Geriatric Medicine for the Primary Care Practitioner. New York, Springer, 1981

Escamilla R: Physical diseases which cause disturbances of sexual development and function. Medical Aspects of Human Sexuality 9(11):47, 1975

Exton-Smith AN, Overstall PW: Guidelines in Medicine. Volume 1—Geriatrics. Baltimore, University Park Press, 1979

Finkle AL, Moyers TG, Tobenken MI, Karg SJ: Sexual potency in aging males. Journal of American Medical Association 170(12):1391, 1959

Finkle AL, Prian D: Sexual potency in elderly men before and after prostatectomy. Journal of the American Medical Association 196(2):125, 1966

Freeman E: The respiratory system, in Brocklehurst JC (ed), Textbook of Geriatric Medicine and Gerontology, 2nd ed. Edinburgh, Churchill Livingstone, 1978

Friedeman JS: Sexuality in older persons: Implications for nursing practice. Nursing Forum XVIII(1):92, 1979

Gibbon M: Caseload over seventy-five. Canadian Nurse 75(3):20, 1979

Griggs W: Sex and the elderly. American Journal of Nursing 78(8):1352, 1978

Gosnell DJ: How available are health care services to the elderly? Journal of Gerontological Nursing 3(3):65, 1977

Gronim SS: Helping the client with unstable angina. American Journal of Nursing 78(10):1677, 1978

Haimovici H: The peripheral vascular system, in Rossman I (ed), Clinical Geriatrics, 2nd ed. Philadelphia, Lippincott, 1979

Harris R: Ischemic heart disease, in Reichel W (ed), Clinical Aspects of Aging. Baltimore, Williams and Wilkins, 1978

Hellerstein HK, Friedman EH: Sexual activity and the postcoronary patient. Archives of Internal Medicine 125:987, 1970

Hennessey MJ, Gorenberg B: The significance and impact of the home care of an older adult. Nursing Clinics of North America 15(2)351, 1980

Herndon CN: Medical genetics, in Steinberg FU (ed), Cowdry's The Care of the Geriatric Patient, 5th ed. St. Louis, Mosby, 1976

Jacobs MM, Bowers B: Protocol: Chronic obstructive lung disease. Nurse Practitioner 4(6):11, 1979

Kahana E, Kahana B: Special aspects of geriatric care, in Steinberg FU (ed), Cowdry's The Care of the Geriatric Patient, 5th ed. St. Louis, Mosby, 1976

Kimbel P, Kaplan AS, Alkalau I, Lester D: An in-hospital program for rehabilitation of patients with chronic obstructive pulmonary disease. Chest 60(2) (Suppl):65, 1971

King PA: Foot problems and asessment. Geriatric Nursing 1(5):182, 1980

Kleiger R: Cardiovascular disorders, in Steinberg FU (ed), Cowdry's The Care of the Geriatric Patient, 5th ed. St. Louis, Mosby, 1976

Kohn RR: Heart and cardiovascular system, in Finch C, Hayflick L (eds), Handbook of the Biology of Aging. New York, Van Nostrand Reinhold, 1977

Krizinofski MT: Human sexuality and nursing practice. Nursing Clinics of North America 8(4):673, 1973

Lawson R, Starr A: Cardiac surgery in the elderly, in Caird FI, Dall JLC, Kennedy RD (eds), Cardiology in Old Age. New York, Plenum, 1976

Lowe CR: Industrial bronchitis. British Medical Journal 1:463, 1969

Massie E, Rose E, Rupp J, Whelton R: Sudden death during coitus—Fact or fiction? Medical Aspects of Human Sexuality 3(6):22, 1969

Masters WH, Johnson VE: Human Sexual Response. Boston, Little, Brown, 1966

Masters WH, Johnson VE: Human sexual response: The aging female and the aging male, in Neugarten BL (ed), Middle Age and Aging. Chicago, University of Chicago Press, 1968

Masters WH, Johnson VE: Human Sexual Inadequacy. Boston, Little, Brown, 1970

Morris R: The development of parallel services for the elderly or disabled. Gerontologist 14(1):14–19, 1974

Motomiya M, Oizumi K, Ariji F, Konna K: Biochemical, histological and structural changes of the lung with aging, in Orimo H, Shimada K, et al. (eds), Recent Advances in Gerontology. Amsterdam, Excerpta Medica, 1979

Myers BA: Provisions of medical care for the aged, in Field M (ed), Depth and Extent of the Geriatric Problem. Springfield, IL, Charles C. Thomas, 1970

Naughton J: Effect of chronic illness in sexual performance. Medical Aspects of Human Sexuality 9(10):110, 1975

Nielson M, Blenknor M, et al: Older persons after hospitalization: A controlled study of home aide services. American Journal of Public Health 62(8):1094, 1972

O'Brien CL: Exploring geriatric day care: An alternative to institutionalization? Journal of Gerontological Nursing 3(5):26, 1977

Pathy MS: Clinical features of ischemic heart disease, in Caird FI, Dall JLC, Kennedy RD (eds), Cardiology in Old Age. New York, Plenum, 1976

Peabody SR: Implications for nursing service of major national health insurance proposals. Journal of Gerontological Nursing 3(2):37, 1977

Pepper C: New Perspectives in Health Care for Older Americans: Recommendations and Policy Directions of the Subcommittee on Long-Term Care. Washington, D.C., Government Printing Office, 1976

Petty TL: Chronic respiratory disease, in Steinberg FU (ed), Cowdry's The Care of the Geriatric Patient, 5th ed. St. Louis, Mosby, 1976

Pfeiffer E: Sexuality and aging, in Rossman I (ed), Clinical Geriatrics, 2nd ed. Philadelphia, Lippincott, 1979

Phillips HT: Public health aspects of geriatrics, in Field M (ed), Depth and Extent of the Geriatric Problem. Springfield, IL, Charles C. Thomas, 1970

Pierotte DL: Day health care for the elderly. American Journal of Nursing 25(8):519, 1977

Rorem R: The economics of health care, in Field M (ed), Depth and Extent of the Geriatric Problem. Springfield, IL, Charles C. Thomas, 1970

Rossman I: Environments of geriatric care, in Rossman I (ed), Clinical Geriatrics, 2nd ed. Philadelphia, Lippincott, 1979

Rossman I: Sexuality and aging: An internist's perspective, in Solnick RL (ed), Sexuality and Aging, revised ed. Los Angeles, University of Southern California Press, 1978

Sadoughi W, Leshner M, Fine HL: Sexual adjustment in a chronically ill and physically disabled population: A pilot study. Archives of Physical Medicine and Rehabilitation 52(7):311, 1971

Scheingold LD, Wagner NN: Sound Sex and the Aging Heart. New York, Human Sciences Press, 1974

Shanas E, Townsend P, et al: Old Age in Three Industrial Societies. New York, Atherton, 1968

Steffl BM: Sexuality and aging: Implications for nurses and other helping professionals, in Solnick RL (ed), Sexuality and Aging, revised ed. Los Angeles, University of Southern California Press, 1978

Trimble GX: The coital coronary. Medical Aspects of Human Sexuality 4(5):64, 1970

Tuttle WB, Cook LW, Fitch E: Sexual behavior in postmyocardial infarction patients. The American Journal of Cardiology 13(1):140, 1964

Villaverde MM, MacMillan CW: Ailments of Aging. New York, Van Nostrand Reinhold, 1980

Wedgewood J: Remediable heart disease, in Caird FI, Dall JLC, Kennedy RD (eds), Cardiology in Old Age. New York, Plenum, 1976

Weg RB: The physiology of sexuality in aging, in Solnick RL (ed), Sexuality and Aging, revised ed. Los Angeles, University of Southern California Press, 1978

Widmer G, Brill R, Schlosser A: Home health care: Services and cost. Nursing Outlook 26(8):488, 1978

Woods JA: Drug effects on human sexual behavior, in Woods NF (ed), Human Sexuality in Health and Illness, 2nd ed. St. Louis, Mosby, 1979

Woods NF, Miner HJ: Sexuality and chronic illness, in Woods NF (ed), Human Sexuality in Health and Illness, 2nd ed. St. Louis, Mosby, 1979

Wynne JW: Pulmonary disease in the elderly, in Rossman I (ed), Clinical Geriatrics, 2nd ed. Philadelphia, Lippincott, 1979

Yeaworth R: Political issues and health care to America's elderly citizens. Journal of Gerontological Nursing 4(2):38, 1978

15

Nursing the Client
Experiencing Reduced Mobility

SIGNIFICANT PROBLEMS

Stresses that alter mobility are particularly significant for the elderly because for many older people mobility is a prerequisite to their feelings of good health and well-being. This chapter explores the nursing care of older clients who are at Adaptation Level Three due to chronic alterations in mobility. Any stress that affects muscles, bones, joints, or the nervous system may stimulate adaptations that threaten mobility. This chapter discusses arthritis, Parkinson's disease, and osteoporosis, three stresses that affect the elderly more often than any other age group. Because these health problems are characterized by a progressively deteriorating course, many older clients eventually lose their independence and enter nursing homes, thereby moving to Adaptation Level Four.

An important area of nursing care for clients with impairments of mobility is to help them maintain their independence as long as possible. In particular, this chapter explores how the nurse can help clients manage pain and maintain regular activity programs. Although neither of these strategies halts the disease process, both can slow the process of disability and improve the older client's quality of life.

Arthritis

In the strict sense, arthritis refers to any inflammatory change in a joint. In actual practice, arthritis includes a wide range of conditions. This section discusses three of those conditions—rheumatoid arthritis, degenerative joint disease, and gouty arthritis. Each condition is a consequence of different stresses, but they all have adaptations in common.

Rheumatoid Arthritis. Rheumatoid arthritis is an extremely disabling systemic disorder that affects the synovial tissues lining tendons, bursa, and joints. Inflammation of synovial membranes occurs when immune complexes consisting of IgG and anti-IgG (rheumatoid factors) are deposited in synovial membranes and phagocytized by leukocytes. The resulting complexes activate complement and cause the release of lysosomal enzymes from leukocytes. Inflammation with edema, vascular congestion, fibrin exudate, cellular infiltrates, and an increase in synovial fluid results. The inflamed tissue hypertrophies and develops a swollen, edematous, red, thickened mass, called pannus. These extend over cartilage and tendons and burrow into bone. Eventually joints consist of naked bone and are painful and difficult to move. Muscles, tendons, and ligaments weaken. The end result is instability and subluxation of joints. Because rheumatoid arthritis is a systemic disease, damage may also occur to the heart, lungs, kidney, eyes, skin, and peripheral nerves (White, 1976).

The stresses responsible for the inflammatory response are unclear. The most widely held theory is that an immunological reaction is involved (Hahn, 1976). It has been postulated that a microorganism, possibly a virus, triggers the onset of rheumatoid arthritis by stimulating the development of antibodies that attack connective tissues as well as the invading microorganisms (Bonner, 1974). Because gold is an effective treatment for rheumatoid arthritis, another theory has proposed that the stress responsible for rheumatoid arthritis is the abnormal metabolism of trace metals.

Rheumatoid arthritis is a prevalent chronic disorder. Of the 3.6 million Americans who have rheumatoid arthritis, half are over age 50 (Kolodny and Klipper, 1976). It affects women twice as often as men (Calin, 1981; Bonner, 1974). Its onset may occur at any age. However, when rheumatoid arthritis manifests itself for the first time in old age, its effect is somewhat different from that in younger persons. Perhaps because older people have less efficient immunological systems, rheumatoid arthritis in the elderly has a particularly relentless and severe course.

Degenerative Joint Disease. Degenerative joint disease (osteoarthritis or osteoarthrosis) is a much less debilitating form of joint disease than rheumatoid arthritis. Controversy exists about whether this disease process is primarily degenerative or primarily inflammatory. Recent data indicate that degenerative joint disease has an inflammatory component that is due to the deposition of calcium hydroxyapatite crystals (Calin, 1981).

Degenerative joint disease affects the joint articular cartilage and subchondral bone. The joints most often affected are those subjected to the greatest stresses during a lifetime—the lumbar spine, knees, and hips. It begins as a silent deterioration of cartilage over many years. First, normal cartilage loses its elasticity, splits, and fragments. Eventually, thinning and denuding of cartilage occur. Simultaneously, there is sclerosis of subchondral bone, with thickening and narrowing of the joint spaces and formation of small, bony cysts. Eventually eburnation of subchondral bone occurs. This involves the formation of a layer of rough, thick, irregular bone. In addition, there is a reactive proliferation of new bone and cartilage at the periphery of joints and at sites of tendonous and ligamentous attachments. These characteristic bony spurs are called osteophytes. Because cartilage has no pain receptors, its relentless loss in degenerative joint

disease is not associated with pain. Eventually, pain develops when osteophytes irritate the periosteum or when joint distortion causes spasms of ligaments and muscles (Clark, 1976; Moskowitz, 1979). The synovial lining is not primarily involved in degenerative joint disease. However, secondarily it is thrown into thick folds and becomes fibrotic. Inflammation of synovial membranes (synovitis) can result when synovial membranes are pinched between bony ends and osteophytes.

The stresses responsible for this degenerative process are poorly understood. Primary degenerative joint disease is believed to be related to the aging process. A genetic predisposition may be associated with its development in some cases. Because there is no history of abnormal wear or trauma, damage to joints is believed to be caused by genetically transmitted biochemical abnormalities that impair cartilage metabolism (Pearson and Kotthoff, 1979). This has been considered an exaggerated reflection of the aging process (Grahame, 1978). Secondary degenerative joint disease is the result of any one or a combination of stresses—trauma or wear and tear to weight-bearing joints, endocrine disorders (acromegaly), infection, obesity, metabolic disorders, developmental defects, or rheumatoid arthritis.

Degenerative joint disease is the most common form of joint disease among the elderly (Steinberg, 1976). Its incidence shows a positive correlation with age. Unless trauma is involved, osteoarthritis rarely occurs in persons under age 40 (Bonner, 1974). Eighty percent of persons over age 60 have some signs of degenerative joint disease (Grahame, 1978). By age 70, those signs are universal (Moskowitz, 1979). Debilitating adaptations to degenerative joint disease occur in 25 percent of women and 15 percent of men over age 60.

Gout. Gout is a form of monoarticular arthritis that involves the formation of needlelike monosodium urate crystals that precipitate out of body fluids to deposit in joints, tendons, and bursae. This causes tender, inflamed joints, which, if not treated, may incapacitate the older person.

Gout may be episodic in middle age, but in old age it becomes chronic. As time passes, the attacks tend to recur with increasing frequency and involve an increasing number of joints (Agus, 1979; Hahn, 1976). Eventually, deformities develop. Gout affects men more often than women. The peak incidence is the fifth or sixth decade. In women the incidence of gout increases after menopause.

Genetic factors are believed to play a role in the development of gout. About 60 percent of clients with gout report a family history of gout. Although not all people with hyperuricemia develop gout and not all people with gout have hyperuricemia, there is a clear association between the two conditions. Monosodium urate crystals usually develop in an environment of hyperuricemia. Attacks of gout have also been associated with abrupt changes in the uric acid level (McCarty, 1979). Uric acid comes from dietary sources, the breakdown of nucleoproteins in body tissues, and direct synthesis from simpler compounds in the body, such as ammonia and carbon dioxide (Boykin, 1977).

Primary and Secondary Gout.   Gout has been divided into two types, according to the nature of the stress associated with its development. Primary gout is due to an unknown stress or to an inborn error of metabolism. The increased uric acid levels may result from an increased rate of purine biosynthesis, an underexcretion of uric acid, or both (McCarty, 1979; Bonner, 1974). In these individuals, a number of environmental stresses, including trauma, fatigue, cold, alcoholic beverages, foods high in purines, foreign proteins in the body, and surgery, have been known to precipitate an acute attack of gout (Anderson, 1976).

When the hyperuricemia is due to a known disorder, the result is secondary gout. Many stresses have been implicated in the development of secondary gout. Some diuretics, including the thiazides and ethacrynic acid, cause secondary gout because they interfere with the tubular secretion of urates or cause dehydration. Certain neoplastic diseases, such as lymphoma and leukemia, and hematological disorders, such as thalassemia, psoriasis, and pernicious anemia, increase purine turnover and result in secondary gout. Acidosis, whether due to alcohol ingestion, decompensated diabetes, regular ingestion of salicylates, starvation, renal failure, or any other factor, causes secondary gout by interfering with the tubular secretion of urates. Some other disorders, such as Paget's disease, and hypo- or

hyperparathyroidism are known to be associated with secondary gout, but the mechanisms responsible for its development are unclear. In both types, monosodium urate crystals are deposited in a joint and trigger an acute inflammatory response (Agus, 1979; McCarty, 1979).

Pseudogout.   Pseudogout is a form of inflammatory arthritis that is similar to gout in both its adaptations and its management. It involves the deposition of calcium pyrophosphate dihydrate crystals in the cartilage of joints and the synovial fluid, causing inflammation (Anderson, 1976). Older people with osteoarthritis, myxedema, and hyperparathyroidism are at high risk for the development of pseudogout (Bluhm et al., 1977). It occurs most often in persons over age 60; there is no sexual preference (Pearson and Kotthoff, 1979).

Osteoporosis

Osteoporosis is one of the major problems of our inactive older population. It results in cosmetic and functional disabilities. A progressive decline in bone density is a normal process in aging men and women. Therefore, a clear distinction between normal bone loss with age and osteoporosis is difficult. Osteoporosis refers to a reduction in bone mass below what is normal for the client's sex, age, and race. The chemical composition of bone remains unchanged. Bone demineralization in osteoporosis is so severe that it results in "crush" fractures, particularly of the vertebrae.

Incidence.   In the United States, 15 million people have osteoporosis. Clinical osteoporosis with its attendant fractures affects 25 percent of women over age 55 (Pont, 1981). Osteoporosis occurs five times more often in women than in men. Seventy percent of all fractures in women over age 45 are incurred by women with osteoporosis. The incidence of osteoporosis is lower in blacks and higher in whites, especially those originating from or living in northern Europe and in persons from China and Japan (Wallach, 1978; Gregerman and Bierman, 1981).

Stresses.   The adult skeleton is composed primarily of two types of lamellar bone: compact (cortical) and cancellous (trabecular). The adult skeleton contains 80 percent compact bone and 20 percent trabecular bone. Trabecular bone is fine and branching and makes up 90 percent of the skeletal surface. Different bones contain varying amounts of cortical and trabecular bone. The vertebrae, femur and tibia, for example, have large amounts of trabecular bone. As bone loss occurs with age, trabecular bone is lost more rapidly than cortical bone. Likewise, when this process is accelerated, as in osteoporosis, loss of bone is proportionately greater in trabecular bone. Once bone loss reaches a critical level—about one-half of trabecular bone—the client is at high risk to develop fractures as a consequence of only mild trauma (Gregerman and Bierman, 1981).

The primary process responsible for osteoporosis is poorly understood. In early adulthood, the skeleton is in a relative steady state and bone formation equals bone resorption. Then, some time after age 40 in women and age 50 in men, bone resorption exceeds bone formation and bone is lost, especially from the vertebrae, skull, femoral neck, midshaft of the femur and tibia, and metacarpals. Whether the decrease in bone is due to an increased rate of resorption, a decreased rate of formation, or both is controversial (Pont, 1981). In susceptible persons, the process of bone loss is excessive and osteoporosis results. Although its density is low, osteoporotic bone is normal chemically and microscopically.

Some individuals are more susceptible than others to the process of demineralization. The amount of bone in the skeleton at maturity varies with sex and race. Blacks have more than whites and men more than women. Factors including childhood nutrition, exercise patterns, general health, and endocrine function influence the amount of bone at maturity. Individuals with the lowest bone mass (particularly white women) are at highest risk for osteoporosis because they have less bone mass to begin with.

The stresses that stimulate the process of bone demineralization are unclear. However, it is clear that multiple, interrelated stresses are associated with the process of demineralization. No single stress appears sufficient to explain the bone loss of osteoporosis.

Hormones. Loss of estrogen may be the most important stress associated with osteoporosis. Research studies have indicated that length of time since menopause, not chronological age, correlates best with the development of osteoporosis in women. In addition, surgically induced menopause in women under age 45 is associated with the development of osteoporosis in 80 percent of cases (Gregerman and Bierman, 1981). Estrogen appears to decrease the sensitivity of bone to the demineralizing effects of parathyroid hormone (PTH). Evidently, when estrogen secretion in women ceases, PTH becomes more active. No increase in the amount of PTH in clients with osteoporosis has been demonstrated. Without the protection of estrogen, there is rapid bone loss, especially in the first 10 years after the menopause. Estrogen is also known to influence calcium absorption in the elderly; therefore, the absence of estrogen may adversely affect the older client's calcium balance. Although estrogen deficiency may be an important stress, it is not the only stress associated with the development of osteoporosis. Men, too, lose bone after age 50 but do not have an estrogen deficiency.

Calcitonin, a hormone secreted by the C cells of the thyroid, is known to inhibit bone resorption when administered in pharmacological doses. It has been suggested that calcitonin levels decrease with age, resulting in increased bone resorption. In fact, men have higher levels of calcitonin than women and a lower incidence of osteoporosis. More research is needed to support this theory (Pont, 1981).

Another theory proposes that hormonal changes, possibly involving an imbalance of anabolic hormones and corticosteroids, affect collagen synthesis or breakdown and result in osteoporosis by altering the collagenous matrix of bone (Kolodny and Klipper, 1976). The fact that clients with osteoporosis tend to have thin, wrinkled skin, compatible with a problem in collagen metabolism, is used to support this theory (Pont, 1981; Green, 1981).

Osteoporosis is a well-known consequence of Cushing's disease and of treatment with corticosteroids. However, hyperadrenocorticism is not believed to be an important factor in the development of osteoporosis among most elderly people (Exton-Smith, 1978).

Dietary Factors. Lifelong dietary patterns may play a role in the development of osteoporosis. Research into the relationship between calcium intake and osteoporosis has yielded conflicting data. Clients with osteoporosis do have a negative calcium balance. This may be the result of increased sensitivity of bone to PTH, or to a reduced calcium intake. It is known that the ability to absorb calcium from the intestines decreases with age. Concomitantly, many older people reduce the amount of calcium in their diet.

Vitamin D deficiency may be an indirect factor in the development of osteoporosis. The active vitamin D metabolite, 1,25 dihydroxyl vitamin D_3, is necessary for intestinal calcium absorption. Food contains 25 hydroxy vitamin D, an inactive precursor to vitamin D_3 that the body changes to vitamin D_3. One theory proposes that older people with osteoporosis undergo an age-related alteration in vitamin D metabolism and are unable to convert vitamin D from an inactive to an active form (Pont, 1981; Gregerman and Bierman, 1981). Another theory suggests that older people suffer from a vitamin D deficiency because they consume fewer vitamin D-enriched dairy products and, if homebound, have less exposure to the sun (Exton-Smith, 1978). In either case, a lack of vitamin D prevents calcium absorption and results in a negative calcium balance.

Deficiencies in ascorbic acid and protein, needed for the development of connective tissue, have also been suggested as stresses responsible for osteoporosis. There is little evidence that they are important factors in its development. An inadequate intake of trace elements that harden bone (strontium, vanadium, and molybdenum) may also be a factor in bone demineralization (Schroeder, 1976).

Research studies have demonstrated that women (but not men) living in high-fluoride areas have a lower incidence of osteoporosis than women in low-fluoride areas. Fluoride stimulates osteoblastic activity in humans. Evidently, it exerts a protective influence during the period of bone growth in childhood and may be an important factor in the prevention of osteoporosis in old age (Exton-Smith, 1978). It appears that a lack of fluoride plays a limited role in the development of osteoporosis, but more research is needed to clarify its role.

Other dietary factors may also be involved in the development of osteoporosis. These include the amount of phosphate and acid–ash foods in the diet. Pont (1981) suggested that when excessive acid is consumed, bone acts as a buffer and is resorbed to neutralize the acid.

Immobility.   Lifelong exercise patterns as well as the decline in activity that accompanies aging have been cited as factors in the development of osteoporosis. It is well known that osteoporosis can be induced by immobilization. If a limb is immobilized due to fracture, joint disease, hemiplegia, or splinting, localized osteoporosis results. When normal young people are placed on complete bed rest, they develop marked negative calcium balance. Many people become increasingly sedentary as they age. This may be a factor that affects the rapidity with which osteoporosis develops and initiates a vicious cycle of bone loss and immobility.

Other Stresses.   Osteoporosis is more common in light smokers than in nonsmokers. The causal relationship between smoking and osteoporosis, if any, is unknown (Pont, 1981).

There is also a high incidence of osteoporosis in clients with rheumatoid arthritis. The incidence is apparently unrelated to corticosteroid therapy. Alcoholism, diabetes mellitus, and COPD have also been associated with an increased incidence of osteoporosis. In all these cases the reasons for the relationship are unclear (Pont, 1981).

Parkinson's Disease

The significance of Parkinson's disease has increased with the extension of the average life span. It is the most common neurological disorder of aging and the third most common chronic disease. Parkinson's disease has an estimated prevalence of 100 to 150 per 100,000 population. Clients usually experience the first adaptations when they reach the sixth decade. The disease shows no preference for sex or race (Yahr, 1981; Burroughs, 1972).

The lesion responsible for Parkinson's disease is situated in the substantia nigra of the basal ganglia in the midbrain and consists of a degenerative loss of pigmented nerve cells. The structures primarily affected are the globus pallidus and corpus striatum. Secondary to the loss of nigral cells, clients have a deficiency of the neurotransmitter dopamine, a compound produced from the amino acid tyrosine and present in the basal ganglia. Studies of clients with Parkinson's disease have established a correlation between the degree of dopamine depletion and the extent of cell loss in the substantia nigra.

Dopamine, a precursor of norepinephrine, is of prime importance to the function of the extra-pyramidal system responsible for posture regulation, righting responses, and autonomic functions. Dopamine acts as an inhibitory substance on the nerve terminals of the striatum, and it balances the excitatory effects of acetylcholine at the neural junc-

TABLE 1. STRESSES, ADAPTATIONS, AND MANAGEMENT OF SECONDARY PARKINSONISM

Type	Stress	Distinguishing Adaptations	Management Principles
Postencephalitic	Its onset has been associated with a history of influenza. It is believed that a virus, other than the influenza virus, remains in the nervous system and eventually causes neurological changes.	Rigidity is more marked. Tremor is less prominent. Autonomic signs, such as profuse sweating and salivation are more prominent. Other distinctive adaptations include oculogyric crisis, impaired pupillary reactions, torsion dystonic posturing, respiratory dysrhythmias, and sleep, personality, and intellectual disorders.	Give L-dopa
Medications	Phenothiazine tranquilizers block dopamine receptors. Reserpine depletes catecholamine stores in the nervous system	Adaptations are temporary. They are believed to be related to the dose and duration of therapy.	Stop medication
Toxins	Carbon monoxide, manganese, mercury, and other toxins affect the basal ganglia.	No distinctive adaptations occur. Adaptations similar to those in idiopathic Parkinson's disease are seen.	Remove toxins Give L-dopa
Arteriosclerosis	Generalized cerebrovascular infarcts occur in area of basal ganglia.	Tremor is usually absent. Adaptations are usually localized with major disability in the lower limbs. Abnormal reflexes and cognitive changes not seen in idiopathic Parkinson's often occur.	Specific treatment

tion. Lack of inhibitory dopamine activity leads to unbridled excitatory acetylcholine activity and to multiple extrapyramidal changes.

The most common type of Parkinson's disease among the elderly is called idiopathic, or primary. The stress responsible for degeneration of the nigral cells in idiopathic disease remains a mystery. There are no data to support theories associated with genetics, viruses, or toxins. Although intriguing, the theory that idiopathic Parkinson's disease represents a premature aging process of dopamine-containing neurons has not been supported.

In secondary parkinsonism, which affects a small minority of clients, the stresses affecting the substantia nigra and the production of dopamine are known. These include encephalitis, medications, toxins, and arteriosclerosis. With some exceptions, the adaptations to secondary Parkinson's disease are identical to those of idiopathic Parkinson's. Table 1 lists the stresses associated with each type of secondary Parkinson's disease, adaptations that differentiate each type from idiopathic Parkinson's, and principles of management.

ASSESSING THE CLIENT'S ADAPTATIONS

Arthritis

Rheumatoid Arthritis and Degenerative Joint Disease. Table 2 describes the similarities and differences between adaptations to rheumatoid arthritis and degenerative joint disease. It is not uncommon for older clients to present with adaptations to rheumatoid arthritis that have been complicated by de-

---

TABLE 2. COMPARISON OF ADAPTATIONS: DEGENERATIVE JOINT DISEASE AND RHEUMATOID ARTHRITIS

Category	Degenerative Joint Disease	Rheumatoid Arthritis
Onset	Slow and insidious.	If it begins in old age, usually explosive with pain and many systemic adaptations. May be insidious.
Location	Most frequently occurs in weight-bearing joints, particularly lumbar and cervical spine, knees, hips, distal and proximal interphalangeal joints, first metacarpal joints, and first metatarsophalangeal joints.	Affects synovial joints, particularly proximal interphalangeal joints (often affected first), metacarpophalangeal joints, small joints of hands and feet, wrists, shoulders, elbows, ankles. Hips, cervical spine, and temporomandibular joints may also be affected.
	Occurs less often in shoulders, elbows, wrists, and metacarpophalangeal joints.	Unlike degenerative joint disease, distal interphalangeal joints are usually spared.
	Usually asymmetrical at first. Eventually, symmetrical involvement occurs.	Usually symmetrical.
Joints	Acute inflammation is *not* a characteristic adaptation, but may occur, particularly in the knees. When present, joints are swollen, tender, warm, and red.	Inflammation with symmetrical joint swelling, tenderness, warmth, and redness is characteristic.
	Joint stiffness occurs briefly, especially in the morning and disappears with joint activity (limbering up).	Morning stiffness lasts longer, from half an hour to several hours is characteristic. It is due to muscle

TABLE 2. (CONTINUED)

Category	Degenerative Joint Disease	Rheumatoid Arthritis
Joints (Continued)		atrophy, muscle weakness and joint involvment. Stiffness is a major complaint of clients with rheumatoid arthritis.
	Crepitation with movement may be felt or heard and is due to cartilage degeneration.	Crepitation is usually not noted.
	Joints are enlarged due to osteophyte formation and less often to synovitis and increased synovial fluid. Osteophytes may be palpated in joint margins. If they develop on the cervical spine they may cause vascular compression. If the vertebral–basilar artery is involved, the client may experience headache, visual disorders, ataxia, dizziness, and loss of leg strength.	Joints are enlarged due to soft tissue thickening or fluid, not to bony overgrowths.
	Heberden's nodes, if present, are usually multiple and appear in women. These are cartilaginous or bony outgrowths on the distal interphalangeal joints. They may be associated with flexion and lateral deviation of the distal phalanx. Although unsightly, they rarely interfere with motion. Bouchard's nodes may develop on the proximal interphalangeal joints.	Subcutaneous nodules develop, especially on elbows and forearms over tendon sheaths, bony prominences, and pressure areas in about 20% of clients.
	Contractures may develop, especially in weight-bearing joints. For example, the client holds the hip in external rotation with hip joints flexed and adducted. Late in the process joints become unstable due to loss of ROM and muscle strength. Occasionally, genu varum or valgum develop.	Eventually, deformities develop. These include: contractures of elbows, hips, and knees; in the hand, ulnar drift of the fingers, Swan neck deformity (distal interphalangeal flexion and proximal interphalangeal extension contracture), Boutonnière deformity (distal interphalangeal extension and proximal interphalangeal flexion contracture); genu varum and valgum, hallus valgus, and hammertoes. Joint instability may develop. Joint subluxation may occur especially in the wrists or in the spine at C_1–C_2, causing occipital headache pain radiating to the eye and neurological deficits.
Pain	May involve one or more joints.	Same as degenerative joint disease.
	In the early stages, pain is aching, intermittent, poorly localized, aggravated by activity, weight bearing,	Joint pain and tenderness are present in varying degrees. Pain is made worse by immobilization.

(Continued)

TABLE 2. (CONTINUED)

Category	Degenerative Joint Disease	Rheumatoid Arthritis
Pain (Continued)	and changes in temperature or humidity, and relieved by rest. Later, pain occurs with minimal joint use and even at rest. Severity of pain does not correlate with the degree of joint destruction.	
	Pain increases as the day progresses. The morning is the client's most comfortable time. Pain at night may occur with joint motion and awaken the client.	In contrast to degenerative joint disease, pain is greatest in the morning.
	Pain causes clients to splint joints to protect them.	Same as degenerative joint disease.
	Characteristics of pain vary with the joint involved. For example, pain due to spine involvement is often referred to the skin. With hip involvement, pain is felt in the outer aspect of the hip, groin, or inner thigh.	Characteristics of the pain vary with the joint involved. For example, when the hip is involved, pain occurs when walking and referred pain to the groin and knee occurs.
Muscle changes	Muscle shortening occurs if motion is consciously restricted to avoid pain.	Same as degenerative joint disease.
	Muscle wasting with loss of muscle strength occurs adjacent to affected joints. For example, if the knee is affected, quadriceps wasting occurs.	Same as degenerative joint disease.
Mobility	Reduced ROM in affected joints develops due to muscle spasm, loss of cartilage and osteophyte formation. For example, when knees are involved, clients have difficulty climbing stairs. If one hip is involved, gait is impaired. The client has a painful limp and difficulty climbing stairs, getting out of the bathtub, and arising from low chairs. With bilateral hip involvement, client has an awkward shuffling gait.	Contractures limit ROM in affected joints. For example, if elbows and wrists are involved, the client has difficulty feeding self. If shoulders are involved, the client has difficulty with abduction and rotation.
Radiographic findings	Narrowing of joint spaces, sclerosis of subchondral bone, bony hypertrophy of joint margins (osteophyte formation), characteristic lipping of bone, bony cysts, and deformity.	In early stages, demineralization around the involved joint, and soft tissue swelling. Later, erosion of marginal bone, loss of cartilage, bone deformity, and osteoporosis.
Laboratory testing	In general blood work is unremarkable but aids in ruling out other forms of arthritis.	Laboratory findings may aid in establishing the diagnosis.

TABLE 2. (CONTINUED)

Category	Degenerative Joint Disease	Rheumatoid Arthritis
Laboratory testing (Continued)	ESR—rarely increased.	ESR—Increased
	Rheumatoid factor—usually negative.	Rheumatoid factor—present in 80% of clients.
	CBC—normal.	CBC—mild anemia, usually normochromic or hypochromic, microcytic or normocytic.
	C-reactive protein—normal.	C-reactive protein—increased.
	Lupus erythematosus cell preparation—normal.	Lupus erythematosus cell preparation—elevated in up to 10%–20% of cases.
	Synovial fluid—low WBC, high viscosity.	Synovial fluid—high WBC, low viscosity.
Skin	No characteristic change.	Changes may occur resembling those seen in osteoporosis: skin becomes thinner with increased translucency, increased pigmentation, and easy bruisability.
Systemic involvement	None	Because it is a systemic disease, involvement of heart, lungs, vessels, kidneys, eyes, skin, and peripheral nerves may occur.
	None	Adaptations include fever, fatigue, malaise, poor appetite, weakness, weight loss, nutritional deficiencies, enlargment of spleen, enlargment of lymph glands, vasculitis of small and medium-sized vessels (telangiectasis, skin ulceration, digital gangrene and neuropathy), and changes in mucous membranes of eye.
	None	Folic acid deficiencies may occur and cause mental and neurological adaptations.
	None	Peripheral neuropathy may develop in the lower or upper limbs or digits and may involve motor or sensory deficits. It is usually asymmetrical. Sensory deficits compound the motor problems of arthritis. Neuropathy is believed to be a consequence of vasculitis and anemia.
Overall level of functioning	May progress slowly and need not severely incapacitate client.	May progress continuously and rapidly in older clients and may severely incapacitate clients.

generative joint disease. When these conditions are suspected, the nurse should focus on the adaptations that characterize arthritis and their effects on the client's ability to function. The initial assessment forms a base line against which later changes can be measured.

When taking the client's history, the nurse should pay particular attention to the client's complaints of pain and stiffness. These adaptations are associated with both rheumatoid arthritis and degenerative joint disease but they manifest themselves in different ways in each condition. The history also provides information about the onset of pain and stiffness and a picture of which joints are involved. If rheumatoid arthritis has been long-standing, the inflammation has usually subsided by old age, but the client has varying degrees of deformity. If the onset of rheumatoid arthritis was

recent, it is likely that joint inflammation will be apparent and the client will have more systemic adaptations and pain than younger clients.

The nurse should conduct a thorough musculoskeletal assessment. For each joint, active and passive range of motion should be measured and recorded and remeasured at regular intervals. Pain on motion should be noted. The nurse should observe and palpate each joint for swelling, tenderness, heat, redness, effusions, osteophyte formation, subluxation, and deformity. Hands and large weight-bearing joints deserve special attention. The small joints of the hands are usually the first place to show evidence of rheumatoid arthritis (Fig. 1), while the weight-bearing joints—hips, knees, spine, and distal interphalangeal joints—are most commonly involved in degenerative joint disease (Fig. 2). Palpation elicits joint tenderness early in the

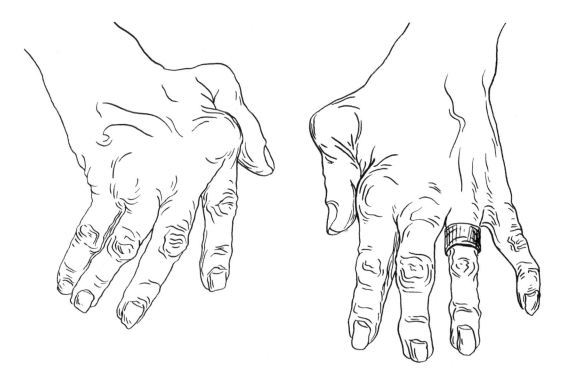

Figure 1. Adaptions to rheumatoid arthritis. Classic deformities of the rheumatoid hand pictured here include severe ulnar deviation on the right hand. On the left hand, note fifth finger with "swan-neck" deformity and third and fourth fingers with "boutonnière" deformity. On both hands, thumbs show "Z" deformity and index fingers show marked swelling.

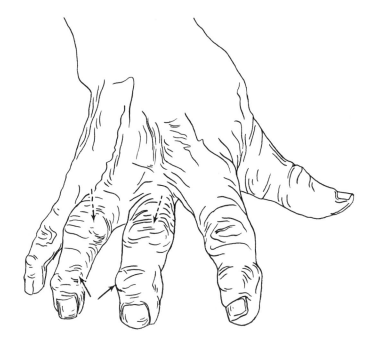

Figure 2. Most common in women, Heberden's nodes are enlargements of distal finger joints (solid arrows) that may cause lateral deviation of distal phalanges; they sometimes occur with Bouchard's nodes (dashed arrows), which involve proximal interphalangeal joints.

disease process, while joint deformities are later adaptations. The nurse should use a stethoscope to auscultate joints for crepitus, a coarse grating sound. Joint instability can be determined by moving the joint through all planes. Muscle size and strength should be assessed because of the likelihood of muscle wasting adjacent to involved joints. Loss of grip strength is a common finding when the hand is involved and affects the client's ability to perform ADLs. If lower extremities are involved the nurse should evaluate the client's gait, ability to climb stairs, and ability to get into and out of a chair. If severe deformities are present, it may be impossible to test muscle strength in adjacent areas. The nurse should also observe for characteristic subcutaneous nodules and skin changes indicative of rheumatoid arthritis.

Because musculoskeletal changes have important implications for the client's overall ability to function, the nurse should assess the client's activity patterns (pp. 303–307) and ability to perform activities of daily living. The nurse can obtain valuable information by making a home visit and observing a portion of the client's daily routine. This allows the nurse to assess the client's ability to carry out personal activities (toileting, feeding, bathing,

washing, dressing), domestic activities (cooking, cleaning, doing laundry), and other essential activities such as the ability to bend over, grasp, pinch, negotiate stairs, and use public transportation.

Elkowitz (1981) has identified four functional classes of arthritis:

1. Completely able to carry on all usual duties without handicap.
2. Able to perform normal activities despite handicap of discomfort or limited motion of one or more joints.
3. Limited to few or none of the duties pertaining to usual occupation or self-care.
4. Bedridden or confined to wheelchair; little or no self-care.

The nurse should also identify any systemic adaptations to rheumatoid arthritis. These have implications for the client's ability to function. Fatigue and malaise, associated with the inflammatory response, have a negative impact on the client's motivation to remain active. Anemia compounds fatigue and further reduces exercise tolerance. Anemia is the most common systemic manifestation of rheumatoid arthritis in the elderly and is almost universal in this age group (Grahame, 1978). The anemia may be a consequence of the inflammatory response, a defect in the ability of individuals with rheumatoid arthritis to transport iron to bone marrow, or gastric bleeding associated with aspirin treatment (Anderson, 1976; Hyams, 1978). The nurse should observe for the other systemic manifestations of rheumatoid arthritis (Table 2), but these are less likely to occur in the elderly.

The limited mobility, chronic pain and deformities associated with arthritis place the client at risk for alterations in body image and depression. The client's psychological adaptation to arthritis should be determined, using techniques described in Chapter 16. If the client has rheumatoid arthritis, emotional status is of particular concern because emotional upheavals have been associated with flareups of the condition in some clients. No particular personality pattern seems to be associated with this phenomenon (Williams, 1979).

If arthritis is suspected, the nurse should refer the client to a physician for diagnostic testing. This involves assessment of blood, synovial fluid, and radiographic findings. Laboratory findings in older people may be confusing. For example, many older people have an increased erythrocyte sedimentation rate in the absence of rheumatoid arthritis. About 15 percent of clients with rheumatoid arthritis are negative for rheumatoid factor, while about 30 percent of people over age 60 who do not have rheumatoid arthritis are seropositive for rheumatoid factor (Pearson and Kottoff, 1979; Calin, 1981). There are no laboratory tests available to confirm the diagnosis of degenerative joint disease. The x-ray is the most specific diagnostic procedure available (Williams, 1978). For these reasons, the detailed history and physical examination remain the most effective ways to assess arthritis.

Gout. Because its adaptations can be controlled with medication, there is no reason why any older person should be immobilized by gout. Consequently it is of paramount importance that the nurse makes an accurate assessment and refers the client for medical management.

Clients at risk for gout include those who are obese and those who overindulge in alcohol. Clients often relate a family history of gout, arthritis, tendonitis, bursitis, or kidney stones. About one-third of those with gout also have hypertension (McCarty, 1979). A history of typical, brief, acute attacks with relief of adaptations between attacks is indicative of gout (Brewerton, 1979).

Characteristically, gout affects the joints of the big toe, but in older people it may also affect the joints of the finger, hand, or wrist and less often the joint of the instep, ankle, knee, and elbow (Grahame, 1978). Before the acute attack, clients may note prodromal symptoms, including mood changes, diuresis, pruritis or discomfort in the affected joint. Clients usually complain of excruciating, throbbing pain in the joint. Often, the pain comes on suddenly. The pain is usually so severe that it is impossible to bear weight on the joint or bend it. The pain is aggravated by the slightest pressure, such as that of light bedcovers.

The nurse should assess the involved joint for tenderness, heat, and asymmetric swelling. The inflammation may be so severe that the skin appears dark red and peels off during the healing phase. The clients may have a mild fever. An acute attack lasts from a few days to 6 weeks, with the average length being 2 weeks. Clients recover whether or not they are treated (Bluhm et al., 1977). Gout is usually monoarticular; as one joint gets better, another gets worse.

Chronic or untreated gout is associated with the development of tophaceous deposits in the involved joints, elbows, and pinna of the ear. These collections of uric acid crystals take up to 10 years to develop and are found in 40 percent of clients. They are not associated with inflammation but may be disfiguring, interfere with motion in tendons and joints, cause neuropathies, or become infected. The tophi act as reservoirs for uric acid crystals for the initiation of acute gouty attacks. The nurse should palpate and illuminate the pinna of the ear. Tophi appear opaque when transilluminated, whereas cysts are translucent (Agus, 1979).

If a nurse suspects gout, the client should be referred to a physician who will perform laboratory and diagnostic tests. The most important laboratory test is the serum uric acid. A concentration higher than 7 mg/dl in females and 8 mg/dl in males indicates hyperuricemia and strongly suggests the diagnosis of gout (Hahn, 1979). However, this laboratory test must be interpreted with caution in older people having nonspecific joint pain because of the high incidence of diuretic-induced hyperuricemia which is not related to gout in the elderly (Calin, 1981). The physician may also order 24-hour urine tests to determine whether or not the excretion of uric acid is sufficient. Laboratory examination during the acute phase also shows the presence of leukocytosis.

The diagnosis can be confirmed only by arthrocentesis to aspirate synovial fluid or tissue. Using the polarized lens of the microscope, the unique needlelike crystals of monosodium urate can be identified. Often, synovial fluid tests are deferred and the diagnosis of gout is made on the basis of a triad of manifestations—monoarticular arthritis, hyperuricemia, and relief with medication. X-ray examination may also be performed. If gout is present, it shows asymmetrical soft tissue swelling and joint changes (Bluhm et al., 1977). In late stages, bony erosions and punched out areas on bones appear (Pearson and Kotthoff, 1979).

Osteoporosis

The History and Physical Examination. Identifying the client with osteoporosis may be difficult. Because osteoporosis develops slowly, effects exist on a continuum. Although some clients experience no negative effects, others are almost totally incapacitated. Some clients have no complaints, even when vertebral fractures are present. Others present with a variety of vague complaints such as easy fatigability, general weakness in the limbs, headache, a feeling of insecurity when walking, weight loss, and depression. At first, these complaints may cause the nurse to suspect a psychological rather than a physical problem. In fact, bone thinning alone does not produce adaptations in clients with osteoporosis. Most of the adaptations are related to fractures.

When taking the client's history, the nurse should obtain an accurate picture of the client's pain, if any. Localized back pain is a cardinal sign of osteoporosis. Usually, the pain is a constant, dull ache located on one or both sides of the midline of the lower thoracic or lumbar region. Clients may believe the pain is due to "rheumatism" or "old age." The pain is usually exacerbated by sitting, standing, or performing the Valsalva maneuver (sneezing, coughing). It is relieved by lying down.

Chronic back pain may be associated with sudden, serious exacerbations, which may or may not be related to trauma or muscle strain. The nurse should palpate the paravertebral muscles. Usually, chronic back pain is associated with muscle spasm.

Less often the pain associated with osteoporosis is sharp, spasmodic, and severe, with a sudden onset. It is located directly over a vertebral process and may radiate to the abdomen, anterior chest, buttocks, legs, and pelvis. It is aggravated by movement and relieved by rest. Pain of this nature is due to a vertebral fracture and develops immediately or several days after the fracture occurs. Radiographic examination will confirm the presence of spinal fracture. Usually this pain subsides gradually in 3 to 4 weeks. In between fractures, the client is often completely free of pain.

Pain often has serious consequences. It may cause the older client to restrict daily exercise and activities of daily living. Some clients may resort to bed rest because immobility relieves the pain. These practices are dangerous for clients with osteoporosis since generalized inactivity may be one of the factors that aggravates bone loss.

Because dietary habits throughout the life span have been associated with the development of osteoporosis, the nurse should take a dietary history. Many of our current older population lived through the depression years and suffered dietary deprivations that may place them at risk now for osteoporosis.

The history may also reveal a loss of height over months or years. This is due to vertebral fracture and vertebral compression. Many older people do not remember their maximum height. If this is the case, loss of height can be determined by comparing arm span to height. At maturity, these two measurements are about equal. A difference of up to 5 or 6 inches may be noted in clients with osteoporosis. The loss of height in the vertebrae can be demonstrated by subtracting the crown to pubis distance from the pubis to heel distance. A difference of several inches indicates osteoporosis.

The nurse should also question the client about a history of fractures and the circumstances surrounding them. Usually, fractures occur in the wrist (Colles' fracture), vertebrae (T_{12}, L_1), and hip. In clients with osteoporosis fractures may be related to minor trauma as well as excessive force. Older women with osteoporosis have been known to fracture vertebrae when sneezing while lying in bed, when attempting to force windows open, when stepping off a high curb and when sitting down too hard in a low chair. A client may fracture the femur when falling while exiting a bus and the radius when bracing a fall.

Fractures are important because they are usually accompanied by severe pain. Consequently, older clients are no longer able to dress, feed themselves, get to the toilet, or perform other essential ADLs. Fractures of the femoral neck may directly threaten life. Care of the client with a fracture is discussed in Chapter 19.

The physical examination should focus on changes in the client's skeleton, skin, gait, and range of motion. The nurse should take serial measurements of the client's height to assess the progression of osteoporosis. Lower dorsal kyphosis ("dowager's" or "widow's hump") with abdominal protrusion appears fairly early in the process of osteoporosis and is due to the wedging of midthoracic vertebrae. Loss of height together with the development of a hump on the back can be debilitating and depressing. These two manifestations are the most reliable clinical signs of the progression of the osteoporotic process (Avioli, 1976). They gradually lead to a downward angulation of the ribs and the iliac crest. Eventually, the client may complain that the iliac crest and ribs rub together. Once the costal margins abut the iliac crests, measurable reductions in height will cease. Changes in the vertebrae and ribs may cause a diminution in the vital capacity of the lungs and place the client at high risk if respiratory infection develops (Exton-Smith, 1978).

Accompanying the skeletal changes, a transverse band of keratinized skin and prominent skin creases appear over the upper abdomen. These result from the accordian-like folding of the torso. Osteoporosis is also associated with generalized skin changes. The skin appears prematurely aged, lax, wrinkled, thin, dry, and transparent. Underlying veins and tendons are visible. Transparent skin is especially noticeable on the backs of the hands and forearms (Hanna and MacMillan, 1978). Skin changes may be due to generalized, age-related changes or defects in collagen metabolism (Pont, 1981).

The client should be assessed for a shuffling, unsteady gait and a broad stance. When the osteoporotic process is severe, the anterior lumbar curve is lost, producing a posterior pelvic tilt, hamstring contractures, and characteristic gait changes.

The spine should be assessed for range of motion. If back pain is present, some immobility of the spine usually occurs. When the pain is severe, the immobility increases. When the client is pain free, spinal movement is usually normal, even if crush fractures and spinal deformity are present (Exton-Smith, 1978). Since nerve root compression is rare and spinal cord damage does not occur with osteoporosis, the client's reflexes should be normal.

If the nurse suspects the presence of osteoporosis, the client should be referred to a physician for diagnostic testing and treatment.

Diagnostic Data. The physician usually performs an extensive laboratory investigation to eliminate conditions that masquerade as osteoporosis and to detect stresses that lead to it. These conditions include osteomalacia, hyperparathyroidism, multiple myeloma, metastatic carcinoma, thyrotoxicosis, malabsorption, renal failure, and Cushing's syndrome. Laboratory test results in clients with age-related osteoporosis are generally unremarkable. Serum calcium, inorganic phosphorus, and alkaline phosphatase are normal in osteoporosis. Usually a moderate rise in serum alkaline phosphatase occurs following fractures (even small fractures) and remains elevated for several weeks. Urinary calcium excretion is usually normal or slightly elevated. Tests for endocrine function are also usually normal.

Unfortunately, there are no simple, uniformly accepted methods for measuring the mineral content of bone. In addition, there are no techniques in widespread use to measure early bone loss. As a general rule, clients with suspected osteoporosis undergo conventional radiographic studies of the spine and hips. This is a somewhat insensitive measure of bone loss, since 30 to 50 percent of the mineral content of bone must be lost before diminished radiographic density can be detected by the eye (Pont, 1981; Bonner, 1974). Consequently, radiographic examination is not useful for the early detection or prevention of osteoporosis. When increased translucency of bone is visible on x-ray, the trabecular bone of the spine is usually affected most. Characteristic changes occur in the vertebral bodies and discs. The femur, distal radius, and metacarpals may also show decreased radiographic density. X-ray films are useful in ruling out some but not all of the conditions with effects similar to osteoporosis. Bone scans may also be used to rule out other osteopenic states. Findings of a bone scan are normal in osteoporosis. The diagnosis of osteoporosis can be differentiated from similar conditions such as osteomalacia and established with certainty only by a bone biopsy, usually of the rib cage or iliac crest. However, this procedure is rarely done. Once the diagnosis has been determined, CT scanning or bone densitometry (using a photon absorptiometer) may be used to follow the client's progressive bone loss (Pont, 1981).

Parkinson's Disease

In 1817 James Parkinson wrote an essay meticulously describing the adaptations associated with Parkinson's disease. Since then, little has been added to knowledge of the clinical picture Parkinson described.

Classic Adaptations.   Parkinson's disease is characterized by a classic triad of adaptations: tremor, rigidity, and akinesia. These three adaptations, together with adaptations in balance, posture, and cranial and autonomic nerves, account for the characteristic changes in motor control, body movement, appearance, facial expression, speech, and functional abilities exhibited by the client with parkinsonism (Table 3).

A *tremor* is a series of involuntary rhythmic movements of a body part. Parkinsonian tremor occurs at rest, diminishing or disappearing upon movement or during sleep. It is a coarse tremor and occurs at a rate of 4 to 7 oscillations per second. The tremor usually affects the hands, especially the fingers, first. Eventually it may spread to the wrist, forearm, tongue, jaw, and lower limbs, especially the ankle. The tremor often begins on one side of the body, advancing later to both sides. The alternating contractions of opposing muscles is best seen as the characteristic "pill rolling" movement of the thumb and forefinger. Tremor is the most common and conspicuous adaptation to Parkinson's disease,

but it is the least disabling. Nevertheless, it may embarrass clients, contributing to their social withdrawal and depression.

Muscle rigidity, or resistance to passive movements, is an almost universal adaptation to parkinsonism. It may begin in only a few muscle groups, but as the disease progresses, rigidity spreads. Muscle rigidity is responsible for the client's complaints of muscle fatigue and loss of endurance. Rigidity is also believed to be related to the client's complaints of muscle aches and cramps and bone pain.

The muscle rigidity noted in parkinsonism may be of two types: cogwheel and plastic. Cogwheel, or fluctuating, rigidity reflects the effects of tremor. It does not contribute significantly to disability. Plastic, or lead-pipe, rigidity is much more disabling, contributing to the client's difficulty with voluntary motions.

Akinesia (or its related condition hypokinesia) is the loss or reduction in the capacity to initiate, maintain, and perform voluntary motor activities with ease and rapidity. Clients may not be able to initiate motions or may have a complete blocking ("freezing") of an ongoing movement. Akinesia is the most disabling of the adaptations associated with parkinsonism because it interferes with the most basic activities of daily living. Clients have difficulty buttoning buttons, tying knots, eating, and brushing the teeth. Akinesia, together with rigidity, is responsible for the slow, stiff movements, expressionless, masklike face, changes in posture, and gait disorders of the client. In walking, the feet look as if the client is standing in soft tar and cannot lift the feet from the ground. Akinesia also interferes with a variety of reflex motor activities, including periodic eye-blinking, arm-swinging while walking, and body-shifting when standing or sitting. These activities, once performed spontaneously, now require conscious and deliberate effort.

Balance and Posture.   As degeneration of the globus pallidus continues, balance may be impaired and righting reactions are lost. When parkinsonism is severe, clients may be unable to stand without assistance. Poor posture contributes to the loss of balance. Postural changes associated with parkinsonism are characterized by a forward displacement of the center of gravity, making it difficult to stand

TABLE 3. PARKINSON'S DISEASE: ASSESSMENT TECHNIQUES AND FINDINGS

Adaptation	Specific Observation	Assessment Technique
Tremor	Pill-rolling of thumb, forefinger. Extension and flexion of ankle. Tremor of wrist and forearm. Tremor of lips, tongue, jaw, causing slurred speech. Tremor is apparent at rest, particularly if client is upset or fatigued. It diminishes or disappears during activity and sleep.	Observe all extremities and face. Note tremor's rate, rhythm, distribution, relation to movement or rest. During conversation, assess speech and enunciation.
Rigidity	Cogwheel rigidity: alternating contraction and relaxation of the muscle being stretched. Plastic rigidity: constant, uniform resistance to the muscle being stretched.	Test ROM of large joints of upper and lower extremities. Ask client about presence of bone pain, muscle aches and cramps.
Akinesia (hypokinesia)	Gross movements slow and deliberate: Difficulty sitting up, turning in bed, rising from chair. Pauses for several seconds between instruction and action. Difficulty performing movements requiring fine muscle coordination: Difficulty with ADLs such as shaving, brushing teeth, buttoning buttons, tying knots, handling money. Writing may be smaller, illegible. Client may print rather than using script. Voice loses amplitude, develops a monotonous quality. Speech may be blocked or explosive. Gait disturbances include slowing, shortened stride, tendency to drag one or both heels, complete halts (freezing), rapid, propulsive steps (festination), difficulty turning, absence of arm-swinging. Face lacks expression or rarely changes expression. Eyes may stare. Blinking is infrequent. Facial muscles are smooth.	Observe general speed and quality of movement. Note parts of body where movement is slow and deliberate, shows hesitation on initiating movement, or shows arrest of an ongoing movement. Assess fine movements. Ask client to tap thumb to each finger in rapid succession for 20 seconds. Observe both hands for ability and speed. Assess alternating movements. Ask client to tap knee alternately with palm and back of hand for speed. Ask client to write one or two sentences and observe size of letters, legibility, and use of script or print. During conversation, assess spech patterns. Observe client walking up and down hall and turning. Note a burst of short shuffling steps as client turns. Observe facial expression and changes as topic of conversation and client's mood change.
Balance and posture	May sway while standing. May fall spontaneously. Loss of righting reaction during fall. Appears immobilized in an anteriorly shifted overhanging position (Simian posture). Head is bowed, trunk bent forward,	Test for Romberg sign. Be prepared to support client. If Romberg sign is negative, gently push client on sternum. Note tendency to fall into festinating gait to avoid falling. Be prepared to support client.

TABLE 3. (CONTINUED)

Adaptation	Specific Observation	Assessment Technique
Balance and posture (Continued)	shoulders drooped, elbows, hips, and knees flexed, hands held in front of body at or above waist. Postural changes result in diminished height. Difficulty standing erect without toppling. If trunk rigidity is asymmetrical, a scoliosis may develop.	Observe client's posture.
Autonomic function	Orthostatic hypotension.	Take blood pressure while client sits and stands. Ask about a history of falls.
	Urinary disturbances.	Ask about difficulty starting urinary stream, hesitation, dribbling, frequency, burning or pain.
	Increased salivation, drooling.	Observe for pooled saliva in mouth. Ask about history of drooling in bed at night.
	Seborrhea.	Observe forehead, lid margins, crevices of ears and nose, lower scalp for crusty, greasy scales, dermatitis, erythema.
	Increased perspiration. Heat intolerance.	Observe skin for moisture. Ask client about tolerance to temperature changes.
Cranial nerve changes	Changes in blinking. Difficulty chewing and swallowing.	Tapping of the client's forehead may produce rapid uncontrolled blinking. Determine if client has history of choking when swallowing food or water. Ask client if swallowing is difficult.
Cognitive and emotional function	Emotional and personality changes. Dementia may increase in severity as other adaptations progress.	Assess orientation, memory and mood. See Chapter 7 for mental status and emotional assessments.

erect without toppling. Body posture is characterized by flexion of the trunk, neck, elbows, hips, and knees.

Autonomic Functions. Changes in autonomic functions are frequent, but they vary widely from one client to another. Drooling, a common problem, may be due to increased saliva production associated with autonomic changes. Other factors that contribute to drooling include akinesia and muscle

weakness, with a concomitant inability to handle secretions and the forward flow of secretions that occurs with the postural changes of parkinsonism. Autonomic changes are also responsible for the oily forehead (seborrhea) of many clients with parkinsonism. A potential stress with seborrhea is infection of the eye or lid. Changes in bladder function are associated with autonomic dysfunction and exacerbated by the immobility and inadequate hydration of clients with parkinsonism. Consequently, these clients have a high incidence of urinary tract infections (Langan, 1976). Orthostatic hypotension is a particularly important consequence of autonomic changes because it accounts for a significant proportion of falls in clients with Parkinson's disease (Pathy, 1978). Constipation is a frequent problem for these clients and is due not only to autonomic changes but to the sedentary life-style that accompanies the disease. The client may also experience increased perspiration and an intolerance to heat, due to flushing.

Cranial Nerve Changes. Impairment of the ocular, facial and oropharyngeal nerves may occur. These contribute to the characteristic changes in facial expression, eye movement, blinking and voice associated with parkinsonism (Steinberg, 1976). Cranial nerve changes are also responsible for dysphagia. The client may complain of difficulty chewing or swallowing solids or liquids. Poor muscle tone exacerbates this problem. Dysphagia is of particular concern, not only because it may result in aspiration pneumonia, but because it contributes to chronic problems with hydration and nutrition. Cranial nerve dysfunctions are also responsible for changes in the convergence of the eyes and in blinking and for oculogyric crisis.

Cognitive and Emotional Changes. The cognitive and emotional consequences of parkinsonism are still controversial. Some authorities believe there are no direct intellectual changes associated with parkinsonism (Davis, 1977; Langan, 1976). These authorities believe emotional changes such as depression and frustration are a response to the stress of chronic disability. They believe confusion and intellectual deterioration are secondary to a variety of organic stresses, such as arteriosclerosis, medications, and the aging process. Other authorities believe dementia is an intrinsic characteristic of parkinsonism and increases in severity as the disease progresses. Impairments of recent memory, calculation ability, and ability to use new concepts have been noted in clients with parkinsonism (Sweet, 1975; Sweet and McDowell, 1975). Clients with severe akinesia are particularly likely to develop cognitive defects (Yahr, 1981; Palkovitz, 1978).

The clinical course of Parkinson's disease varies widely from one client to another. Normally, adaptations begin so insidiously that clients cannot remember when they first noticed changes. They usually begin unilaterally and eventually become bilateral, progressing slowly but steadily until eventually they become a stress that immobilizes the client.

In advanced parkinsonism, the clinical adaptations are unmistakable and diagnosis is straightforward. The classic triad—tremor, rigidity, and akinesia—have diagnostic significance. However, in its early stages, parkinsonism can be mistaken for normal aging or for a variety of disorders, with adaptations similar to parkinsonism. These include involutional depression, senile dementia, thyroid and parathyroid disorders, essential (familial) tremor, and disorders of the basal ganglia such as drug intoxication and tumors.

Assessment Techniques. The most important tools for assessing the client with parkinsonism are the comprehensive history and knowledgeable observation. The key to accurate assessment is the skilled interview. A detailed history of the client's ADL pattern and recent changes in that pattern is especially useful. The neurological component of the physical examination also provides important information. While sensory status and deep tendon reflexes are usually normal, many other neurological signs are abnormal. Table 3 identifies assessment techniques useful in eliciting the adaptations associated with Parkinson's disease.

No reliable laboratory tests or x-ray or electrodiagnostic procedures have been developed to confirm the presence of Parkinson's disease. Clients being assessed for parkinsonism are given the usual laboratory tests to assess overall health. Blood chemistries are done to rule out other stresses such as thyroid and parathyroid dysfunction. If drug therapy is being considered, studies of cardiac, liver, and kidney function are done to assure that the pathways for drug metabolism and excretion are intact.

Detection of Early Parkinsonism. Although the early adaptations to parkinsonism are not diagnostic their detection can lead to early diagnosis and treatment. The early adaptations to parkinsonism are usually so subtle that clients do not report them unless they are brought to their attention by specific questions. Consequently, careful history taking is essential if Parkinson's disease is to be detected before adaptations are full blown. Involving a spouse, relative, or close friend in the interview can be helpful because clients are usually not aware of all the subtle changes in their own behavior. For example, a relative may be more likely to notice that the client smiles less often or no longer swings one or both arms while walking.

Specific questions, likely to elicit information about the early changes of parkinsonism include:

- Have you slowed down a bit in the last year or two?
- Does it take you longer to do routine housework?
- Is knitting or mending more difficult?
- Is letter writing more difficult?
- Does it take you longer to dress in the morning?
- Do you have trouble buttoning your collar? Tying your shoes? Getting your arm into the second sleeve of your jacket?
- Do you often cut yourself while shaving?
- Do friends ask you why you don't smile any more or look depressed?
- Do you have a feeling of weakness in an arm or leg?
- Do you tire easily?
- Do you have neck or shoulder pain? (probably due to loss of arm swing)
- Is your gait unsteady?

During the physical examination, the nurse should look for the earliest signs of Parkinson's disease. These include:

- Marked slowing of body movements
- Reduced facility in movement
- Disturbances of balance
- Disturbances of posture
- Changes in facial expression

Clients sensing a subtle deterioration of function may show feelings of tremulousness or reactive depression with accompanying psychomotor retardation.

NURSING INTERVENTIONS

Arthritis

Rheumatoid Arthritis. Because the stresses associated with rheumatoid arthritis are not fully understood, management of the client is aimed at the adaptations. The specific treatment program varies somewhat according to the stage of the disease. In any case, it is rigorous and comprehensive and involves a combination of elements: emotional support, education, medications, an activity program, modification of ADLs, and, in some instances, surgery.

The goals of treatment include the following:

- Fostering adjustment to chronic disease
- Educating the client about the disease and its management
- Minimizing pain, stiffness, and, if present, inflammation
- Arresting and/or reversing functional losses
- Preserving as much function as possible
- Preventing crippling deformities

Convincing clients to obtain or continue with appropriate treatment is an important nursing action. Often the nurse identifies victims of arthritis who have been treating themselves or have ignored their adaptations for years. Such clients often suffer needless, irreversible joint damage. Older clients with rheumatoid arthritis are particularly vulnerable to quackery. Not only is little known about rheumatoid arthritis, but it is characterized by spontaneous remissions. It is not surprising that when faced with a severe and crippling chronic disease, many clients become depressed, desperate, and ready to resort to quack remedies. In such cases, innumerable methods of treatment, all unproven, are readily available.

The nurse's educative and supportive roles with the client are important contributions to client care. The client's compliance is critical if the treatment program is to succeed. Education about the disease process and the goals and elements of the treatment program helps the client to adhere to the program. Clients need to understand that they cannot expect a cure but that much can be done to make them comfortable and minimize functional loss.

When clients learn their diagnosis, they need psychological support. Older clients living alone or with friends or family are conscious of their vulnerability. They may perceive their actual or impending loss of function as a calamity. It is true that rheumatoid arthritis is a painful and crippling disease and there are no answers for clients who ask *why* they have been affected. Nevertheless, the nurse should allay clients' fears and reassure them that crippling deformities may not occur. In fact, only 10 to 15 percent of older clients with rheumatoid arthritis are severely disabled (White, 1976). Most clients can manage their disease and their treatment program. Nursing interventions should be aimed at helping clients maintain self-confidence and self-respect as they learn to do so. The nurse can also serve as a sympathetic and caring listener as clients begin to cope emotionally as well as physically with limited function and pain, and learn to readjust their life-style.

Medication Therapy. Medications are an integral part of the treatment program at every stage of the disease (Table 4). No matter which drugs are ordered, clients should take them as prescribed. The nurse should advise clients not to stop the drug or reduce the dosage when they feel better. If clients take the medication irregularly or at less than optimal doses, the dosage may be enough to suppress pain but not the joint-damaging inflammation. When a new drug is prescribed, clients should be advised to be patient since improvement may not be noted for weeks or months. The nurse should gather data of therapeutic effectiveness by monitoring reductions in pain, stiffness, and swelling of affected joints, improved mobility and grip strength and reduction of sedimentation rate. Many medications for arthritis are more toxic in older people than young ones and associated with characteristic side effects. Because many of these side effects are significant, clients should know of their possibility and be advised to report them to the physician. Medications used to treat rheumatoid arthritis and nursing implications are summarized in Table 5.

Despite their hazards, salicylates remain the first choice for rheumatoid arthritis. Clients may feel that aspirin is such a common drug it could not possibly work. However, older clients with mild

---

TABLE 4.   RELATION OF MEDICATIONS TO OTHER ELEMENTS OF RHEUMATOID ARTHRITIS TREATMENT PROGRAM

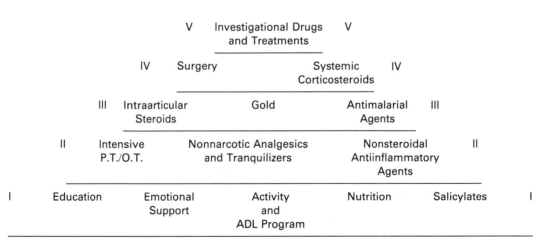

Medications are related to other elements of the treatment program for rheumatoid arthritis from Stage I (mild adaptations) to Stage V (severe disability). If medications at the first stage are not effective, those at the next stage will be tried.

TABLE 5. MEDICATIONS COMMONLY USED FOR RHEUMATOID ARTHRITIS

Drug Group	Action	Nursing Implications
Salicylates		
Aspirin	Reduce inflammation. Provide analgesia.	Adverse effects are more common with the elderly and include dyspepsia, gastrointestinal bleeding, peptic ulcer, tinnitus, hearing loss, headache, dizziness, irritability, mental confusion, bleeding tendencies. Salicylate intoxication is most likely when renal function is poor. Teach client to check for black tarry stools, petichiae, and ecchymoses. Check for tinnitus, which may be insidious in the elderly. Check client's hearing regularly against watch. Advise client to take aspirin simultaneously with food, large amounts of water, or antacids to reduce gastric irritation. Potentiate the anticoagulant effect. Do not give to clients receiving warfarin or dicoumarol. Advise client to purchase lowest cost product.
Nonnarcotic Analgesics		
Acetaminophen (Tylenol)	Relieve mild and moderate pain.	Side effects are rare when recommended dose is used, and include blood dyscrasias, hepatic and renal damage, and psychological changes. Advise clients on long-term therapy to have hepatic, renal, and blood functions monitored regularly.
Dextropropoxyphene hydrochloride (Darvon)		Adverse reactions include tremulousness, restlessness, euphoria, dizziness, lightheadedness, drowsiness, headache, nausea, and vomiting. If adverse effects occur, advise client to lie down. Institute safety precautions.
Tranquilizers and Muscle Relaxants		
Diazepam (Valium) Meprobamate (Equinil)	Reduce anxiety and consequently muscle tightness and pain due to muscle spasm.	Side effects that are more common in the elderly include drowsiness, confusion, ataxia, constipation, and urinary retention.

(Continued)

TABLE 5. (CONTINUED)

Drug Group	Action	Nursing Implications
Tranquilizers and Muscle Relaxants (Continued)		If necessary, supervise ambulation or institute safety precautions. Warn client to avoid use of alcohol. Advise client to have periodic CBC and liver function tests.
Nonsteroidal Antiinflammatory Agents		
Pyrazolones: Phenylbutazone (Azolid, Butazolidin) Oxyphenbutazone (Tandearil)	Reduce inflammation during short-term flare-ups.	Should be used cautiously in older people because of the increased incidence of side effects. These agents reduce the GFR, causing an increased accumulation of drug and side effects. Side effects include elevated BUN, bone marrow depression (most common in the elderly), gastrointestinal distress or bleeding, peptic ulcers, liver dysfunction, skin rash, mouth ulcers, hematuria, fever, sore throat, tachycardia, fluid retention causing cardiac failure, visual disturbances, and dizziness. These agents also potentiate the action of coumarin anticoagulants. Institute safety precautions if CNS effects develop. Advise client to take with milk or meals to reduce gastrointestinal distress. Instruct client to take daily weight, observe for black tarry stools and notify physician if weight gain, tarry stools, sore mouth, bruising, rash, fever, sore throat, blurred vision, or jaundice develop. Advise client to have CBC and urinalysis checked frequently. Contraindicated if client has a history of peptic ulcer, heart failure, hypertension or blood dyscrasias.
Indole derivatives: Indomethacin (Indocin) Tolmetin (Tolectin)	Reduce inflammation during brief, subacute exacerbations. Reduce fever, stiffness, pain, swelling, and tenderness.	Used sparingly in the elderly because of increased incidence of side effects. Side effects include aplastic anemia, elevated BUN, peptic ulcer, gastrointestinal bleeding, fluid retention causing cardiac failure, hematuria, allergic rash, nausea, vomiting, diarrhea, depression, anxiety, and confusion.

Drug	Action	Nursing Considerations
Propionic acid derivatives: Ibuprofen (Motrin) Naproxen (Naprosyn) Fenoprofen calcium (Nalfon)	Believed to inhibit formation or release of certain prostaglandins found in great quantity in inflamed rheumatic joints, thus reducing swelling, stiffness, and pain.	Teach client to monitor weight, observe for edema and tarry stools, and notify physician if weight gain, bruising, or tarry stools develop. Caution client to avoid aspirin-containing products. Advise client to have CBC and urinalysis checked regularly. Observe client closely for CNS effects, which are easily overlooked in the elderly. Advise client to take with meals or antacids to reduce gastric distress. Contraindicated in clients with peptic ulcer, colitis, or diverticulitis. Side effects include dyspepsia, gastrointestinal bleeding, transient headache, dizziness, drowsiness, rash, visual changes, tinnitus, sodium retention, and edema. Teach client to identify black tarry stools, weight gain, skin rash, and report these as well as blurred vision and headache to physician. If dizziness or drowsiness occur, institute safety precautions. Advise client to have periodic eye examinations. Advise client to take with milk or on a full stomach to lessen the possibility of gastrointestinal distress. Contraindicated in clients with a history of peptic ulcer and asthma.
Gold Salts Gold sodium thiomalate (Myochrysine) Aurothioglucose (Solganal)	Provide long-term suppression of joint inflammation by an unknown action. May arrest or slow the disease process.	Used with caution in the elderly because of an increased incidence of toxic effects. Toxicity may occur to gold or the medium in which it is suspended. Reactions to the media include flushing, weakness, dizziness, palpitations, and urticaria. The most dangerous signs of toxicity to gold include bone marrow suppression, causing aplastic anemia, pruritic rashes (the most common), and stomatitis with metallic taste.

(Continued)

TABLE 5. (CONTINUED)

Drug Group	Action	Nursing Implications
Gold Salts (Continued)		Other adverse effects include kidney damage with proteinuria and hematuria, pulmonary edema, asthma, cardiovascular collapse, hepatitis, peripheral neuritis, visual problems, vomiting, diarrhea, giddiness, and headache. Advise client to have urine and feces monitored regularly for proteinuria and leukopenia. Observe for side effects with special care during first 6 months of treatment when most side effects appear.
Antimalarials		
Chloroquine phosphate (Aralen) Hydroxychloroquine (Plaquenil)	Effectively reduce inflammation by an unknown mechanism for short periods of time. Effectiveness declines with long-term use. May be used in combination with aspirin.	Used with caution in older people because of the increased incidence of undesirable effects. Side effects include blood dyscrasias, nausea, vomiting, abdominal cramps, weight loss, alopecia, change in hair color, photosensitivity, dermatologic lesions, anorexia, nausea, weakness, irreversible pigmentary changes of the retina, and reversible corneal lesions that impair vision. Assess client's vision regularly. Advise client to have ophthalmologic examination every 6 months. Warn client that hyperpigmentation of the skin may occur if exposed to the sun.
Intraarticular Steroids		
Hydrocortisone, methylprednisolone acetate	Local antiinflammatory and analgesic actions.	Because injections mask joint pain, advise client not to overuse joint or weight bear until physician advises. Then assist client with posttreatment exercises. Systemic effects are rare. Observe client for joint infection, the major complication.

Systemic Corticosteroids

Prednisolone, Prednisone	Suppress the inflammatory response. May be given with aspirin.	Side effects include osteoporosis with fractures, necrosis of bone, gastrointestinal bleeding, peptic ulcer, fragility and easy bruising of skin, hirsutism, moon face, acne, hyperglycemia, hypertension, sodium retention, cataracts, glaucoma, increased susceptibility to infection, and emotional changes. If possible, give in one morning dose to minimize suppression of pituitary–adrenal axis. Take with food to reduce gastric irritation. Advise client to be fastidious about personal hygiene and give special attention to the skin. Advise client to have regular eye examinations and to monitor weight.

Investigational Drugs

Penicillamine (D-penicillamine)	In client who can tolerate it, effectively reduces inflammation by an unknown mechanism, possibly related to the inhibition of collagen formation.	Rarely used in the elderly because of high incidence of side effects. Side effects include bone marrow depression, severe renal damage with proteinuria, hepatic dysfunction, changes in taste and smell, peripheral motor instability, optic neuritis, rashes, bleeding into the skin, friable skin, gastric distress, and vitamin B_6 deficiency. Administer on an empty stomach. Advise client to check skin for bruising or other changes.
Cytotoxic and immuno-suppressive agents: Cyclophosphamide (Cytoxin) 6-Mercaptopurine	May exert their antiinflammatory action by affecting circulating or cellular immune reactions.	Side effects include bone marrow suppression, alopecia, sterility, nausea, diarrhea, and hemorrhagic cystitis.
Azathioprine (Imuran)		Side effects include herpes zoster, increased incidence of malignant changes, bone marrow depression, nausea, diarrhea, and liver damage (increased serum transaminase).

rheumatoid arthritis often respond well to a regimen of aspirin and a comprehensive activity program. To obtain optimum antiinflammatory effects, a salicylate blood level of 15 to 30 mg/dl must be achieved. The dose required to reach this level varies widely from one client to another, and may range from 1600 to 4800 mg/day taken in four divided doses. Because analgesia is achieved with much lower doses, clients must understand that the prescribed dose is necessary if inflammation as well as pain is to be reduced. In younger clients with rheumatoid arthritis, the optimal dose is usually achieved by increasing the dose to toxicity, defined as "tinnitus," and then reducing it slightly. A special problem exists when this practice is used with the elderly, since adequate inner ear function is required to perceive tinnitus. If the client's inner ear function is poor, the client may not hear tinnitus. Therefore, toxicity may not be noted and may continue and destroy the vestibular apparatus, resulting in vertigo and loss of balance (Calin, 1981). The nurse should advise clients who are to begin aspirin therapy to obtain a base line audiogram before beginning the medication and to have regular follow-up hearing tests.

Nonnarcotic analgesic agents that do not have antiinflammatory properties may be useful in relieving pain. Narcotic analgesic agents should be avoided since therapy will continue for an extended period of time. Muscle relaxants and tranquilizers are sometimes used to relieve pain and stiffness, especially when they are associated with paravertebral muscle spasm. Widespread use of these agents is not advocated because they tend to cause confusion and drowsiness in the elderly.

Because rheumatoid arthritis usually progresses, sometimes at a rapid rate, many clients require antiinflammatory agents that are stronger than aspirin. Several nonsteroidal antiinflammatory agents are available for use, but some of them are more appropriate than others for use in the elderly. The pyrazolones and the indole derivatives are older drugs that are used primarily for short-term treatment of exacerbations of rheumatoid arthritis. Because these drugs have an increased incidence of serious side effects in older people, they are not widely used with the elderly. If the older client is taking one of these drugs, the nurse should assess carefully for side effects. Drugs in the propionic

acid group are newer preparations that are valuable agents in older clients who cannot tolerate aspirin or do not respond to it. Advantages of these drugs are that they have a lower incidence of gastrointestinal toxicity than aspirin, the pyrazolones, and indole derivatives and do not affect platelet function. A disadvantage is their relatively high cost.

When antiinflammatory drug therapy has been used for several months but has not been effective in reducing joint inflammation, the physician may prescribe gold, antimalarial drugs, or intraarticular injections of corticosteroids. Gold salts were first used to treat rheumatoid arthritis in the 1920s and are one of the most effective therapeutic agents available in clients who tolerate them. Gold is used for the long-term treatment of arthritis. It is administered in weekly intramuscular (IM) injections. The dose is gradually increased for 3 or 4 weeks until a dose of 50 mg is achieved. Then weekly or biweekly injections are given until the client has received 1000 mg of gold. If a remission of the disease is to occur it does so within the first 6 months of treatment (Bonner, 1974). Gold therapy is expensive. There are some data that it may not be as effective in the elderly as in younger clients (Grahame, 1978).

Antimalarial drugs have produced significant improvement in clients who did not respond to aspirin and could not tolerate gold. These drugs are easily administered by the oral route. They require 2 to 6 months to achieve full effectiveness. Unfortunately, they are most effective for short periods and lose effectiveness over time. Intraarticular corticosteroid injections are given during the acute stage of rheumatoid arthritis because of their beneficial effects on joint inflammation. Strict sterile technique must be observed when preparing the injection for elderly clients because their resistance to infection may be impaired.

The use of systemic corticosteroids for the treatment of older clients with rheumatoid arthritis is controversial. Some physicians condemn their use because of serious side effects. Others believe that systemic corticosteroid therapy is warranted in older clients when dosage is carefully individualized. Steroid therapy is justified, they say, on the premise that most of the complications are long-term ones and in older people, steroid therapy is usually required for a short time (Grahame, 1978). Steroid therapy is reserved for clients who have not responded to salicylates, gold, and antimalarials and who are in danger of developing major disabilities. Steroid use in some older clients who were virtually immobile enables them to become fully mobile and active. Improvement occurs rapidly within 48 hours. Unfortunately, once steroids are begun, they usually cannot be discontinued because the arthritis flares up. Steroids with a short half-life are prescribed on a daily basis. Although taking steroids on an alternate-day schedule protects the pituitary–adrenal axis, most clients with rheumatoid arthritis cannot tolerate this schedule because the arthritis flares up on the day the drug is omitted.

A number of other potent medications are being investigated for use with clients who do not respond well to the usual treatment for rheumatoid arthritis and have life-threatening or crippling disease. These include cytotoxic agents, immunosuppressive agents, and penicillamine. Although trials with these drugs indicate that they may be more effective than gold, they have a high incidence of serious adverse effects, particularly in the elderly (Hahn, 1976; Grahame, 1978).

A variety of medications are available for use with rheumatoid arthritis. They have revolutionized the treatment of this disease. When they are coupled with a well-planned activity program, the medication regimen remains one of the most effective ways to manage the client with rheumatoid arthritis.

Modifying Activity and ADLs. Success in living with arthritis depends as much on adherence to an activity and ADL regimen as on adherence to the medication regimen. A discussion of the client's activity program begins on page 304. In addition to an activity program, the nurse should assess the client's ADLs to see what potentially dangerous situations should be eliminated and what activities could be facilitated. Many devices can be inexpensively made or bought to assist clients with severe handicaps to function independently. For example, if contractures limit grip, handles on eating utensils, toothbrushes, and combs can be built up and Velcro fasteners or snaps can replace buttons on clothing. Special implements or plans for making them can be obtained from local chapters of the Arthritis Foundation or from The Independence Factory, P.O. Box 597, Middletown, Ohio 45042. Included are devices to turn water taps, hold playing cards, manipulate keys for doors and auto ignitions, and retrieve objects from the floor. Other aids for dressing and grooming include a long-handled sponge for back washing and a long-handled shoe horn. The household may need to be rearranged to promote the client's independence in ADLs. Changes may include altering the levels of bed, tables, counters, and chairs, applying rails to help the client rise from the bath and toilet and negotiate stairs, raising the toilet seat, and obtaining a nonslip mat for the bathtub. If clients are to succeed in doing things for themselves, counseling of family members may be necessary. Some clients also benefit from retraining, done through participation in formal occupational therapy programs or more informal programs. Other clients benefit from provision for an outsider (home health aide, companion) to come into the home for a period of time to help with ADLs.

Nutrition. There is no evidence that diet plays a role in the onset of rheumatoid arthritis. Although no special diet is usually required, clients should be advised to avoid fad diets and irrational vitamin and mineral consumption. Clients with rheumatoid arthritis have an increased need for nutrients, probably because of cellular proliferation in synovial membranes and impaired intestinal absorption. Deficiencies in folic acid and pyridoxine and anemias can develop. Clients should be encouraged to eat a varied diet with adequate amounts of meat, fish, eggs, spinach, potatoes, and whole meal flour (Hyams, 1978).

Surgical Interventions. The nurse provides pre- and postoperative care for clients for whom surgical intervention is warranted. Surgery is performed when more conservative treatment has failed. Goals include correcting deformity, relieving pain and restoring motion. Advanced age is not a contraindication to surgery unless significant disease of major organs is present (Hahn, 1976). When active synovitis is present without gross destruction of the joint, a synovectomy to remove thickened synovial membrane may be performed. The purpose is to relieve pain, swelling, and disability. This procedure is used most often for a single joint, usually the knee, but may also be used with hands, wrists, elbows, and shoulders. Older people tolerate this procedure well and experience significant pain relief. It is unclear whether synovectomy halts or slows destruction of cartilage (Grahame, 1978). Following this procedure the nurse should encourage mobility as early as possible to reduce stiffness in the affected joint.

When joint destruction and deformity have occurred, other types of surgical procedures are required. A fusion of the spine may be done for the client with an unstable cervical spine. This procedure relieves pain and nerve root compression (Charlesworth and Baker, 1978).

Arthrodesis is sometimes performed on unstable or dislocated joints to reduce pain and improve function. When done on large joints, such as the hip, this procedure requires a long period of immobilization, a disadvantage for older people (Habermann, 1979). In addition, in some joints such as the hip, the older person does not tolerate the reduction in movement created by fixation of the joint. Today, there is a movement away from arthrodesis toward the use of arthroplasty. This procedure involves the replacement of a badly affected joint with a prosthesis that is mechanically sound and provokes no tissue reaction. Arthroplasty is used frequently with the hip, as well as with the knee, elbow, shoulder, ankle and fingers. Total replacement arthroplasty is available for the hip, knee, and small joints of the fingers. Arthroplasty improves mobility and relieves pain in severely disabled clients.

In the preoperative period, attention must be paid to the client's nutrition and general health. Arthroplasty is a more extensive surgical procedure than arthrodesis, and necessitates that the client be in good health. To prevent postoperative infection, clients must be carefully assessed to assure they are free of infection. Postoperative care can vary widely, depending upon the procedure that was done and the preferences of the physician. Following the surgical procedure, the nurse must obtain information of what was done and detailed orders about what activity is allowed. Information is needed about the exact positioning of the extremity, turning, transferring, standing, and ambulating with or without weight bearing. Most physicians want the older client to be active and ambulatory as soon as possible.

Following hip arthroplasty a brief period of rehabilitation is essential. The nurse implements a prescribed program that progresses from isometric and passive exercise to weight bearing and gait training. Infection is one of the most common complications following arthroplasty. During the postoperative period, the nurse uses care to prevent infection. Strict aseptic technique is required when changing the dressing.

Degenerative Joint Disease. Although the nursing care of clients with degenerative joint disease is similar in most respects to that of clients with rheumatoid arthritis, some differences deserve to be mentioned. The goals of the treatment program for the two conditions are identical. Like the program for rheumatoid arthritis, the treatment program for degenerative joint disease includes some or all of the following elements: emotional support, education, medication, an activity and ADL program, nutrition, and surgery. Clients who have learned that they have degenerative joint disease should be reassured that it does not produce the widespread and disabling adaptations of rheumatoid arthritis. They also need to know that the pain of degenerative joint disease is episodic and can be controlled with medication.

The basic treatment for degenerative joint disease consists of a judicious program of activity and ADLs plus diet. Activity should be balanced with rest and avoidance of overuse of involved joints. The activity program is discussed in detail on page 304. When the client is obese weight reduction is an essential part of the treatment plan, as it is one of the best ways to minimize strain on affected joints.

When this basic program fails to relieve the client's adaptations, drug therapy may be used. No drugs are available that alter the progression of degenerative joint disease, but analgesics may be required to relieve pain. Salicylates are especially useful because they have antiinflammatory as well as analgesic properties. Stronger analgesics and muscle relaxants may also be prescribed. Nonsteroidal antiinflammatory agents are also useful in relieving pain. Local intraarticular administration of corticosteroids is highly effective. The effects are temporary, however, and repeated injections are usually required. Injections are repeated every few months, but should not be repeated too frequently because they cause further atrophy of cartilage and an increase in joint destruction (Clark, 1976). Because degenerative joint disease does not have a significant inflammatory component, systemic corticosteroids are contraindicated. Gold, antimalarial agents, and investigational drugs used to control rheumatoid arthritis are not indicated in the treatment of degenerative joint disease (Hahn, 1976).

Because the usual course of degenerative joint disease is a gradually worsening one, surgical intervention is indicated when clients are disabled. The nurse cares for older clients undergoing a variety of reconstructive procedures, including osteotomy, arthrodesis, and arthroplasty. Osteotomy is performed most often in the early stages of osteoarthritis of the hip joint. In most cases it reduces pain and arrests cartilage degeneration. If it is performed early enough, cartilage regeneration may occur. Arthroplasty is performed on a variety of joints, including the foot, knee, and hip. Replacement prosthetic devices take pressure off joint surfaces, stabilize the joint, relieve pain, and restore motion to the joint. Total replacement arthroplasty is most successful with the hip joint and is widely performed in older people with hip involvement.

Although degenerative joint disease is one of the most common problems of the aged, pain relief and protection against disability are possible. The key to success is client participation in all elements of the treatment program. The nurse helps clients adhere to the therapeutic regimen by providing education, support, and supervision as well as direct care.

Gout. Medications. The keystone to the management of acute and chronic gout is medication. Table 6 summarizes the medications most often used to treat acute and chronic gout and their nursing implications.

During acute attacks, colchicine, phenylbutazone, and indomethacin are the drugs of choice. Colchicine is given orally or intravenously in a dose of 0.5 to 0.6 mg every hour or 1.2 mg every 2 hours until side effects begin to appear or the adaptations subside. Phenylbutazone (200 mg every 6 hours for 48 hours) or indomethacin (50 mg every 6 hours for 48 hours) may be used instead and both have fewer gastrointestinal side effects. Usually these medications effect complete relief in 24 hours. If an arthrocentesis has been performed the physician

may at that time inject corticosteroids into the affected joint. Doing so usually reduces inflammation within 12 hours. The administration of systemic steroids and ACTH is not recommended (McCarty, 1979). Other medications that may be used during an acute attack are nonsteroidal antiinflammatory agents such as oxyphenbutazone, naproxen and fenoprofen. See Table 6 for actions and nursing implications.

During the acute phase, nursing care is directed at reducing pain and monitoring fluid and electrolyte balance. During this period, clients must avoid weight bearing on the involved joint. They are often placed on bed rest. A bed cradle should be positioned at the foot of the bed. Pain medications, such as codeine, may be ordered (Anderson, 1976). Clients taking colchicine need ample fluids in order to effectively excrete uric acid. They must also be observed carefully for the side effects of colchicine, the most common of which are abdominal cramps and diarrhea.

Once the acute phase has subsided clients may be maintained on daily doses of 0.5 mg to 1.5 mg colchicine for several months. In addition, once acute inflammation has ceased, clients with chronic gout may be given either of two types of medication to reduce serum uric acid levels and prevent future acute attacks. If the high serum uric acid level is believed to be due to an underexcretion of uric acid, uricosuric medications, such as probenecid and sulfinpyrazone, are given. Uricosurics are effective in dissolving tophi, but because they remove already formed urate rather than interrupting uric acid formation at an earlier stage, they increase urinary urate concentration with the consequent risk of stone formation. If urolithiasis is present or if there are other reasons to believe the client is overproducing uric acid, medications such as allopurinol are given to inhibit uric acid synthesis. These help protect the kidney from chronic renal disease secondary to urate deposition. They also dissolve tophi, but so gradually that 6 to 12 months are required before changes are noticeable (Bluhm et al., 1977). Older clients tolerate medications to reduce uric acid and the incidence of side effects is very low (Grahame, 1978).

If the client has chronic gout, joint inflammation persists after the acute phase. In these cases, the physician also prescribes continual therapy with

TABLE 6. ANTIHYPERURICEMIC AGENTS USED FOR GOUT

Drug	Action	Contraindications	Nursing Implications
Agents for Acute Gout			
Colchicine	Indirectly inhibits leukocyte migration and phagocytosis to gouty joints, thus decreasing the inflammatory response. In addition, may decrease urate crystal deposition. Does not affect uric acid metabolism.	Use with caution in the elderly. Do not use if liver, kidney, or bone marrow function is impaired or if client is hypersensitive to this drug.	Administer with meals. Assure client maintains a fluid intake of at least 2 liters per day. During first 12 hours of administration observe for early side effects: nausea, stomach cramps, and mild diarrhea. Warn client to discontinue medication as soon as these appear. Observe client for serious side effects: gastroenteritis, diarrhea, prostration from fluid loss, and bone marrow depression. If client develops diarrhea, monitor diet carefully to prevent conditions linked with excess loss of water-soluble nutrients. If given IV, check IV site for severe tissue irritation. Side effects are less common when drug is given intravenously.
Phenylbutazone (Azolid, Butazolidin)	Reduces serum uric acid and inflammation.	Do not give if client has gastric irritation, peptic ulcer, congestive heart failure, hypertension, or blood dyscrasias. Discontinue in elderly clients if edema appears.	Side effects occur more often in older clients. Observe client for fluid retention, elevated BUN, bone marrow depression, gastritis, fever, sore throat, and CNS changes. Administer with food or milk. Instruct client to record daily weight and check legs and face for edema. Give antacids to prevent gastritis.

Indomethacin (Indocin)	Has antiinflammatory, analgesic, and antipyretic effects due to ability to block prostaglandin biosynthesis.	Do not administer if client is taking aspirin or has had colitis, gastrointestinal ulcers, diverticulitis, or allergy to indomethacin.	Give with food, milk, or antacids. Observe for aplastic anemia, elevated BUN, liver dysfunction, headache, upset stomach, diarrhea, gastric ulcers and bleeding, dizziness, psychic disturbances, giddiness, and fluid retention. Institute safety precautions if CNS side effects develop. Side effects decrease if drug is used in combination with colchicine. Incidence of side effects is particularly high in the elderly. Give with meals or antacids to reduce gastric distress.
Oxyphenbutazone (Tandearil, Oxalid); Naproxen (Naprosyn); Fenoprofen Calcium (Nalphon)	Nonsteroidal antiinflammatory agents.	Do not use if client has a history of asthma, gastrointestinal inflammation, or ulcer. Discontinue if edema appears.	Observe for gastrointestinal irritation and bleeding, fluid retention, skin rash, dizziness, headache, drowsiness, and changes in vision and hearing. Administer with milk or before and after meals.

Agents for Chronic Gout

Colchicine	(See under *Agents for Acute Gout* above)		
Allopurinol (Zyloprim)	Used for overproducers of uric acid. Lowers serum uric acid level by inhibiting action of xanthine oxidase essential for the production of uric acid from xanthine. Serum uric acid levels are lowered to normal within 48 hours. Colchicine is often given concurrently during first 6 months of treatment.	Do not use if client is hypersensitive to the drug. Use cautiously if client has impaired liver or kidney function. Discontinue at first sign of skin rash.	Administer with meals. Monitor intake and output. Assure fluid intake of at least 2 liters per day. Encourage client to eat alkaline–ash foods low in purine to maintain urine with alkaline or neutral pH. Alternatively, client may be asked to take sodium bicarbonate or potassium citrate to alkalinize urine.

(Continued)

TABLE 6. (CONTINUED)

Drug	Action	Contraindications	Nursing Implications
			Observe for skin rash, itching, other hypersensitivity reactions, gastrointestinal irritation, vasculitis, liver dysfunction (rare), and bone marrow depression (rare). Warn client that drowsiness may occur and, if necessary, institute safety precautions.
Probenecid (Benemid)	A uricosuric agent. Competitively inhibits renal tubular reabsorption of uric acid, thus promoting uric acid excretion. No antiinflammatory or analgesic properties.	Do not use if client's GFR is less than 50% of normal, or if client is hypersensitive to the drug, has kidney stones, or blood dyscrasias. Salicylates block the effects of uricosuric drugs and should not be used concurrently.	Administer drug with meals or antacid. Maintain fluid intake of 2 liters per day. Teach client to eat an alkaline–ash diet of fruits and vegetables low in purines. Sodium bicarbonate or potassium citrate may be given instead to alkalinize urine. Instruct client not to take aspirin. Observe for allergic dermatitis, gastrointestinal irritation, peptic ulcers, headache, dizziness, skin rash, and kidney stones.
Sulfinpyrozone (Anturane)	A uricosuric agent. Competitively inhibits renal tubular reabsorption of uric acid, thus promoting uric acid excretion. No antiinflammatory or analgesic properties.	Same as probenecid. In addition, do not use if client has active peptic ulcer.	Same as probenecid.

an antiinflammatory agent. Phenylbutazone and indomethacin are both used in this group of clients (Hahn, 1976).

Dietary Modifications.   Since the advent of effective medication therapy, severe dietary restrictions to treat gout are not usually necessary. However, clients are sometimes required to modify their food and fluid intake because the metabolism of uric acid can be altered by dietary means, resulting in changes in serum uric acid levels. The nurse often teaches and counsels clients to assist them to make and maintain necessary modifications in diet. Principles of diet therapy with older clients were described in Chapter 16.

Excessive purine loads aggravate gout. Although diet is not the only source of uric acid, a diet low in purines helps to reduce blood levels of uric acid by 1 to 2 mg/dl (Boykin, 1977; Agus, 1979). Table 7 lists foods high in purines and others with moderate and slight purine content. In addition to modifying purine intake, clients are usually advised to eat adequate, but not excessive, amounts of protein, to avoid fatty foods, and to eat a diet high in carbohydrates to maintain their desired weight levels. Limiting protein intake from animal sources restricts the intake of nitrogen-dependent purines. Although a high-fat diet retards the flow of uric acid and may trigger an attack of gout, a diet high in carbohydrates increases the excretion of uric acid.

Clients with gout should also learn to control their caloric intake. Because gout is associated with obesity, those who are obese are placed on weight reduction diets until the ideal weight is obtained. To prevent hyperuricemia, however, weight loss must be gradual. In some cases, salt restriction may help control gout; therefore, clients may also be placed on sodium-restricted diets (McCarty, 1979).

To prevent kidney damage from urate crystals, clients must maintain a high fluid intake (usually 2 liters/day). Since tea and coffee do not contain uric acid in a form converted to tophi, they need not be restricted (Boykin, 1977). Because alcohol increases uric acid levels, alcoholic intake should be limited to one cocktail per night.

Other Interventions.   Other interventions for clients with gout include surgery and physical therapy. Tophi may be removed surgically for cosmetic reasons or if they compromise the blood supply or result in ulcers or infections (Bluhm et al., 1977). Physical therapy, using regimens similar to those for rheumatoid arthritis, may be ordered if joints are deformed (Anderson, 1976).

Because clients with gout are at risk for a number of potential stresses, they should be reevaluated on a regular basis. Due to the amount of uric acid they excrete, the incidence of renal lithiasis in these clients is one thousand times higher than in healthy older clients. Clients with gout are also at high risk for hypertension, strokes, diabetes mellitus, and atherosclerotic vascular disease (Agus, 1979; Hahn, 1976; Bluhm et al., 1977).

Osteoporosis

Accurate assessment of the client with osteoporosis is important because treatment can mean a new lease on life. Often, relief is noted in only a few days. The therapeutic regimen for the client has two goals:

1. Prevention of bone loss and fractures due to bone loss

2. Rehabilitation of the client with fractures

TABLE 7.   SELECTED FOODS AND THEIR PURINE CONTENT

Foods Rich in Purines

Any meat extract	Rabbit
Organ meats	Duck
Kidney	Bear
Sweetbreads	Goose
Liver	Shellfish
Brains	Anchovies
Tripe	Sardines
Wild Game	Heavy wines
Venison	

Foods with Moderate Amounts of Purines

Red meat	Lentils
Poultry	Dried beans
Herring	

Foods Low in Purines

Vegetables	Eggs
Asparagus	Grain and grain
Cauliflower	products
Mushrooms	Oatmeal
Spinach	Whole wheat breads
Legumes	Cereals
Dairy products	Sugar
Cheese	
Milk	

This chapter focuses on the nurse's role in helping the client meet the first goal. Care of the client with fractures is discussed in Chapter 19. The therapeutic regimen has the following components:

- Psychological support
- Medication therapy
- Dietary management
- Activity modification

Psychological Support. The diagnosis of osteoporosis may be a shock because it is an insidious process. In the early stages, adaptations are nonexistent or deceptive and the condition can be easily overlooked. Clients who have just learned their diagnosis need nursing support as they learn to cope with a chronic illness.

The client with osteoporosis often responds with depression, pessimism, and irritability. The diagnosis and use of lay terms such as "crumbling spine" have a negative, sinister connotation. Nevertheless, the outlook for a full life as well as life expectancy are good if the condition is properly treated. The nurse needs to help clients maintain an optimistic outlook and support them as they modify their activity patterns and adjust to their new treatment regimen. Adherence to treatment, particularly to the medication therapy, has been associated with an improvement in the client's psychological adaptations (Bonner, 1974).

Medication Therapy. Medication therapy for clients with osteoporosis has not been fully defined in regard to optimal combinations of medications, schedules, or doses. Some medications now used for osteoporosis have not been approved yet for that purpose by the FDA. Consequently, the nurse should expect to work with clients on a variety of different regimens. Hormone administration in combination with vitamin D or vitamin D and calcium is currently the most widely accepted medication regimen. In addition, fluoride, calcitonin, and growth hormone may also be used.

Hormones in one form or another are usually prescribed for clients with osteoporosis. In postmenopausal women, bone resorption decreases significantly with short-term use of estrogen and to a lesser extent with its long-term use. Estrogen also prevents the bone loss that follows surgical men-

opause in younger women. Estrogen therapy may correct, at least partially, calcium malabsorption in the elderly (Gregerman and Bierman, 1981). Estrogens such as diethylstilbesterol, ethinylestradiol, and mestranol may be used. Estrogen therapy is usually prescribed in courses of 4 weeks with a 1-week gap in between. Clients need to know that withdrawal bleeding may occur after each course. Although estrogen does not entirely arrest the process of bone demineralization, it is extremely useful in preventing osteoporosis and in reducing the fracture rate (Pont, 1981). Estrogen therapy remains controversial in part because it is associated with serious adverse effects. These include sodium and water retention, hypertension, heart disease, blood clots, and breast and endometrial cancer (Elkowitz, 1981). The client on estrogen therapy needs close follow up and ongoing reevaluation.

Hormones other than estrogen are being investigated for use in the prevention of bone demineralization. Based on the assumption that the age-related loss of adrenal androgens might be a factor in bone demineralization, synthetic anabolic steroids, such as methandrostenolone, have been used and found to have effects similar to those of estrogen therapy. Androgens alone may be prescribed for men with osteoporosis. Combined androgen/estrogen therapy may be used for women. Combination therapy helps negate the troublesome virilizing side effects of androgens in women. Other side effects include liver dysfunction, sodium and water retention, nausea, and other gastrointestinal disturbances. Progestogen has also been used for periods of up to 1 year in clients with osteoporosis and found to be effective (Kolodny and Klipper, 1976; Wallach, 1978).

Hormone therapy is used in conjunction with vitamin D and calcium supplementation. Supplements are used because it is difficult for older clients to consume a diet that is high enough in vitamin D and calcium without exceeding an appropriate calorie range. Hormone therapy is not used alone because it is believed to be self-defeating. Calcium is removed from the blood to remineralize bone, but the resulting slight hypocalcemia stimulates the production of PTH, which in turn stimulates bone resorption and the release of calcium into the blood to correct the hypocalcemia (Wallach, 1978).

Studies of estrogen in combination with 25

hydroxy vitamin D indicate that this form of vitamin D is rapidly converted to the active vitamin D metabolite. Therapy is effective in reducing the negative calcium balance of osteoporosis. Studies using the active metabolite of vitamin D plus estrogen in women or testosterone proprionate in men have been found to be highly successful in restoring a positive calcium balance (Nordin, 1980; Gregerman and Bierman, 1981). Usually 1000 to 2000 IU of vitamin D are given to clients with minimal sun exposure or with diets low in dairy products (Pont, 1981; Wallach, 1978). Vitamin D alone or with only calcium supplementation is not advocated because bone is sensitive to the resorbing action of vitamin D (Nordin, 1980).

Oral calcium given with hormones or with hormones and vitamin D has been shown to prevent bone loss in some and perhaps all bones. Usually 1500 mg daily of calcium is advised for postmenopausal women. What is not obtained from food sources can be obtained from supplements. These include Os-Cal (500 mg tablets, two to three times a day) or liquid Neo-Calglucon (one tablespoon three to five times daily) (Wallach, 1978; Pont, 1981). Clients taking high doses of calcium should be observed for toxic signs, including increased thirst, polyuria, anorexia, nausea, headache, and increased nervousness (Peck et al., 1977). Intravenous doses of calcium, once used to treat osteoporosis, are now known to be ineffective as a treatment (Pont, 1981; Avioli, 1976).

Fluoride therapy for osteoporosis is experimental and will remain so until studies demonstrate or disprove its efficacy. If it is used, sodium fluoride (50 mg per day) is administered with vitamin D and calcium. Preliminary data indicate that osteoblastic activity is increased and bone resorption is decreased. Some questions have been raised about the strength of bone when fluoride therapy is used. Fluoride alone should never be used because it increases the crystallinity of bone and the risk of fractures (Exton-Smith, 1978; Pont, 1981).

Limited trials with calcitonin therapy have yielded conflicting results. In some cases, use of porcine calcitonin reduced bone resorption (Exton-Smith, 1978), whereas other reports have indicated that calcitonin therapy was ineffective. More studies are needed. Growth hormone has been used alone and in combination with calcitonin to reduce bone demineralization. To date, this treatment has been only marginally effective (Pont, 1981).

Dietary Management. Osteoporosis may be the by-product of lifelong dietary patterns, not merely the poor eating habits of some older people. The nurse who counsels members of the younger generation about sound dietary practices is making an important contribution toward the prevention of osteoporosis. At this time, a diet high in calcium and vitamin D, with adequate amounts of fluoride, ascorbic acid, and protein is advocated for the development of healthy new bone and the prevention of osteoporosis. Dietary modifications for clients with osteoporosis are discussed in Chapter 16.

Activity Modification. The institution of a regular, active exercise program is an essential part of the therapeutic plan. Regular activity slows the process of demineralization and allows the client to maintain an independent life-style. Because of its critical importance, activity modification is discussed in detail on page 307.

When clients with osteoporosis are assisted to follow a comprehensive therapeutic care plan their mobility can be preserved and even improved. Consequently, their prognosis is excellent.

Managing Pain

Pain is a universal human experience. For the elderly, it often becomes a fact of everyday life. As people age, they are increasingly likely to develop multiple chronic illnesses, and with illness comes pain. Older people know the sharp, suffocating tightness of angina, the burning sensation of peripheral vascular occlusion, the aching joints of arthritis, and the deep pain of cancer. Older people know other types of pain as well: the pain of loss, rejection, failure, and hardship.

Defining Pain. There is no one universally accepted definition of pain. Pain is a complex phenomenon that involves the total person, including sensation, perception of sensation, and response. The process of perceiving painful sensations is complex. Perception is modulated by anxiety and other emotions, expectations, past experiences, attitudes about pain, the presence or absence of other simultaneous sensations, the meaning of the painful sensation, and the attention paid to it. Likewise, the client's responses to pain are complex. Zborowski (1969) demonstrated that the norms of the individual's cultural group affect behaviors used to deal with the painful experience. There are wide variations from the cultural pattern by members of each cultural group. Fordyce (1978) proposed that conditioning affects responses to pain. Positive reinforcement of an individual's behavior in response to pain causes those behaviors to persist. Eventually, pain behaviors become a way of life. Other variables also influence response to pain: life-style, personality, and the nature and extent of the pain (Luce et al., 1979; Butler and Lewis, 1977).

Theories of Pain.   Although there is no comprehensive, unified theory of pain, many theories have been proposed to explain the pain experience and to serve as rationales for interventions to relieve pain. Both specificity theory and pattern theory (Melzack and Wall, 1965) focus on the sensory dimensions of pain, including the presence of a noxious stimulus and pain pathways involving sensory nerve fibers, the thalamus, cortex, and other areas of the brain. Pattern theory also seeks to explain a phenomenon often associated with chronic pain, that is, the perception of pain without the presence of an obvious noxious stimulus, trauma, or tissue damage. The thalamic neuron theory is a relatively new theory proposing that pain can develop when normal sensory stimuli pass through abnormal, hyperexcitable neurons, usually located in the thalamus. This theory explains the presence of chronic pain, such as osteoarthritis, even when the source of trauma cannot be identified or has been removed (Lee, 1977).

There are also a number of biochemical theories of pain. One theory stresses the potential significance of interaction between brain opiate receptors and recently discovered enkephalins (endogenous, morphinelike brain hormones) to suppress pain (Basbaum and Fields, 1978). Other theories involve the role that prostaglandins and histamine may play in stimulating the nociceptors and contributing to pain reception (Luce et al., 1979). The gate control theory includes the sensory dimensions of previous theories and adds new dimensions to the pain experience (Melzak and Wall, 1965). According to this theory, mechanisms in the spinal cord and the brain can be called upon to alter the pain experience, either increasing or decreasing the perception of pain. This theory explains why level of arousal, anxiety and other emotions, memory of past experiences, attention, anticipation, and suggestion influence pain perception and reaction to pain. This theory has been used to develop many creative interventions to manage pain.

Types of Pain.   The nurse encounters older clients with three types of pain:

1. *Acute pain* lasts from a few minutes to a few days. This pain has a useful purpose, serving as a warning that tissue damage is present.
2. *Chronic pain* lasts for months or years. It may be present constantly or intermittently. The reason for chronic pain may or may not be known. If after thorough examination no organic reason can be found to explain the pain, the pain is suspected to be psychic. In either case, neither the pain nor the stress responsible for it is life threatening. This type of pain no longer serves a useful purpose and may deplete the client's energy reserves.
3. *Progressive (terminal) pain* is a constant pain associated with a life-threatening stress, such as cancer. It is experienced most often by dying clients. Although the intensity of progressive pain varies, it is never totally relieved. This pain once served as a warning of tissue damage but no longer serves a useful purpose.

Because the characteristics of each type of pain are different, the nursing assessment needs to be comprehensive enough to identify each type and differentiate them.

Aging and Pain.   Very little is known about the pain experience, and even less is known about how this experience might differ in the elderly. Much of the research related to pain in the elderly has yielded contradictory findings. So many variables influence perception of and response to pain that it is understandable why it is difficult to isolate just how age affects the pain experience. The free, peripheral nerve endings undergo very little change with age; consequently, dermal sensation of pain should remain relatively intact (Goldman, 1979). Speed of response does slow with age, however.

Age may also affect the individual's ability to process sensory data. These changes may affect the ability of older people to protect themselves when faced with an immediate noxious stimulus; for example, to remove the hand if accidentally placed on a hot burner. The pain threshold (the lowest intensity at which pain is felt) may remain unchanged with age. Some clinical data have indicated that older people may have a higher pain threshold than the young, but this has been explained as a hesitancy on the part of older people to report the presence of pain (Storandt, 1979). Older people may delay reporting the pain they feel for fear of raising a false alarm. Data on differences in the ability of old and young people to tolerate the pain they feel are also conflicting. The elderly may quietly accept the pain they feel, believing it to be an unavoidable part of aging. They may have conditioned themselves to the experience of pain and found ways to mask their pain response.

On the other hand, it is known that older people complain of pain more often than younger people. This behavior may simply be a function of the increased incidence of illness in old age. It may also be a manifestation of "body monitoring." This activity of old age has been described by Butler and Lewis (1977). They have noted that as a group, older people concern themselves with their body and its functions in a more concerted way than younger people. This absorption with their body becomes a compelling preoccupation for older people and may explain their increased complaints of pain.

We also know that the pain experience in older people is often atypical. This is true of acute and chronic pain. Pathy (1967) demonstrated that chest pain was absent in 81 percent of elderly clients with myocardial infarction. Clinical data indicate that the severe pain commonly associated with acute inflammation and abdominal emergencies, such as appendicitis, cholycystitis, pleurisy, and pericarditis, is frequently muted in older people. The reason for these differences is unknown. The differing presentations of acute illness in older clients means that pain is not a reliable indicator of the extent of trauma or tissue damage experienced by the elderly.

Chronic pain has unique implications for older people, who have fewer energy reserves and a reduced capacity to adapt to stress. Chronic pain can deplete the older client's energy reserves, resulting in emotional or mental disorganization or an inability to participate in usual ADLs. It can reduce the client's pain tolerance, making any new pain more difficult to bear. Immobility is a common response to pain by young and old. Clients with widespread pain go to bed or seek rest. Clients with local pain splint or guard involved body parts. In the elderly, this normal response is particularly hazardous. Chronic pain is preoccupying. Many clients tend to withdraw from social interactions to focus their attention and energy on the experience of pain. Family and social relationships can be disrupted (Shealy, 1980). This tendency is especially dangerous in the elderly, many of whom are already at risk for social isolation.

Assessing the Older Client's Pain. Sternbach (1974) says that pain is whatever the person says it is and exists whenever the person says it does. This broad definition is a useful basis for directing the client assessment. Pain is very real to the person experiencing it, but there is no direct, objective means of assessing its existence. The only way the nurse can understand the client's pain is indirectly— by listening to what the client has to say and by observing physical signs and behavioral responses to it.

Older clients in pain may not complain about their experience. Some accept pain as a natural concomitant of growing old. Others have ceased talking about their pain, having been told too often that nothing could be done about it. Even when directly asked, some older clients deny that pain exists in order to avoid a physical examination and discovery of functional problems.

A good way to obtain data about pain is to use a combination of directive and nondirective questions. Direct questions should be used to obtain data about the site, radiation, duration, quality, intensity, and temporal characteristics of pain. Some clients are not knowledgeable enough to report accurately their perception of pain. It may help if the nurse suggests words to describe the quality of the pain. Intensity can be measured by having the client describe the pain as mild, moderate, severe, or agonizing. If the pain is chronic or progressive, clients may have difficulty pinpointing the location and quality of the pain. The nurse also needs information about what the client feels has precipitated the pain, and what aggravates and alleviates it. The nurse should question older clients about how they cope with the pain. If the client takes analgesics, the response to the medication and duration of relief should be determined. Information about other relief measures, including heat, cold, massage, pressure, movement, distraction, and rest should be gathered. The nurse should also determine what effects pain has on the client's sleep patterns and food intake. Insomnia and fatigue increase pain perception. A diet that lacks essential nutrients is of little help in managing the stress of pain (Shealy, 1980). An excellent way to obtain data about the client's pain pattern and its effect on functioning is to ask the client to keep a daily log of pain severity, activity, and relief measures. Once interventions are instituted, the log is useful in evaluating their effectiveness.

Assessing the client's personal responses to pain is best done by using open-ended questions. Common emotional responses to pain, including fear, anxiety, and tension, should be identified. Fear is often found in older clients who view pain as a threat to their independence. Anxiety is a special problem with chronic pain. Most people view pain as a warning that something is wrong. Although their instinct is to avoid the pain and correct the problem, clients in chronic pain cannot do so. This failure is frustrating, anxiety producing, and creates a cycle that increases the pain.

All pain has an emotional component. Negative emotions increase the perception of pain and reduce pain tolerance. When assessing a client's emotional responses to pain, it may be necessary to include a complete mental status assessment. Pain can cause disorganized thought processes, incoherent speech, inability to concentrate, irritability, and mood swings, as well as the emotions discussed earlier. Depression frequently accompanies chronic pain, possibly because chronic pain depletes the client's supply of normal coping mechanisms. The mental status assessment also provides data about the presence of psychic pain. The stresses of poverty, weakness, poor health, and loss make older people especially vulnerable to psychic pain.

The nurse should also determine how pain affects the client's normal routine and ability to function. Does the pain interfere with ADLs or daily

exercise routines? What effects does pain have on the client's social relationships? Does the client withdraw and refuse to participate in social activities or visit with friends? What, if any, secondary gains are associated with the pain? For example, does the pain serve as an excuse that keeps the client from participating in anxiety-producing activities? Is it a means for getting recognition or attention from nurses or physicians that is not given unless the client complains? Is it a way of obtaining protection from the family? If clients with chronic pain derive secondary gains, these tend to reinforce the pain response and make pain management more difficult (Fordyce, 1978). Does the pain interfere with the older client's safety? For example, if the client experiences dizziness or hypotension with pain, the risk of falls or fractures is increased. If the client's safety is in jeopardy, the nurse can institute appropriate precautions. The nurse should encourage the client to talk about previous experiences with pain and the coping measures instituted at that time, as these influence current reactions to pain. What does pain mean to the client? Is it a form of punishment, a source of shame, or an unavoidable part of living? What is the client's attitude about the current pain? Clients who believe that pain is short lived and explainable exhibit different responses from clients who perceive their pain as chronic or life threatening. The nurse should also obtain information about what the client believes are appropriate pain behaviors. The client's beliefs are, in part, a function of culture, socioeconomic group, sex, and age. It is especially helpful if older clients can express what they feel to be appropriate pain behaviors for people in their own age group. This is an area that deserves research attention.

Finally, what expectations does the client in pain have of those who are providing care? For example, some clients may expect that because of their age, health care providers will ignore their complaints. Others may expect that because of their age they have earned a right to immediate attention and pain relief.

Most pain, whether acute, chronic, or progressive, has an organic component. The first purpose of the physical assessment is to identify the physical basis for the pain. Then, management can be aimed at eliminating the stress when possible. The physical assessment is particularly important when assessing pain in older people not only because they are sometimes reluctant to report pain but because their perception of pain may not correlate with the extent of pathology. Special attention should be given to examining the areas that the client pinpoints as painful. The nurse should also perform a neurological assessment, giving special attention to the sensory assessment. The musculoskeletal assessment should include evaluation of joints for swelling, stiffness, and guarding behaviors and assessment of muscle strength in involved areas. The condition of the skin should be determined, with particular attention given to bony prominences. The nurse should observe the client's outward appearance, noting facial expressions such as grimacing and body movements such as writhing, restlessness, clenched hands, and guarding or splinting. Outward appearance does not always correlate with the client's perception of pain. Some clients do not believe it is appropriate to manifest these outward signs of pain. Others, especially clients in chronic pain, have learned to control these responses to pain. Consequently, if clients do not exhibit these responses, the nurse should not necessarily assume that they are not in pain.

When pain is severe, it may stimulate the autonomic nervous system and produce weakness, hypotension, increased respiratory rate, tachycardia or bradycardia, nausea, vomiting, diarrhea, sweating, ashen or pale face, disorientation, or confusion. The nurse should determine whether or not these adaptations are present. Although these responses are likely to accompany acute pain, they are usually not observed in clients with chronic pain, even when it is severe.

Fordyce (1978) has identified two problems often seen in older people that mimic pain. The two problems, depression and functional impairment, make assessing pain in older people a complicated process. If the older client complains of pain that is puzzling in its distribution, onset, or temporal characteristics, it is possible that the client's complaints of pain are mislabeled. The client's real problem may be depression, a frequent problem in the older population as well as a frequent companion to pain, especially chronic pain. If the nurse suspects that depression is the client's main problem or a major component of the problem, a complete mental status assessment should be performed.

Chapter 16 describes many useful tools for assessing depression. Another problem that complicates the assessment of pain is the possibility that the older client has invented the complaint of pain in order to hide a functional impairment, such as short-term memory loss, difficulty performing fine motor skills, or sensory losses. Older clients may find it more acceptable to use pain as the reason they no longer participate in ADLs, social activities, or other tasks than to risk revealing their functional loss to other people.

Interventions for Pain Relief. The most direct measures to relieve pain are those aimed at the stress responsible for it. However, this is not always a realistic approach, particularly with older clients who have multiple chronic illnesses. For them, pain relief is one of several elements of a therapeutic program aimed at helping them adapt to chronic illness. Most of the techniques available for pain management can be used for older clients. Many of them have been developed as a consequence of pain theories, especially the gate control theory. The nurse can provide older clients with information about the array of pain management techniques and help them make decisions about which techniques might be most suitable.

Because of the strong psychic component associated with pain, much attention has been directed toward management techniques that modify the client's mental and emotional responses and reduce pain perception. Anxiety and fear increase perception of pain. Nursing efforts should be directed toward reducing these emotions. One important way to do so is to instill confidence in the client that the care-givers can be effective in reducing pain.

With older clients who have gone from one professional to another seeking relief in vain, instilling confidence can be a real challenge. Nurses need to communicate the belief that the pain is real and its management is a priority. When providing relief measures, they need to convey confidence that those measures will be effective. Other nursing actions that reduce anxiety include answering questions, dispelling myths and fears about pain, staying with the client in pain and helping the client to find effective coping strategies for management of pain. Older clients can be active participants in the process of pain management. They should be involved in making decisions on specific techniques to be used to control their pain. As clients begin to experience success in managing their pain, their sense of helplessness and fears about pain are reduced and they experience a sense of control over the pain.

The gate control theory serves as the rationale for a variety of stimulation control measures. These include cutaneous stimulation techniques, electrical stimulation, and distraction. They are aimed at decreasing noxious stimuli by increasing other types of sensory input that close the gate and inhibit pain transmission. Cutaneous stimulation includes the use of touch, backrubs, moderate massage, heat, cold, menthol rubbing agents, and contralateral stimulation. Because older clients vary widely in their response to touch, the nurse should assess each client's response. Although some clients respond to minimal or moderate amounts of touch, others withdraw and do not want to be touched when in pain (Burnside, 1978). Massage is an excellent technique because it reduces tension and increases mobility while providing cutaneous stimulation (Shealy, 1980).

Menthol rubs close the pain gate by providing a sensation that overrides pain. They may also release pain inhibitors (endorphins) (McCaffery, 1980). The nurse should assess clients who receive these rubs for signs of skin irritation. When an area is too sensitive to touch or inaccessible due to a cast or bandage, contralateral stimulation with cold, massage, or menthol may be effective (McCaffery, 1980).

Electrical stimulation relieves many types of pain, including spinal disc pain, sciatica, headache, cancer pain, and arthritis pain. Several methods of electrical stimulation are available (Gaumer, 1974). The transcutaneous method (TENS) is the safest and easiest. It relieves pain by delivering an electrical charge to electrodes, positioned over the painful area or a peripheral nerve pathway. Stimulation closes the gating mechanism. Currently, at least 75 models of TENS devices are available. Clients select the one that provides maximum relief. In one program, 50 percent of clients received 50 to 100 percent relief using a TENS device (Shealy, 1980).

Peripheral nerve implants and dorsal column stimulators are two devices that work on the same principle. Clients who are to be given dorsal column stimulators undergo a laminectomy to attach elec-

trodes to the dorsal column at the level of the pain. Candidates for this procedure are evaluated first for emotional stability and undergo a trial period with a TENS device to assure they can achieve success with an implanted stimulator. After the device is implanted clients are withdrawn from their analgesic drugs and placed on a program of physical activity. The nursing care plan includes teaching clients how to use and maintain the device. Despite its long-term effectiveness in 25 percent of chronic pain clients, this procedure is associated with a high rate of complications and is performed only in selected cases (Shealy, 1980).

The use of distraction and redirecting of attention to other considerations is based on the premise that cognitive processes can be manipulated to close the pain gate and reduce the pain experience. These techniques are aimed at reducing the client's attention to and anticipation of pain. Distraction is effective even with severe pain by shielding the client from full awareness of pain (McCaffery, 1980). The nurse can suggest reading, watching television, needlework, listening to music, and involvement in hobbies. Redirecting attention involves dissociating some aspects of the noxious stimulus complex and reinterpreting some of these aspects (Blinchik and Grzesiak, 1979). For example, in a technique called "wakened imagined analgesia" clients learn to imagine a pleasurable sensation involving the painful part and to relive that sensation when in pain (Siegele, 1974). Group programs are available to help clients master these techniques (Blinchik and Grzesiak, 1979).

To minimize the client's tendency to focus inward on the pain experience, the nurse can use strategies to redirect the client's interests and energies outward. One way to do this is to provide for a progressive exercise program that includes limbering and aerobic exercises. Most clients can increase their physical activity if they do so slowly. Walking, if not contraindicated, is valuable because it provides diversion as well as direction of energies (Wolf, 1980). Exercise programs have other benefits. They elevate mood and help convince concerned family members that the client is not helpless. Many of the group programs for pain management use exercise as one component of their therapeutic regimen.

The nurse may also be involved in behavior

modification programs. These use a system of rewards for nonpain behaviors to teach clients to disregard their pain (Fordyce, 1978; Luce et al., 1979). Family, friends, and health professionals help the client by providing support and reinforcement of nonpain behaviors such as using distraction, relaxation, physical activity, or social activity. Pain behaviors, such as complaining or resting, are ignored. The nurse who schedules frequent home visits on a regular basis rather than visiting only after the client telephones with complaints of pain is applying behavior modification theory. Behavior modification has been criticized because it may teach clients to ignore new pain that signals tissue damage as well as chronic pain.

Because tension increases pain perception, relaxation techniques have been devised. These reduce anxiety and emotional tension, ease muscle tension and enhance the action of analgesics. Relaxation techniques range from the use of yoga and meditation to special breathing techniques. Some of these may be difficult to master, but their benefits may make the older client's efforts worthwhile (McCaffery, 1980).

Fatigue intensifies pain. Providing opportunities for uninterrupted sleep and rest periods helps older people cope with pain. Nighttime is one of the most difficult times for clients in pain. Isolation is intensified and the usual distractions, such as household activities and television are not readily available. The nurse can help the client devise a plan that promotes sleep. A judicious plan of relaxation techniques, diversionary techniques, analgesics, and other medications may be helpful.

When discussing pain management, medications may be the first intervention that comes to mind. However, drug therapy can be hazardous in the elderly. When the origin of pain can be traced to a specific site, medications can be given to reduce the pathology. This is the rationale for giving nitroglycerin to clients with angina or colchicine to clients with gout. However, when the stress responsible for the pain cannot be determined or eliminated, analgesics are used. Data regarding the effects of analgesics in older people are limited. Rossman (1979) reports that in one study the effectiveness of both placebos and morphine sulfate was greater in the elderly than in the young. On the other hand, some older clients have had frightening experiences with medications and fear drug use. When considering whether or not to use medications to control pain, the physician should consider a variety of variables: the advantage of freedom from pain, the need to preserve alertness and physical strength, and the risk of side effects (Butler and Lewis, 1977). Older clients who receive medications for pain require close supervision to assure that they provide the expected relief and to minimize the risk of adverse effects.

Drugs used for pain relief include nonnarcotic and narcotic analgesics, tranquilizers, antidepressants, and muscle relaxants, used singly or in a variety of combinations. The type of pain (acute, chronic, progressive) and its severity determine what analgesic is to be used. Most physicians believe that unless the client has severe, progressive pain, the mildest analgesic in a minimum dose should be prescribed on a fixed dose schedule. This plan avoids the risk associated with the p.r.n. schedule that pain responses are being positively reinforced (Fordyce, 1978). The philosophy guiding the management of terminally ill older clients is more aggressive. Older clients who are dying have the same right as younger clients to be free of actual pain as well as the fear of future, uncontrollable pain. The fear that the older client will become addicted is misplaced (Kastenbaum, 1979). The nurse should give medications on an as-needed basis before the pain becomes severe. The client should not have to waste limited energy resources worrying about whether or not sufficient pain medication will be available. At first, mild, less addicting narcotics are prescribed to relieve pain. The risk of the client developing a tolerance is reduced by carefully controlling dosage and time intervals between drugs. When working with the terminally ill client the nursing care plan should include a mix of other pain management strategies in addition to analgesics.

Narcotics are potent analgesics that should be used with extreme caution in older people. Codeine is not recommended because it tends to cause dizziness and drowsiness in the elderly. It may also cause retention of bronchial secretions with a resultant possibility of infection. Morphine sulfate is also associated with hazards, including respiratory depression, constipation and urinary retention. Morphine sulfate should be reserved for elderly clients in severe pain, for example, clients with myocardial infarction or advanced cancer (Davison, 1981). Hospice programs have reported the successful use of narcotic analgesics in elderly, dying clients to produce analgesia and euphoria without impairing consciousness.

Older clients may be candidates for surgical interventions to relieve pain. These include cordotomy, rhizotomy, neurectomy, and sympathectomy. Neurosurgery abolishes intractible pain by destroying the nerve pathways that carry painful sensations. These procedures are irreversible and are performed only as a last resort.

No matter which techniques are used, effective pain management requires that the nurse be caring and understanding. Objective assessment and individualized management of the client in pain are essential. Nurses may have attitudes and values about pain that differ from those of the older client. They may observe responses to pain that are at variance with their own. It is important for nurses to gain insight into their own feelings about pain so that they can put them in the background and help older clients cope in ways they find most effective. Pain is a holistic concept, and pain relief is achieved when the nurse considers the whole person.

Parkinson's Disease

Management of the client with Parkinson's disease is lifelong and requires ongoing medical and nursing intervention. Because there is no cure, the aim of treatment is to keep the client as functional and productive as possible. Doing so slows the process of deterioration.

Medical Intervention. Medical interventions include medication, surgery and rehabilitation.

Medications. Pharmacological intervention is the cornerstone of medical management of clients with Parkinson's disease. The aim of drug therapy is to correct the disturbed relationship between dopamine and acetylecholine that underlies the major adaptations associated with the disease. This can be accomplished by using drugs that decrease cholinergic activity or increase dopaminergic activity (Table 8). The various antiparkinson medications mix well and are often given in combination because they have synergistic effects (Sweet, 1975).

The physician usually bases the decision to prescribe drugs on the stage of the disease, the client's functional capacity, and an evaluation of the expected risks and benefits of the antiparkinsonism agents. Often, medications are not prescribed until the adaptations become stresses that interfere with the client's ability to function or are a source of emotional distress to the client.

During the early stages of the disease, when dopamine deficiency in damaged nigral cells is partially compensated for by increased dopaminergic activity in undamaged cells, the role of drug therapy is to enhance biosynthesis of dopamine. The drugs of choice in this phase include anticholinergic agents, antihistamines, and tricyclic antidepressants that have anticholinergic properties in addition to their primary mode of action. Dosage must be carefully adjusted if these agents are to relieve adaptations without causing disturbing side effects.

Levodopa, or L-dopa, has revolutionized the management of Parkinson's disease. Usually the physician does not prescribe L-dopa until the adaptations are well established and the client experiences difficulty carrying out physical or social activities. At this point, most nigral cells are destroyed and dopaminergic drugs to enhance the productivity of the few remaining cells are not effective. Since dopamine does not cross the blood–brain barrier, L-dopa, its immediate precursor, is given instead. L-dopa is converted to dopamine in the brain, where it exerts its therapeutic effect, and at peripheral sites, where it is wasted. L-dopa does not prevent deterioration but allows optimal functioning at every stage of the disease.

When L-dopa was first introduced, it was rarely used with elderly clients because experts believed the incidence of side effects was higher in the elderly. Subsequent research has demonstrated that when dosage is carefully adjusted, undesirable side effects in the elderly are no more frequent than in the young (Caird, 1974). In fact, the elderly require lower initial and maintenance doses than do the young. If side effects develop, the dosage is temporarily reduced until they disappear. Then the client is returned to the original dose.

The most desirable form of medication is Sinemet. Because Sinemet contains Carbidopa in combination with levodopa, the conversion of L-

TABLE 8. DRUGS USED TO TREAT PARKINSON'S DISEASE

Drug	Action	Side Effects	Nursing Implications
Anticholinergic Agents Benztropine mesylate (Cogentin) Trihexyphenidyl (Artane) Biperiden (Akineton) Atropine	Act by virtue of their anticholinergic properties. Partially block the nerve receptors in the striatum stimulated by acetylcholine. Improve muscle control, tremor and salivation.	Early: dry mouth, blurred vision, and vertigo. Late: vomiting, mental confusion, and hallucinations. Others: memory lapse, aggravates glaucoma, urinary retention, constipation, nausea, and nervousness.	Teach client about potential side effects. Chewing gum and sucking hard candy may alleviate dry mouth. Encourage high fiber, high liquid diet to reduce constipation.
Antihistamines Orphenadrine (Disipal) Disphenyhydramine (Benadryl) Chlorphenoxamine (Phenoxeme)	Supplement the anticholinergic agents. Inhibit uptake of dopamine at the synapse. Reduce tremor and rigidity.	Drowsiness, euphoria, headache, tachycardia, hypotension, weakness, and tingling of hands. Others similar to anticholinergics.	Teach client about potential side effects.
Antidepressants Amitriptyline (Elavil) Imipramine (Tofranil) Proriptyline (Vivactil)	Act by virtue of their anticholinergic properties.	Dry mouth, perspiration, insomnia.	Warn client about possible side effects.
Antiviral Agents Amantadine Hydrochloride (Symmetrel)	Mode of action unknown. Reduce adaptations in many clients but lose their effectiveness in very short time.	Side effects rare. If taken with levodopa or anticholinergic agents, side effects of those drugs may be exaggerated.	
Dopamine Agents Amantadine (Symmetrel) Levodopa (Dopar)	Cross the blood–brain barrier and are converted to dopamine in basal ganglia. Improvement begins in 1.5–2 weeks and may not peak for 16 weeks. Akinesia responds first, then rigidity and last tremor.	Mental overactivity; insomnia; sedation; behavioral disturbances; confusion; anorexia; nausea; vomiting; cardiac arrhythmias; hypotension; syncope; phlebitis; dyskinesia of tongue, face, and mouth; coughing; breathing disturbances; mild anemia; mild elevations of BUN, SGOT, creatinine.	Observe for side effects, especially behavioral changes. Encourage client to reduce total amount of protein in diet and avoid alcohol and excessive dietary pyridoxine. These are antagonists to levodopa. For hypotension, encourage client to get up slowly to reduce dizziness and wear elastic stockings.

(Continued)

TABLE 8. (CONTINUED)

Drug	Action	Side Effects	Nursing Implications
Levodopa (Dopar) (Continued)		Because these drugs are metabolized more slowly in the elderly, older clients are at high risk for side effects even with low doses of the drug. Enhance excretion of K^+, increasing risk of digitalis intoxication if client also takes digitalis.	Clients who are dizzy or drowsy should be advised not to drive. Counsel client that color of urine, saliva and perspiration may darken and is not harmful. Clients must understand the importance of taking medications regularly. An alarm wrist watch may assist forgetful clients. Give after meals or with milk to reduce nausea.
Levodopa/Carbidopa (Sinemet)	This combination blocks the peripheral metabolism of levodopa, reducing severity of many side effects (especially nausea and vomiting) and increasing the amount of levodopa available for transport to the brain. Because levodopa is not broken down to dopamine in the GI tract, a lower dose of medication is needed.	Same as above. Less nausea and vomiting and hypotension. Dyskinesias may occur sooner and at lower dosages.	If necessary, institute safety precautions for hypotension. Observe for side effects. Assure client takes medication regularly.

dopa to dopamine at peripheral sites is inhibited. Therefore, fewer side effects develop and the drug is effective much more quickly (7 to 10 days versus up to 16 weeks with levodopa).

Clients need to know that their improvement may be gradual. Effectiveness of the drug varies widely and clients with intellectual impairments and depression often show the least improvement. The nurse should observe clients on long-term L-dopa therapy for continued effectiveness of the drugs. Studies indicate that L-dopa may be most effective during the first three years, after which effectiveness declines (Davis, 1977; Yahr, 1981). In particular, akinesia may appear. The client may experience hypotonic "freezing," especially when exposed to stress, akinesia shortly before the time the next dose of medication is scheduled, or episodic akinesia (called "on–off phenomenon") that ceases as quickly as it began. These phenomena are safety hazards for older clients as they may lose all mobility and fall during an episode.

The nurse should monitor the client for signs

of side effects that may develop in gastrointestinal, cardiovascular, and nervous systems. L-Dopa is known to have multiple, sometimes contradictory side effects. Most are believed to be due to the peripheral conversion of L-dopa to dopamine. Therefore, side effects vary, depending upon what form of medication is taken and fewer side effects develop when L-dopa is combined with Carbidopa. Some side effects, such as incontinence and postural hypotension, are not dose related and often disappear spontaneously. Others, such as nausea, dyskinesia and mental disturbances are dose related and improve when dosage is reduced. Nursing implications for clients receiving L-dopa are summarized in Table 8.

Surgery. In the 1960s many surgical procedures were performed to relieve parkinsonian tremor and rigidity. Usually, freezing (cryosurgery) or thermocoagulation was used to place lesions in the medial globus pallidus or the lateral thalamus. Although initial benefits were good, they were only temporary. Surgical techniques were never used as often with elderly clients as with their younger counterparts. Today, because surgery does not seem to prevent the relentless progression of the disease, it is rarely performed (Sweet, 1975; Sambrook, 1976).

Rehabilitation. For the client with parkinsonism, rehabilitation may involve a comprehensive approach with a physical therapist, occupational therapist, speech therapist, social worker, and psychiatrist. Goals of rehabilitation include improving the client's ability to function in the environment and increasing communication skills and self-esteem. Specific activities vary according to the client's needs, but may include speech therapy, group exercise sessions, gait training, and training in activities of daily living (Davis, 1977; Sweet, 1975). Clients often participate as outpatients in rehabilitation programs. By being familiar with the client's rehabilitation program, the nurse can coordinate activities and assure that activities learned are reinforced in the client's daily life.

Nursing Care. All clients with Parkinson's disease need to participate in a total self-care regimen. Through teaching, counseling and providing direct care, the nurse plays an important role in initiating

and maintaining such a regimen and in modifying it as changes in the client's abilities warrant. Clients in the early stages of the disease who have not yet been placed on medication can maximize their strengths by active involvement in such a self-care regimen. Although it is true that medication therapy is the mainstay of treatment for clients with advanced Parkinson's disease, they also benefit greatly from full participation in a self-care regimen. In fact, if attention is not given to the client's physical and psychosocial needs, it appears that many clients fail to respond optimally to drug therapy (Yahr, 1981).

The key to a successful self-care program is that it be individualized, using the client's adaptations and functional abilities as the guide. The self-care regimen for the client involves three main elements: psychosocial care, maintenance of mobility, and nutrition.

Psychosocial Care. The client with Parkinson's disease lives with a chronic, incurable, fluctuating condition that is responsive to physical and psychological stresses. The negative prognosis and bizarre adaptations are a threat to clients and expose them to many stressful and embarrassing situations. Withdrawal, embarrassment, and anger are often the result of tremor, lack of expression, and speech difficulties. Clients may become depressed and discouraged. Clients need support and reassurance from the nurse if they are to remain motivated to participate in self-care activities. In addition, the nurse must provide teaching, counseling, and reassurance to the family who must learn to cope with a chronically handicapped member. A major burden falls on the spouse or companion who must care for an immobile, stiff person. Families should be urged to require clients to be as independent as possible without exceeding their capabilities. The family should understand that mobility varies from time to time; thus, the client may normally be more dependent at some times than at others.

Clients have difficulty communicating their feelings and emotions because of facial immobility and speech difficulties. Consequently the nurse may overlook depression, a frequent accompaniment of Parkinson's disease. The nurse should be alert for cues to depression and give support. At times, depression may mimic intellectual deterioration.

Depression can contribute to the disability, and when it is alleviated, the client's functional abilities often improve.

As a consequence of their disabilities, many clients withdraw from interpersonal relationships. Whenever possible, clients should be encouraged to socialize. If speech is a problem, clients should be encouraged to practice by singing and reading aloud, coordinating articulation with expiration to increase the volume of sound. Exercises of the facial muscles and lips to improve phonation can be instituted. Clients with severe speech deficits should be referred to a speech therapist.

Maintenance of Mobility. In addition to participation in formal physical and occupational therapy, clients with Parkinson's disease benefit from meticulous attention to every aspect of their mobility. Clients need help establishing a regular activity regimen (pp. 307–308) and help with their activities of daily living. Because of poverty of movement, clients have difficulty carrying out ADLs, including hygiene activities, dressing, and toileting. At best, clients perform ADLs slowly. The nurse can suggest that the client establish a daily routine to avoid being rushed. Clients who "freeze" during motor tasks should be encouraged to relax and then initiate the proper movement for the attempted task. The nurse can explain that "freezing" does not last long.

HYGIENE. Safety measures should be instituted in the client's living areas, including the tub and toilet areas (Chapter 8). If clients are unsteady standing, a stool can be placed in the tub to allow them to sit while showering. Meticulous skin care is essential, especially for inactive clients. All clients should bathe daily and inspect pressure areas for redness. Oral care is important to counteract the effects of dysphagia and drooling. Mouth care (brushing teeth and rinsing mouth with water) after meals increases the client's comfort and removes remaining food particles, which may be aspirated. Clients can also be taught to use a bulb syringe to remove food and saliva from the mouth. Clients who drool may fear choking and should be taught to lie on their side to decrease the pooling of saliva in the back of the mouth.

Because clients with Parkinson's disease blink infrequently and may have severe seborrhea, they are subject to corneal drying and external eye dis-

ease. Clients can use sterile wetting agents to prevent inflammation of the eyes. Clients with seborrhea should be taught to use moist Q-tip swabs daily to remove greasy scales from lid margins.

DRESSING. Many devices are available to assist clients with hypokinesia who have difficulty dressing. Slip-on shoes instead of shoes with laces, clothing with zippers or Velcro fasteners instead of buttons, and elastic waistbands increase the client's independence. Because many clients with Parkinson's disease complain of feelings of suffocation, clothing should be lightweight and loose fitting.

TOILETING. Elimination problems are common in older clients with Parkinson's disease due to aging changes, immobility, muscle weakness, autonomic changes that accompany the disease, and medication therapy. Clients with mobility problems may benefit from having a urinal or commode placed near the bedside. To minimize constipation, clients should be urged to exercise daily, maintain a high intake of fluids and fiber-containing foods, and set aside a regular time for evacuation. Laxatives, especially lubricants, may be prescribed, but mineral oil should be avoided because aspiration pneumonia is a potential stress for dysphagic clients.

Urinary incontinence may be a problem when clients begin L-dopa therapy, but this adaptation usually disappears spontaneously. Urinary retention is another, more lasting, side effect of L-dopa. In addition, these clients have a high incidence of urinary tract infections. The nurse should monitor clients for adaptations of hesitancy, frequency, burning or pain with urination, and, when indicated, refer the client to a physician. To maintain optimal urinary function, the importance of adequate hydration should be stressed.

Nutrition. Clients with Parkinson's disease must have their nutritional status carefully supervised. Not only do they have difficulty swallowing, but drug therapy may adversely affect appetite or result in nausea and vomiting. If tremor and rigidity interfere with getting food to the mouth, clients should be urged to use spoons for eating. Flexible drinking straws may help clients who have difficulty handling cups. Clients with hypokinesia may need help cutting food.

Dysphagic clients are at risk for malnutrition and dehydration. The importance of adequate fluid intake should be stressed. Clients should be taught to eat foods that are easily chewed and swallowed, to take small bites, and to chew thoroughly.

Clients taking L-dopa need special diet counseling since the intake of protein, alcohol, and large amounts of pyridoxine interferes with the drug's action. Drinking may be an important social function for some clients. They should be advised to limit alcoholic intake to one or two small drinks per day and to avoid alcohol whenever possible. The client should decrease the total amount of protein in the diet and should spread protein intake over the entire day by eating four smaller meals, instead of three. Limiting protein in the diet is known to reduce the amount of levodopa needed to control the client's adaptations (Langan and Cotzias, 1976). Clients are not placed on low pyridoxine (B_6) diets because doing so can be dangerous. Instead, they should be instructed to avoid excessive intake of pyridoxine-containing foods. These dietary restrictions are not necessary when clients are placed on combination medications such as Sinemet. Clients who are overweight should be encouraged to go on a low-calorie diet. Weight loss not only makes medication regulation easier but enhances mobility and reduces the risk of cardiovascular disease.

Summary. Parkinson's disease is a motor disorder characterized by tremor, rigidity, and akinesia. Elderly clients with Parkinson's disease must live with the threat of loss of mobility and, thus, loss of independence. Medication therapy is important in maintaining client functioning at an optimal level. To be most efficacious, medication therapy should be supplemented with a total self-care regimen. By helping the client to maintain such a regimen the nurse can help the client attain a more normal life.

Modifying Activity

In the midst of our hurried society, one is struck by the paradox of older people sitting passively and motionless. Our society has created a stereotype that older people should sit back and take a well-deserved rest, since they have worked all their lives. Because many of the current generation of older people have never participated in sports or recreation, they can easily drift into a life-style of inactivity. Indeed, it sometimes appears quicker to do things *for* older people than to encourage them to

do things for themselves. In addition, it may seem less risky to see that older people are sitting, safe but inactive, in restrictive chairs than to encourage them to get up and about. Nevertheless, the belief that physical activity for older people is an important aspect of maintaining optimal adaptation is gaining widespread acceptance. Although the nurse should promote activity in the well elderly (Chapter 8) it is at least equally important to encourage the chronically ill elderly to remain as active as possible. DeCarlo et al. (1977) demonstrated that a regular activity regimen for elderly clients with arthritis, diabetes, and heart disease improved their health status. A matched group who did not participate in the program demonstrated no improvement in health. Activity stimulates and maintains bone tissue, muscle strength and endurance, joint flexibility, and work capacity. It enhances gastrointestinal, cardiovascular, and nervous system function. Exercise may well have a preventative effect against diseases, including heart disease, hypertension, and osteoporosis.

Many older people have health problems that make it difficult to participate in an exercise program. The nurse can be instrumental in planning appropriate programs for this group. Individual and group programs can be useful.

Any exercise regimen for the chronically ill elderly must be preceded by a careful assessment. What are the client's stresses and adaptations? Are there any physical impediments to exercise? What is the client's current daily schedule? What is the client's current activity pattern?

Exercise regimens will differ widely, depending upon the client's stresses and adaptations, abilities and disabilities. They should be modified to include necessary safety precautions. The program must be a balanced regimen of rest and activity. It must fit with the client's life-style and preferences. Exercise becomes a habit only when it fits comfortably with both the client's abilities and lifestyle.

The challenge is to provide sufficient activity to prevent the hazards of immobility and the adverse adaptations of chronic disease and simultaneously to avoid undue stress that might precipitate injury. To accomplish these goals, the exercise regimen should be initiated gradually, beginning at the client's current level of ability. It should be performed regularly, and gradually increased. The nurse should make regular assessments of the client's exercise tolerance and gains. A record of the client's activity throughout the day can be a useful assessment tool. The client should be told to record the amount of time spent performing relevant activities, such as lying down, sitting, ADLs, and specific exercises.

The nurse must also deal with the older client's feelings about beginning a structured activity regimen. If an exercise program is to be successful, the nurse must gain the client's cooperation. To do so, the nurse should include the client in planning and ask the client for suggestions on how best to structure specific aspects of the program. If clients resist the exercise program because of fear of harming themselves, the nurse should explain the benefits of exercise and the risks associated with inactivity. The client needs to know that a pattern of inactivity can initiate a vicious cycle that may contribute to the development of new health problems and eventual immobility. For example, with osteoporosis, inactivity increases the rapidity of bone loss and may increase the risk of fractures with even minimal daily activity. Many clients have negative feelings about exercise. It can be lonely, boring, and even painful. Clients need opportunities to discuss their feelings as well as encouragement to continue being active in spite of their feelings. Eventually, maintenance of a regular exercise regimen often has positive effects on emotions and may elevate mood.

All of the health problems discussed in this chapter alter mobility status. At the same time, they require that clients adopt an exercise and activity regimen, specifically designed to their strengths and limitations, if they are to reach and maintain their highest level of mobility. The details of activity regimens for clients with arthritis, osteoporosis, and Parkinson's disease are discussed below.

The Client with Arthritis. A regular activity program is the single most important therapeutic measure for clients with degenerative joint disease and rheumatoid arthritis. Unfortunately, it is often the most neglected measure. Clients who adhere to an exercise program retard the crippling adaptations of arthritis and prevent the development of adaptations to immobility. Clients who adhere to their medication regimens but fail to adhere to their exercise

programs do not make maximum gains in their mobility status.

The goals of an activity program for clients with arthritis are to:

1. Reduce joint stiffness and pain
2. Maintain or improve joint ROM and function
3. Increase muscle function and strength to aid in stabilizing involved joints

If these goals are to be reached, an individualized program of activity should be designed. The program includes the following elements:

- Active and passive exercise
- Rest periods
- Measures to protect joints
- Use of modalities and supports (such as heat, splints, and special shoes) to promote activity

A regular exercise regimen is the mainstay of the activity program. Chronic arthritis is associated with weakness and atrophy of muscles that move the involved joints. This initiates a vicious cycle. Muscles and tendons support and stabilize joints, and muscle action serves to brake joint motions. If muscles are weak, they add to the wear and tear on joints and increase pain. The pain of arthritis reduces joint range of motion. A program of graded exercise improves muscle and joint function and reduces the stiffness and aching pain that follow inactivity.

Each client needs an individually prescribed regimen of daily exercise that considers the stage of the disease and the involved joints. The nurse should design an exercise program in collaboration with a physician or physical therapist. Exercises should be carried out two to four times a day. They should neither hurt nor fatigue the client. The extent of effort can be increased gradually as the client's ability increases. In general, clients should begin with only a few repetitions of each motion per session, gradually increasing to 10 or 15 repetitions.

The exercise program should involve full range of motion exercises for all joints, not just arthritic joints. Even if clients are active, performing regular ADLs and other tasks is not likely to provide joints with sufficient range of motion. Active exercises are better than passive exercise for this purpose. Resistive exercises should be avoided. The client should also perform stabilizing exercises to strengthen supporting muscles around involved joints. Isometric exercises are preferred to isotonic. For example, if the knee is involved, the nurse should instruct the client in exercises that strengthen the quadriceps muscle group. If the lumbar spine is involved, the client should strengthen the abdominal muscles. Special attention should also be given to strengthening muscles that will be needed later to maintain the client's independence. For example, if multiple joints are involved, it is helpful to develop strong arm muscles to make future use of crutches easier. If involvement of either hand is likely to become incapacitating, the nurse can teach the client to develop a degree of ambidexterity. Periodically, the nurse should observe clients as they perform their exercises to assure they are doing them correctly.

Crafts may also be used as a form of exercise for specific joints. Weaving and needlework promote flexion of fingers. Pottery promotes extension of fingers. Similar programs can be devised to exercise wrists, elbows, knees, and hips.

The nurse should encourage the client to maintain the exercise program faithfully. The client needs to understand the reasons for making exercise a daily habit. As clients progress their exercise, the nurse needs to assess their exercise tolerance. If clients experience pain lasting more than half an hour or increased stiffness on the following day, they are doing too much. If this occurs, the nurse should encourage the client to spread the exercise program over shorter, more frequent periods. If the client complains of persistent pain, the nurse should revise the exercise program. Overeager or stoic clients may need to be cautioned about too ambitious an exercise program. On the other hand, the nurse needs to encourage overly sensitive clients to maintain the exercise regimen.

Rest periods are important for clients with arthritis. For the client with rheumatoid arthritis, fatigue is one of the most demoralizing aspects of the condition. Flare-ups of this disease have been associated with overfatigue and stress. The more inflamed the joints, the more rest is needed. The nurse can make a home visit to evaluate the environment and suggest ways to reduce energy expenditure.

Clients need to learn to incorporate rest into their life-style. They need to become attuned to their own responses to activity and stop an activity before they become overtired. Some clients find that an afternoon nap or a rest of $\frac{1}{2}$ to 1 hour at midday helps them get through the day.

As a general rule, clients with arthritis should be advised to interrupt sustained physical activity with short rest periods of 10 to 15 minutes. They should also schedule several rest periods at regular intervals throughout the day. Although rest is essential, too much rest for involved joints can be dangerous. Clients should not keep a joint in one position for too long, and they should not sit without moving for more than 20 minutes.

The treatment program includes measures to protect the involved joints by reducing the mechanical stress on them. Doing so prevents deformity and minimizes loss of function. Protective measures vary, depending upon which joints are involved. If the large joints of the hip are involved, clients may benefit from using a cane in the contralateral hand, using a walker or crutches, or elevating the ipsilateral foot with a shoe lift. If the client uses a mobility aid, the nurse must assess the client's ability to use it. The nurse should not assume that the client who has used the aid for a prolonged period is using it correctly. Incorrect use of an aid can lead to excessive weight bearing and trauma to involved joints. The nurse should also determine whether or not the aid is functioning correctly and is equipped with needed safety features. Supporting collars are useful in cervical arthritis to decrease motion and relieve pressure on nerve roots. Lumbar corsets or light braces may be used if the lumbar spine is involved; however, many older people do not tolerate braces and corsets as well as younger people.

The nurse should teach clients how to avoid doing unnecessary work with involved joints. Activities can be simplified by analyzing tasks and eliminating unnecessary steps. Clients should alter their activities to favor involved joints in order to avoid placing undue stress on vulnerable joints. For example, clients with involvement of the hands should avoid scrubbing, use both hands, not one, when working, and carry a heavy purse from the shoulder or elbow instead of the fingers. Clients with lumbar spine involvement should not lift heavy objects or wear heavy coats. Household equipment should be put on wheels. Clients with hip and knee involvement can relieve these joints by sitting as much as possible when working, avoiding climbing stairs and walking for long distances, and taking frequent rest periods. If arms are involved, clients should push, not pull, heavy objects. Some clients tend to use joint positions that foster deformity when performing routine activities. For example, when getting out of bed, they flex their fingers in a fist and push up, straining the knuckles. The nurse should teach the client to push up with the palm open. Opening jars and using manual can openers stress fingers. The nurse should suggest that the client install mechanical devices. Clients should also learn to be more aware of which joints they use when performing an activity and, when possible, using the strongest joint available for the job. When the hands are involved, pinching movements should be avoided. For example, heavy pots can be removed from the oven by putting the hands under the pan and placing the weight on the wrist and elbows, rather than by gripping with fingers and thumbs. Plates should not be held at the edge but with the hand underneath to provide a wider base of support. Because the elderly are particularly likely to develop contractures in inflamed joints, especially the knee and wrist, lightweight splints may be used to protect and support the joint in a functional position (Anderson, 1976; Grahame, 1978). Often, these are used at night and removed during daily activities (Williams, 1979). The nurse should determine if the client is wearing the splint as required and check the splint at periodic intervals to assure that it is in good condition and still fits the client. Alterations in the disease process may make wearing a splint uncomfortable. Splints should not be worn on a continuous basis because they cause muscle weakness.

The nurse should advise the client that using good body mechanics also protects joint mobility and relieves trauma on joints. Clients should maintain good posture when walking, standing or sitting. Clients should not slouch. Women should not wear high-heeled shoes. Work surfaces should be adjusted to convenient heights that promote good posture. Chairs with high seats, not low ones, should be used.

The nurse can advise clients about the use of a number of simple adjuncts to their activity program. Heat, especially moist heat, is a most important adjunct. It helps relieve muscle spasm and pain and ease motion in arthritic joints. Using heat before exercise helps clients limber up and improves the results of the exercise program. Use of heat at night reduces pain so clients can sleep. In the hospital settting, short-wave diathermy, ultrasound, and wax baths are used (Green, 1981; Knapp, 1978). If clients live at home, the nurse can suggest that they soak in a warm bath, stand under a hot shower, or apply hot washcloths. Some clients find that their ability to perform exercises improves if they do them when soaking in a hot bathtub. Hydrocollator packs obtained from pharmacies, heating pads, and infrared lights are also useful but more expensive. In some clients, heat seems to aggravate pain. These clients may benefit from cold applications.

When using heat or cold with older clients, the nurse should take special precautions. Because the elderly often have diminished perception of heat and cold, they lack the protection of normal sensation and risk trauma to tissues when using these modalities. If occlusive vascular disease is present, the older client's ability to tolerate local heat safely is further reduced. If the older client's cardiovascular system is compromised, soaking in a hot bathtub may result in dangerous hemodynamic changes that cause hypotension or syncope. In addition, because the older person's thermoregulatory mechanisms may be inefficient or impaired, prolonged exposure to heat may result in hyperpyrexia and to cold may result in hypothermia (Tobis, 1979).

Clients with arthritis need supportive shoes to increase mobility and reduce pain. They should use bedboards or invest in a firm mattress to assist in the maintenance of posture. Spring seats may be purchased to help them arise from chairs without straining joints. Clients with Heberden's nodes may find that wearing nylon spandex gloves, especially at night, affords relief of pain, throbbing, stiffness, and paresthesias.

Even during the acute phases of degenerative joint disease and rheumatoid arthritis, inactivity is dangerous. Use of bed rest during acute phases is controversial because it is associated with rapid muscle wasting and places the older client at high risk for decubiti and thrombi (Grahame, 1978). When a client in the acute phase of rheumatoid arthritis is placed on bed rest, passive and sometimes active exercises are prescribed appropriate to the client's condition (Williams, 1979). Excellent nursing care is required to minimize deformity and other consequences of immobility. Bed cradles, padded foot boards, and light splints are used to maintain joints in functional positions. The nurse should position the client carefully and support joints. Pillows to flex the knees are not permitted. Passive exercise is also prescribed during the acute phase of degenerative joint disease to minimize osteophyte formation (Hudak, 1977). Once the acute phase subsides and the fever disappears exercise is progressed according to the client's tolerance.

The Client with Osteoporosis. Immobility, particularly bed rest, must be avoided, as it aggravates bone loss and promotes osteoporosis. Bed rest is appropriate only occasionally during acute phases of the disease. Even when the client has a painful spine and collapsed vertebrae, efforts are made to avoid immobility if possible.

With younger clients who are susceptible to osteoporosis but have not yet exhibited its adaptations, the nurse should encourage maintenance of a physical fitness program throughout life. Regular exercise helps postpone and slow the demineralization process (Wallach, 1978).

The nurse should encourage the client with osteoporosis to develop a planned daily exercise program. Exercise improves the strength and endurance of atrophied muscles so that they can bear weight and increases range of motion. Exercise does not correct existing postural deformities.

An initial assessment is mandatory to avoid placing clients with severe osteoporosis on an exercise program that is too strenuous for their depleted skeletons. Doing so may cause additional vertebral collapse. The exercises should be carefully selected and matched to the condition and capacity of the client. Compressive forces on the spine should be decreased, not increased. Swimming and walking up to 3 miles per day are recommended. To assure safety when walking, shoes with broad flat heels should be used. A cane may help reduce compressive forces on the spine. The pace should be slow and the client encouraged to stand erect. Rid-

ing a stationary bicycle is also helpful. A real bicycle on a bumpy road or in traffic may involve the client in an accident and break vertebrae and bones. Other exercises to condition muscles should be performed daily while lying on the back on the floor. These will not strain the spine.

The use of heavy spinal braces should be avoided at all costs. The use of light, elastic corsets and spinal braces is controversial. If the client cannot tolerate them, they should not be used. In some cases, they reduce back pain and give clients the support and encouragement they need to remain active (Exton-Smith, 1978; Anderson, 1976).

Clients who are active need education regarding ways to promote safety and prevent accidents. They should avoid lifting heavy objects, making sudden movements, carrying much weight, bending over a great deal, and riding in cars at high speeds or on rough roads. These activities produce compression forces on the spine. If the client lives at home, the nurse should advise the client on ways to remove safety hazards. It is especially important to safeguard against falls. Loose rugs and extension cords should be tacked down. Stairs and hallways should be well lit. Clients should be told to use handrails when climbing stairs. With a regular program of exercise, clients with osteoporosis can return to a higher level of mobility and retard the progression of the disease.

The Client with Parkinson's Disease. The nurse should instruct clients to remain as physically active as possible. Exercise does not reverse rigidity but loosens stiff muscles, maintains muscle strength, and prevents contractures. Clients should participate in some form of exercise every day. Active and passive ROM exercise, stretching, and reciprocal movements control rigidity and improve mobility (Davis, 1977). Using a stationary bike or arm pulleys and squeezing a soft rubber ball also accomplish these purposes. If respiration is affected, clients should be taught breathing exercises. Any period of physical inactivity, however brief in duration, has severe negative consequences for the client with Parkinson's disease. If the client is bedridden, decubiti, contractures, and infections are special risks (Pathy, 1978; Steinberg, 1976; Anderson, 1976). Although clients complain of weakness and fatigue, they need to realize that prolonged rest only exacerbates this feature of basal ganglia disease (Fischback, 1978).

Gait and Posture.   The nurse needs to give careful attention to the client's safety during ambulation. Medication therapy gives the client increased mobility, but that mobility places the client at high risk for fractures, especially of the femur, as well as for angina and cardiac failure in clients with attendant cardiac disease (Anderson, 1976). The client should practice walking, taking long strides with feet apart and lifting the feet as though stepping over obstacles. Arm swing should be practiced. Clients should be taught to reach upward with the head for erect posture and balance when walking. When turning, clients should learn to take a series of small steps or raise their toes and place weight on their heels (pivotal turning). To help clients balance and reverse the tendency to fall backward when standing, the heels of the shoes can be elevated. Walkers can be provided to supply important stability during ambulation. Clients should be monitored carefully for fatigue and shortness of breath during practice sessions. "Freezing" may occur when clients ambulate or engage in many other activities and is often precipitated when clients are faced with motor decisions or minor obstacles. To prevent "freezing," clients should not be rushed or given too much physical assistance.

Other Activities.   Clients should be encouraged to use straight-backed chairs instead of low, easy chairs. Some clients need to learn transfer techniques or balance techniques to enable them to get up from a chair. Clients can be independent in moving about in bed if a rope is attached to the foot of the bed to enable clients to pull themselves to a sitting position. Adherence to an exercise regimen is an important part of the therapeutic regimen that can retard the onset of the immobility that occurs in advanced Parkinson's disease.

SUMMARY

Because of normal aging changes in bone, muscle, joints, and nerves, older people are especially vulnerable to stresses that threaten to alter mobility. Many older people believe that a diagnosis such as arthritis or Parkinson's disease consigns them to a life of dependence upon others to meet their basic needs. Although new medications have done much to slow the course of disease and improve the quality of life for clients with impairments in mobility, it is their own efforts that ultimately determine the success or failure of the plan of care. Nursing roles include teaching clients and supporting them as they learn effective strategies for managing pain and maintaining an activity regimen that maximizes independence.

REFERENCES

Agate J: Common symptoms and complaints, in Rossman I (ed), Clinical Geriatrics. 2nd ed. Philadelphia, Lippincott, 1979

Agus B: Hyperuricemia—What to do about it? Consultant 19(12):19, 1979

Anderson F Sir: Practical Management of the Elderly, 3rd ed. Oxford, Blackwell, 1976

Avioli LV: Aging, bone and osteoporosis, in Steinberg FU (ed), Cowdry's The Care of the Geriatric Patient, 5th ed. St. Louis, Mosby, 1976

Basbaum AT, Fields NL: Endogenous pain control mechanisms: Review and hypothesis. Annals of Neurology 4:451, 1978

Benoliel JO, Crowley DM: The patient in pain: New concepts. Nursing Digest 5(2):41, 1977

Blinchik ER, Grzesiak RC: Reinterpretative cognitive strategies in chronic pain management. Archives of Physical Medicine and Rehabilitation 60:609, 1979

Bluhm GB, McCarty DJ, Wallace SL: "Live with it" is out for gout. Patient Care 11(6):18, 1977

Bonner CD: Medical Care and Rehabilitation of the Aged and Chronically Ill, 3rd ed. Boston, Little, Brown, 1974

Boykin L: Controlling gout through diet. Nursing Care 10(10):18, 1977

Brewerton DA: Rheumatic disorders, in Rossman I (ed), Clinical Geriatrics, 2nd ed. Philadelphia, Lippincott, 1979

Brown-Skeers V: How the nurse practitioner manages the rheumatoid arthritis patient. Nursing 79 9(6):26, 1979

Burnside IM: Psychosocial caring: Touch, sexuality and cultural aspects, in Burnside IM, Ebersol P, Monea HE (eds), Psychosocial Caring Throughout the Life Span. New York, McGraw-Hill, 1978

Burroughs Wellcome Co. Medical Notes on Parkinsonism and Pseudoparkinsonism. Research Triangle Park, NC, The Company, 1972

Butler RN, Lewis MI: Aging and Mental Health: Positive Psychosocial Approaches. 2nd ed. St. Louis, Mosby, 1977

Caird FI: Parkinsonism, in Anderson F Sir, Ferguson W, Judge TG (ed), Geriatric Medicine. London, Academic, 1974

Calin A: Gerontology—Aspects of Rheumatology, in Ebaugh FO (ed), Management of Common Problems in Geriatric Medicine. Menlo Park, CA, Addison Wesley, 1981

Charlesworth D, Baker RH: Surgery in old age, in Brocklehurst JC (ed), Textbook of Geriatric Medicine and Gerontology, 2nd ed. Edinburgh, Churchill Livingstone, 1978

Clark H: Osteoarthritis—An interesting case? Nursing Clinics of North America 11(1):199, 1976

Davis JC: Team management of Parkinson's disease. The American Journal of Occupational Therapy 31(5):300, 1977

Davison W: Medical treatment in the elderly, in Folmer ANJR, Schouten J (eds), Geriatrics for the Practitioner. Amsterdam, Excerpta Medica, 1981

DeCarlo TJ, Castiglione LV, Caousoglu M: A program of balanced physical fitness in the preventive care of elderly ambulatory patients. Journal of the American Geriatrics Society XXV(7):331, 1977

Devas M: Orthopedics, in Steinberg FU (ed), Cowdry's The Care of the Geriatric Patient, 5th ed. St. Louis, Mosby, 1976

Durnin JVGA: Nutrition, in Brocklehurst JC (ed), Textbook of Geriatric Medicine and Gerontology, 2nd ed. Edinburgh, Churchill Livingstone, 1978

Eland JM: Living with pain. Nursing Outlook 26(7):430, 1978

Elkowitz EB: Geriatric Medicine for the Primary Care Practitioner. New York, Springer, 1981

Exton-Smith AN: Bone aging and metabolic bone disease, in Brocklehurst JC (ed), Textbook of Geriatric Medicine and Gerontology, 2nd ed. Edinburgh, Churchill Livingstone, 1978

Exton-Smith AN, Caird FI (eds): Metabolic and Nutritional Disorders in the Elderly. Chicago, Year Book, 1980

Fischback FT: Easing adjustment to Parkinson's disease. American Journal of Nursing 78(1):66, 1978

Fordyce WE: Evaluating and managing chronic pain. Geriatrics 33(1):59, 1978

Frankel LJ, Richard BB: Be Alive As Long As You Live. Charleston, WV, Preventicare Publications, 1977

Gaumer WR: Electrical stimulation in chronic pain. American Journal of Nursing 74(3):504, 1974

Gibherd FB, Page NGR, Spencer KM, et al: Controlled trial of physiotherapy and occupational therapy for Parkinson's disease. British Medical Journal 282:1196, 1981

Goldman R: Decline in organ function with aging, in Rossman I (ed), Clinical Geriatrics, 2nd ed. Philadelphia, Lippincott, 1979

Gore I: Physical activity in old age. Nursing Mirror 142(7):49, 1976

Grahame R: Disease of the joints, in Brocklehurst JC (ed), Textbook of Geriatric Medicine and Gerontology, 2nd ed. Edinburgh, Churchill Livingstone, 1978

Green MF: Metabolic emergencies, in Coakley D (ed), Acute Geriatric Medicine. Littleton, MA, PSG Publishing, 1981

Gregerman RI, Bierman EL: Aging and hormones, in Williams RH (ed), Textbook of Endocrinology. Philadelphia, Saunders, 1981

Gresh C: Helpful tips you can give your patient with Parkinson's disease. Nursing 80 10(6):26, 1980

Habermann ET: Orthopaedic aspects of the lower extremities, in Rossman I (ed), Clinical Geriatrics, 2nd ed. Philadelphia, Lippincott, 1979

Hahn BH: Arthritis, bursitis and bone disease, in Steinberg FU (ed), Cowdry's The Care of the Geriatric Patient, 5th ed. St. Louis, Mosby, 1976

Hanna MJD, MacMillan AL: The skin, in Brocklehurst JC (ed), Textbook of Geriatric Medicine and Gerontology. 2nd ed. Edinburgh, Churchill Livingstone, 1978

Hardin WB: Neurological aspects, in Steinberg FU (ed), Cowdry's The Care of the Geriatric Patient, 5th ed. St. Louis, Mosby, 1976

Harris E: Extrapyramidal side effects. American Journal of Nursing. 81(7):1324, 1981

Hawker M: Keep-fit exercises for geriatric patients. Nursing Mirror 142(7):50, 1976

Hudak CM: A pyramidal treatment plan for the patient with arthritis. Nurse Practitioner 2(5):19, 1977

Hyams DE: The blood, in Brocklehurst JC (ed), Textbook of Geriatric Medicine and Gerontology, 2nd ed. Edinburgh, Churchill Livingstone, 1978

Jacox AK: Assessing pain. American Journal of Nursing. 79(5):895, 1979

Kastenbaum R: The physician and the terminally ill old person, in Rossman I (ed), Clinical Geriatrics, 2nd ed. Philadelphia, Lippincott, 1979

Knapp ME: Managing osteoarthritis: The role of physical medicine. Consultant 18(7):82, 1978

Kolodny AL, Klipper AR: Bone and joint diseases in the elderly. Hospital Practice 11(11):91, 1976

Langan J: Parkinson's disease: Assessment procedures and guidelines for counseling. Nurse Practitioner 2(6):13, 1976

Langan RJ, Cotzias GC: "Do's and don'ts for the patient on levodopa therapy." American Journal of Nursing 76(6):917, 1976

Lee TN: Thalamic neuron theory: A hypothesis concerning pain and acupuncture. Medical Hypothesis 3(3):113, 1977

Low AW: The patient's view of osteoporosis. Nursing Times 75(1):38, 1979

Luce JC, Thompson TL, Getto CJ, Byyny RL: New concepts of chronic pain and their implications. Hospital Practice 14(4):113, 1979

McCaffery M: Relieving pain with noninvasive techniques. Nursing 80 10(12):55, 1980

McCarty DJ: The management of gout. Hospital Practice 14(9):75, 1979

McMahon MA, Miller P: Pain response: The influence of psycho-social-cultural factors. Nursing Forum XVII (1):58, 1978

Melzack R: The Puzzle of Pain. New York, Basic Books, 1973

Melzack R, Wall PD: Pain mechanisms: A new theory. Science 150:3699, 1965

Moskowitz RW: Management of osteoarthritis. Hospital Practice 14(7):75, 1979

Nordin BEC: Calcium metabolism and bone, in Exton-Smith AN, Caird FI (eds), Metabolic and Nutritional Disorders in the Elderly. Chicago, Year Book, 1980

Palkovitz HP: Parkinson's disease: An update on diagnosis and treatment. Consultant 18(10):54, 1978

Pathy MS: Clinical presentation and management of neurological disorders in old age, in Brocklehurst JC, (ed), Textbook of Geriatric Medicine and Gerontology, 2nd ed. Edinburgh, Churchill Livingstone, 1978

Pathy MS: Clinical presentation of myocardial infarction in the elderly. British Heart Journal 29:190, 1967

Pearson LJ, Kotthoff ME: Geriatric Clinical Protocols. Philadelphia, Lippincott, 1979

Peck WA, Recher RR, Saville PD: Osteoporosis: Exploring options and odds. Patient Care 11(18):72, 1977

Pont A: Management of osteoporosis, in Ebaugh FG (ed), Management of Common Problems in Geriatric Medicine. Menlo Park, CA, Addison Wesley, 1981

Pratt MA: Physical exercise: A special need in long term care. Journal of Gerontological Nursing 4(5):38, 1978

Price JH, Luther SL: Physical fitness: Its role in health for the elderly. Journal of Gerontological Nursing 6(9):517, 1980

Rossman I: The anatomy of aging, in Rossman I (ed), Clinical Geriatrics, 2nd ed. Philadelphia, Lippincott, 1979

Sambrook MA: Parkinsonism. Nursing Times 72(12):454, 1976

Schroeder HA: Nutrition, in Steinberg FU (ed), Cowdry's The Care of the Geriatric Patient, 5th ed. St. Louis, Mosby, 1976

Schwald MC: Advice to arthritics: Keep moving. American Journal of Nursing 78(10):1708, 1978

Shealy CN: Chronic pain intervention techniques. Topics in Clinical Nursing 2(1):1, 1980

Siegele DS: The gate control theory. American Journal of Nursing 74(3):498, 1974

Smith SE: Drugs and parkinsonism. Nursing Times 71:1828, 1975

Steinberg FU: Rehabilitation medicine, in Steinberg FU (ed), Cowdry's The Care of the Geriatric Patient, 5th ed. St. Louis, Mosby, 1976

Sternback RA: Pain: Patients, Traits and Treatment. New York, Academic, 1974

Storandt M: Psychological aspects of aging, in Rossman I (ed), Clinical Geriatrics, 2nd ed. Philadelphia, Lippincott, 1979

Sweet RD: Parkinson's disease: Current diagnosis and treatment, in Fields WS (ed), Neurological and Sensory Disorders in the Elderly. New York, Stratton Intercontinental, 1975

Sweet RD, McDowell FH: Five years treatment of Parkinson's disease with levodopa: Therapeutic results and survival of 100 patients. Annals of Internal Medicine 83:456, 1975

Tobis JA: Rehabilitation of the geriatric patient, in Rossman I (ed), Clinical Geriatrics, 2nd ed. Philadelphia, Lippincott, 1979

Vaterlaus E: A holistic approach to nursing the patient in pain. Canadian Nurse 75(6):22, 1979

Wallach S: Management of osteoporosis. Hospital Practice 13(12):91, 1978

Weg RB: Changing physiology of aging: Normal and pathological, in Woodruff D, Birren J (eds), Aging: Scientific Perspectives and Social Issues. New York, Van Nostrand, 1975

Weissman G: Clinical strategy in the arthritides. Hospital Practice 14(6):11, 1979

White A: Rheumatoid arthritis. Nursing Mirror 143(18):i, 1976

Williams RC: Rheumatoid arthritis. Hospital Practice 14(6):57, 1979

Wolf ZR: Pain theories. Topics in Clinical Nursing 2(1):9, 1980

Wright V: Rheumatoid arthritis—Conservative management. Nursing Times 73(48):1878, 1977

Yahr MD: Early recognition of Parkinson's disease. Hospital Practice 7:65, 1981

Zborowski M: People in Pain. San Francisco, Jossey-Bass, 1969

16

Nursing the Client Experiencing Problems of Regulation

Regulation enables the organism to maintain cells, tissues, and organs within a normal range of function. Regulatory mechanisms prevent either excessive or diminished functioning that would be incompatible with safety or survival. Body systems essential to the maintenance of regulation include the nervous, endocrine, and immunological systems. Although the ego cannot be described in physiological terms, there are many who would add it to the list of behavioral regulators.

The mechanisms of regulation may be either internal or external to the cell. Genes, enzymes, and vitamins, for example, operate internally; hormones circulate outside the cell as messengers, providing the key that unlocks the cell to outside regulation.

This chapter reviews four major disturbances in regulation prevalent in aging populations:

- Hearing loss
- Depression
- Acute and chronic brain disorders
- Diabetes mellitus

All of these problems threaten the elderly person's ability to adapt. Most older people with these problems can function at Adaptation Level Three provided they learn to use appropriate supports, such as therapeutic diets, medications, or a hearing aid.

As in the preceding chapters, description of all four problems is followed by sections on assessment and sections on nursing interventions. Two interventions that are emphasized are the nurse's role in diet therapy and therapeutic interaction.

SIGNIFICANT PROBLEMS

Hearing Loss

The prevalence of handicapping hearing impairments increases with age. Hearing problems are at least ten times as common in old age as in young adulthood (Oyer and Oyer, 1979). As many as 50 percent of people over age 65 in the United States possess some degree of hearing impairment (Hull, 1977). About 30 percent of the elderly experience significant adaptations that impair communication and require aural rehabilitation (Butler and Lewis, 1977). Although hearing loss is common it is not universal among the aged. Consequently, the nurse should evaluate each older client individually rather than assume that all older people are hard-of-hearing.

Extent of Hearing Loss. Hearing loss exists on a continuum from mild to profound. The term "hard-of-hearing" describes persons in whom hearing is defective but functional, with or without a hearing aid. Most older people fall into this category. The term "deaf" denotes a loss that is so profound that hearing is not functional (McCartney and Nadler, 1979).

Types of Hearing Loss. Hearing loss involves a deterioration in acuity for pure tones (hypacusis) and deterioration in acuity, reception, and discrimination for speech (dysacusis). There are three types of hearing loss: conductive, sensorineural, and mixed. *Conductive losses* are caused by abnormalities of the external auditory canal, tympanic membrane, or middle ear space that obstruct the transmission of sound to the inner ear fluids. *Sensorineural losses* are caused by abnormalities of the cochlea, eighth cranial nerve, or its central connections. These prohibit the transduction of mechanical to electrical impulses and the transmission of neural responses to the auditory central nervous system. Combinations of conductive and sensorineural losses are called *mixed losses* (Gacek, 1975).

Stresses Associated with Hearing Loss. Hearing loss is an adaptation. For many older people, however, it becomes a stress that stimulates serious psychological and social difficulties. The same factors that cause hearing loss in the young can do so in the old. Hearing loss may be a direct consequence of normal or pathological changes in the auditory system itself or a manifestation of a disorder in another body system.

Outer Ear. The most common cause of conductive hearing loss in the elderly is cerumen that occludes the external auditory canal (Ruben, 1977). Generally, the result is only a negligible hearing loss. However, if the older person already has another conductive or sensorineural loss, the combination of stresses may significantly impair hearing. External otitis, due to bacterial or fungal infection, rarely impairs hearing, but may do so, especially in older, diabetic persons, if the ear canal is blocked.

Middle Ear. Stresses of the middle ear account for hearing loss in only 3 percent of the elderly (Alberti, 1977). Secretory otitis media, chronic otitis media, perforation of the tympanic membrane, tympanosclerosis, cholesteatoma, middle ear tumors, and head injury are potential stresses. Otosclerosis, a genetic disease, may affect hearing as early as the third decade, but the hearing loss may not become noticeable until the client reaches old age and hearing losses from other stresses are superimposed.

Hearing loss that involves the middle ear may be due to a number of systemic processes. For example, acute otitis media may result from the impaired immunity that accompanies leukemia and other carcinomas. Serous otitis media may occur when a nasopharyngeal tumor blocks the Eustachian tube. Paget's disease of the bone, which affects about ten percent of people over eighty, causes a progressive, bilateral mixed hearing loss in those with skull involvement (Margolis and Sherman, 1981).

Inner Ear. Stresses that affect the cochlear or retrocochlear portions of the inner ear and result in sensorineural hearing loss include environmental factors, pathological processes, and aging. Ototoxic medications (Table 1) can damage either the vestibular or cochlear portion of the eighth cranial nerve, or both. Often, ototoxicity is dose related. Older persons with impaired renal function are especially vulnerable. Except for aspirin, discontinuing the drug rarely reverses the neurosensory loss. Sound trauma is another environmental stress that may have neurosensory consequences. Vascular disorders, including arteriosclerosis, hypertension, and vascular accident may cause gradual or sudden unilateral hearing losses if the essential blood supply is compromised. Ménière's disease, viral labyrinthitis, syphilis, and acoustic neuroma are other factors responsible for sensorineural hearing loss in the elderly. Diabetes and other degenerative diseases may be associated with gradual, bilateral sensorineural hearing loss.

Presbycusis is the gradual, progressive, permanent, bilateral hearing loss due to age alone. Chapter 5 describes the physiological changes associated with presbycusis. As early as the third decade, the degenerative changes of presbycusis begin in all portions of the auditory system. These are believed to affect about 60 percent of all those over age 65 in the United States (Hull and Trainor, 1977). Presbycusis is the most common cause of hearing loss in older people (Gacek, 1975). Its prevalence has not been established to a satisfactory degree because it is difficult to determine whether the sensorineural losses exhibited by so many older people are due only to aging or to a combination of factors,

TABLE 1. **MEDICATIONS WITH POTENTIAL OTOTOXICITY**

Medication	Potential Adaptation
Aminoglycoside Antibiotics	
Amikacin sulfate	Adaptations vary depending on specific drug. Hearing
Capreomycin sulfate	loss is usually bilateral, sensorineural, beginning in high
Dihydrostreptomycin	frequencies and progressing to lower frequencies.
Gentamicin	Speech discrimination may be affected. Tinnitus may
Kanamycin	precede hearing loss. Damage to the vestibular portion
Neomycin	may occur first. Look for vertigo, ataxia, nausea, and
Paromomycin	changes in the ability to ambulate. Hearing loss may not
Streptomycin	appear until after cessation of medication.
Tobramycin	
Vancomycin	
Viomycin	
Diuretics	
Ethacrynate sodium	Hearing loss may involve all frequencies. Speech
Ethacrynic acid	discrimination may be inordinately poor. Loss may be
Fenoprofen calcium	transient or permanent. Vestibular involvement may also
Furosemide	occur.
Acetylsalicylates and Salicylates	
Aspirin	Decreased hearing, especially in high frequencies.
Chloroquine phosphate	High-frequency tinnitus.
Quinine	
Miscellaneous	
Polymixin B	Progressive hearing loss.

such as heredity and noise, which produce adaptations similar to presbycusis. The etiology of presbycusis is unclear. It may be related to metabolic or vascular changes that occur with aging and affect the sensory and neural structures of the ear and the brain (Senturia et al., 1976). Oyer and Oyer (1979) cite research that questions whether presbycusis is in fact a normal aging process or a function of diet, noise, anxiety, and other stresses. In their studies of various primitive cultures, these researchers found a much lower incidence of presbycusis than in this culture.

Several different forms of presbycusis have been identified. Each has unique physiological characteristics and effects on hearing ability (Schuknecht, 1964; Gacek, 1975). *Sensory presbycusis* results from progressive atrophy of hair cells of the organ of Corti. *Neural presbycusis* is associated with loss of nerve fibers, especially in the auditory pathways and cochlea. *Metabolic presbycusis* re-

sults from changes in the stria vascularis. The pathology of *mechanical presbycusis* is unclear but appears to be associated with the cochlear partition. Many other forms of presbycusis are believed to exist. Changes in the brainstem and auditory cortex are likely to be significant in their development. More research needs to be done to determine what physiological changes occur in the aging auditory system and how these influence hearing.

Classifying the various forms of presbycusis draws attention to the widespread nature of the degenerative changes that occur in the aging auditory system. However, the nurse should bear in mind that many older people exhibit manifestations of not one, but several types of presbycusis. The resulting adaptations are additive. Other otological conditions may exist coincidentally. Because the resulting picture of adaptations reflects each process, it may be complex. Consequently it is important not to take a simplistic approach when assessing and managing the older client with hearing loss.

Depression

Regulatory mechanisms of the brain are subject to defective development, which may be of genetic origin or result from a deficiency or excess of brain amines (i.e., catecholamines). An extra X or Y chromosome can cause a mild intellectual or personality disorder (Kety, 1979). In Down's syndrome, an extra autosomal chromosome (number 21) causes mental and physical retardation. An excess of the neurotransmitter norepinephrine is thought to be responsible for manic behavior, while a deficiency is thought to cause depression. In like manner, a deficiency of acetylcholine has been found in cases of dementia—both presenile and senile types. Disturbances of regulation may also arise from an individual's perception of the situation, that is, the state of ego functioning, and give rise to anxiety, which also affects behavior.

In addition to genes and neurochemicals, a number of other stresses disturb the regulatory system of the brain. Among them are infectious agents, trauma, vascular insufficiencies, poisons, neoplasms, developmental defects, and psychogenic disorders (Beland, 1965). The brain is especially sensitive to trauma, neoplasm, and disturbances in blood supply. All of these regulatory disturbances result in physical and psychological adaptations.

Depression is the most prevalent psychiatric disorder of the later years. This finding is hardly unusual if one considers that social losses, ageism, and the deterioration of the family are commonly superimposed upon the degenerative diseases associated with the aging process. In addition, the older person's reduced responsiveness to stress may also contribute to vulnerability to feelings of depression.

Recent studies indicate that persons over the age of 65 show higher rates of psychopathology in general and depressive adaptations in particular than are found in younger population groups (Eisdorfer, 1980). The Duke Longitudinal study reported that as many as 20 percent of 209 community-based older subjects experienced significant depressive episodes during the course of a 3-year period. Prevalence data on depression among the institutionalized aged or those with significant illness are considerably higher. Some argue that these higher rates

result from studies that use symptom checklists rather than clinical evaluations. However, in a cross-national study that reviewed clinical evaluations, it was found that American psychiatrists tend to diagnose depression with less frequency than the British (Copeland et al., 1974).

Theories of Depression. Why do the aged become depressed so frequently? Many theories have been advanced, ranging from those that focus on the increasing social losses experienced by the elderly to those that look at genetic and biological substrata. There is also speculation that depression may be related to changes in brain structure or function or the body's decreased ability to respond to stressful events. Depression has also been linked to social and psychological changes in the later years. Refer to Table 2 for the terminology used in discussing depressive illness.

Genetic. Most genetic theories have been based on the incidence of depressive illness within families. Familial patterns of inheritance are seen in clients exhibiting manic-depressive illness (Cadoret and Winokur, 1975). Recently researchers (Weitkamp et al., 1981) reported locating one or more genes on the sixth chromosome that make people susceptible to severe depression. A nearby cluster of genes controls a part of the body's immune system (HLA system). The newly located genes are not necessarily specific for depression but may be involved with susceptibility to depression and other diseases. The researchers doubt there will be any simple explanation of the cause of depression.

Biological. Much evidence for a biological substratum comes from the success of drugs in altering mood—especially lithium, reserpine, and the tricyclics. Drugs as well as metabolic problems can affect the transmission of impulses across the synapse from one nerve cell to the next. Levels of MAO (monoamine oxidase) are higher in the elderly and MAO is known to destroy norepinephrine at neuron ends. The increased levels of MAO may cause low levels of amine at synapses (Lipton, 1976). In addition, changes that occur with age in thyroid and pituitary function may impair or diminish their role in mediating autonomic responses to stress.

Behavioral. The behavioral school sees the depressed client as lacking important sources of pos-

---

TABLE 2. TERMINOLOGY USED IN DEPRESSIVE ILLNESS

Endogenous depression—Etiology uncertain; usually without a precipitating event that explains the onset. Research indicates that neurochemical imbalance contributes to the disorder and that a genetic component may exist.

Reactive (exogenous) depression—Illness follows severe loss or disappointment; it is generally self-limiting.

Psychotic depression—Characterized by an inability to function, often with delusions and hallucinations present.

Involutional depression—Characterized by agitation, delusions of guilt, and hypochondriasis. Tends to appear first in women from 40 to 55, in men from 50 to 65.

Unipolar affective disorder—Depressive illness characterized by a change in mood from normal to "depressed" without a history of mania.

Bipolar affective disorder—Characterized by mood shifts of both mania and depression. Bipolar disease is thought to have a strong genetic component and is generally responsive to lithium therapy.

Neurotic depression—Affective disorder in a client with a long-standing personality problem.

Primary affective disorder—Affective disorder of a client with prior history of mania or depression.

Secondary affective disorder—Affective disorder in client who had or currently has another psychiatric disorder.

Source: Eisdorfer C: Unit 6, Multi-Media Medicine. American College of Physicians, 1980, with permission.

itive reinforcement either because of environmental change (e.g., death of a spouse) or personal inadequacy. Lewinsohn et al. (1976) proposed three reasons for depression. If the schedule of reinforcement is too lean, the frequency of behaviors that are likely to be positively reinforced will decrease. Secondly, reinforcements may not be contingent on behavior at all (this is the theory of learned helplessness, in which the individual cannot do anything to get positive reinforcement). Finally, when a change in the environment occurs (loss of a friend or spouse) behaviors that were formerly rewarded no longer are and they stop. The researchers also found that persons who obtain the highest rates of positive reinforcement are active, outgoing people who respond quickly to others and use many opportunities to give others positive reinforcements. Depressed persons manifest fewer of these skills. When a life change occurs, they have fewer skills to develop new sources of stimulation and rewards.

Seligman (1975) offers the theory of "learned helplessness." Dogs in a laboratory were administered shocks from which they were unable to escape. Later the animals were allowed to escape, but they did not try. In a subsequent experiment with

humans, Seligman and his associates found that when individuals were presented with noises that they could not control or problems they could not solve, they behaved much as the dogs did. He concluded that learned helplessness in humans was characterized by passivity, reduced aggressiveness, diminished appetites for food and sexual activity, sadness, anxiety, hostility, lowered self-esteem, decreased learning ability, and depletion of neurotransmitters—all hallmarks of depression. Seligman also found that depressed people tended to adhere to a thinking style that reinforced their depression, that is, they tended to blame themselves rather than others or the environment for their troubles. They also attributed good outcomes to forces outside themselves, thus depriving themselves of a sense of success even when they did succeed. Seligman believes that this negative view, while not the cause of depression, is a predisposing factor that allows depression to persist.

Cognitive Style.   Beck is the leading proponent of cognitive theory (1976). According to Beck, depressed people view themselves, their environment, and their future in an exaggeratedly negative way.

Even neutral events are construed as negative while good things that happen are ignored. In a classic experiment, Beck had depressed and nondepressed persons participate in a ring toss game. The depressed predicted lower scores and afterwards rated their performance as worse, when in actuality the scores did not differ from nondepressed subjects. Beck theorized that something akin to primary process takes place in depressed thinking. Between an event and an individual's reaction to it, there intervenes a cognition or "automatic thought" that dictates the resulting affect. If a friend fails to call, the depressed client infers that the friend no longer cares. The ensuing sadness acts as a stimulus to confirm the original thought. Beck found that therapeutic methods that dealt directly with these negative views, rather than with conflict in the unconscious, achieved improvement rather rapidly. Several studies have already suggested that cognitive therapy may be more effective than antidepressant drugs. The National Institute of Mental Health (NIMH) is currently mounting a study in that direction.

Life Changes. Early studies of depression emphasized its similarity to an exaggerated style of mourning and suggested that the influence of death of parents and traumatic childhood separations might increase a person's vulnerability. Although the relation of childhood losses to depression in adult years is still controversial, a majority of studies suggest higher rates of depression among persons who experience the death of a parent in childhood and adolescence (Zarit, 1980). Although no single category of events consistently predicts depression, studies have shown that depressed clients have experienced significantly more undesirable events in their recent past than control subjects and have more leavetakings from others for various reasons than do controls (Paykel, 1974).

Kay et al. (1955) suggested that illness plays a more prominent role when the onset of depression occurs late in life rather than early in life. Zarit (1979) cautions that recently uncovered biological correlates of depression do not imply causation. Life stresses or habitual patterns of behaving may lead to alterations of the various amines and their precursors. Biological vulnerability and personality and environmental stresses may all influence the development of depression. There may be several pathways leading to a common end stage of altered physiological responses and depressed behavior (Akiskal and McKinney, 1973).

Acute and Chronic Brain Disorders

All of the neurons present in the brain of an elderly person were present at birth (Strehler, 1975). In fact, if neurons were shed like skin or hair, built-in memories would rapidly disappear. To cope with the nonrenewability of the system, tremendous redundancy has been built in, so much so that even with partial destruction of the brain, one side is frequently able to take over for another.

Brain deterioration does eventually occur with age in one of several ways. Shrinkage occurs through normal involution of neurons; a general decline in neural reserve takes place, resembling the decline in other systems like the cardiac and respiratory systems; lasting damage can also occur from a prior insult (such as a cerebrovascular accident); and, finally, deterioration may result from specific disease processes (syphilis, herpes, encephalitis, or the von Economo virus, which has been linked with many cases of parkinsonism in the elderly today).

As the reserve of neurons diminishes, the ability to compensate declines (Laurence and Stein, 1978). When impairment of memory is first recognized it is often difficult to know whether the normal process of involution is occurring or whether it is the early stage of a disease process. Too often an acute disease process is mislabeled "senility." Many acute processes are reversible if recognized in time and properly treated. In fact, however, reversible processes often go unrecognized and progress to cause irreversible or chronic damage. Whatever label is affixed (reversible or irreversible dementia, acute or chronic brain syndrome, delirium or dementia) the primary adaptations seen are those related to intellectual impairment.

Adaptations in Acute and Chronic Brain Disorders. Normally individuals use both abstract and concrete thinking. Abstract thinking is the highest cognitive faculty that allows planning for the future and symbolic thinking. It is also the first cognitive faculty to be lost. It was Goldstein (1942) who first pointed out that brain-injured subjects lost the ability to conceptualize or to focus on thoughts about an object. Instead, they become bound to their immediate experience. Ideation tends to be impoverished, concrete, and associated with perseveration (the stereotypical repetition of words or phrases). The next cognitive faculty to be lost is memory, starting with recent events. Impairment in orientation is most marked for time, less for place and person. Judgment, along with the ability to plan for the future is also markedly impaired and the affect becomes shallow and labile, changing from laughter to tears or from anger to euphoria in a matter of seconds. In brain disorders, whether acute or chronic, impairment invades all spheres of functioning.

Brain Disorders in the Elderly—An Overview.
Delirium. This describes a set of adaptations in which impaired memory and orientation figure prominently. Delirium is characterized by a clouding of the sensorium with reduced level of consciousness and a reduction in the ability to shift focus and sustain attention (Sloane, 1980). It represents a temporary change in brain cell functioning. Illusions, delusions, hallucinations, and incoherent speech are also seen, and there is increased or decreased motor activity, that is, lethargy or agitation. Unlike dementia, delirium is characterized by its suddenness of onset, usually developing over the course of a few hours or days.

Dementia. This is the term given to a group of adaptations involving a global decline in intellectual ability that is sufficiently severe to interfere with a person's daily functioning (Mace and Rabins, 1981). The person is awake and alert but unable to think in abstract terms, do simple calculations, or make sound judgments. The impairment, which begins insidiously, may extend to speaking ability, coordination, and eventually involve severe personality changes.

Dementia has and continues to be called by many names (e.g., senile dementia, chronic brain syndrome, chronic confusional state, senility, reversible and irreversible dementia, arteriosclerotic dementia, and primary or endogenous metabolic encephalopathy). The adaptations can be caused by many stresses, some of which are treatable and some of which are not (Table 3). In some cases, dementia can be stopped; in others, it can be reversed; in still others, no amount of intervention can change the underlying process.

To complicate the distinction further, people with dementing illness may also develop delirium as a result of superimposed illness, infection or the introduction of a new drug. Findings also indicate that depression may be superimposed upon dementia, especially early in the process as the client begins to notice a change in intellectual functioning. Depression is also frequently confused with dementia by clinicians because the depressed client looks and acts demented. In a study of clients at the Johns Hopkins Hospital, about one-quarter of those who had adaptations of dementia were actually depressed and 82 percent recovered with proper treatment (Mace and Rabins, 1981). The Burke Rehabilitation Center (connected with Cornell Medical Center), which also studies dementia, reports similar findings (McDowell, 1980).

Most research data on dementia today indicate that about 50 percent of cases are caused by Alzheimer's disease, an irreversible condition, another 20 percent by multiinfarct disease, and another 10 to 20 percent by a combination of the two diseases. Still another 10 percent of cases of dementia are attributable to treatable causes, either metabolic disorders, structural problems of the brain (i.e., tumors, subdural hematomas, trauma), infections (syphilis, tuberculosis, meningitis or encephalitis), toxins (drugs or alcohol), or autoimmune diseases and depression.

Pseudodementia. This is a functional psychiatric disorder that mimics dementia (Wells, 1979). Clients present similar adaptations and give responses to mental status examination questions that are much like those seen in dementia. The condition was first discussed by Kiloh (1961), who described 10 clients with functional disorders, yet who manifested the classic changes of dementia—impairment of orientation, memory, judgment, and intellectual functions such as comprehension, calculation, and knowledge. He noted that in pseudodementia, the dysfunction was often of somewhat abrupt onset and short duration. Since then, other differentiating features have been suggested (Roth and Myers, 1975). The depressed client with pseudodementia often communicates a sense of distress, whereas with true dementia, the emotions are often shallow; such a client also does poorly on some tests of memory and intelligence but unexpectedly well on others. In addition, there is often a personal or family history of depression. Post (1975) pointed out that the adaptations of depression usually precede cognitive failure. He also observed that "near miss" answers

TABLE 3.   CAUSES OF REVERSIBLE DEMENTIA

Intracranial conditions
  Meningiomas
  Subdural hematomas
  Hydrocephalus
    Communicating
    Noncommunicating
  Epilepsy
  Multiple sclerosis
  Wilson's disease
Systemic illnesses
  Pulmonary insufficiency
  Cardiac arrhythmia
  Severe anemia
  Polycythemia vera
  Uremia
  Hyponatremia
  Portosystemic encephalopathy
  Porphyria
  Hyperlipidemia
Deficiency states
  B_{12} deficiency
  Pellagra
  Folate deficiency
Endocrinopathies
  Addison's disease
  Panhypopituitarism
  Myxedema
  Hypoparathyroidism
  Hyperparathyroidism
  Recurrent hypoglycemia
  Cushing's disease and steroid therapy
  Hyperthyroidism
Drugs
  Methyldopa and haloperidol
  Clonidine and fluphenazine
  Disulfiram
  Lithium carbonate
  Phenothiazines
  Haloperidol and lithium carbonate
  Bromides

Drugs (Continued)
  Phenytoin
  Mephenytoin
  Barbiturates
  Clonidine
  Methyldopa
  Propranolol hydrochloride
  Atropine and related compounds
Heavy metals
  Mercury
  Arsenic
  Lead
  Thallium
Exogenous toxins and industrial agents
  Trichloroethylene
  Toluene
  Carbon disulfide
  Organophosphates
  Carbon monoxide
  Alcohol
Infections
  General paresis
  Chronic meningitis
  Cerebral abscess
  Cysticercosis
  Whipple's disease
  Progressive multifocal leukoencephalopathy
Collagen–vascular and vascular disorders
  Systemic lupus erythematosus
  Temporal arteritis
  Sarcoidosis
  Cogan's syndrome
  Behcet's syndrome
  Carotid artery stenosis (?)
"Potentially recoverable dementia"
  Cerebral anoxia
  Trauma
  Excessive electroconvulsive therapy
  Encephalitis

Source: Cummings JL, Benson DF, L. Verne F: Reversible dementia. Journal of the American Medical Association 243:23, 1980, with permission.

on tests of cognitive function suggest organic deficit, whereas "don't know" answers are typical of pseudodementia.

Acute Brain Disorders. Adams et al. (1978) view delirium as part of a continuum beginning with a confusional state, progressing to disorientation, and, with-

out intervention, ending in delirium. Disorientation begins with time, then place, and finally involves orientation to person. Trockman (1978) believes the time to look for confusion in older hospitalized clients is on the second or third day following admission when they begin to react to an unfamiliar environment. Nighttime, with its decreased stimuli, is another time when the client with marginal reserve is likely to become confused, a phenomenon long recognized in nursing homes as "sundowning." Clients in the community may undergo an acute confusional state after a change in residence.

Stresses Associated with Delirium. In the elderly, delirium may result from any number of pathophysiological stresses, including metabolic imbalance, infection, drug intoxication or withdrawal, cardiac or respiratory conditions, or trauma. The emotional stress of illness or surgery can also trigger delirium. When an elderly client becomes delirious, however, there is rarely a single cause. More commonly the client is undergoing many interrelated stresses at the same time. As an example, a person with mild congestive heart failure and anemia may be given diuretics and a sedative for the agitation induced by the hypoxic state. Not infrequently the end result is an electrolyte imbalance.

According to Libow (1977) medications are one of the most frequent causes of delirium. All drugs that act on the central nervous system, especially sedatives, can cause delirium. L-Dopa, indomethacin, steroids, digitalis, propranolol, cimetidine, diuretics, the anticholinergics (especially found in over-the-counter cold preparations and sedatives), and aspirin have all been implicated. The so-called "salicylate jag" is similar to ethanol intoxication in that it produces varying degrees of confusion, stupor, and delirium.

Hamilton (1966) concluded that it was the loss of neurons with aging that was primarily responsible for altered reactivity and sensitivity to drugs. Not only does the aging central nervous system respond more sensitively but, as mentioned earlier, with declining liver and kidney function, the detoxification process is much slower. Thus, the introduction of any new drug is likely to interact unfavorably with drugs the client is currently taking.

Withdrawal from drugs or alcohol is another stress. Delirium tremens is a well-known phenomenon in clients hospitalized for medical or surgical conditions. Generally it takes from 48 to 72 hours for it to develop but the process may be delayed up to 10 days by exposure to anesthesia. Since alcoholism is not an uncommon problem among the lonely aging (Mishara and Kastenbaum, 1980) the nurse should be on the alert for this phenomenon even in the most unlikely candidates.

Sleep deprivation is another cause of delirium in the elderly client, especially in an intensive care setting where one is subjected to constant interruption of normal sleep. Adams et al. (1978) point out that REM sleep has a restorative function that maintains optimism, attention, and self-confidence and is especially important after periods of stress, worry, or new learning. Deprivation of REM sleep can result in hallucinations and psychotic episodes. Deprivation of non-REM sleep—the anabolic phase of sleep when RNA and proteins are synthesized in the central nervous system—produces lethargy and depression.

Sensory deprivation or overload may also lead to delirium. Deprivation may occur because of impaired vision or hearing, the absence of familiar surroundings or a clock or too little light. Overload, on the other hand, may result from pain or a noisy hospital environment. At times even the action in television programs may proceed too quickly for the elderly person with some degree of organic deficit to process.

Sloane (1980) lists a number of other conditions that can precipitate delirium. Decreased cardiac output, whether caused by an arrhythmia or heart failure, profound anemia, emphysema, or any hypoxic state, can all produce delirium. Hyper- and hypoglycemia, myxedema, hyperthyroidism, azotemia, uremia, and hepatic encephalopathy are some of the metabolic disturbances that produce delirium. Infections of the urinary tract, tuberculosis, pneumonia, inadequate fluid intake leading to an electrolyte imbalance, and urinary obstructions caused by benign prostatic hypertrophy have also been known to produce delirium. Finally, malnutritional states, especially deficiencies in thiamine, riboflavin, ascorbic acid, and vitamin A, all of which are commonly seen in the elderly, can also cause delirium.

Chronic Brain Disorders. Dementia, as indicated earlier, may involve reversible or irreversible conditions. Many of the reversible conditions have already been mentioned in the discussion of delirium. For a full list of reversible conditions, see Table 3. Once these conditions have been ruled out, there are only a handful of degenerative and vascular diseases identified as irreversible dementia. Of these, the two most common are Alzheimer's disease and multiinfarct dementia.

Alzheimer's Disease. This was named for a German neuropathologist who noted shrinking of the brain with nerve cell changes in a 51-year-old woman and called it presenile dementia. Until recently it was considered a rather uncommon disease. Senile dementia, on the other hand, was viewed as a less dramatic condition afflicting only clients over the age of 65. The prevailing view now holds that the two conditions—Alzheimer's presenile dementia and senile dementia, Alzheimer's type (SDAT)—are both clinically and pathologically indistinguishable and should be considered as a single disease entity (Katzman, 1976).

By combining all clients within a single category, the importance of this disease is highlighted. The disease is thought to affect anywhere from 500,000 to a million and a half Americans, contributing to as many as 100,000 deaths a year (Karasu and Katzman, 1976; Blass, 1980). Victims of the disease have only one-half to two-thirds the life expectancy of their peers.

Pathological findings in Alzheimer's disease include atrophy of the brain, minor loss of neurons, neurofibrillary tangles, granulovacuolar changes, and neuritic (senile) plaques. On microscopic examination the plaques appear as dying nerve endings (a center of debris) with proteins folded in a particular way (amyloid core). Recent studies using sophisticated microscopic and neurochemical techniques indicate that the real pathological process is the deterioration in the presynaptic portions of the basal and horizontal dendrites in the cortical neurons (Torack, 1979). The clumping of neurofibrils in the axons (the classic neurofibrillary change described by Alzheimer) and the formation of senile plaques are later changes. Perhaps the most exciting development has been the discovery that it is the cells utilizing the neurotransmitter, acetylcholine, that are principally affected by the disease.

Stresses Producing Dementia. Research is continuing in a number of areas to find the specific stresses that produce both the presenile and senile types of Alzheimer's disease and multiinfarct dementia.

STRUCTURAL BRAIN CHANGES. Neuritic senile plaques and neurofibrillary tangles are found in small quantities in the brains of normal older people. Scientists are analyzing their structure and chemistry for clues to their formation and role since they are found in abundance in the client with Alzheimer's.

BIOCHEMICAL. In clients with Alzheimer's researchers have discovered a striking reduction (as much as 90 percent less than normal) of the enzyme choline acetyltransferase, which is necessary to produce the neurotransmitter acetylcholine. Research is under way to find a way to increase acetylcholine in the brain or find a drug that mimics it. Since the body uses both lecithin and choline in making acetylcholine, research has been conducted using both these nutrients in the diet. Although the results to date have been disappointing—subjects appear brighter but perform no better on tests—the research goes on in these areas. Some short-lived improvement in memory has also been noted in Alzheimer's clients when parenteral physostigmine in low doses was used.

GENETIC. An adult's chances of developing Alzheimer's disease are 1 or 2 in 100 at age 65 but the odds increase fourfold if a close relative has the disease (Mace and Rabins, 1981). Alzheimer's is considered to be multifactorially inherited, with the HPI[1] gene serving as the facilitative factor. It is known that people with Down's syndrome have a good chance of developing Alzheimer's disease if they survive beyond 40. Heston and Mastri (1977) point to a unitary genetic etiology for Alzheimer's disease, Down's syndrome, and leukemia.

VIRUSES. Brain disorders such as Kuru and Creutzfeldt–Jacob disease are caused by slow viruses and accompanied by brain plaques like those seen in senile dementia, Alzheimer's type. There is no evidence at present to support the hypothesis that Alzheimer's disease is caused by a slow virus, but active research is under way in this area. Slow viruses cannot be detected by ordinary laboratory procedures and do not manifest signs of antibody formation, pus, or inflammation, which characterize most infections. They can exist in harmless latent states for many years, becoming pathological when the internal environment changes. Aging may activate these slow viruses.

AUTOIMMUNE SYSTEM. Some of the proteins used to fight infection are seen in abnormally high levels in Alzheimer's disease. Scientists suspect that the body's immune system may go awry and begin attacking brain cells.

MULTIPLE INFARCTIONS. Multiple infarctions are another cause of irreversible dementia. Formerly termed "hardening of the arteries," multiinfarct dementia is the result of repeated strokes within the brain that destroy small areas of brain tissue. Adaptations to multiinfarct dementia depend to some extent on the area of brain damage, although memory, coordination, and speech are generally affected. The progress of the disease occurs in stepwise fashion. Some multiinfarct dementias progress; others may not worsen for years. Some can be stopped by preventing further infarcts with anticoagulants, while others proceed to dementia. Bishydroxycoumarin, an anticoagulant, has been reported to have positive effects on intellectual functioning in clients with multiinfarct dementia (Walsh and Walsh, 1974).

Adaptations to Dementia. Apart from failing memory, some of the first adaptations to dementia are serious errors made in judgment. Early in the disease process, the client with dementia has insight into the problems that are occurring and often feels depressed. The person may, at first, attempt to cover the memory loss by changing the subject or avoiding certain social situations where familiar names must be remembered. When memory loss is gradual, there is a devastating loss of personal dignity and confidence. As memory loss increases, insight disappears. A poignant picture of dementing illness is told in the letters of a mother to her daughter, a nurse, as the woman monitors and reports on her own mental decline until she finally loses touch with her deteriorated state (Hagerty, 1980).

One of the first adaptations that brings the client to medical attention is wandering. Frequently, relatives complain that the person has gotten lost on a familiar walk through the neighborhood. Inappropriate behaviors, pointing to deteriorating judgment, also produce calls for help.

During the second stage there is increasing restlessness at night and an inability to recognize the meaning of stimuli (agnosia). The person finds it increasingly difficult to recognize familiar objects by touch (astereognosis) or by sight (alexia). In the third, or terminal, stage, irritability increases, speech becomes garbled as the client chooses the wrong word to express meaning (paraphasia), and cerebral seizures occur.

Diabetes Mellitus

Diabetes mellitus in the elderly deserves special consideration. More people who developed diabetes as youths are now surviving to old age. More people are living into their sixties, when the incidence of diabetes is highest. An estimated 17 percent of 65-year-olds have diabetes. Adiposity, an important risk factor for diabetes, occurs normally with age as the proportion of fat to lean body mass increases (Keen and Thomas, 1978; Gitman, 1974; Williams, 1978).

Diabetes involves a number of processes, all of which are characterized by abnormally high circulating levels of blood glucose. Two basic types of diabetes have been identified:

1. Juvenile-onset diabetes, or insulin-dependent diabetes, usually develops before age 25 but may develop in the elderly as well. The client does not produce insulin and is prone to ketosis. The onset of insulin-dependent diabetes is rapid and occurs in people of normal weight. Stresses believed to be associated with its onset include genetic predisposition, virus, or autoimmune factors.

2. Adult-onset diabetes, or insulin-independent diabetes, usually develops after age 40 and is the type most often seen in the elderly. Clients are usually ketosis resistant. They retain the ability to produce insulin but it is either insufficient or ineffective in preventing hyperglycemia. Stresses associated with the development of adult-onset diabetes include a genetic predisposition to diabetes, age over 65, obesity, infection, and other stresses such as surgery, myocardial infarction, cerebrovascular accident, or emotional distress, all of which increase the body's need for insulin to control the blood glucose.

Glucose intolerance is a normal adaptation to aging. Stresses associated with its development may include a delayed insulin response to a glucose load, reduced tissue responsiveness to insulin, an increase in the secretion of proinsulin and increased levels of insulin antagonists (see Chapter 5). Hyperlipemia, common in the elderly, acts as an insulin antagonist and may contribute to hyperglycemia. The decreased exercise levels of most elderly persons may also be a factor, since exercise potentiates the effect of insulin in lowering the concentration of blood sugar. Medications taken by the elderly, including thiazide diuretics, furosemide, ethacrynic acid, nicotine acid, estrogen, cortisone, and levodopa also contribute to a deterioration of glucose tolerance (Rifkin et al., 1979).

Because glucose intolerance is a normal concomitant of aging the question arises: When is the elevated blood glucose level an adaptation to normal aging and when does it signal the onset of diabetes? The fasting blood sugar, oral glucose tolerance test, and the presence of physical adaptations to diabetes are the criteria used to determine whether or not the older person is diabetic. Fasting hyperglycemia (a blood glucose level above 130 to 140 mg/dl) is considered diagnostic in the elderly when this finding is confirmed by a second test (Williams, 1978; Fitzgerald, 1978; Gitman, 1974). Prior to collection of a specimen for fasting blood sugar, the nurse gives the client nothing by mouth except water for 10 hours. However, the fasting blood sugar alone is unreliable since it does not correlate well with the presence of physical adaptations to diabetes in the elderly (Gitman, 1974; Williams, 1978).

The oral glucose tolerance test (OGTT) is used to determine the client's ability to maintain a normal blood sugar after a glucose challenge. It is the best means to diagnose diabetes in the elderly. Because severe carbohydrate restriction reduces glucose tolerance, the client must have a carbohydrate intake of at least 150 g daily for each of 3 days preceding the test, provided the client has consumed a normal diet prior to this period. In elderly clients with poor nutritional status, an intake of 250 to 300 g of carbohydrate daily for 3 days is more appropriate. Since physical inactivity and acute illness also decrease glucose tolerance, a minimum of 3 to 4 weeks should elapse following illness or bed rest before performing the test to produce accurate results. All drugs that might modify the test results should be stopped 2 weeks before the test. On the morning of the test, a fasting specimen is drawn, the client is given an oral glucose load of 50, 75, or 100 g, and specimens are drawn after 1 and 2 hours. During the test the nurse observes for signs of hyperglycemia such as mental confusion.

There is disagreement about the interpretation of the OGTT. Since oral glucose tolerance is a result of absorption, storage, and peripheral utilization of glucose, any age-related impairment of one of these processes, whether or not related to diabetes, may produce abnormal curves. Other factors, including

the time of testing, the size of the oral glucose load, ingestion of a regular meal as compared with pure glucose intake, the activity of the client during the test and the sampling and analysis procedures may alter the findings. It is best to use age-related norms to interpret the glucose tolerance test. The use of norms established for younger populations leads to the diagnosis of many false positives, that is, people with abnormal fasting blood glucose levels and no other physical adaptations. The nomogram developed by Andres (page 73) permits comparison of the client's 2-hour plasma glucose value with others in a similar age group. The diagnosis of diabetes is based on a decision about what proportion of the population should be considered diabetic at any age.

The Report of the Workshop on Definition and Diagnosis of the National Commission on Diabetes (1976) has recommended criteria for the determination of diabetes in the elderly (Figs. 1 and 2). Normal levels, borderline levels, and values that would be considered diagnostic of diabetes are indicated in relation to age. Although there is still dispute about what blood glucose values following a glucose load constitute diabetes, there is increasing evidence that treatment of hyperglycemia tends to reduce the frequency of many of its complications, including arterial disease and retinopathy. For this reason, it is not unusual for older clients with blood sugar values of 120 to 200 mg/dl 2 hours after a glucose load to be treated for diabetes (Anderson et al., 1979).

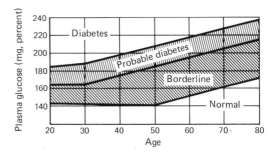

Figure 1. Diagnostic levels of plasma glucose 2 hours after glucose challenge for various ages. From Report of the Workgroup on Definition of Diabetes Mellitus. Washington, D.C., Department of Health, Education, and Welfare, 1976

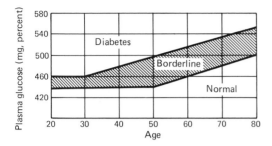

Figure 2. Diagnostic levels of sum OGTT/2 hour (F + 1 + 2) after glucose challenge for various ages. From Report of the Workgroup on Definition of Diabetes Mellitus. Washington, D.C., Department of Health, Education, and Welfare, 1976

ASSESSING THE CLIENT'S ADAPTATIONS

Hearing Loss

The nursing assessment is used to detect clients with hearing losses, to gather data about the loss, and to identify the impact of the loss on the client's ability to function. An important nursing responsibility is the determination of whether or not the client should be referred to specialists for further evaluation and aural rehabilitation.

If hearing loss is suspected, it is important that the nursing assessment be comprehensive. Adaptations vary widely depending on many variables: age at which the loss occurred, extent of loss, type of loss, frequencies affected, and communicative demand on the hearing system (McCartney and Nadler, 1979). In the older person, hearing loss is only one of many interrelated sensory changes. Together, these may have a profound impact on the client's perception, personality, and behavior. In addition, hearing loss in older people may be a consequence of a serious, even life-threatening stress. Many of these are amenable to medical or surgical intervention. Only when all other potential stresses have been ruled out should the nurse assume that hearing loss is due to age alone.

Detection of Hearing Loss. Cues to Hearing Loss. Although early detection is an important first step in the treatment of hearing loss, it may be difficult. Older people are at high risk for hearing loss, but they may not be aware of an actual loss because it has occurred so gradually that they have adapted over time. Other older people may be aware of their loss, but may not be aware of its serious psychological consequences. Some may accept the loss as a natural part of aging, believing nothing can be done about it. Other older people may view deafness as a stigma and deny their condition or resist efforts by others to have their hearing evaluated. Consequently, the nurse must be alert to subtle cues of hearing loss in older clients. These include inappropriate responses to questions, failure to respond to questions, difficulty following verbal directions, inattention, withdrawal, asking for clarification or repetition frequently, turning one ear to the speaker, watching the speaker intently, poor articulation, or speaking in a voice that is too loud or too soft, monotonous, harsh, or of unusual quality.

The History and Physical Examination. The history and physical examination identify clients with hearing deficits and provide information about the type of loss, its extent, and the reasons for it. When taking a nursing history from a client with a suspected hearing loss, it is important to gather data in the following areas: characteristics of the hearing loss, associated adaptations, related medical history, and family history. Table 4 outlines important information to be obtained in the history.

Conductive and sensorineural losses can be distinguished because each is associated with a unique pattern of adaptations. Many of these can be identified during the nursing history.

Conductive Losses. Clients with conductive losses exhibit a loss of hearing sensitivity, which is usually the same for all frequencies. Speech discrimination is relatively unimpaired as long as speech is loud enough to be heard. Low-frequency tinnitus may accompany conductive losses. The client may tolerate loud noise and hear better in the presence of noise than a person with normal hearing. The client may speak in a quiet voice because the conductive blockage enhances bone conduction of sound. Thus the client perceives sound as louder than without the loss.

**TABLE 4.   GUIDELINES FOR TAKING A
NURSING HISTORY FROM A CLIENT
WITH A SUSPECTED HEARING LOSS**

Characteristics
  Date of onset
  Nature of onset: sudden, gradual, fluctuating
  Unilateral or bilateral
  Ability to identify the direction of sounds
  Loss of hearing sensitivity
  Reduced speech discrimination
  Effect of noise on hearing
  Ability to understand telephone
    conversations, radio, television
  Ability to talk with one person; with a group

Associated adaptations
  Aural pain
  Itching
  Drainage
  Feeling of fullness in ear
  Tinnitus
  Nausea
  Vertigo

Related medical history
  Earache
  Head cold
  Allergy
  Ear drainage
  Ménière's disease
  Otosclerosis
  Viral and bacterial disease (mumps,
    encephalitis, bacterial meningitis)
  Perforated ear drum
  Tinnitus
  Head injury (broken nose, skull fracture,
    concussion)
  Degenerative diseases (diabetes, etc.)
  Hypertension
  Noise exposure
  Drug history (Table 1)

Family history
  Family members with hearing loss
    Nature of loss
    Reason for loss

Sensorineural Losses.   The client with sensorineural hearing loss usually manifests dysacusis as well as hypacusis. Most important, the client experiences less than normal understanding of speech and other sounds, even when they are loud enough to be heard easily. In addition, clients are sensitive to sounds presented above the threshold of hearing. They may complain that loud noise causes discomfort or makes them anxious, a phenomenon called "loudness recruitment." If present, tinnitus is usually high pitched. The client may speak with an inappropriately loud voice because the cochlea and eighth cranial nerve are impaired. The client usually hears best in a quiet environment, and in a noisy setting may complain of not understanding what is said.

Assessment Techniques.   Two of the most important components of the physical examination are the otoscopic examination and the tuning fork test. If the otoscopic examination reveals abnormalities of the external auditory canal or tympanic membrane, these are indicative of a conductive hearing loss. The otoscopic examination may be normal in clients with sensorineural losses.

Tuning fork tests are especially useful in providing information about the state of the auditory mechanism and the client's hearing sensitivity. Because hearing sensitivity from 500 to 2000 Hz is important for speech reception, it is important that 512-, 1024-, and 2048-Hz tuning forks be used for a complete examination. Testing air conduction gives information about the entire auditory system. Testing bone conduction measures only the integrity of the cochlea, eighth cranial nerve, and its central connections. The Schwabach test indicates whether or not the client's bone conduction and air conduction sensitivity are better or worse than the examiner's. The Weber test indicates whether or not the client's ears are affected to different degrees and whether or not a conductive component is present. In the Weber test, a lateralized tuning fork response indicates that hearing sensitivity between the two ears is different. The tuning fork will lateralize to the ear with a conductive loss. Lateralization to one ear does not eliminate the possibility that a less severe conductive component may exist in the opposite ear. If a sensorineural component is present, the fork lateralizes to the better ear. The nurse must explain the examination carefully to the client. Because it may be difficult for older clients to understand that the buzz of the tuning fork can be heard in the poorer ear, clients may become confused during the examination and respond falsely that they hear the tone in the better ear.

When used with the Weber test, the Rinne test adds valuable information about hearing ability. Air-conducted tones are heard longer than bone-conducted tones in a normal or sensorineural ear. If bone conduction is greater than air conduction, a conductive loss is indicated. Specific assessment techniques and findings for the client with presbycusis are discussed in Chapter 7.

Assessing Psychosocial Adaptations. The psychosocial implications of hearing loss can be vast. However, because hearing loss carries little status in the hierarchy of disabilities, these may be difficult to appreciate. Hearing loss is associated with many negative stereotypes, such as slowness. Because older people are already a part of one group (the elderly) that is negatively valued, they may be profoundly affected by this additional deficit. Ultimately, the adaptations may be so severe that clients may lose their independence altogether.

The nurse who identifies a client with impaired hearing must be aware of potential psychosocial adaptations. Most of these are known because they have been observed in hard-of-hearing older clients. Little research has been directed toward the identification of the psychosocial consequences of hearing loss.

Hearing plays a critical role in helping the individual feel a part of the environment. Three psychological levels of hearing have been identified: symbolic, signal, and auditory background. The symbolic level involves communication with words. The signal level involves the use of warnings or signals, such as bells and sirens, that communicate impending safety hazards. Auditory background functions on a primitive, subconscious level and includes background sounds such as rain, chirping birds, and traffic sounds. Because these sounds are usually faint, they are often the first to be lost. Because people take these sounds for granted, their loss is believed to be responsible, in part, for the feelings of depression, isolation, and withdrawal from the environment experienced by so many persons with hearing loss.

The inability to hear and understand makes it easy for the client to withdraw from communication situations that are potentially difficult. Withdrawal and avoidance occur on the part of the hearing-impaired person who is discouraged by communication failures and fears being misunderstood, and on the part of others who avoid those with hearing impairments because of the difficulty involved in communicating with them. Because the hearing impaired cannot grasp what is said, they are not a part of the ongoing stream of human events. Social isolation can cause bitterness due to feelings of exclusion. If social isolation continues, emotional problems may develop. Repeated communication failures can lead to low self-esteem in the older person. If others are not aware of the hearing deficit, they may label the isolated older person as "senile." Older people who do not understand their hearing problems may fear they are losing their mental faculties.

Butler and Lewis (1977) suggest that one of the most serious psychosocial adaptations to hearing loss is a reduction in ability to reality test, which can lead to suspiciousness and paranoia. For example, older people who see others talk but cannot hear what is being said may suspect they are being talked about. Hearing-impaired people may also experience frustration, anger, irritability, unhappiness, and tension due to the failures they experience in social situations. Even talking in a quiet room with one or two others may become impossible. Their loud, harsh, poorly articulated speech may have a negative impact on their social relationships. Tensions may spill over and affect relationships with friends and family (Oyer and Oyer, 1979).

Clients often feel embarrassed when they respond inappropriately in social situations because they have misunderstood directions or questions. Boredom is another adaptation of the hard-of-hearing person whose channels of communication are cut and of the audience who is subjected to a monologue by a hard-of-hearing person who is threatened by the loss and trying to avoid questions. Difficulties in hearing well and in rapidly processing information they do hear lead to fatigue. Finally, the safety of older clients with impaired hearing is at high risk. Loss of hearing may prevent clients from hearing warning signals (fire alarms, horns) or from localizing the warning if it is heard.

Depression

Depressive Adaptations.   Older depressed clients manifest an atypical pattern of depression, with less dysphoria or sadness and more depressive equivalents, such as somatic complaints, together with apathy, listlessness, and a quiet attitude of self-depreciation (Epstein, 1976). Pfeiffer and Busse (1973) found that excessive feelings of guilt or repressed anger are less frequently observed. Gurland (1976) also found that, unlike younger subjects, the older client tends to emphasize somatic complaints, such as insomnia, excessive sleep, loss of libido, headache, diminished appetite, and other gastrointestinal problems, particularly constipation. At times the level of somatic preoccupation may approach hypochondriasis. Somatizing may be viewed as an adaptive mechanism that allows the client to seek treatment within the medical arena, which is generally less threatening than asking for psychiatric help or emotional support (Eisdorfer, 1980).

In addition to somatic complaints, depressive adaptations cover a range of affective, behavioral, and psychological disturbances. The behavioral manifestations are readily recognizable—easy fatigability, apathy, social withdrawal, and loss of interest in previously enjoyed activities. Some clients may exhibit psychomotor retardation, an obvious slowing of speech and body movements that may result in social withdrawal, neglect of self-care, and refusal to eat or speak. Others become agitated, with adaptations ranging from restlessness, hand-wringing, and obsessive worrying to compulsive, repetitious behaviors. Another hallmark of depression is that the severity of adaptations may vary on a daily basis. Clients often appear more depressed in the morning and improve as the day wears on.

The psychological adaptations seen in the elderly include feelings of despair, pessimism, inadequacy, hopelessness, anger, and worthlessness. Disturbances of memory, attention, and orientation are usually prominent features. In cases of severe depression the client may exhibit nihilistic or somatic delusions (Table 5).

Assessment of the Depressed Client.   *Evaluating Suicidal Risk.*   Depressive illness has been the context for many suicide attempts, especially among the elderly. Except for extreme old age, suicide

---

TABLE 5.   CLUES TO LOOK FOR IN ASSESSING DEPRESSIVE ILLNESS IN THE ELDERLY

A recent major loss (e.g., loved one, employment, independent status)

Feelings of rejection by family or friends

Feelings of isolation from family members

Hostility toward those in a position to help (housekeeper, storekeeper, etc.)

Feelings of hopelessness

Absence of an identifiable role in life

Loss of sexual function, particularly one involving the loss or availability of a sexual partner

---

rates tend to increase among people as they grow older. The rate among males increases with each decade; in the eighth decade it is three times as frequent as in the third decade. Loss of health, death of a spouse, retirement, and children marrying and moving away are frequent precipitants of depressions of suicidal proportions.

Two independent investigations carried out in Scotland and the United States during the 1950s focused on suicide attempts involving the elderly and reported similar findings (Batchelor and Napier, 1953; O'Neal et al., 1956). About half of those studied had had previous mental illness, usually depressive in character, and those who had not been mentally ill were often limited in social adaptation, with shyness, dependency, anxiety, hypochondriasis, and restricted interest predominating. About 17 percent of the cases studied had a family history of suicidal acts, pointing to an apparent familial manic-depressive illness.

Suicide among the elderly is rarely an impulsive act, although it may at times be associated with alcoholism. Most attempts are not gestures or threats but rather failed attempts. The methods tend to be even more lethal than those used by the young—ranging from overdoses of hypnotic drugs, poisons, and gas to cutting, drowning, leaping, hanging, or shooting (Batchelor, 1957).

In evaluating an elderly client with a recent history of personality change, assessment of suicide potential is a priority (Havens, 1965; Murphy, 1975). The following risk factors should be carefully reviewed by the nurse.

DEMOGRAPHY. Depressed clients who are single, divorced, widowed, or living alone are at higher risk for suicide. There is often a temptation on the part of the nurse to empathize, "If I were in that person's shoes, I wouldn't have much to live for." It helps to remember that treatable depression is common among the elderly and there are an increasing number of programs available that make the outlook seem less grim.

REACTION OF THE NURSE. How does the client make the evaluator feel? This is often the single most important factor in the evaluation of suicide potential. If the client's life circumstances and affect make the nurse feel depressed, it would be unwise to send the client home. Some clients make the nurse angry, frequently the case with alcoholics; the nurse must be careful not to react with anger or send the client away without a complete evaluation.

EVENTS. The client should be evaluated for recent losses—death of a spouse or relative, a divorce, loss of a job, or financial loss.

COMMUNICATION. How well does the client communicate with the evaluator? Has the client been able to communicate with others recently? Withdrawal from relationships increases the risk of suicide. The client should be asked rather directly if suicide has been considered. Older clients tend to discuss suicidal thoughts more openly than their younger counterparts.

SUPPORT SYSTEM. A clear picture of the client's support system is invaluable. Frequently one finds a single or widowed person with no support system or with children who live at some distance. Their situation appears hopeless. An alternative reliable support system must be arranged with neighbors, friends, or the church and the nurse must continue to keep in frequent touch via the telephone.

ALCOHOL. The incidence of alcoholism among the elderly is much higher than most professionals imagine (Mishara and Kastenbaum, 1980). Alcohol is a solace to the lonely and the depressed but it is also a precipitant to suicides.

HOSTILITY. How hostile or angry is the client? Some clients may be so angry and hostile toward those around them that they truly wish to die in order to show how badly they have been treated.

Hostility is often a key factor in a contemplated suicide.

LETHALITY. If a client admits to suicidal intent, what method is being considered? The client with a well-thought-out plan that includes a lethal method (weapon, toxic substance, hanging) is at higher risk for suicide.

Client History. A good history will include a thorough review of systems since many diseases can exacerbate or produce depressive adaptations. For example, endocrine problems such as hypo- or hyperthyroidism, diabetes, hypo- or hyperparathyroidism, Cushing's disease, and Addison's disease, Alzheimer's disease, pernicious anemia, carcinoma, systemic lupus erythematosus, infections, and congestive heart failure can all produce depressive adaptations (Eisdorfer, 1980).

A thorough drug history should be included since many drugs produce depressive-like symptoms (Table 6). Are there any medications the client is receiving now or has received in the recent past that have been associated with a change in mental status? Have any relatives of the client developed similar adaptations when using the same drugs? Familial patterns to drug response have been noted. Reus (1979) reminds us that medication may carry a symbolic meaning for an individual that can produce adaptations not directly attributable to the drug's actions. For example, a man who is diagnosed as hypertensive becomes depressed shortly after receiving a prescription for reserpine. Is the mood change a direct effect of the medication or the diagnosis? If a drug produces constipation, it may result in feelings of anxiety, particularly for the older client for whom regularity of bowel function commonly serves as the barometer of good health. Elderly clients are particularly at risk for mental side effects to the following medications:

DIGITALIS. Approximately one out of every five clients receiving digitalis will experience some signs of central nervous system intoxication. Adaptations can range from fatigue and slight drowsiness to depression. At times, an acute confusional psychosis may occur. Labeling the client a "reactive depressive" may preclude consideration of medication as a focal stress.

PROPRANOLOL. This commonly prescribed beta-blocking agent has been employed for treatment of

---

TABLE 6.   DRUGS THAT CAUSE DEPRESSIVE ADAPTATIONS

Alcohol
Amphetamines
Antianxiety agents
Antidiabetic agents (oral)
Antihypertensives
Barbiturates
Corticosteroids
Digitalis
Estrogen preparations
Immunosuppressive or cytotoxic agents
Insulin
Major tranquilizers
Sedative hypnotics

---

hypertension, arrhythmia, and angina pectoris but a wide range of side effects, including toxic psychosis, insomnia, and depression, have been reported. The incidence of depression is unclear, one investigator reporting a 50 percent incidence in clients receiving 120 mg per day while another reported an incidence of less than 5 percent (Reus, 1979).

ANTIHYPERTENSIVE AGENTS. Many drugs used in the treatment of hypertension may affect sexual functioning. As many as 25 percent of male clients receiving methyldopa, clonidine, or guanethidine report experiencing episodes of impotence, retrograde ejaculation, and/or decreased libido. Female clients have noted difficulty in achieving orgasm. Methyldopa, in particular, has also been noted to cause amnesia like episodes and to affect concentration in cognitive tasks. Depression and/or a history of marital difficulty may be seen as indirect adaptations.

CORTICOSTEROIDS. Elderly and severely ill clients have been noted to be especially sensitive to the arousing, "vitalizing" effects of corticosteroids. With long-term treatment, however, the reverse is often true. Clients who initially show psychomotor activation, increased appetite, decreased sleep patterns and express feelings of well-being, may progress to signs of a depressive affect, drowsiness, and decreased cognitive ability.

HORMONES. In many cases hormones appear to act physiologically as neuromodulators of central nervous system activity, and there is growing evidence of endocrine involvement in many aspects of cognitive function and affective state. Thyroid hormones may produce thyrotoxicosis, with adaptations of anxiety, restlessness and a maniclike syndrome characterized by excessive hyperactivity, pressured speech, and euphoria. A female client receiving estrogen supplement may be at greater risk since estrogen increases iodine uptake and thyroxine levels in plasma.

Acute and Chronic Brain Disorders

Assessing Brain Disorders.   The early stages of delirium and early dementia may present with very similar adaptations. The client may simply look confused and be unable to follow simple directions or perform simple tasks like eating, bathing, and dressing. As confusion progresses to disorientation, the picture may still be perplexing. It is well to keep in mind that dementia is a more insidious process, which is gradual and progressive, whereas delirium occurs rather rapidly. Once the client has reached a stage of acute delirium, the clouded sensorium, diminished level of awareness, and the lethargy and exhaustion—or agitation—will be sufficient clues. Dementia is usually marked by an obtundity or slowing of mental grasp. As it progresses, it is often difficult to differentiate from a serious depression, although in depressive illness there is usually a clearer history of recent deterioration. Depression is also characterized by the vegetative signs—loss of appetite, weight loss, constipation, poor sleep, and early morning awakening. Late dementia is marked by a number of additional adaptations—alexia, apraxia, astereognosis, and agnosia.

It is important to remember that the elderly client with an acute infectious process—pneumonia or appendicitis—often does not exhibit pathognomonic adaptations like pain and fever. The first sign of illness may be a clouded sensorium. The client who becomes forgetful may be demonstrating the first adaptation of an underlying metabolic disorder. These situations make it mandatory that any client exhibiting a change in mentation or personality be thoroughly evaluated for an underlying reversible condition.

Interviewing the Client.   In interviewing the client, Trockman (1978) suggests the use of open-ended questions initially to reveal the extent of confusion.

Instead of a standard question, "How are you to-day," which produces the inevitable "Fine," try asking "What are your plans for today?," a question that requires some degree of organization to produce a response. If the client is unable to cooperate in the history taking, one or more family members should be enlisted. However, it is suggested that the client be present at the interview to affirm or deny the information elicited.

In taking the history, it is advisable to ask about headaches, nausea, vomiting, fainting, falling, ataxia, seizures, incontinence, memory loss, and lack of concern for personal care or the surrounding environment. The presence of these factors generally suggests an organic etiology.

To rule out a drug-induced delirium, a thorough history of medications should be elicited. Not only is it important to know what drugs the client is taking but whether they have been taken as prescribed. Most studies on compliance outside the hospital setting suggest that few clients really understand or follow the physician's instructions. Since many elderly clients take over-the-counter drugs, which they consider harmless, the nurse should look for the possibility of a drug interaction. It is also useful to ask if relatives have any known drug intolerance since the client may be reacting in the same way. Normally all drugs that are not necessary for life support will be stopped, and the dosage of even critical drugs will be reassessed.

A good nutritional history is also critical to find out the adequacy of food, fluid, and vitamin intake. Nutritional deficiency in the elderly may lead to brain disorders or may develop in those with brain disorders. In taking a dietary history, the client's current eating habits should be determined, as well as how those habits have changed with aging. Death of a spouse, retirement, or departure of children from the home should also be determined. Are three meals taken each day? What kinds of food predominate—meats? cereals? tea and toast? How often does the client shop for groceries? Some clients may be afraid to leave home to shop or their ability to prepare food may be impaired because they suffer from reduced mobility.

The Physical Examination.   A good mental status examination will detect the extent of impairment in mentation, memory loss, disorientation, and judg-

ment. The Mini Mental State Exam is useful in differentiating dementia from depression (Folstein et al., 1975). The test provides a formal measure of memory and orientation as well as cognitive and language abilities. Out of a possible score of 32, depressed but nondemented clients usually score 24 to 30; clients with Alzheimer's disease and senile dementia generally score below 20.

The neurological examination will also be helpful in differentiating dementia from depression. To rule out depression, the examiner should look for the reemergence of primitive reflexes—snout, sucking, and grasp reflexes—which are usually seen in dementia. Some authorities believe that primitive reflexes are more likely to be evident in late dementia; others have identified them in relatively early stages.

To test for the grasping reflex, stroke the palmar surface of the client's hand; the fingers will flex and pull against your hand. To test for the snout reflex, place a tongue blade vertically over the median portion of the lips and tap it lightly at the vermilion border of the upper lip; the response will be a pouting or puckering of the lips.

If confusion and disorientation have passed into the third stage of frank delirium, the neurological exam will reveal some focal weakness or abnormal movements. Posner (1975) found a coarse, irregular tremor on exertion which is absent at rest. Asterixis and multifocal myoclonus may also be seen. *Asterixis* is the involuntary jerking movement elicited when the wrist is dorsiflexed and fingers are extended. *Multifocal myoclonus* is the sudden, nonrhythmic, nonpatterned gross muscle contraction commonly seen in the face and jaws of a person at rest. It is frequently seen in uremia, penicillin overdose, and metabolic encephalopathies.

If peripheral neuropathy is detected, it may be associated with a thiamine deficiency. Cameron et al. (1977) suggest that in looking for severe malnutrition, the most telling signs can be found in the mouth, teeth, and gums. Fissures around the mouth suggest a combined riboflavin and nicotinamide deficiency; this condition is fairly common to clients in some nursing homes and extended care facilities. The tongue is also very revealing. With a severe riboflavin deficiency, the surface will be a magenta color; a niacin deficiency produces a fiery red color. With pellagra or a B_{12} deficiency, the normally rough-looking papillae on the surface will be smooth in appearance. Sore mouth and bleeding gums point to a vitamin C deficiency. Cameron and his associates also point out that a self-perpetuating cycle is established wherein the client becomes less tolerant of rough, fibrous foods and begins to utilize soft, starchy foods, often winding up with the "tea and toast" syndrome. Loss of teeth further complicates the problem.

A physical examination should always include an eye and ear evaluation, since impaired vision and hearing are frequently implicated in delirium.

Laboratory Tests for an Organic Workup. Wells (1977) offers the following procedures for a routine diagnostic work-up in clients suspected of organic brain disease:

1. Urinalysis
2. Chest x-ray
3. Blood studies
   a. Complete blood count
   b. Serological test for syphilis
   c. Standard metabolic screening battery
   d. Serum thyroxine by column (CT_4)
   e. Vitamin B_{12} and folate levels
4. CAT scan

Not all of these tests are required in all clients, since a diagnosis might be reached through selected tests without needing to use them all. When the diagnosis is uncertain, however, a thorough laboratory evaluation is needed.

CAT (computerized axial tomogram) scanning is quick, safe, and painless and provides much detail about intracranial structures. It has largely replaced the pneumoencephalogram and, to a lesser extent, cranial angiography. It has proved helpful in finding evidence of a stroke, multiinfarct dementia, tumors, changes in the flow of fluid surrounding the brain, hematomas, and cerebral atrophy. The latest scanning technique is positron emission transaxial tomography (PETT scan). The PETT scan enables the physician to see just which parts of the brain are active when the brain does specific tasks. The equipment is extremely costly, however, and not yet widely used.

Recording Changes in Mentation. Ludwick (1981) has devised an assessment tool for the delirious client that reflects the level of consciousness, memory, mood, and the ability to recognize self, location, and time. The tool is designed to be used for frequent assessment in order to establish patterns and trends of behavior over time as well as to avoid mislabeling the client.

Diabetes Mellitus

Assessment of the elderly diabetic is difficult because the classic adaptations to elevated blood glucose may not appear. Usually the older diabetic is obese, with mild or moderate hyperglycemia. Urine tests for glucose may be misleading since the threshold for urinary glucose excretion usually rises with age. Glycosuria may not appear until the blood glucose exceeds 300 mg/dl (Williams, 1978; Anderson, 1976). Therefore, there may be no polyuria or polydipsia since these result when the kidneys excrete the extra water load and the body attempts to replace that lost fluid. Classic polyphagia and weight loss may not develop because of normal aging changes in taste sensation as well as the fact that the elderly diabetic continues to produce some insulin and does not break down large amounts of fats, producing ketoacidosis. Instead, the onset is gradual or mild. The nurse should question the older client to identify the presence of any risk factors of diabetes—in particular, weight gain. Over 50 percent of diabetics are obese and many report a sudden weight gain prior to the onset of adaptations (Gitman, 1974).

Assessing Acute Adaptations. The nurse assesses the elderly client with diabetes for acute conditions that indicate a failure to adapt. These include hyperosmolar nonketotic coma, diabetic ketoacidosis, lactic acidosis, and hypoglycemia.

Hyperosmolar Nonketotic Coma. Hyperosmolar nonketotic coma is a serious adaptation to diabetes seen most often in elderly diabetics who are insulin independent. The mechanisms of development are not fully understood. It is probably precipitated by a stress such as diuretic therapy, surgery, or concurrent illness such as renal insufficiency or infection. In some older persons, hyperosmolar coma is the first indicator of diabetes. Adaptations develop slowly over several weeks. The first adaptation is hyperglycemia, which causes glycosuria and eventually dehydration and even shock. Glucose levels may rise as high as 1000 mg percent. The result is hyperosmolarity (serum osmolarity above 350 mOsm/L). Since hyperosmolarity diminishes insulin release in response to a glucose stimulus, this sets up a vicious cycle of increasing hyperglycemia and decreasing insulin responsiveness. Even if clients increase their water intake, this is usually insufficient to compensate for fluid losses. Due to water loss, serum sodium is elevated. Serum potassium is usually decreased due to total body potassium depletion. Serum chloride, bicarbonate, and urea are also elevated. Usually, the client develops hypotension, but hyperventilation, acetone on the breath, and other signs of ketoacidosis are absent. Because there is not an absolute absence of insulin, lipolysis does not occur and ketoacids are not formed.

Assessment of urine for ketosis is not a reliable indicator of hyperosmolar nonketotic coma, since ketonuria is not present. Therefore, clients who are ill or who have had surgery need periodic blood glucose determinations. Any change in mental status should alert the nurse to the presence of hyperosmolar nonketotic coma. As the client becomes dehydrated, lethargy develops and may progress to unconsciousness.

Hyperosmolar nonketotic coma constitutes a life-threatening emergency necessitating the replacement of fluids, insulin, and possibly potassium to restore normal plasma volume and reduce blood sugar. During the administration of saline the nurse observes the elderly client for signs of overhydration and cardiac failure. The serum potassium must be carefully monitored especially if the client is receiving digitalis or if coronary artery disease is present. Because of the increased viscosity of the blood the client is at high risk for the development of thromboemboli.

Diabetic Ketoacidosis. In the elderly, infection of the urinary tract and pulmonary tuberculosis are the most common stresses precipitating ketoacidosis. A small group of insulin-dependent elderly diabetics are at risk to develop ketoacidosis as a result of emotional or physical stress or omission of insulin. The mechanisms of ketoacidosis development and

its adaptations are the same for the elderly as for the young, but the events have a much greater impact on the adaptation of the elderly client. If the nephron population has been reduced by chronic disease, the kidneys do not readily handle the increased load of hydrogen presented. Hypotension may further reduce renal blood flow. Ketoacidosis and hypotension may also interfere with cerebral blood flow, reducing cerebral function and possibly causing a cerebrovascular accident. Following ketoacidosis, the elderly are at high risk to develop arterial occlusion.

Treatment of ketosis in the elderly is individualized, depending upon the client's cardiopulmonary and renal status and on the presence of infection. The goals are to stop endogenous production of acid and restore fluid volume and electrolytes. Hypotonic saline solutions are often administered to the elderly if the client is at risk for congestive heart failure. Insulin, sodium, potassium, and phosphorous may also be given. During fluid and electrolyte replacement the nurse monitors the client for signs of fluid overload and electrolyte imbalance. Many clients have central venous pressure lines to monitor fluid balance.

Lactic Acidosis. Elderly diabetics are more likely than their younger counterparts to develop lactic acidosis, especially following a major illness, such as myocardial infarction, pulmonary embolus, or diabetic ketosis, with consequent increased tissue production and decreased hepatic utilization of lactate. Adaptations develop rapidly and include Kussmaul respirations and stupor. Treatment of lactic acidosis is controversial and involves correction of dehydration, shock, and hypoxemia, if present. Bicarbonate is administered to correct the acidosis (Rifkin et al., 1979).

Hypoglycemia. Hypoglycemia may occur in elderly clients taking oral hypoglycemic agents or insulin, particularly if they omit meals or do not eat the required amounts. Adaptations to severe, even fatal, lowering of blood sugar in the elderly are not always heralded by the usual signs of increased epinephrine output exhibited by the young. Older clients may become unconscious without warning. Adaptations in the elderly may be mistaken for advanced arteriosclerosis or cerebrovascular accident. Confusion, disorientation, convulsive seizures, somnolence, slurred speech, and bizarre psychotic episodes may occur. At night, older clients with hypoglycemia may experience restlessness, headaches, nightmares, sleep disturbances, or unusual sleep postures; they may cry out in their sleep or be difficult to arouse. If the older client has cerebral arteriosclerosis, profound central nervous system adaptations may result. If hypoglycemia is repeated and unrecognized, chronic organic mental syndrome may occur. Although hypoglycemia seldom causes serious problems in young diabetics, the release of catecholamines triggered by hypoglycemia may lead to cardiac arrhythmia and death in the elderly. Myocardial infarction or cerebrovascular accident with permanent neurological deficit may also follow hypoglycemia.

Immediate treatment to correct hypoglycemia is important. Clients should know the adaptations to hypoglycemia and be instructed to drink orange juice or soft drinks or eat sugar cubes or honey if they experience a hypoglycemic episode. If the client does not improve within 10 minutes, the concentrated sugar should be repeated. If the client does not improve after 30 minutes, medical care should be obtained. If clients live with others, they can be taught how to administer intramuscular Glucagon if the client is unable to take anything by mouth.

Assessing Long-Term Adaptations. The first indication that the older client has diabetes may be the presence of vascular or neurological changes, infection, or other serious long-term adaptations of diabetes (Table 7). These adaptations develop as a consequence of the metabolic derangements, especially prolonged hyperglycemia, that are associated with diabetes. The older client is at particular risk to develop these adaptations because the degenerative changes of aging intensify their likelihood.

Vascular Adaptations. Vascular adaptations are the most common and serious changes that occur in the diabetic. The development of atherosclerotic plaques in large- and medium-sized vessels is influenced by disorders of carbohydrate metabolism (Gitman, 1974). Plaques develop more rapidly and at a younger age in diabetics, especially women.

TABLE 7. CHRONIC ADAPTATIONS TO DIABETES MELLITUS

Vascular
  Macrovascular
    Coronary artery disease
    Cerebrovascular accident
    Peripheral vascular disease
  Microangiopathy
    Nephropathy
    Retinopathy
Neuropathy
  Peripheral nerve degeneration
  Amyotrophy
  Cranial nerve lesions
  Autonomic neuropathy
    Nocturnal diarrhea
    Gastric autonomic neuropathy
    Urinary retention
    Sweating
    Orthostatic hypotension
    Sexual dysfunction
Infections
  Pulmonary tuberculosis
  Urinary tract; renal
  Skin lesions
Others
  Cataract
  Glaucoma
  Dupuytren's contracture
  Itching

Assessment of the large vessels includes palpation of pulses, auscultation of the carotid arteries for bruits, auscultation of heart sounds, and electrocardiogram. Dependent edema may be present if coronary or renal circulation is impaired.

Because the large and small vessels of the legs may be involved, a vascular assessment of the lower legs is essential. Both arteries and veins may be affected. Because the management of arterial and venous insufficiency is different, the nurse must differentiate these two conditions. A cold foot with atrophic, hairless, and pale skin, thick, layered, dystrophic nails, and a temperature gradient at some point on the calf is ischemic. Pallor on elevation of the leg and discoloration on dependency also indicate arterial vascular changes. Determining which pulses are absent and where claudication occurs indicates the level of arterial occlusion. The client should be questioned about nocturnal leg cramps, rest pain, and cold feet. If clients also have peripheral neuropathy, they may be unaware of cold feet. If venous insufficiency is present, edema, dryness, scaling, brownish discoloration, aching, and tenderness of the lower leg may occur. The management of arterial and venous insufficiency is discussed in Chapter 14.

Microvascular disease involves the capillaries and is characterized by basement membrane thickening. Its clinical significance is uncertain but it may affect the permeability of capillary walls. Basement membrane changes are associated with the diabetic's increased susceptibility to infection. Leukocytes may have difficulty transversing a thickened basement membrane and be unable to reach the infected area in adequate numbers. Microvascular changes can occur in the kidney and the eye.

The incidence of renovascular changes is highest in young, insulin-dependent diabetics, but such changes can also occur in the elderly (O'Malley, 1980). Microscopic changes occur in the glomeruli and their basement membranes. There are two types of nephropathy: diffuse and nodular (Fitzgerald, 1978). Usually, adaptations are not apparent until glomerular damage is extensive. Urine should be tested periodically for protein, the first sign of nephropathy. Edema may also be present. Hypertension is rare (Caird, 1980). Eventually, chronic renal failure may occur. Unfortunately, hemodialysis is poorly tolerated because the elderly client usually is susceptible to infection and has peripheral vascular disease, making vascular access for hemodialysis difficult to maintain (Feinstein and Friedman, 1979).

Retinopathy is noted in about 45 percent of diabetics over age 60 and results in severe visual impairment (Rifkin et al., 1979). In fact, visual changes may be the reason the older client seeks health care. Routine urine testing for glucose in eye clinics would be a useful screening mechanism for diabetes. Because of the frequency of retinopathy, ophthalmoscopic examinations must be an integral part of the health assessment of the aged. If the client is diabetic, an ophthalmic examination is indicated every 3 to 6 months. The nurse should refer all newly diagnosed diabetics to an ophthalmologist.

The two main types of diabetic retinopathy are nonproliferative and proliferative. With nonproliferative retinopathy, fundoscopic changes are confined to the retina. If these occur in the macula, they impair visual acuity. Over 60 percent of diabetics with impaired vision have nonproliferative retinopathy. In proliferative retinopathy, new vessels form near the optic disk, break through the membrane of the retina, grow on the surface and infiltrate the vitreous. Hemorrhage of these vessels can result in scarring, retinal detachment, or loss of vision (Eddy, 1978; Fulton et al., 1974).

Retinopathy is usually bilateral. Retinal vessels become tortuous and engorged and aneurysms that leak blood develop on capillaries. Viewed through the ophthalmoscope, the earliest manifestation of retinopathy is seen as tiny clots around the macula or close to a main vein. Next, blot hemorrhages appear and the retinal veins look full and irregular. The appearance of exudates of a hard waxy or white character, often in a ring around the macula, are especially characteristic in the elderly and indicate visual impairment. These changes are called background retinopathy. Eventually, the areas of hypoxia stimulate the formation of new vessels and these leak blood into the retina, preretinal space, or vitreous.

Clients with retinopathy should avoid heavy lifting and straining. As the retinopathy worsens, the nurse must help the client cope with the prospect of decreasing vision or blindness. Photocoagulation, or argon laser therapy, is used to treat retinopathy, with good results. It creates a scar, occluding friable new vessels and microaneurysms, thereby reducing the incidence of retinal and vitreous hemorrhages (Fulton et al., 1974). For clients with advanced retinopathy, vitrectomy is performed, removing opaque vitreous and preretinal hemorrhages (O'Malley, 1980).

Neurological Adaptations. Diabetic neuropathy is most common in clients over age 50. It may be the presenting adaptation to diabetes or it may not develop until many years after the diabetes is discovered. Neuropathy may be a consequence of microscopic changes in the myelin sheath and Schwann cells of nerves (Fitzgerald, 1978). Microangiopathy of the vasculature supplying nerves may also be involved (Rifkin et al., 1979).

The most serious form of neuropathy is sensory or peripheral polyneuropathy, which usually affects the lower extremities symmetrically. Assessment of peripheral neuropathy is difficult because many of its adaptations also occur normally in old age. These include the loss of vibration sense and ankle and knee reflexes. Physical findings that confirm the presence of neuropathy are loss of pain, temperature, and touch sensation, loss of proprioception, and nocturnal pain. The client may complain of burning sensations, severe hyperesthesias, or a feeling that the foot is "dead." Unlike the pain associated with ischemic vascular disease, there is relief with movement but not when the legs hang over the side of the bed. If the pain is severe, the physician may prescribe salicylates or codeine (Whitehouse, 1979). With loss of sensation, the foot becomes extremely vulnerable to injury. Foot drop may also be noted if the condition is advanced. The nurse should emphasize to the client that acidosis worsens neuropathy. Using a foot cradle in the bed may reduce painful sensations on the foot. The client should be advised to exercise the feet, ankles, and legs to preserve range of motion and prevent hemostasis.

Weakness and wasting of the hip and thigh muscles may also be noted. This adaptation, known as diabetic amyotrophy, is especially significant for the elderly diabetic because it limits mobility. Amyotrophy is usually asymmetrical. The involved area is painful, and the deep knee reflex is absent. Sensation is preserved. Amyotrophy is usually observed in diabetics who are newly diagnosed or poorly controlled. The client should be told that once the diabetes is brought under control, muscle power should gradually return to normal (Anderson, 1976).

Extraocular muscle palsies are another manifestation of diabetic neuropathy. Usually, the third and sixth cranial nerves are involved. Adaptations include pain behind the orbit, nausea, dizziness, difficulty walking, and ptosis of the lid. Pupillary function usually remains normal. This palsy disappears spontaneously in 3 to 6 months.

The diabetic client should also be assessed for autonomic neuropathy. Afferent degeneration of baroreceptor reflexes may result in postural hypotension. Syncope may develop when the client stands up. In the elderly, especially those with atherosclerosis of the coronary or cerebral vasculature, syncope is a stress that may lead to falls and fractures. The blood pressure should be auscultated with the client sitting and standing and the pulse assessed at rest and after deep breathing. The heart rate is usually fixed and does not change with respiratory changes. The nurse should advise clients with postural hypotension to wear firm, full-length elastic stockings. The physician may prescribe fludrocortisone or indomethacin for postural hypotension (O'Malley, 1980).

Because the incidence of hypotonic dilated bladder is especially high in diabetics over age 60, the older client should be assessed for a distended bladder. Eventually, overflow retention develops. This form of neuropathy is especially serious because it may result in urinary tract infections and eventually kidney dysfunction. Clients should be taught to void at least every 4 hours and to attempt to empty the bladder completely at each voiding. The nurse can also teach the client to perform Credé's method, applying pressure over the bladder to help empty it completely. Cholinergic medications such as Bethanechol (Urecholine) may be prescribed to facilitate voiding.

Neuropathies of the gastrointestinal system take several forms. The nurse should be particularly alert to these conditions in clients with retinopathy or other types of neuropathy. Some forms of gastrointestinal neuropathy may alter absorption and lead to nutritional inadequacies, vitamin deficiencies, anemia, and fluid and electrolyte imbalances. Therefore, the nurse should conduct a comprehensive nutritional assessment of the client with gastrointestinal neuropathy (see Chapter 10). Episodic or continuous diarrhea, nocturnal incontinence of feces, and loud borborygmi are adaptations to diabetic diarrhea. The physician usually prescribes tetracycline for this condition since it is believed to be associated with bacterial colonization of the small bowel (Caird, 1980). Nausea, vomiting, gastric dilation, retention of food, and difficulty controlling blood glucose levels are adaptations to gastric autonomic neuropathy (Straus, 1979).

With increasing age and increasing duration of diabetes, neuropathy can also lead to the distressing problem of impotence and retrograde ejaculation in the male and to decreased orgasms in the female. Nursing care of the client with sexual dysfunction is discussed in detail in Chapter 14.

Infection. Since the introduction of chemotherapy, the incidence of pulmonary tuberculosis in diabetics has been reduced. Nevertheless, the prevalence of tuberculosis is higher among diabetics of all ages than among nondiabetics. A chest x-ray should be a part of the health assessment of every newly discovered elderly diabetic and performed on a regular basis thereafter. Tuberculosis is dangerous to the elderly diabetic because it may precipitate ketosis.

Urinary tract infections in the diabetic can be dangerous because they may lead to serious renal complications. Regular urinalysis is indicated to detect their presence.

The skin, nails, and mucous membranes of the diabetic should be inspected regularly for evidence of bacterial or fungal infections, such as furuncles, carbuncles, paronychia, candidiasis, and other skin lesions. Clients with infections should be referred to a physician for treatment because systemic infection is a serious threat to the adaptation of the elderly diabetic.

Other Adaptations. A comprehensive eye examination is an essential component of the assessment of the elderly diabetic. Although lens opacities are no more common in older diabetics than nondiabetics, the rate at which opacities develop and cataracts mature is much more rapid in diabetics. The clinical appearance of cataracts in elderly diabetics is identical to those of nondiabetics. The elderly diabetic with cataracts should be referred to a physician for their surgical removal. Periodic tonometry is also an important component of the assessment since glaucoma may be a manifestation of prediabetes or latent diabetes (Rifkin et al., 1979). Changes in refraction error and optic neuritis have also been associated with diabetes (Fulton et al., 1974).

Dupuytren's contractures occur often in older women and even more frequently in diabetics. The hands should be observed for overgrowth and contracture of the palmar fascia that progressively involve the ring and other fingers and may restrict function of the hand (Elkowitz, 1981).

Skin problems are common in the elderly diabetic. Generalized itching is a frequent complaint. Pruritis vulvae is also a common finding. Chapter 8 discusses nursing interventions for these problems. The nurse should assess the feet with care. The elderly are more susceptible to foot problems than their younger counterparts. Three stresses—ischemia, neuropathy, and sepsis—singly or in combination, are involved in the development of foot lesions. Since treatment of the lesion depends on the specific stress involved, an accurate assessment is important. Arterial ulcers are circular, with a "punched out" appearance located on the lateral aspect of the limb, especially the lateral malleolus. Venous ulcers are usually irregular in shape, with circumferential brownish discoloration. They are usually located on the medial surface of the leg. Ischemic lesions may result in the development of gangrene.

The sensory loss associated with neuropathy may result in trophic or neuropathic ulcers at pressure or friction points on the feet. These ulcers may develop even when blood supply is adequate; therefore peripheral pulses will be present. The lesions are painless at first, but if infection spreads to the fascial web spaces of the foot or bone, pain occurs. These lesions respond to drainage of abscesses, antibiotics, removal of involved bone, and control of diabetes (Anderson, 1976). Because infections exacerbate ulcers, they must be controlled.

The nurse also assesses adaptations that affect the older client's ability to assume self-management. The ability to learn and perform manual skills associated with diet, medication, and urine testing is vital. The nurse assesses the client's mental status, including understanding, ability to process new information, recent memory, and readiness to learn. The client's economic status should also be determined because it relates to the cost of medications and special diet. Physical adaptations common in older people must also be assessed so that they can be considered when teaching self-management. Fine motor skills, coordination, and speed of performance, which may be affected by aging, arthritis, and other neuromuscular problems, influence the client's ability to handle insulin syringes and vials. If sensory neuropathy has affected the hands, the client's tactile sensitivity and dexterity may be reduced. Visual impairments reduce the client's ability to read calibrations on the insulin syringe. Yellowing of the lens influences the ability to discriminate blue–green colors used to detect glycosuria when testing urine. Consequently the client may have difficulty using Tes-Tape or a Clinitest color chart. The assessment of the client's resources and limitations is used to individualize goals.

NURSING INTERVENTIONS

Hearing Loss

If the nursing assessment confirms the presence of a significant hearing deficit, the nurse should persuade the client to seek specialized help. A great deal can be done to improve the communication ability and quality of life of older people with hearing losses. The nurse should refer clients to an otologist or otolaryngologist who identifies and treats problems amenable to medical and surgical intervention, and to an audiologist or a speech and hearing clinic for an audiological examination.

A small percentage of hearing disorders afflicting elderly clients can be successfully treated by medical or surgical intervention. Many conductive disorders are treated surgically, and hearing is partially or completely restored. If drainage is present, it must be treated first, either medically or surgically (Ruben, 1977). If the nurse suspects that hearing loss may be due to otitis media, cholesteatoma, otosclerosis, mastoiditis, Ménière's disease, vascular disorders, viral labyrinthitis, syphilis, or an acoustic neuroma, the client should be referred promptly to a physician.

Sensorineural hearing losses such as presbycusis, the kind most often found in the elderly, are usually not amenable to medical or surgical intervention. Hormones, vasodilator drugs, lipoproteolytic drugs, and vitamins have been widely used to treat presbycusis but there are no data to demonstrate their usefulness (Fisch, 1978). If the source of the hearing loss cannot be treated, the problems created by it can be through a nonmedical process called aural rehabilitation.

The nurse needs to understand the roles of the otologist and audiologist in evaluating and treating hearing disorders. Because nurses play a major role in identifying clients with hearing disorders, they must be able to recognize clients who would benefit from referral and counsel clients about what to expect during otological and audiological examinations. In addition, nurses must be able to give support to older clients who are involved in long-term programs of aural rehabilitation.

The otologist makes an objective appraisal of the hearing loss, integrating the findings with those of other health practitioners working with the client. The otologist identifies the reason for the hearing loss and, if possible, initiates medical or surgical intervention. The main concern is to eliminate or control any stresses that may be affecting the client's hearing. If successful, intervention may obviate the need for further treatment or for aural rehabilitation.

Audiologists can be found in many settings, including hospitals, speech and hearing clinics, and private offices. The audiologist assesses auditory function using audiometric testing, evaluates whether or not the client would benefit from amplification, provides guidance in the selection and use of a hearing aid if indicated, and participates in other aspects of aural rehabilitation.

Audiometric Testing. Basic audiometric testing for purposes of assessment and hearing aid evaluation is the same. It involves pure tone air and bone conduction tests, speech reception threshold tests, and speech discrimination tests. Clients should know that all tests are painless and involve the use of an audiometer. Pure tone tests identify the type and degree of hearing loss. Speech audiometry scores provide an indication of the effect of the hearing impairment on communication. Speech tests are especially important because communication depends on speech, and speech involves a combination of frequencies, not single tones. Additional, more specialized, tests may also be performed by the audiologist. These include impedance audiometry and others that further localize the pathology (Pearson and Kotthoff, 1979).

If the client has any form of presbycusis, results of pure tone bone conduction and air conduction audiograms are essentially the same. Losses are bilateral. In sensory presbycusis, major losses are high frequency and hearing may be near normal in speech frequencies. Speech tests remain near normal as long as presbycusis is limited to the high frequencies. In neural presbycusis, speech scores are inordinately poor in relation to the degree of hearing loss present. This pattern indicates that speech communication is significantly impaired and hearing aids may have limited value. Metabolic presbycusis is characterized by pure tone losses approximately equal in all frequencies and by excellent speech discrimination scores. Mechanical presbycusis is associated with near normal pure tone scores in the speech frequencies and a gradually changing pattern of poorer scores in higher frequencies.

Aural Rehabilitation. It is the audiologist who decides whether or not the client would benefit from the use of a hearing aid or from other aspects of an aural rehabilitation program. The purpose of aural rehabilitation is to improve communication skill through auditory training, speech reading, speech conservation, hearing aids, and education and counseling. The nature of the hearing disorder determines which aspects of the program are appropriate. Audiologists and speech therapists are usually involved in implementing the aural rehabilitation program.

Auditory Training. Auditory training involves practice sessions to develop the hearing impaired client's ability to discriminate sounds. If the client has dysacusis, which interferes with speech discrimination, and only mild hypacusis, auditory training may be used in lieu of a hearing aid. Depending upon the client's loss, auditory training involves helping clients distinguish between grossly different sounds or make fine distinctions. It makes the client more alert and attentive to clues that may improve hearing. If the client has a hearing aid, training involves learning to interpret the sounds received with the aid.

Speechreading. Speechreading, or lipreading, helps the client derive clues to what another person is saying from movements of the eyes, tongue, cheeks, throat, lips, and other body parts. Because it requires profound concentration, speechreading can be fatiguing, especially for older clients. Although it does not improve hearing, speechreading improves visual perceptual ability. Unfortunately many older clients are visually impaired and speechreading is impractical.

Speech Conservation. The purpose of speech conservation is to prevent deterioration of speech and voice patterns or to improve them if deterioration has occurred. These problems occur because clients are unable to monitor their own voices.

Hearing Aids. Hearing aids are amplifiers of sound. They can assist many, but not all, older clients with hearing impairments. Newer, more sophisticated models are now available with selective amplification. Therefore, the nurse should not assume that the client's hearing deficit is too profound or too complex to benefit from a hearing aid. All clients should be evaluated before such a decision is made.

The decision to fit an older client with a hearing aid should be made on the basis of the audiological examination and an assessment of other factors associated with successful hearing aid use. The objective appraisal of the audiological examination provides important data because the nature and extent of hearing loss are factors related to success. Hearing aids amplify sound but do not correct the distortion of sound associated with many sensorineural losses, including neural presbycusis. Therefore, hearing aids are most successful when clients have pure tone losses rather than inordinately poor speech discrimination scores. Amplification may further distort sound, reducing speech discrimination to a point that the beneficial effects of amplification are offset. Clients who experience loudness recruitment may find that the level of sound delivered by the hearing aid is harsh and uncomfortable. In addition, if the loss is in the high frequencies, the hearing aid may not appreciably improve the intelligibility of the important consonant sounds.

Other factors must also be present if the client is to be a successful hearing aid user. The operation and maintenance of the aid requires some manual dexterity and the ability to understand the instrument itself. Client motivation and expectations are also related to successful hearing aid use. Clients should not be talked into purchasing a hearing aid. Many come for audiological testing merely to please relatives or friends. Some, quite honestly, are not bothered by the hearing loss and do not wish to have it corrected. An important factor to consider is the client's need for amplification in daily living. Other clients are resistant because they feel the hearing aid is a visible sign of old age or that there is a stigma attached to its use. Clients may have had previous unsuccessful experiences with hearing aids or they may have friends who have had negative experiences. These clients need sensitive guidance. Potential hearing aid users must have realistic expectations of the instrument or they will become disappointed and discard it. Clients need to know that the hearing aid will not restore hearing to normal. It will amplify all environmental sound, not merely those sounds the client wants to hear. Because their hearing loss was gradual, many older people have heard environmental sounds at reduced intensities and are distressed when these sounds are amplified. Familiar sounds will be heard in unfamiliar ways. The client needs to know that in some situations, such as in group conversations or when the speaker is a long distance away, the hearing aid will have limited usefulness. The client also needs to know that the hearing aid is only one aspect of a comprehensive aural rehabilitation program and adjustment to it will be a slow process.

Only after a careful appraisal by the otologist and audiologist should a client be sent to a hearing aid dealer. A 1977 decision by the Federal Trade Commission makes audiological examination prior to hearing aid dispensation mandatory. Unfortunately, older people can waive this requirement, and many still purchase hearing aids without professional consultation. Hearing aids are expensive (average cost $600), and costs are not reimbursed by Medicare. Therefore, the decision to purchase one should be based on careful, clinical judgment.

There are no hearing aids designed especially for the elderly. Older people may be fitted with any one of the four types of hearing aids: body-worn aids, eyeglass style, behind-the-ear style, and the newer, in-the-ear model. Usually, the audiologist uses data from the examination to make recommendations about hearing aid type. Hearing aids may be fitted in one or both ears, depending on the client's needs. Each type has advantages and disadvantages for the older person, and these should be taken into consideration when selecting a hearing aid. Body-worn hearing aids provide a large amount of amplification and are necessary if the client has a severe hearing loss. Because they are large, their controls are easy to manipulate. However, noise may be induced by clothing and be bothersome to the client. In addition, the cord from the hearing aid to the earphone can be easily tangled or broken.

The other types of hearing aids are smaller and, therefore, are limited in the amount of amplification provided and the frequencies that are picked up. These models are lightweight and inconspicuous. Because they are very small their switches and batteries may be difficult to manipulate, especially for the older person with diminished fine touch, arthritis, or tremors. The eyeglass model is useful for clients who require eyeglasses on a full-time basis. The behind-the-ear model is currently the most popular with older people. The in-the-ear model is best for clients with mild or moderate hearing loss. It is least helpful for clients with presbycusis (Oyer and Oyer, 1979).

Once a hearing aid has been selected, the client should rent it, not buy it, for a period of about 4 weeks. Most reputable hearing aid dealers have rental policies. All new hearing aid users undergo a period of adjustment to the instrument. They should be urged to see their audiologist for formal training and counseling in hearing aid use during this adjustment period. The nurse should give the client as much encouragement as necessary during this period to bring about a successful adjustment. Some older clients believe they will be unable to adjust to the new sounds heard with the hearing aid. Others lack confidence in their ability to learn the skills needed to operate and maintain the instrument.

Practice and patience are required during the adjustment period. Older clients may need repeated instruction in how to handle, insert, remove, and maintain the hearing aid. Hearing aids are delicate instruments that are easily damaged by excessive heat, cold, or moisture. Clients also need help to interpret the unfamiliar sounds they are receiving. New hearing aid users should wear the hearing aid initially at home and in controlled, quiet environments for short periods. Gradually, the client should increase the time the hearing aid is worn and the types of situations in which it is worn. If the client feels nervous or fatigued, the hearing aid should be removed temporarily. Eventually, the client should wear the instrument consistently, removing it at night or when bathing.

Nurses not only help new hearing aid users adjust to the instrument, but participate in follow-up assessments of clients who have used hearing aids for a period of time. Even successful hearing aid users need help from time to time. Consequently, nurses need to know about the types, uses and maintenance of hearing aids. Table 8 provides guidelines for hearing aid use and maintenance. Many of the problems that cause hearing aid users to discard their hearing aid have simple solutions. The earmold may become clogged with cerumen, the batteries may run down, or the earmold may be improperly fitted. Clients who have hearing aids should be encouraged to undergo reevaluation by an audiologist regularly every 1 to 2 years. The client's hearing status or the shape of the ear canal may change, necessitating changes in the type of hearing aid or the earmold. Most hearing aids have

a limited life span and must be replaced every 3 to 5 years. Earmolds need replacing every 2 to 3 years. Changes in the client's physical status, especially neuromuscular coordination or vision, may necessitate a change to a larger hearing aid or retraining in how to manipulate the hearing aid. Nurses also need to know that it is not uncommon for successful hearing aid users to experience a temporary regression in ability to use their hearing aid after illness or surgery. If this occurs, teaching and counseling may be needed until the client is once again able to function (Margolis and Sherman, 1981).

The nurse should inform the hard-of-hearing

TABLE 8. GUIDELINES FOR HEARING AID USERS

Applying the hearing aid
1. Turn volume control off when inserting.
2. Insert when relaxed.
3. Insert earmold firmly in ear.
4. Turn hearing aid on slowly to one-third to one-half volume.
5. With someone talking at a distance of 3 to 4 feet, adjust volume to a comfortable level.
6. If there is an M–T–O (microphone-telephone-off) switch, turn to M.

Routine maintenance
1. Store in dry, cool place away from extreme heat or cold.
2. Turn off or remove battery when not in use.
3. Do not drop on hard surface. Handle over a bed or table.
4. Do not apply hairspray when wearing aid.
5. Clean earmold of wax and other debris by washing in mild soapy water once a week.
6. If earmold is plugged with wax, gently clean with toothpick.
7. Change battery every 1 to 2 weeks. If feedback (a whistle) is not heard when volume is fully on, a new battery is needed.
8. Buy only 1 month's supply of batteries at a time.

Trouble-shooting
1. If whistling or squeaking occurs check for:
   — earmold poorly fitted, cracked or clogged.
   — earmold incorrectly inserted.
   — volume too loud.
   — tubing cracked or leaking.
2. If signal flutters or goes on-off in rapid succession check for:
   — internal dysfunction.
3. If signal is weak or instrument nonfunctioning check for:
   — earmold clogged with wax.
   — batteries dead.
   — batteries inserted incorrectly.
   — battery contacts need cleaning.
   — cord damaged.
   — volume control not adjusted.
   — telephone switch is not in the M (microphone) position.

client about a number of other devices besides the hearing aid that can be of assistance. These include radio, television, and telephone amplifiers, a light-flashing doorbell or door mat, and alarm clocks that vibrate the pillow or flash a light. These devices can be purchased from hearing aid dealers, the telephone company, and electronic shops.

Teaching and Counseling. Whether or not the older client is fitted with a hearing aid, teaching and counseling are considered to be essential to any successful aural rehabilitation program. Audiologists frequently conduct formal teaching and counseling programs for clients who are involved in aural rehabilitation. Nurses may participate in these programs and are also involved in informal, ongoing teaching and counseling with hearing-impaired clients.

Education about the hearing process, the nature of the hearing loss and the frequencies affected helps clients to understand how the loss affects communication. Clients may be reassured by understanding the three psychological levels of hearing and the impact of hearing loss on the ability to hear auditory background sounds and signals.

Interested family members or friends should be included in counseling. Commercially made records are available that can simulate what is heard by the client and help others understand what the client is experiencing. There is a great deal that those who communicate with the client can do to help the client cope with the loss and to improve communication. Clients with hearing losses also need to be familiar with these guidelines so that they can structure conversations in ways that enhance communication (Table 9). Family members may have unrealistic expectations of a hearing aid. They need to understand the limitations of the instrument and how to enhance communication with the client. Although operation and maintenance of the hearing aid is usually the wearer's responsibility, family members need to learn these skills, especially if the older client has motor, vision, or memory problems that limit the ability to handle the instrument.

Summary. Hearing loss is not an inevitable consequence of old age. For clients who develop only mild presbycusis, there is usually no need for any-

TABLE 9. HOW TO TALK WITH THE ELDERLY HEARING IMPAIRED CLIENT

1. Sit face-to-face with a light falling on your mouth, not behind your head.
2. Sit close enough to the client so your lips can be seen.
3. Position yourself near the client's better ear or on the aided side.
4. If in a group, have the client face as many people as possible.
5. Reduce or eliminate background noise.
6. Be certain client is wearing eyeglasses, if used.
7. Get the client's attention before beginning to speak.
8. Use normal tones when speaking.
9. Do not shout.
10. Do not whisper.
11. Pronounce words distinctly.
12. Do not overarticulate or use exaggerated lip movements.
13. Talk at a moderate or slow rate, with somewhat longer pauses between sentences.
14. Avoid long sentences.
15. Do not eat, smoke, or chew gum, or obstruct your face when speaking.
16. Use appropriate gestures.
17. Allow enough time for the client to respond.
18. Alert client when topic of conversation changes.
19. If it is necessary to repeat a comment that has not been heard, rephrase it rather than repeating the same words.
20. Evaluate and verify client's ability to understand what was said.
21. Supplement conversation with written material.

thing other than speech reading. The use of a telephone amplifier and buzzer, a loud door buzzer, radio and television earphones, and an understanding of the psychosocial consequences of hearing loss on the part of significant others may also be helpful. Understanding and knowledge of how to maximize communication with the client will solve most of the problems of older people with mild sensorineural hearing problems. For those with more profound losses, a comprehensive program of aural rehabilitation, coupled with ongoing support from the nurse, can help older clients improve their communication abilities and safeguard their independence.

Depression

Pharmacotherapy. In recent years, drug treatment has received a great deal of attention based upon new theories—specifically, the biogenic amine hypothesis. The amines are a group of chemical transmitters of electrical impulses that maintain homeostasis in the nervous system and include norepinephrine, dopamine, and serotonin (5-hydroxytryptamine, or 5HT). In the absence of these transmitters, clinical depression may occur (Wiener et al., 1979). By the same token, in the event their metabolism is suppressed, their release enhanced, or there is an alteration at their receptors, mania or psychotic behavior may result.

The tricyclic antidepressants are the drug of choice for unipolar depression (Eisdorfer, 1980). They are presumed to enhance the bioavailability of serotonin or norepinephrine by several mechanisms. First, these agents may enhance the activity of norepinephrine by blocking its reuptake into the storage granules of nerve endings. Second, they may potentiate serotonin (5HT) by blocking its reuptake or its metabolism. The biogenic amine hypothesis is now undergoing reappraisal in view of new evidence that may make it appear somewhat oversimplified.

Until recently, all tricyclic antidepressants were considered equally efficacious. From various studies it now appears that some tricyclics exhibit variable selectivity in the ability to block norepinephrine and serotonin (5HT) reuptake. Other studies, utilizing biogenic amine metabolites that are thought to reflect the turnover of norepinephrine and serotonin (5HT), have suggested that two subtypes of unipolar depression exist (Eisdorfer, 1980). The norepinephrine-deficient client displays low pretreatment levels of the metabolite MHPG and responds well to imipramine. The serotonin-deficient client with low cerebrospinal fluid levels of the metabolite 5HIAA has a good response to amitriptyline. Although these are only preliminary findings, they suggest that, in the future, the selection of a specific tricyclic will be made on a more rational pharmacological basis. At present, the choice is largely determined by potential side effects. The choice of an antidepressant with sedative properties (such as amitriptyline) may be more appropriate for an agitated client with a pronounced sleep disturbance. Similarly, the selection of the least anticholinergic antidepressant—desipramine—may offer an advantage for older men in whom prostate enlargement threatens urinary obstruction.

For older clients, regardless of the choice of drug, all tricyclic antidepressants should be used in doses lower than those prescribed for the young adult. A typical starting dose is one-third to one-fourth of the usual adult dose (Table 10). Administration of antidepressants in divided doses reduces

---

TABLE 10. DOSAGE OF TRICYCLIC ANTIDEPRESSANTS SUITABLE FOR THE OLDER CLIENT

Generic Name	Trade Name	Average Daily Dose During First 2 Weeks in Divided Doses (mg)	Usual Range of Daily Dose After First 2 Weeks in Divided Doses (mg)
Amitriptyline hydrochloride	Elavil	50	75–150
Doxepin hydrochloride	Sinequan Adapin	50	75–150
Imipramine hydrochloride	Tofranil	50	75–150
Desipramine hydrochloride	Norpramin Pertofrane	50	75–150

Source: Eisodorfer C, 1980, with permission.

the likelihood of postural hypotension from a single dose. The client and the family should be informed that treatment for 5 to 6 weeks may be required to achieve the maximal therapeutic effect although some adaptations, such as sleep disturbances, may respond rapidly.

In elderly clients, drug elimination is often slowed by compromised liver, kidney, and lung function. With aging, the total body ratio of fat to protein increases. Since psychotropic drugs are more lipophilic than other agents, they tend to accumulate in the elderly person and elimination time is prolonged.

Older clients also suffer a higher incidence of side effects to tricyclic antidepressants. Among the more common adaptations seen are sedation, anticholinergic effects (dry mouth, urinary retention), adrenergic hyperactivity (tremulousness and sweating), and vivid dreams. Of major concern, however, are the complex cardiovascular effects of the tricyclics. Clients with evidence of preexisting conduction abnormalities or who are already receiving antiarrhythmic drugs with quinidinelike properties, must use the tricyclics with great caution. Clients with poorly compensated congestive heart failure or who have had a recent myocardial infarction must also avoid the tricyclics. Narrow-angle glaucoma, urinary obstruction, seizure disorders, or a history of postural hypotension are also contraindications to use of the tricyclics.

Monoamine Oxidase Inhibitors. Use of MAO inhibitors in the elderly is generally limited by their adverse effects. Ingesting tyramine-containing food (Table 11) while taking these agents can produce hypertensive crisis, hyperpyrexia, seizures, and death. The MAO inhibitors are also known to cause postural hypotension. Although they produce a more rapid remission of depression than tricyclics, most physicians are reluctant to use them with an elderly population because of the potential hazards involved. When MAO inhibitors are used with the elderly, their dosage must be reduced (Table 12).

Nursing Responsibilities in Pharmacotherapy. As mentioned earlier, a good drug history is a basic nursing responsibility. With a variety of prescribed and over-the-counter drugs that some elderly clients

---

TABLE 11. MEDICINES AND TYRAMINE-CONTAINING FOODS THAT MAY PRECIPITATE HYPERTENSIVE CRISIS

Foods		Drugs
Alcohol	Fish	Amphetamines
Beer	Pickled herring	diet pills
Red wine, especially Chianti	Canned fish	Ephedrine
Caffeine	Smoked salmon	nasal sprays
Coffee	Snails	Epinephrine
Tea	Licorice	L-Dopa and dopamine
Cola	Meat tenderizer	Narcotics
Cheeses, especially aged	Sour cream	Phenylpropanolamine
Chicken, chicken liver	Soy sauce	cold remedies
Chocolate	Vegetables	Tricyclics
Fruits	Broad beans	
Avocados	Pickles	
Bananas	Sauerkraut	
Canned figs		
Citrus fruits		
Pineapples		
Raisins		

TABLE 12. DOSAGE RANGE OF MONOAMINE OXIDASE INHIBITORS FOR THE OLDER CLIENT

Generic Name	Trade Name	Approximate Outpatient Dosage Range (mg/d)*
Isocarboxazid	Marplan	10–30
Phenelzine sulfate	Nardil	15–75
Tranylcypromine sulfate	Parnate	10–30

*Dosage in the elderly should rarely exceed the lower end of this range (Source: Eisdorfer C, 1980, with permission.)

are likely to take, there is the ever-present danger of drug interaction. The nurse is also responsible for teaching the client about side effects. For the client who is reluctant to take any medication—and many of the elderly fit this category—it is a mistake to overdramatize the side effects but all clients should be aware of the possibility of hypotension. Clients should be advised to sit up and rise slowly to avoid syncope. Whether hospital or community based, the nurse should be alert for side effects of medications while listening to the complaints of the client. Dry mouth, blurred vision, constipation—the anticholinergic effects—are probably least serious yet the most disturbing to the client. They can generally be handled with reassurance and simple nursing measures. Gastrointestinal effects, anorexia, diarrhea, stomatitis, and a peculiar metallic taste are also disturbing but they tend to remit with continued therapy. What is of more consequence is the occasional hematological problem that occurs with the antidepressants. Clients who complain of sore throats or fever should have leukocyte and differential counts and the drug should be stopped if abnormal results are obtained because eosinophilia, leukopenia, purpura, and agranulocytosis have been reported.

Therapeutic Interaction

Therapeutic interaction is a primary nursing intervention used with clients experiencing many adaptations. This section focuses on interactions with the depressed client and is followed by discussions of interactions with clients experiencing brain disorders. However, the principles can be applied to interactions with other clients in a variety of settings.

The many theories of depression offer the nurse a wide range of therapeutic interventions beyond participation in drug therapy. In working with a depressed client, it is not uncommon for the nurse to feel depressed and frustrated. When this occurs, three things need to be remembered: depressions are contagious; they are also self-limiting; and aggressive interventions can produce results—despite the helplessness and hopelessness expressed by the depressed client.

If the nurse accepts the Freudian view that depression is the result of anger turned inward, then angry feelings must be brought to the client's conscious awareness so they can be dealt with in a healthy manner. After helping the client identify angry feelings (which may be masked as sadness) and the losses or disappointments that have contributed to these feelings, the client can be encouraged to seek alternative behaviors that allow for the expression of underlying anger. Barnard and Banks (1967) describe a method of ego enhancement called motor psychotherapy. In this approach, the therapist functions as a role model who describes to the client safe, effective ways to express aggression. In general, the therapist attempts to elicit aggressive behavior on a graduated scale, beginning with activities such as tossing a ball back and forth, then throwing it harder and harder. Finally, the client is requested to cry out in a loud voice when throwing the ball.

Anger often stems from resentment and feelings of being "put upon" by others. If so, the nurse can help the client approach the problem more assertively. Clark (1978) has developed specific strategies to teach assertiveness. She points out that the alternatives—aggression and withdrawal—represent two sides of the same problem, which is basically a lack of self-esteem and respect. Teaching assertiveness enables the client to stand up for personal rights without denying the rights of others. By learning respect for self, the client can gain the respect of others. Assertiveness also teaches one to express anger in appropriate ways, rather than repressing it, which can cause much physical and psychic damage.

If the nurse chooses to use a behavioral framework, there are several methods that can increase the client's level of positive reinforcement. The first approach attempts to increase the client's activity level. Using high-frequency behaviors (those especially enjoyed by the client) the nurse can reinforce low-frequency behaviors (activities the client is reluctant to perform). First the client is helped to identify the kinds of activities that were formerly enjoyed. Perhaps it was window shopping, visiting a museum, or dining out at a restaurant. These behaviors are then used to reinforce ones that the client is reluctant to undertake, such as leaving the house. Another version of this is simply to reinforce any activities the client likes to do, thus making sure the activities will happen more often.

Burgess (1969) describes "shaping" as a process of breaking down the target behavior into small steps and then successively rewarding the client for performing the simplest steps no matter how remote they may be from the target behavior. One community nurse utilizes a shaping technique for clients who are homebound. Little by little she mobilizes the client, first to get dressed for her visits, then to be groomed, then to leave the house with her for a short walk, then to visit a neighborhood coffee shop, and finally to undertake a full-blown shopping trip. At times the nurse can enlist a spouse or friend as an auxiliary therapist to provide this kind of positive reinforcement.

Physical exercise also contributes to feelings of well-being and control. Research has shown that depressed individuals come out of their depression sooner if they jog every day than if they receive traditional treatment (Griest, 1978). Although all elderly clients cannot be expected to jog, the nurse should have the expectation of an increased level of aerobic activity.

Two modalities that involve movement as a way of getting in touch with one's body and adding vitality to life are T'ai Chi Ch'uan and aerobic exercises. T'ai Chi, one of the ancient martial arts, is ideal for the elderly. Although the movements appear deceptively simple, they require much concentration, forcing one to integrate body and mind. Aerobic exercise, which is aimed at improving cardiorespiratory function, is also most appropriate for

older persons if the exercise is tailored to meet individual needs. Walking, hiking, swimming, and dancing are considered best for the older person (Morse and Smith, 1981).

Another modality to relieve depression in the elderly and change attitudes is the use of touch, which can range from hugs and kisses to body massage. One of the best "touching techniques" according to Alford (1982) is a beauty makeover. Feeling good about oneself begins when people look their best and others tell them how nice they look.

If cognitive therapy is utilized, the nurse must become actively involved in the interview situation to identify the misconceptions and thought patterns of the depressed client. The client must then be trained to become aware of automatic thoughts. Knowles (1981) indicates that with years of practice we learn to telescope our thoughts into instantaneous emotion. For example, a client may watch two people dancing on television and become sad. The nurse then intervenes by asking what thought accompanied the feeling of sadness. "They're so young and I'm so old" or "They're having such a good time and I'm not" might be the response. Sometimes the reminder of lost youth and attractiveness can automatically make the client feel sad. By recognizing automatic thoughts, the client can learn to seek emotional distance and view them from a more critical and realistic perspective. Knowles (1981) suggests that the client be encouraged to replace the thought that provokes sadness with one that is pleasant.

Still another technique used to overcome depression is to induce affects that are incompatible with depression. This can occur by using the technique of reminiscing. Getting the client to remember happier times—childhood, or the early years of marriage—can produce the kind of happy memories that compete favorably with the depressive overlay.

Freud did not consider individual psychotherapy appropriate for clients over the age of 45. He believed that after that age a person's character was too inflexible to make changes brought about by insight therapy. Memory disturbances were also thought to represent an obstacle to treatment because the elderly might not remember details of childhood (Freud, 1924). His successors have been far more optimistic. Alexander (1944) deemed supportive therapy more important to the elderly than insight. Meerloo (1953) emphasized the decreased resistance of the elderly to therapy rather than their rigidity. Goldfarb introduced the idea of brief therapy (Goldfarb and Turner, 1953). He pointed out that the dependency seen in the elderly is a function of somatic changes, intellectual impairment, socioeconomic status, and personal losses. Whereas others discouraged dependency, he attempted to use the increased dependency as a therapeutic tool. Goldfarb's treatment cast the client in the parental role and the therapist in the filial role; he then supported the illusion in order to give the client a sense of power.

Today, psychotherapy with the elderly is performed by several professional disciplines (psychiatrists, psychologists, nurses, and social workers) utilizing a variety of modalities. During the 1960s, behavior therapy was introduced to geriatric psychiatry by the psychologists. In the 1970s, Goldstein (1973) designed a comprehensive program to train psychiatric nurses to serve as psychotherapists with the elderly. Known as "Structured Learning Therapy," it involves significant others as a potential source of help.

The concept of the "Life Review" was first discussed by Butler (1963), who noted the tendency of the elderly to return to a consciousness of past experiences, particularly those unresolved conflicts that could be reassessed and integrated. This concept has since been developed into a special therapeutic approach that is action oriented and psychoanalytically influenced (Butler, 1975; Lewis and Butler, 1974). Butler devised several methods of evoking memory in older persons: written or taped autobiographies and pilgrimages to the past (trips to one's birthplace or the scene of one's childhood or young adult life); family reunions and geneologies (fears of death can often be resolved by gaining a sense that other family members have died before them); and by preserving one's ethnic identity (first-generation Americans are often so involved in establishing themselves, they have not always facilitated the transmission of their heritage to children). Evoking positive memories that ward off despair is an adaptive strategy that nurses might well promote. Ryden (1981) discussed how to select clients and initiate strategies when using this technique.

In his review of psychotherapy, Gotestam (1980) states that age should not be regarded as a contraindication. Mental outlook of the client is far more important. He points out that one of the greatest obstacles to psychotherapy may be lack of motivation. If the person has lost the supportive environment of spouse, job, and friends, no motivation for treatment may exist. Motivation can only be increased by rebuilding the supporting environment. Treatment must, of course, be adapted to the individual's resources—physical and psychic capacity, memory, and motivation.

Pfeiffer (1971) has described some of the modifications necessary in the psychotherapeutic approach with the elderly. First, more activity is needed on the part of the therapist in delineating and clarifying the client's problem; second, losses the person has sustained (income, prestige, associates, or friends) must be identified and replacement sources must be found; and finally, realistic goals must be defined that center around increased functioning, striving for more independence and a lesser degree of care.

In replacing or supplementing social contacts, the purpose is not simply to fill in gaps but to design strategies for clients to do this on their own. It may mean the therapist actively advises the elderly client what clubs to seek, what courses to attend, or what methods can be used to make new contacts. Since apathy and emptiness are commonly found following the death of a spouse, and the remaining partner frequently dies within the same year, it is important to replace losses with new social contacts.

Since the 1970s, an increasing number of studies have used environmental change to improve the well-being and behavior of the institutionalized elderly. Loew and Silverstone (1971) conducted a controlled study on the effect of intensified stimulation with two groups displaying confusion and disorientation. The physical environment of the experimental group was colorfully decorated with mobiles, curtains, paintings, live plants, family pictures, and mementos. A large visible clock and daily calendars provided orientation. Auditory stimulation was provided by live and recorded music periods during which wine was served. Religious services were conducted with the hope of recalling earlier cultural experiences. The researchers found a significant improvement in the experimental group as evaluated by tests of cognitive, affective, and social attitudes. Clients improved both their interaction with staff and their time orientation. A spin-off was the staff members' increased sensitivity to the clients' needs. These observations continued to be true in a follow up conducted 10 months later.

Acute and Chronic Brain Disorders

Nursing Interventions in Acute Brain Disorders. Trockman (1978) suggests that it is most important to give the delirious client help in perceiving the environment correctly. He offers a number of specific orienting suggestions, such as checking on the need for eyeglasses, a hearing aid, or even a foreign language interpreter. Touching is another important sensory modality. The client should be positioned for optimal reception of stimuli; for example, the client with a CVA and associated hemianopsia must be approached from the intact side. Simple orienting devices like calendars, clocks, radios, or a chart listing the day's activities posted at the bedside can be helpful. Primary nursing, which reduces the client's exposure to unfamiliar personnel, can prevent further disorientation.

In communicating with the delirious client, short simple statements are best. Protect the client from questions that are difficult to answer. Identifying information should be provided with each contact, for example, "Mrs. Smith, I'm your nurse, Mr. Davis. Here is your medication." Nurses should give more frequent explanations of what they are doing. During routine procedures, reference should be made to the client's occupation, status, hobbies, or interests. Reminding one of areas of competent functioning can be ego supportive and maintain self-esteem. Another way to enhance self-worth and prevent regression is to encourage the client to perform as much self-care as possible.

In handling the anxiety associated with memory impairment, Trockman advises a calm, unhurried approach that is supportive and caring. It is not recommended that the nurse encourage any exploration of anxiety with a confused client. It is best to simply acknowledge the client's anxious feelings and move on to a more familiar esteem-building subject. The client's expressions of realistic hope or optimism should be reinforced. Other support can be provided by the presence of family members, provided they focus on concrete, observable, familiar things. A clergyman can be of help to those for whom religion is important.

Once diffuse anxiety begins to subside and confusion lessens, the client may completely deny any emotional concern about the experience. Trockman notes that partial denial is a natural and adaptive response to stress. Feelings will emerge when the client is ready to handle them. When the time comes to reintegrate the experience, enough information should be provided for orientation, without giving specific details about the disoriented phase, which can always be offered when the client specifically asks for them. Levine (1969) points out that depression is a normal sequel to the delirious experience and should be recognized as adaptive in that it allows for more effective conservation of energy and healing.

Delusions, hallucinations, and hostile behavior often accompany delirium. In responding to these disturbances, nurses should acknowledge the fear that the client is experiencing, and at the same time provide reassurance that they do not share these perceptions in any way. This approach presents the reality of the situation yet allows for empathy. Morris and Rhodes (1972) point out that delirious clients seldom form extensive or highly symbolic delusional systems. The confused client is simply trying to impose familiar, commonplace explanations on a world that is frightening and incomprehensible.

Confusion that occurs in the evening, called sundowning, is due to a stimulation input below the level needed to maintain contact with reality. The older client with less cerebral reserve to adapt to this situation is at higher risk. Bringing the client nearer to the nurses' station, using a night-light, or leaving the radio on all tend to increase stimulation and reduce the sundowning effect.

Working with the Family. As a counselor to the family, the nurse has an important role to play. A client who comes into the hospital in an acute stage of delirium or who develops delirium following surgery needs an advocate with the family. A supportive, familiar home environment would be the most conducive to recovery. The nurse working in the hospital can provide both education and support to the family. The community-based nurse can continue the role and provide necessary follow up. If assured of follow up, the family will be less apprehensive about taking the member home. Recovery may take from a few days up to a month.

Nursing Interventions in Chronic Brain Disorders.

Once the diagnosis of Alzheimer's disease is made, little can be done to alter the clinical course. What can be done is to change the course of the individual's and the family's day-to-day living. Family members find themselves overwhelmed, bewildered by an illness they do not understand, and unable to cope with the day-to-day situation of care. As a result, they often cut themselves off from the very social contacts that are most needed at the time. They literally become captives in their own home. Coping requires the special help of a professional.

The nurse who works with the demented client has a multifaceted role to play with the family. As a teacher, the nurse can inform the family about the disease process and its expected course and help in solving the more perplexing problems that arise. The nurse can also act as a role model for therapeutic interaction with the demented client.

There are a number of excellent publications that might be recommended to the family to expand their information and ability to cope. One of the newest, *The 36-Hour Day* (Mace and Rabins, 1981), can be obtained through the local chapter of the Alzheimer's Disease and Related Disorders Association at the current cost of $6.95. The book is replete with suggestions, ranging from how to secure medical help and deal with problematic behaviors to advice on financial and legal issues and a current review of the state of dementia research. Not only is the book comprehensive but it is also highly practical in its approach to a wide range of frustrating problems with which the family must cope. *Managing the Person with Intellectual Loss at Home* (McDowell, 1980) while not as comprehensive, is another good resource that can be obtained in pamphlet form from the Burke Rehabilitation Center, 785 Mamaroneck Avenue, White Plains, NY 10605 at a current cost of $1.25.

There are five major concepts that the nurse can teach and role model for families:

- *Structured environment:* Many of the most frustrating problems that arise in dealing with the demented client are brought about by lack of structure in the environment. The environment must be kept as simple as possible and routines must be firmly established. Catastrophic reactions occur when the client becomes excessively upset by a strange situation, new people, noise, or simply the request to do something that is too difficult. Helping the family develop specific routines for feeding, toileting, exercising and socialization can be most beneficial. Structuring includes frequent orientation to time, place, and person. Mace and Rabins (1981) describe the wife of a demented client who orients him each day by saying, "Good morning John, I'm your wife, Mary. It's breakfast time. We're going to have orange juice, cereal, toast, and coffee and then we'll call our daughter Susan on the telephone."

- *Safety:* Clients with dementia have lost the ability to judge dangerous situations. The family must often take the same precautions they would to secure the safety of a young child. If the client wanders, an identifying tag can be worn around the wrist. Gates may need to be installed at the top of the stairs if the client wanders at night. Locks may be needed on windows. Most accidents occur in the bathroom or kitchen. Often the client with dementia has problems with coordination. Holding bars may be needed in the shower or rails to provide access to the tub. Locks may have to be removed from bathroom doors. In the kitchen, the stove is a particular hazard, especially when empty pans are left on a hot burner. Knobs on the stove may have to be removed, or the gas company consulted on ways to make the stove safer. Latched cabinets may be required for cleaning solutions and poisonous houseplants may have to be discarded.

- *Activity:* Maintaining normal activities of daily life is essential to the well-being of the client with dementia. It goes without saying that eating and rest must be maintained but grooming, bathing, exercise and socialization all contribute to the client's sense of well-being. Not only is grooming important for self-esteem but it is also essential if any level of socialization is to continue. Exercise is important for tension relief and to produce sleep. *The 36-Hour Day* offers many suggestions for exercise suitable to the client's abilities.

- *Respite:* The escalating problems of the dementia client place a great physical and emotional burden on the care-giver, who can become totally exhausted. Often the care-giver must devote the entire day and part of the night to the client and, without adequate rest, the behaviors become more difficult to tolerate. Giving relief to the family has been found to reduce the rate of institutionalization (Bergman et al., 1979). The care-giver needs encouragement to take breaks away from home for shopping trips or visits with friends. A part-time homemaker, another relative, or a competent sitter could provide needed relief for a few hours. Family members should also be encouraged to take vacations away from home. Since the client suffering dementia is usually upset by new surroundings, it is better to have another close relative or friend care for the client at home.

● *Support:* Experts say support groups are the most important tool in relieving family burdens. As adjuncts of treatment and evaluation clinics they offer families both help and reassurance. In some communities, self-help groups have been organized and can be called on for assistance (e.g., Project Assist in Seattle, one of the oldest support groups, now numbering 600 members). Additional support is provided by the Alzheimer's Disease and Related Disorders Association (ADRDA). This association focuses on education, client care, research, and advocacy. It is headquartered at 292 Madison Avenue, 8th Floor, New York, NY 10017. There are 25 chapters around the country. When writing for information, enclose a stamped, self-addressed, legal-size envelope.

Counseling.   When important decisions about the client must be made by the family, the nurse can step in as a counselor. Families often need a professional ear at a time of crisis. They may also need information on which decisions can be based as well as alternatives they may not have considered. Families also need help in expressing feelings, especially if they are considering alternative forms of care—either day care, hospitalization, or nursing home placement. The nurse can lend objectivity to the situation and raise important questions: "How would you feel if your husband goes to a nursing home?" or "What do you plan to do when your finances no longer permit the present type of care to continue?" Counseling can play an important supportive role for the family in crisis situations.

Advocacy.   There is an alarming amount of physical abuse and neglect directed toward the aged by those closest to them. Lau and Kosberg (1979) found that of the 404 elderly in a chronic illness center, nearly one in ten was a victim of physical abuse or neglect by a family member. Most abuse by family members is not premeditated, but precipitated by crisis situations and often related to the fact that sometimes professionals do not provide adequate support, leaving relatives to cope unaided (Burstone, 1975). Testifying before the U.S. Senate in 1980, the wife of an Alzheimer's victim told a story that is far from unique. In the hospital waiting room filled with people, she was informed that her husband had progressive, irreversible brain deterioration, for which there was no known cause or treatment. "That's the way it is. You'll have to go on from there," her doctor said. He then excused himself and left to see another client without any explanation of the disease, what to expect, how to cope, and without referral to someone who might be of help (Getze, 1981). The nurse is in a position to recognize the potential for abuse and step into the advocacy role. By linking the client and the family with additional supports (whether medical, social services, or respite care) the potential for abuse can be minimized.

Referral.   Referral may be needed to provide respite, in which case day care placement can be recommended. The nurse can also refer the care-giver to a self-help group for support and assistance. When care becomes too difficult, nursing home placement can be suggested. Haycox (1980) says the absolute criterion for nursing home placement is that time when people are less important to the client than the service they provide. When physical needs and their satisfaction are the *only* things that matter, a nursing home may be preferable.

Selecting Long-Term Care Facilities

Sometimes a family is unable to care for a person with a dementing or other debilitating illness at home, even if relief services are available. The decision to place the client in a nursing home often comes about as family or friends realize the consequences of decline in level of adaptation. The adult who lives alone but forgets to eat, does not or cannot keep clean, leaves the stove turned on, neglects to pay utility bills, or wanders and becomes lost cannot be allowed to continue living alone. Either a full-time care-giver, or a relative or friend must be willing to assume responsibility. If neither of these arrangements can be made, then nursing home placement is necessary.

Choosing a nursing home is always a difficult experience for the family. Most family members harbor guilt at the thought of placing a loved member in a home, equating it with abandonment. Many will recall the numerous exposés on nursing homes that have pointed up glaring deficiencies—to the extreme of having residents nailed into their rooms! Some will even know of more subtle abuses—excessive bills, charging for services not rendered, providing kickbacks to physicians or pharmacists. Few, however, will have experience with the rather complex process involved in selecting a good nursing home.

The nurse can serve both as an adjunct to the family undergoing this process and as a resource person, providing information and direction to family members. Equally important, the nurse can encourage family members to become more assertive in their search for the best facility. When the family members feel they have left no stone unturned in securing the best facility, some of the guilt they are experiencing is relieved.

There are excellent resources to guide the nurse in this process (Department of Health and Human Services, 1980; Mace and Rabins, 1981; McDowell, 1980). The Department of Health and Human Services publication *How to Select a Nursing Home* discusses all aspects of nursing home selection and includes a checklist suitable for comparing facilities under inspection. It can be obtained from the U.S. Government Printing Office, Washington, D.C. 20402 at the current cost of $3.50. The Mace and Rabins publication and the McDowell publication are specifically aimed at families who have a member with Alzheimer's disease.

Since the search can be a lengthy one, the family should be advised to look into all possible alternatives well in advance of the time when placement is needed. By submitting applications to several homes, the family will have the opportunity to evaluate the quality of program offered in each setting. They should also be informed that professional help can be sought from the County Department of Social Services, the County Public Health Nursing Service, the local Office of the Aging, any mental health facility, or one of the many family services agencies with strong geriatric programs. Other families that have faced and dealt with a similar experience can also be helpful. However, it is important that hearsay evaluations be followed up with an in-person inspection and evaluation to be certain that family expectations are met.

Initially, contact with the nursing homes can be made by phone to ascertain whether the home can provide the appropriate care needed and if it is approved for participation in Medicare or Medicaid programs. The family member can also find out about specific admission criteria and how long the waiting list is for admission. The family should then be advised to make an appointment with the administrator and, if possible, with the director of nursing services and social services. The Department of Health and Human Services advises family members to meet with key personnel not only for specific information about criteria and cost, but also to get a feeling for the kind of people they are and their attitudes toward their work. The meeting can also be used to verify vital points of information. Who owns the nursing home? Is it a profit or nonprofit institution? Is the home state-licensed or operating under a letter of approval from the licensing agency? As a further check, the local Social Security Office can be consulted for the most recent Medicare survey report on the home which will list any deficiencies. If Medicaid is involved, this information can be obtained from the State Welfare Department. Obviously no serious deficiencies can exist if Medicare and Medicaid approval are to be continued.

The nurse can advise the family member to secure a copy of the statement of residents' rights. Under federal regulations, residents must be kept informed about services available and related charges, their medical condition, and they must have the opportunity to participate in the treatment plan. They must also be free of mental and physical abuse as well as abuse from chemical or physical restraint unless authorized in writing by a physician. They also have the right to free association and participation in social, religious, and community groups as well as to privacy during visits from a spouse. Moreover, they can file grievances or a request for change with the staff or an outside representative (ombudsman).

In touring the home with a staff member, the family should be encouraged to investigate the following areas:

- *Patient Comfort:* How much privacy is permitted? To what extent are physical restraints being used? What criteria are used to select roommates? Is it by cultural background, special interest, or some other criteria? Are visiting hours convenient for residents? Does each resident have a reading light, comfortable chair, closet, and drawers for personal belongings? Do bathing and toilet facilities provide privacy? Is a telephone accessible? Are personal furnishings allowed?

- *Environment:* The general appearance and atmosphere should be pleasant. The home should be attractively furnished and decorated and reasonably free of unpleasant odors.

- *Safety:* Safety should be a prime consideration. Are handrails available along corridors? Are safety devices in place in bathrooms? Are emergency call buttons located at the bedside and in bathrooms? Are smoke detectors and automatic sprinkler systems in place? What provision has been made for emergency exodus of residents in the event of fire? Are exits clearly marked? Are they unobstructed and unlocked? Are there wet spots on floors, loose rugs, or other hazards in view?

- *Medical Services:* Is there a physician on duty or on call? How often are residents seen and records reviewed? How are emergencies handled? Is there an arrangement with a nearby hospital? Is emergency transportation available? Does the home have an arrangement with an outside dental service to provide residents with dental care when necessary?

- *Nursing Services:* What is the ratio of registered nurses to clients? Does a registered nurse serve as director of nursing services? What role does the nursing director play in overall operation of the home? Is at least one registered nurse on duty at all times?

- *Food Services:* Is the kitchen clean? Are three meals served? At normal hours? Are nutritious between-meal and bedtime snacks available? Are special meals prepared for residents on therapeutic diets?

- *Rehabilitation and Resident Activities:* Are rehabilitation and activities programs established?—a weekly schedule should be available. Well-rounded programs generally include both individual and group activities as well as social gatherings, such as parties, dances, and outside trips. Is there suitable space for resident activities? Are activities offered to residents confined to their rooms? Are activities provided each day and are some scheduled in the evenings? Is the program varied? Do residents have an opportunity to attend religious services and talk with a clergyman?

- *Pharmaceutical Services:* Are pharmaceutical services supervised by a qualified pharmacist? Does a qualified pharmacist maintain and monitor a record of each resident's drug therapy? Is a room set aside for storing and preparing drugs?

- *Social Service and Financial Matters:* Are social services available to aid residents and families? Do estimated monthly costs compare favorably with the cost of other homes? Is a refund made for unused days that are paid for in advance? Are these matters specified in the contract?

The checklist provided by the Department of Health and Social Services pamphlet will allow families to compare nursing homes visited and come up with the best choice.

Diabetes Mellitus

Control of diabetes in the elderly prevents long-term vascular and neuropathic adaptations and lens opacities or retards their progress if they are already established (Anderson, 1976; Cahill et al., 1976; Caird, 1980). There is still some debate about what constitutes "good" control in the elderly and the best way to achieve it. Some clinicians still advocate "rigid" control of diabetes in the elderly. Many clinicians take a more flexible approach with elderly clients than with younger ones. Fasting plasma glucose values near 140 mg/dl and 2- or 3-hour postprandial values of 160 to 180 mg/dl are considered acceptable for the elderly as long as other adaptations to diabetes are relieved. Occasionally spilling small amounts of sugar in the urine is also considered acceptable for the elderly diabetic (Williams, 1978; Fitzgerald, 1978). Efforts are made to avoid wide swings in blood glucose in elderly diabetics. Attempting to reduce the blood glucose values of the elderly to the same levels as in younger diabetics is not always possible and may be dangerous because the elderly are at high risk to develop hypoglycemia.

Principles of management differ somewhat in the elderly diabetic from those of younger clients. Simplicity is the key to successful treatment. The main goal is to achieve a satisfactory level of control through a regimen built around the older client's established patterns of living. It is unrealistic to expect older clients to alter the patterns of a lifetime when told they have diabetes. Both the client and health professionals must make some compromise regarding the treatment regimen. The elderly client with diabetes usually has other stresses to cope with as well, and diabetes adds additional burdens. The imposition of a rigid treatment regimen may cause fear and anxiety and emotional and socioeconomic conflicts and is usually unwarranted.

In the elderly, management of the long-term adaptations to diabetes is often the most difficult part of the treatment regimen. Other elements of the program include:

1. Diet
2. Medications
3. Exercise
4. Urine testing
5. Hygiene

The nurse teaches the client the elements of the therapeutic regimen. Modifications are made on the basis of the client's self-management abilities.

Diet. Glucose tolerance in the elderly can often be improved by diet alone, especially in elderly diabetics who are obese or who have glucose tolerance levels below 300 mg/dl (Levin, 1976). Provided ketosis is not present, many elderly new diabetics are placed on a low-calorie diabetic diet and observed for changes in glucose levels and glycosuria over several weeks. The diabetic diet and the nurse's role in diet therapy are discussed later in this chapter.

Medications. If diet alone is not sufficient for adequate control, oral hypoglycemic agents or insulin may be necessary. Oral agents are used pri-

marily in adult-onset diabetics who are not ketosis prone and who, therefore, have pancreatic insulin reserves. The only oral agents currently approved for use in the United States are the sulfonylureas (Table 13). Of these, diabinese is not recommended for elderly clients because its effects are too potent and protracted and may precipitate heart failure or hyponatremia. There is debate over whether the sulfonylureas and diet are any more effective than diet alone in controlling blood glucose levels. There is also evidence that an increase in the cardiovascular mortality rate may be associated with their use (Rifkin et al., 1979; Meinert et al., 1970). Oral hypoglycemic agents are the main cause of hypoglycemia in clients over age 60 (Levin, 1976). In order to avoid the risk of hypoglycemia, clients who take these medications must be knowledgeable about their actions and risks and about adaptations to hypoglycemia.

Insulin is required for 20 percent of older clients, including those who have juvenile-onset diabetes or who no longer respond to oral agents (Williams, 1978). Insulin is also indicated to assure close control whenever the elderly diabetic develops a concurrent illness. If insulin must be used, it is best if an acceptable diet plan is identified first, with the type and amount of insulin then adjusted to the meal plan. Because of the hazards of hypoglycemia in the elderly, older clients who take insulin are often allowed to spill a small amount of sugar (Levin, 1976).

Medication therapy complicates the treatment regimen of the older diabetic who may have difficulty understanding or implementing a complex regimen. When possible, medications should be selected that require only one dose per day. Because impairments of short-term memory are frequent among the elderly, the nurse should always provide the client with a written schedule of medications. Impairments of vision and mobility are the most common problems of elderly insulin-dependent diabetics. The nurse must assess clients and then judge whether they can safely draw up the correct dose and administer the injection. If not, family members can be taught to draw up and administer injections. If vision is impaired, brighter lighting, a white background, long glass syringes, magnifying devices, aids for needle insertion into the insulin bottle, or

TABLE 13. THE ORAL HYPOGLYCEMIC AGENTS (SULPHONYLUREAS)

Agents	Maximum Daily Dose	Onset-Duration of Action	Actions	Side Effects	Nursing Implications
Tolbutamide (Orinase)	2–3g	$\frac{1}{2}$–12 hr	Reduce blood glucose and improve glucose tolerance by stimulating release of insulin from beta cells	Gastric upset Skin rash Jaundice Intolerance to alcohol	Observe for hypoglycemia. Agents may produce prolonged hypoglycemia especially in elderly confused clients who forget to eat.
Acetohexamide (Dymelor)	1–1.5 g	$\frac{1}{2}$–24 hr	May also:		Assess client's medications: Diuretics, steroids, and nicotinic acid antagonize action.
Chlorpropamide (Diabinese)	750 mg	1–60 hr	Act on skeletal muscle and adipose tissue Inhibit gluconeogenesis		Sulfonamides, salicylates, phenylbutazone, antithyroid drugs, probenecid, MAO inhibitors, propranolol, and coumarin potentiate action and increase risk of hypoglycemia.
Tolazamide (Tolinase)	1 g	4–24 hr	Increase insulin binding to cells		Sulphonylureas may potentiate effects of barbiturates and alcohol. Since these agents are excreted primarily through the kidneys, use with caution in older clients with decreased renal function.

preset syringes may be helpful. Alternatively, the visiting nurse can draw up, label, and refrigerate a week's supply of syringes for the client.

Exercise. Sustained regular daily exercise is second only to diet in the management of diabetes in older people. Even a modest increase in exercise, if maintained, helps to achieve and maintain weight reduction, increase glucose utilization, and lower blood sugar (Williams, 1978). Clients should be told why exercise is necessary. Those who are sedentary should be cautioned against suddenly undertaking vigorous exercise but encouraged to participate in mild forms of exercise such as walking and swimming. The nurse plans an exercise program that is individualized. Any exercise program needs strong reinforcement by the nurse if long-term changes in exercise levels are to be maintained.

Urine Testing. If older diabetics are to be motivated to test their urine on a regular basis they must understand the relationship between blood glucose and urine. Urine testing several times each day is unnecessary for the older diabetic unless the client's condition is unstable. In those who show no glycosuria, a single daily urine test or a test twice a week serves to detect any potentially serious change such as insidious infection that might result in hyperglycemia (Williams, 1978; Anderson, 1976). It is useful to schedule such a single test when plasma glucose is likely to be highest, that is, after the major meal. The client should be instructed to test the second voided specimen. If glucose is present, the client should test for acetone. The client should be instructed to keep a written record of urine testing to share with the nurse and physician.

Urine testing in the elderly may not accurately reflect blood glucose because the renal threshold for glucose increases as age advances. Drawing blood and urine samples for sugar simultaneously is helpful for interpreting the results of subsequent urine sugar tests. If the client has a neuropathic bladder, the atonic bladder empties incompletely and collects large amounts of urine that do not accurately reflect the blood glucose level. In addition, a neuropathic bladder masks the polyuria of hyperglycemia. If the nurse suspects that the client is not completely emptying the bladder, the client can be catheterized for residual urine immediately after voiding. Large

numbers of elderly people take medications, including cephalothin, levodopa, probenecid, salicylates, and phenazopyridium, that invalidate the urine test. Clients taking these medications should be informed about how they affect urine testing. Because of the likelihood that the test for urine sugar may be inaccurate in older people, they should not rely on urine sugars alone as evidence that their diabetes is under control (Hayter, 1981).

Normal and pathological changes in vision make accurate urine testing difficult for the elderly. Many methods of urine testing, including Clinitest, Diastix, and Tes-Tape, rely on the client's ability to accurately perceive subtle changes in blue-green tones. This ability declines with age. If clients have poor vision or arthritis, extra large dipsticks can be obtained.

Hygiene. For the diabetic, scrupulous hygiene prevents infections which, once acquired, are difficult to manage because of the client's high blood glucose and diminished circulation. The nurse should instruct the client and family in appropriate hygiene measures, demonstate correct techniques, and evaluate return demonstrations. Clients and family should know which problems require prompt reporting or prompt intervention. At each visit the nurse should assess the client's skin. Doing so reinforces the importance of this practice.

Mouth care should be performed at least twice daily. Dentures should be removed and the mouth inspected regularly. The diabetic client is prone to fungal infections, such as candidiasis (moniliasis), which grows under dentures and at the angle of the mouth. Because oral infections may adversely affect the client's appetite, they must be treated promptly.

The client should inspect all parts of the body, especially the feet, every day. The client can use a mirror to see the soles of the feet and back. Swelling, discoloration, blisters, pustules, breaks in the skin, calluses, corns, ingrown nails, and other lesions should be noted. Clients should also note the presence and location of any pain. When infection and other injuries occur, the client should seek care promptly. Inspection is important because the older client with reduced sensation or with peripheral neuropathy may not feel potentially serious changes, especially on the feet or hands. Faulty vision and obesity make inspection difficult for some clients.

In this case a family member, nurse, or other responsible person should make regular inspections.

Diabetic clients should bathe daily, using mild soap. The client should use lukewarm water and gentle cleansing motions. All body parts should be dried thoroughly, especially between the toes. Daily foot care is essential to maintain healthy, unbroken skin. The client with diabetes should be taught correct foot care. The procedures identified in Chapter 14 for clients with peripheral vascular disease should be followed.

Diet Therapy

Therapeutic diets are an important component of the treatment regimen of many chronic illnesses. Because the elderly often have multiple chronic illnesses, each requiring diet modifications, diet therapy for the elderly is complex. Although the principles of diet therapy remain the same for the elderly as for the young, some principles deserve special emphasis. This section applies the principles of diet therapy to the aged and discusses the specific diet modifications associated with diabetes, obesity, hypertension, and osteoporosis, some of the chronic conditions that most often necessitate diet modification among the elderly.

A therapeutic diet of any kind involves changing the client's eating patterns. If the reason for the diet is chronic illness, the change is permanent. Eating habits are established by constant repetition over long periods of time. The longer the habit has gone on, the more deeply ingrained it becomes into the very personality of the individual and the more difficult it is to change. Therefore, the modification of habitual diet can be much more difficult for the elderly.

Diet therapy is a time-consuming and complex process that involves the use of teaching and counseling. The process often begins in the hospital when the client's new health problem is diagnosed and treated. Any qualified professional, including the nutritionist or nurse, may be involved in presenting initial information about the new diet. Follow-up teaching and counseling are essential. Usually this is done by the professional nurse, who visits the client at home. Follow up is important because no client can learn to accept a new health problem and manage the therapeutic diet during the brief period of hospitalization. Follow-up visits are used to introduce new information about the therapeutic diet, to validate or correct previous knowledge, to make needed adjustments in the initial diet plans, and to evaluate the client's progress and response to the new diet. Follow up also provides opportunities to rekindle the client's motivation to adhere to the diet.

The first step in assisting the client to cope with a therapeutic diet is assessment. A complete diet history, as discussed previously in Chapter 10, should be taken. If the therapeutic diet is to be successful the nurse must identify the "when, what, and where" of eating as well as who prepares the food. It is necessary to determine the daily patterns and practices of eating, and whether eating habits vary on certain days of the week. For example, some older clients may spend most Sundays at their children's home and eat meals there. The client's energy level, manual dexterity, and memory should be assessed since these influence the ability to prepare adequate meals. The new diet must also consider the client's shopping patterns, cooking facilities, and dentition. Since most therapeutic diets are expensive, the client's economic status must also be determined. If the client cannot afford to buy suggested foods, the diet is useless. Ethnic background and cultural and religious preferences must be incorporated into the prescription if the new diet is to be individualized. The client's knowledge of general nutrition must also be assessed. Often general nutrition education to counteract ignorance of nutritional facts, food prejudices, and fears of unfamiliar foods must precede education about the therapeutic diet.

Motivation is essential if a therapeutic diet is to be successful. Before beginning the education process, the nurse must convince the client that a change in diet is important for good health. The risks of the current diet can be pointed out. The specific reasons for the modified diet should be explained. The nurse should explain exactly what the client may expect in terms of health as a result of adherence to the diet. Many clients who must modify their diet have undergone a recent crisis during which a new health problem was identified. Therefore, they are anxious about their condition and motivated to accept advice about nutrition. Mild anxiety can promote learning. The nurse should also be alert for barriers to learning, such as severe anxiety and denial. If the client has not yet accepted the health problem and is using denial, diet education should be postponed because it increases the client's need to use the denial mechanism.

Principles of nutrition education and counseling are described in Chapter 10. Because of the importance of a therapeutic diet to the client's level of adaptation, family and/or significant others should be included in the educational process. If the client lives with family, care must be taken to assure that the client's dietary needs are met without creating conflicts within the family or disrupting family activities. Even when older clients live alone, they may rely on their family for shopping or visit the family for meals. When the client is sick, the family may temporarily cook for the client.

Setting diet goals and planning specific day-to-day meal plans must be done with the client if the diet is to be individualized. For the elderly, the therapeutic diet should include the minimum of modifications. The diet should be as similar to the client's current eating patterns as possible. Favorite foods should be incorporated in the menus and, if possible, meal times and snack times should remain the same. Specific instructions should be positive and aimed at substitution instead of exclusion. It is easier for the client to accept the advice "use margarine instead of butter" than "never use butter again." Diet education must be specific and involve day-by-day meal planning. The client must be able to translate eating patterns into daily menus. General admonitions, such as "stay away from sweets and starches" are inadequate and may lead to bizarre food choices.

To supplement verbal instructions, the nurse can use food models to help the client visualize portion sizes. The client should also be given written instructions that have been adapted to meet specific preferences and needs. The nurse should also show the client how to keep a log of planned menus and foods eaten. This can be used to identify problems with the new diet and assess the client's progress.

The older client should not be barraged with books, instruction sheets, and exchange lists. Printed menus and diets that do not consider the client's individual preferences should not be used. As the education continues, the nurse can offer written materials in moderation to supplement what the client knows. Cookbooks may be of real practical value.

There are a number of cookbooks on low-salt, low-fat and low-cholesterol, or diabetic diets. Because of the high level of public interest in diet, many of these cookbooks are available in bookstores. Others can be obtained by contacting such health agencies as the American Heart Association, American Dietetic Association, or the American Diabetes Association. The older client can also benefit from participation in small group teaching or counseling sessions to supplement individualized diet education. Group encounters provide opportunities to exchange ideas and experiences and to reinforce personal decisions. If the client is limited in the ability to purchase or prepare adequate meals due to financial, physical, or psychosocial factors, the nurse should arrange for appropriate resources, such as Meals on Wheels or food stamps.

Diabetic Diet. Dietary control is essential for successful control of diabetes mellitus. In some cases, diet alone is enough to control insulin-independent diabetes (Wilson et al., 1980). The goals of the diabetic diet include:

1. To maintain or attain ideal weight
2. To maintain plasma glucose near the normal physiological range
3. To relieve troublesome adaptations to diabetes
4. To prevent or delay the onset of potential stresses associated with diabetes
5. To maintain or attain optimum nutrition
6. To enable the client to live as normal a life as possible.

Because many clients with adult-onset diabetes are overweight, achieving the ideal weight for one's height and sex is the first goal of the diabetic diet. Clients with adult-onset diabetes continue to produce some insulin, though not enough. By losing weight, the client attains a smaller body mass in relation to the available amount of insulin. Weight loss also alters insulin receptors so that the available insulin is more effective. For some clients with adult-onset diabetes, weight loss alone is enough to return the glucose tolerance to normal levels (Greene, 1971). Therefore, obese clients with diabetes are placed on a low-calorie diet until the desirable weight is attained. Principles involved in weight reduction diets are discussed in the next section.

Several variations of the diabetic diet are in use today.

The free or regular diet controls calories only, with or without restriction of refined sugars. Because this diet requires the fewest dietary modifications, it is often prescribed for use with older insulin-independent clients, since it is so difficult to alter lifelong eating patterns in the elderly.

The carbohydrate-restricted diet controls calories and restricts or eliminates carbohydrates, especially refined sugar. Clients are permitted to eat whatever amounts of protein and fats are desired, provided the diet is nutritionally balanced. The client is instructed to avoid all sweets, frosted cakes, pies, sweetened fruit juices and carbonated beverages, honeys, jams, candy, and sweetened fruits. Although this diet is relatively simple to follow, avoiding high-carbohydrate foods and sweets may be a terrible hardship for the elderly. Often these foods are the least expensive and easier to secure and prepare than other foods.

A point system has been devised to facilitate diet planning when only carbohydrates and calories are controlled. All foods are divided into three nutrient groups—proteins, fats, and carbohydrates—with each group assigned points. The diet prescription details the points allowed in each group. Diet plans using this system are available from the Kansas Wheat Commission, Hutchinson, Kansas.

The exchange system provides for day-to-day consistency in the amount of calories consumed and in the distribution of carbohydrates, fats, and proteins. The system is based on six food groups—milk, meat, fat, bread, vegetable A, and vegetable B. The portion size for each group is predetermined. Each group contains many different foods, each of which can be exchanged for another item within the group.

The exchange system, advocated by the American Diabetes Association, is widely used. In 1976, the Association revised the Exchange List for Meal Planning, emphasizing individualization of meal planning under the guidance of an experienced health professional, rather than a fixed diet schedule. Individual recommendations are written out in consultation with the client. Local chapters of the American Diabetes Association can provide information about the exchange system.

The principles of the exchange system may be confusing for older clients, especially if they have little information about normal nutrition. The nurse should use written diet sheets and if necessary provide the client with repeated explanations. Common household measures should be used to illustrate portion sizes. If the elderly person does not understand how to substitute foods from the appropriate group, the meals may become monotonous and conducive to the development of nutritional deficiencies. The nurse must follow up closely to assure that the client is able to use the diet correctly.

When other chronic conditions are present, the diabetic diet must be modified further. The American Dietetic Association provides supplements to the exchange lists modified for bland, low-fiber, or low-sodium diets. The exchange list diet can also be modified for lacto- or lacto-ovo-vegetarians or pure vegetarians, although some iron, vitamin, and mineral supplements may be necessary.

The *weighed diet* requires that all food and fluid be weighed or measured. This diet is the most stringent and least flexible of all diabetic diets. Weighing and measuring prevent any error in the estimation of portion size.

Both the exchange system and the weighed diet are based on an assessment of the client's energy requirement and a determination of the number of calories needed to maintain ideal weight and the proportion of those calories devoted to carbohydrates, fats, and proteins. For the elderly diabetic client who is not overweight, the calorie requirement is the same as for healthy older clients: 2400 calories for men and 1800 for women who exercise moderately.

The American Diabetes Association (1979) recommends the following distribution of nutrients:

Protein	12 to 20 percent
Carbohydrate	50 to 60 percent
Fats	20 to 30 percent
Polyunsaturated	10 percent
Saturated	less than 10 percent
Monosaturated	the remainder

In light of recent research findings, the American Diabetes Association (1979) has increased the proportion of carbohydrates and reduced the proportion of fats allowed. In some ethnic groups, rice, noodles, and potatoes can be used to meet the carbohydrate requirement. Cereals, breads, vegetables, and fruits can also be used. This diet is associated with improved glucose tolerance. It also takes into account the fact that diabetics have a high incidence of hyperlipemia and vascular disease.

Not all experts agree that the high-carbohydrate diet is the most effective (Todhunter and Darby, 1978; Wilson et al., 1980; Reaven et al., 1979). They argue that the evidence has not yet been completely processed and a high carbohydrate diet may cause nutritional deficiencies. Consequently, they recommend a carbohydrate intake of 40 to 50 percent and a slightly higher fat intake of 35 to 40 percent.

The American Diabetes Association (1979) also recommends that the diabetic client restrict the amount of salt in the diet. They also suggest that a high-fiber diet may be advantageous. Foods high in plant fibers include whole grains, fruits, root vegetables, and legumes. A high fiber intake is achieved by substituting unrefined or minimally refined foods for highly refined carbohydrates and fats. Plant fibers are digested or fermented in the colon and their metabolic products are absorbed. An increase in plant fiber intake is accompanied by a lower fasting blood sugar, a lower postprandial plasma glucose value, and lower insulin requirements. In some cases, serum triglycerides and cholesterol values are also reduced (Anderson et al., 1979). Diabetics should record the amount of fiber eaten and endeavor to keep the amount constant. If insulin-dependent clients significantly increase the amount of fiber in their diet, they may require alteration in insulin. In fact, some clients may no longer require insulin (Jenkins et al., 1980).

The foods selected for the diabetic must be carefully chosen. The lower caloric needs of the elderly make it essential that foods be selected with attention to their nutritional density, that is, the ratio of essential nutrients to caloric content. It is important to include in the diet lean meat, eggs, milk, fresh fruits and vegetables, legumes, enriched whole grain cereals and bread stuffs. The nurse must periodically reevaluate the elderly diabetic's nutritional intake. In some cases, the most important goal is to assure that the older person eats something at regular meal times to maintain nutrition.

Stability in the timing, amount, and distribution of food intake is necessary to avoid hypoglycemia if the diabetic client is taking insulin or oral hypoglycemic agents. It is recommended that the client eat three small meals and two snacks, one in the afternoon and one before bed. Many older clients are accustomed to eating only two widely spaced meals each day. For them, the regulation of meals may be a real hardship.

The nurse must be prepared to explain the rationale behind each diet and teach the principles of each. In addition, if clients are to implement appropriate meal plans, they must have information about food selection and preparation and the nutrient composition of foods. The nurse and client work together to develop meal plans that are acceptable to the client and will achieve the therapeutic goals. Personality and life-style should be considered in planning menus. A flexible meal plan may be suitable for some clients, while other, more compulsive persons may desire a more rigid dietary regimen. Expensive dietetic and diabetic foods are not necessary to meet the nutritional requirements of the diabetic diet. The nurse can suggest written materials that will help the client implement menu plans. The American Diabetes Association publishes a cookbook for diabetics and a magazine for clients with information on the disease and recipes based on exchange lists. The nurse and client should review menus regularly and modify them as required to meet the client's needs.

Weight Reduction Diet. Obesity is a major nutritional problem among the elderly. Forty to 50 percent of women and 15 to 20 percent of men over age 60 are obese (Beauchene and Davis, 1979). The frequency of obesity in the elderly is not usually a consequence of "overeating" per se but of failure to gradually reduce the caloric intake with successive decades. With aging, the basal energy requirements are reduced. As the older person gradually reduces physical exercise, the caloric requirement is further reduced.

Obesity is related to the incidence of atherosclerosis, hypertension, diabetes mellitus, gallstones, and cirrhosis. In the elderly, the incidence of obesity has been associated with disease and disability which limit physical activity, the use of eating as a substitute for boredom, loneliness, depression, and a loss of social contacts, and an increase in less vigorous hobbies such as playing cards and watching television (Price and Pritts, 1980). In general, it is not necessary to insist that the elderly obese but otherwise well-nourished client lose weight unless there is a good reason to do so. Any organic damage due to overeating has probably already been done. Clients with arthritis, osteoporosis, fractures, strokes, COPD, and heart disease should be encouraged to lose weight because obesity increases disability associated with these diseases and reduces rehabilitation potential.

When physicians prescribe weight reduction diets for older people, they use the client's age, sex, size, and exercise level to adjust the calorie intake so that the ideal weight can be approached. The weight loss may vary from one-half pound to 2 pounds per week. In general, it is safe to reduce the older client's intake by 500 calories per day, producing a weight loss of 1 pound per week. For the average older adult, this is 1900 calories for a man and 1300 for a woman. The older person should never be restricted to less than 800 calories per day. If the diet is too restricted, it is difficult for the older person to comply. Limitations to 500 calories per day, the starvation level, may compromise the older person's adaptation.

Caring for a client on a weight reduction diet begins with a period of data collection. The nurse should direct the client to collect as much information as possible about present eating in the form of a food record. Doing so helps clients become aware of eating patterns and what influences them. The record should include the amount and type of food eaten, the time it is eaten, situation while eating, level of hunger just before eating, mood, location of eating, persons present, and any other pertinent information. Many overweight clients are unaware of much of their eating.

The nurse should involve the client in setting reasonable short-term goals for weight loss. The nurse must repeatedly stress the time factor involved if the ideal weight is to be achieved. The nurse can help the client make simple diet modifications. Decreasing fats and oils, using leaner cuts of meat and low-fat skim milk and strictly limiting or avoiding confections, nuts, rich pastry, pie, and cakes reduce the caloric intake. Broiling or baking instead of frying is helpful. Using fresh or water-packed fruits

for dessert and increasing the proportion of fruits and vegetables, especially dark green leafy and low-calorie vegetables, improves the overall quality and variety of the diet. The nurse should also help the client include some favorite foods in the diet, since this will increase the chance for success. When possible, the nurse should encourage the client to take daily exercise. Doing so not only burns calories during the period of exercise, but speeds up the metabolic rate for a period of time after the exercise, thus further increasing the energy expenditure.

When working with a client on a weight reduction regimen, the nurse should make frequent follow-up visits to evaluate the client's progress, rekindle motivation, and teach the client new, more healthful eating habits. Clients should be taught to control environmental situations that result in frequent, rapid, or uncontrolled eating. To control the rate of eating, clients can be taught to chew every mouthful 15 times before swallowing, to wait 15 seconds between bites, to set down utensils between bites, and to set the table before beginning to eat. To control frequency of eating the client should eat only in one place, eat only when hungry, keep food out of sight between meals, and identify and participate in activities other than eating that are enjoyable. To control the amount of food eaten, the client can be taught to serve meals on a smaller plate so it appears as if there is more food and to eat half of everything. When eating in a restaurant the client should leave food on the plate. The client should also learn the caloric and nutritional content of frequently eaten foods and beverages. Because the older person on a weight reduction diet has such a limited caloric intake, the risk of an unbalanced diet is high. Periodically the nurse should assess what the client has eaten for nutritional adequacy. Vitamin and mineral supplements may be advisable during the period of weight loss.

Diet Modifications for Osteoporosis. Although dietary management does not cure the disabling skeletal demineralization of osteoporosis, it is important for these clients to maintain an adequate diet. Clients should be advised to follow a diet high in calcium (800 mg daily) with adequate amounts of fluoride and vitamin D (400 IU). They should avoid an excessive intake of phosphorus to maintain a calcium-to-phosphorus ratio of 1:1 or greater (Todhunter and Darby, 1978). Drinking water, tea, and seafood are good sources of fluoride. Eggs, dairy products, fortified milk, and margarine are high in vitamin D. Although some foods, such as milk and cheese, are high in both calcium and phosphorus, dark-green vegetables and dried legumes are high in calcium and low in phosphorus. Although this diet does not dramatically alter adaptations or contribute to remineralization of bone, it provides maximum dietary protection against the progress of the condition.

Sodium-Restricted Diet. Sodium restriction is an effective way of reducing high blood pressure and the sodium retention associated with congestive heart failure. For some clients with hypertension, medication can be reduced or stopped altogether if dietary sodium can be controlled. Clients with heart failure who adhere to a sodium-restricted diet usually require lower doses of diuretics. Unfortunately, the low-sodium diet does pose problems for the elderly who have low incomes, inadequate cooking facilities, or difficulty shopping for or preparing food. Although it may be much easier for the older client to use frozen or canned convenience foods, these have inordinate amounts of sodium. In addition, the fresh ingredients, though lower in sodium than canned or frozen items, may be too expensive, or the effort involved in preparing them may be prohibitive. Many foods that older clients use regularly, such as bouillion cubes, mayonnaise, mustard, bread, breakfast cereals, canned tuna and tomato juice, sugar substitutes, and flavor enhancers such as MSG are high in sodium.

Because of the difficulty complying with a severely restricted low-sodium diet, most clients are allowed 2 to 3 g of sodium per day. No salt should be used at the table, but it may be used lightly in cooking. Foods that are not permitted include peanut butter, cheese, highly salted foods such as crackers, potato chips, corn chips, salted nuts and salted popcorn, salt-preserved foods, bacon, sausage, corned beef, frankfurters, sauerkraut, and sardines. If the client is prescribed a 1 g sodium diet, no salt is allowed at the table or in cooking. In addition to foods listed above, the client should avoid all canned foods, regular bread, and certain specified vegetables.

Because the older person's perception of salt is diminished, a sodium-restricted diet may taste unpalatable at first. After several months the client should notice a difference in the taste appeal of certain foods and a new appreciation for flavors. The nurse can encourage the client to experiment with spices to compensate for the lack of salt. If the diet is to be successful, the client needs to learn which foods are high in sodium and must be avoided, the sodium content of foods most often eaten, how to estimate the total sodium content in a day's menu, and how to read labels and shop for brands of canned and packaged goods that do not contain sodium. Many excellent low-sodium cookbooks are available to help the client plan tasty, well-balanced menus. The American Heart Association has descriptive pamphlets about specific sodium-restricted diets.

Clients need to know that many dental products and nonprescription medications, such as bulk laxatives and antacids, contain large amounts of sodium. Sodium can enter the body by many routes and medications for topical application or rectal or vaginal instillation may also contain unacceptable amounts of sodium. Before buying any over-the-counter products clients on a sodium-restricted diet should consult with the nurse or another health professional to determine whether or not the drug is contraindicated.

SUMMARY

Hearing loss, depression, brain disorders, and diabetes mellitus are four problems of regulation that commonly affect the elderly. If older people with these problems receive adequate support, they are usually able to maintain independent functioning for long periods of time. There are many ways the nurse can support older clients, including using therapeutic interaction techniques or helping clients implement a therapeutic diet. If clients cannot cope, the nurse's role may involve helping older clients and their families select a nursing home.

REFERENCES

Adams M, Hanson R, et al : The confused patient—Psychological responses in critical care units. American Journal of Nursing 78:1504, 1978

Agate J: Common symptoms and complaints, in Rossman I (ed), Clinical Geriatrics, 2nd ed. Philadelphia, Lippincott, 1979

Akhtar AJ, Broe D, et al: Disability and dependence in the elderly at home. Age and Aging 2:102, 1973

Akiskal HS, McKinney WT: Depressive disorders: Toward a unified hypothesis. Science 182:20,1973

Alberti PW: Hearing problems in a geriatric population. Journal of Otolaryngology 6 (Suppl 4):I,1, 1977

Alexander FG: The indication for psychoanalytic therapy. Bulletin of the New York Academy of Medicine 20:319, 1944

Alford DM: Expanding older persons' belief systems. Topics in Clinical Nursing 3(4):35 1982

American Diabetes Association. Principles of nutrition and dietary recommendations for individuals with diabetes mellitus: 1979. Diabetes 28(11):1027, 1979

Anderson Sir F: Practical Management of the Elderly, 3rd ed. Oxford, Blackwell, 1976

Anderson JW, Midgley WR, Wedman B: Fiber and diabetes. Diabetes Care 2(4):359, 1979

Anwar M: Communication difficulties with the elderly hard-of-hearing. Nursing Mirror 145(18):26, 1977

Barnard GW, Banks SH: Motor psychotherapy: A method for ego enhancement. Mental Hygiene 51:604, 1967

Bartol MA: Nonverbal communication in patients with Alzheimer's disease. Journal of Gerontological Nursing 5(4):21, 1979

Batchelor IRC: Suicide in Old Age. New York, McGraw-Hill, 1957

Batchelor IRC, Napier MB: Attempted suicide in old age. British Medical Journal 2:1186, 1953

Bates JF, Elwood PC, Foster W: Studies relating mastication and nutrition in the elderly. Gerontology Clinic 13(4):227, 1971

Beauchene RE, Davis TA: The nutritional status of the aged in the USA. Age 2:23, 1979

Beck AT: Cognitive Therapy and the Emotional Disorders. New York, International Universities Press, 1976

Beck C: Dining experiences of the institutionalized elderly. Journal of Gerontological Nursing 7(2):104, 1981

Beland IL: Clinical Nursing: Pathophysiological and Psychosocial Approaches. New York, Macmillan, 1965

Bergmann K, Foster EM, Justice AW, Mathews V: Management of the demented elderly patient in the community. British Journal of Psychiatry 132:441, 1979

Blass J: Special report: Unraveling the mysteries of dementia. The Chronicle. Publication of the Burke Rehabilitation Center, White Plains, NY, 1980

Bozian M, Clark HM: Counteracting sensory changes in the aging. American Journal of Nursing 803:473, 1980

Burgess EP: The modification of depressive behaviors, in Rubin RD, Franks CM (eds), Advances in Behavior Therapy. New York, Academic, 1969

Burstone G: Granny battering (Editorial). British Medical Journal 6:592, 1975

Busse E: Eating in late life: Physiological and psychological factors. American Pharmacy 20(5):36, 1980

Butler RN: The Life Review: An interpretation of reminiscence in the aged. Psychiatry 119:721, 1963

Butler RN, Lewis MI: Aging and Mental Health: Positive Psychosocial Approaches. St. Louis, Mosby, 1973

Butler RN, Lewis MI: Aging and Mental Health: Positive Psychosocial Approaches. 2nd ed. St. Louis, Mosby, 1977

Butler RN: Psychiatry and the elderly: An overview. American Journal of Psychiatry 132(9):893, 1975

Cadoret RJ, King L: Psychiatry in Primary Care. St. Louis, Mosby, 1974

Cadoret RJ, Winokur G: Genetic studies of affective disorders, in Flach FF, Draghi SC (eds), The Nature and Treatment of Depression. New York, Wiley, 1975

Cahill GF, Etzwiler DD, Freinkel N: Control and diabetes. New England Journal of Medicine 294(18):1004, 1976

Caird FI: Management of diabetes and its complications, in Exton-Smith AN, Caird FI (eds), Metabolic and Nutritional Disorders in the Elderly. Chicago, Year Book, 1980

Cameron I, Frankel J, Savitsky E, Still C: Assessing and managing dementia. Patient Care—The Practical Journal for Primary Physicians II(20):90, 1977

Chandalia HB, Bagrodia J: Effect of nutritional counseling on the blood glucose and nutritional knowledge of diabetic subjects. Diabetes Care 2(4):353, 1979

Chandler PT: Diabetic vascular disease: An update. Consultant 19:43, 1979

Clark CC: Assertive Skills for Nurses. Wakefield, MA, Contemporary Publishing, 1978

Clark C, Mills GC: Communicating with hearing impaired elderly clients. Journal of Gerontological Nursing 5(3):41, 1979

Clarke M, Wakefield LM: Food choices of institutionalized vs. independent living elderly. Journal of American Dietetic Association 66:600, 1975

Copeland JRM, Kelleher MJ, et al. (U.K.), with Gurland BJ, Sharpe L, et al. (U.S.): Diagnostic differences in psychogeriatric patients in New York and London. Canadian Psychiatric Association Journal 19:267,1974

Davidhizar R, Gunden E: Recognizing and caring for the delirious patient. Journal of Psychiatric Nursing and Mental Health Services 16(5):38, 1978

Davison W: The hazards of drug treatment in old age, in Brocklehurst JC (ed), Textbook of Geriatric Medicine and Gerontology, 2nd ed. Edinburgh, Churchill Livingstone, 1978

Department of Health and Human Services Publication HCFA-30043. How to Select a Nursing Home. Health Care Financing Administration, December 1980

Dodd M: The confused patient: Assessing mental status. American Journal of Nursing 78(9):1501, 1978

Eddy DM: "Vitrectomy." American Journal of Nursing 78(4):609, 1978

Eisdorfer C: Common Psychiatric Disorders of the Aged. Unit 6. Multi-Media Medicine. American College of Physicians, 1980

Eliopoulous CE: Diagnosis and management of diabetes in the elderly. American Journal of Nursing 78(5):886, 1978

Elkowitz E: Geriatric Medicine for the Primary Care Practitioner. New York, Springer, 1981

Epstein LJ: Depression in the elderly. Journal of Gerontology 31:278, 1976

Feinstein EI, Friedman EA: Renal disease in the elderly, in Rossman I (ed), Clinical Geriatrics, 2nd ed. Philadelphia, Lippincott, 1979

Fisch L: Special senses: The aging auditory system, in Brocklehurst JC (ed), Textbook of Geriatric Medicine and Gerontology, 2nd ed. Edinburgh, Churchill Livingstone, 1978

Fitzgerald MG: Diabetes, in Brocklehurst JC (ed), Geriatric Medicine and Gerontology, 2nd ed. Edinburgh, Churchill Livingstone, 1978

Folstein MF, Folstein SE, McHugh PR: "Mini-mental state": A practical method for grading the cognitive state of patients for the clinician. Journal of Psychiatric Research 12:189, 1975

Freud S: On Psychotherapy. Collected Papers. London, Hogarth, 1924, vol 1

Fulton M, Schweizer D, Ruhland F, et al: Helping diabetics adapt to failing vision. American Journal of Nursing 74(1):54, 1974

Gacek RR: Degenerative hearing loss in aging, in Fields WS (ed), Neurological and Sensory Disorders in the Elderly. New York, Grune and Stratton, 1975

Gates N: The elderly deaf. Nursing Mirror 144(3):67, 1977

Getze LH: They're coping with senility. Modern Maturity April-May, p 82, 1981

Gitman L: Diabetes mellitus in the aged, in Chinn AB (ed), Working with older people: Guide to practice. Volume IV: Clinical Aspects of Aging. U.S. Department of Health, Education, and Welfare, 1974

Glickman L, Friedman S: Changes in behavior, mood or thinking in the elderly: Diagnosis and management. Medical Clinics of North America 60(6):1297, 1976

Goldberg C, Stanitis MA: The enhancement of self-esteem through the communication process in group therapy. Journal of Psychiatric Nursing Health Services 15(12):5, 1977

Goldfarb AI, Turner H: Psychotherapy of aged persons. American Journal of Psychiatry 109:116, 1953

Goldfarb AI: Aging and Organic Brain Syndrome. Bloomfield, NY, Health Learning Systems, 1974

Goldstein AP: Structured Learning Therapy. New York, Academic, 1973

Goldstein K: After Effects of Brain Injuries in War: Their Evaluation and Treatment. New York, Grune and Stratton, 1942

Goode RL: The effect of aging on the ear, in Enough FG Jr (ed), Management of Common Problems in Geriatric Medicine. Menlo Park, CA, Addison-Wesley, 1981

Goodhill V: Deafness, tinnitus, and dizziness in the aged, in Rossman I (ed), Clinical Geriatrics, 2nd ed. Philadelphia, Lippincott, 1979

Gotestam KG: Behavioral and dynamic psychotherapy with the elderly, in Birren JE, Sloane RB (eds), Handbook of Mental Health and Aging. Englewood Cliffs, NJ, Prentice-Hall, 1980

Greene J: Nutritional care consideration of older Americans. Journal of the National Medical Association 71(8):791, 1971

Grieger OG, Johnson LA: Positive education for elderly persons, correct eating through reinforcement. Gerontologist 14:432, 1974

Griest JH: Running through your mind. Journal of Psychosomatic Research 22:259, 1978

Gurland BJ: The comparative frequency of depression in various adult age groups. Journal of Gerontology 31:283, 1976

Hagerty G: Growing more balmy each day . . . Love, Mom. American Journal of Nursing 80(12):2173, 1980

Hamilton LD: Aged brain and the phenothiazines. Geriatrics 21:131, 1966

Havens L: The anatomy of a suicide. New England Journal of Medicine 272:401, 1965

Haycox J: Late care of the demented patient. The question of nursing home placement. New England Journal of Medicine 303:165, 1980

Hayter J: Diabetes and the older person. Geriatric Nursing 2(1):32, 1981

Heston LL, Mastri AR: The genetics of Alzheimer's disease: Associations with hematological malignancy and Down's syndrome. Archives of General Psychiatry 34(8):976, 1977

Hodkinson HM: Common Symptoms of Disease in the Elderly, 2nd ed. Oxford, Blackwell, 1980

Hogstel MO: Communicating with the elderly, in Hogstel MO (ed), Nursing Care of the Older Adult. New York, Wiley, 1980

Hull RH: Hearing Impairment Among Aging Persons. Lincoln, NE, Cliffs Notes, 1977

Hull RH, Trainor RM: Hearing impairments among aging persons in the health care facility: Their diagnosis and rehabilitation. American Health Care Association Journal 3:14, 1977

Jenkins DJA, Wolever TMA, et al: Diabetic diets: High carbohydrate combined with high fiber. The American Journal of Clinical Nutrition 33(8):1729, 1980

Jernigan J, et al: Diagnosing dementia and its treatable causes. Geriatrics 34(3):79, 1979

Karasu TB, Katzman R: Organic brain syndromes, in Bellak L, Karasu TB (eds), Geriatric Psychiatry: A Handbook for Psychiatrists and Primary Care Physicians. New York, Grune and Stratton, 1976

Katzman R: The prevalence and malignance of Alzheimer's disease. Archives of Neurology 33:217, 1976

Katzman R, Terry R, Bick KL (eds): Alzheimer's Disease: Senile Dementia and Related Disorders. New York, Raven, 1978

Kay DWK, Roth M, Hopkins B: Affective disorders arising in the senium: I. Their association with organic cerebral degeneration. Journal of Mental Science 101:302, 1955

Keen H, Fuller JH: The epidemiology of diabetes, in Exton-Smith AN, Caird FI (eds), Metabolic and Nutritional Disorders in the Elderly. Chicago, Year Book, 1980

Keen H, Thomas B: Diabetes mellitus, in Dickerson JWT, and Lee HA (eds), Nutrition in the Clinical Management of Disease. Chicago, Year Book, 1978

Kety S: Disorders of the human brain. Scientific American 241(3):202, 1979

Kiloh LG: Pseudo-dementia. Acta Psychiatric Scandinavia 37:336, 1961

Knowles RD: Dealing with feelings: Control your thoughts. American Journal of Nursing 81(2):353, 1981

Krasa EJ: Some experiences in feeding the elderly. Journal of Geriatric Psychiatry 9(1):81, 1972

Kroner D: Dealing with the confused patient. Nursing 79 9(11):71, 1979

Lau E, Kosberg J: Editorial. Journal of the American Medical Association 241:18, 1979

Laurence S, Stein DG: Recovery after brain damage and the concept of localization of function, in Finger S (ed), Recovery From Brain Damage: Research and Theory. New York, Plenum, 1978

Levin ME: Diabetes mellitus, in Steinberg FU (ed), Cowdry's The Care of the Geriatric Patient, 5th ed. St. Louis, Mosby, 1976

Levine ME: Introduction to Clinical Nursing. Philadelphia, Davis, 1969

Lewis M, Butler RN: Life Review therapy. Geriatrics 29:165, 1974

Lewinsohn PM, Biglan A, Zeiss AM: Behavioral treatment of depression, in Davidson PO (ed), The Behavioral Management of Anxiety, Depression and Pain. New York, Brunner/Mazel, 1976

Libow LS: Senile dementia and pseudosenility: Clinical diagnosis, in Eisdorfer C, Friedel RO (eds), Cognitive and Emotional Disturbance in the Elderly. Chicago, Year Book, 1977

Lipton MA: Age differentiation in depression: Biochemical aspects. Journal of Gerontology 31:293, 1976

Loeb A, Beck AT, Diggory J: Differential effects of success and failure on depressed and nondepressed patients. Journal of Nervous and Mental Disease 152:106, 1971

Loew CA, Silverstone BM: A program of intensified stimulation and response facilitation in the senile aged. Gerontologist 11:341, 1971

LoGrasso BA: Using words without sound. American Journal of Nursing 80(12):2187, 1980

Ludwick R: Assessing confusion: A tool to improve nursing care. Journal of Gerontological Nursing 7(8):474, 1981

Mace N, Rabins P: The 36-Hour Day. A Family Guide to Caring for Persons with Alzheimer's Disease, Related Dementing Illnesses and Memory Loss in Later Life. Baltimore, Johns Hopkins University Press, 1981

Mahan CK: A sensible approach to the obese patient. Nursing Clinics of North America 14(2):229, 1979

Margolis L, Sherman FT: Hearing disorders, in Libow LS, Sherman FT (eds), The Core of Geriatric Medicine: A Guide for Students and Practitioners. St. Louis, Mosby, 1981

McCartney JH, Nadler G: How to help your patient cope with hearing loss. Geriatrics 34(3):69, 1979

McDowell F (ed): Managing the Person with Intellectual Loss (Dementia or Alzheimer's Disease) at Home. White Plains, NY, The Burke Rehabilitation Center, 1980

McDowell F (ed): Choosing a Nursing Home for the Person with Intellectual Loss. White Plains, NY, The Burke Rehabilitation Center, 1980

Meerloo JAM: Contribution of psychoanalysis to the problem of the aged, in Heiman M (ed), Psychoanalysis and Social Work. New York, International Universities Press, 1953

Meinert CL, Knatterud GL, Prout TE, Klimt CR: University group diabetes program: A study of the effects of hypoglycemic agents on vascular complications in patients with adult-onset diabetes. II. Mortality results. Diabetes 19 (Supp 2):789, 1970

Mishara B, Kastenbaum R: Alcohol and Old Age. (Seminars in Psychiatry) New York, Grune and Stratton, 1980

Moore MV: Diagnosis: Deafness. American Journal of Nursing 69(2):297, 1969

Morris M, Rhodes M: Guidelines for the care of confused patients. American Journal of Nursing 72(9):1630, 1972

Morse C, Smith E: Physical activity programming for the aged, in Smith E, Serfass R (eds), Exercise and Aging: The Scientific Basis. Hillside, NJ, Enslow, 1981

Moses DV: Reality orientation in the aging person, in Carlson CE (ed), Behavioral Concepts and Nursing Intervention. Philadelphia, Lippincott, 1970

Murphy G: The physician's responsibility for suicide. II. Errors of omission. Annals of Internal Medicine 82:305, 1975

O'Malley BC: Recent advances in managing the complications of diabetes. Geriatrics 35(6):51, 1980

O'Neal P, Robins E, Schmidt EH: A psychiatric study of attempted suicide in persons over sixty years of age. Archives of Neurology and Psychiatry 75:275, 1956

Oyer H, Oyer EJ: Social consequences of hearing loss for the elderly. Allied Health and Behavioral Science 2(2):123, 1979

Paykel ES: Recent life events and clinical depression, in Gunderson EKE, Rahe RH (eds), Life Stress and Illness. Springfield, IL, Thomas, 1974

Pearson LJ, Kothoff ME: Geriatric Clinical Protocols. New York, Lippincott, 1979

Perron DM: Deprived of sound. American Journal of Nursing 74(6):1057, 1974

Pfeiffer E: Psychotherapy with elderly patients. Postgraduate Medicine 50:254, 1971

Pfeiffer E, Busse EW: Mental disorders in later life—Affective disorders: Paranoid, neurotic, and situational reactions, in Busse EW, Pfeiffer E (eds), Mental Illness in Later Life. Washington, D.C., American Psychiatric Association, 1973

Posner JB: Delirium and exogenous metabolic brain disease, in Beeson PB, McDermott W (eds), Textbook of Medicine, 14th ed. Philadelphia, Saunders, 1975, vol 1

Post F: Dementia, depression, and pseudo-dementia, in Benson DF, Blumer D (eds), Psychiatric Aspects of Neurologic Disease. New York, Grune and Stratton, 1975

Price JH, Pritts C: Overweight and obesity in the elderly. Journal of Gerontological Nursing 6(6):343, 1980

Rainbow-Wind S: T'ai Chi Ch'uan as a healing art, in Berkeley Holistic Health Center (eds), The Holistic Health Handbook. Berkeley, CA, And/or Press, 1978

Reaven GM, Coulston AM, Marcus RA: Nutritional management of diabetes. Medical Clinics of North America 63(5):927, 1979

Report of the Workgroup on Definition and Diagnosis of Diabetes Mellitus (1976), in Report of the National Commission on Diabetes to the Congress of the United States. Washington D.C., Department of Health, Education and Welfare, vol 3, part 1

Reus V: Behavioral side effects of medical drugs. Primary Care 6(2):283, 1979

Rifkin H, Ross H, Shapiro HC: Diabetes in the elderly, in Rossman I (ed), Clinical Geriatrics, 2nd ed. Philadelphia, Lippincott, 1979

Roth M, Myers DH: The diagnosis of dementia. British Journal of Psychiatry, Special Publication 9:87, 1975

Ruben RJ: Otolaryngologic problems of the old. Hospital Practice 12(8):73, 1977

Ryden M: Nursing intervention in support of reminiscence. Journal of Gerontological Nursing 7(8):461, 1981

Schneideman J: Remotivation: Involvement without labels. Journal of Psychiatric Nursing and Mental Health Services 14(7):41, 1976

Schow RL, Christensen JM, Hutchinson JM, Nerbone MA: Communication Disorders of the Aged. A Guide for Health Professionals. Baltimore, University Park Press, 1978

Schuknecht HF: Further observations on the pathology of presbycusis. Archives of Otolaryngology 80:369, 1964

Seligman MEP: Helplessness. San Francisco, Freeman, 1975

Seltzer B, Sherwin I: Organic brain syndromes: An empirical study and critical review. American Journal of Psychiatry 135(1):109, 1978

Senturia BH, Goldstein R, Hersperget WS: Otorhinolaryngologic aspects, in Steinberg FU (ed), Cowdry's The

Care of the Geriatric Patient, 5th ed. St. Louis, Mosby, 1976

Shraberg D: The myth of pseudodementia: Depression and the aging brain. American Journal of Psychiatry 135:5, 1978

Sloane RB: Organic brain syndrome, in Birren JE, Sloane RB (eds), Handbook of Mental Health and Aging. Englewood Cliffs, NJ, Prentice-Hall, 1980

Steinberg FU: Rehabilitation medicine, in Steinberg FU (ed), Cowdry's The Care of the Geriatric Patient, 5th ed. St Louis, Mosby, 1976

Steury S, Blank ML (eds): Readings in Psychotherapy with Older People. U.S. Department of Health, Education and Welfare. National Institute of Mental Health, DHEW Pub #(ADM), 1978

Straus B: Disorders of the digestive system, in Rossman I (ed), Clinical Geriatrics, 2nd ed. Philadelphia, Lippincott, 1979

Strehler BL: Introduction: Aging and the human brain, in Terry RD, Gershon S (eds), Aging. New York, Raven, 1975, vol 3

Strob RL: Alzheimer's disease—Current perspectives. Journal of Clinical Psychiatry 41(4):110, 1980

Thompson M: Geriatric nutrition. Journal of the National Medical Association 72(8):795, 1980

Todhunter EN, Darby WJ: Guidelines for maintaining adequate nutrition in old age. Geriatrics 33(6):49, 1978

Torack RM: Adult dementia: History, biopsy, pathology. Neurosurgery 4:434, 1979

Trockman G: Caring for the confused or delirious patient. American Journal of Nursing 79(9):1495, 1978

Ventura E: Foot care for diabetics. American Journal of Nursing 78(5):886, 1978

Walsh AC, Walsh BH: Presenile dementia: Further experience with an anticoagulant psychotherapy regime.

Journal of the American Geriatrics Society 22:467, 1974

Weir DR, Houser HB, Davy L: Recognition and management of the nutrition problems of the elderly, in Chinn AB (ed), Working With Older People: Guide to Practice. Volume IV: Clinical Aspects of Aging. Washington, D.C., U.S. Department of Health, Education and Welfare, 1974

Weitkamp L, Stancer H, et al : Depressive disorders of HLA: A gene on chromosome 6 that can affect behavior. New England Journal of Medicine 305(22):1301, 1981

Wells CE: Diagnostic evaluation and treatment in dementia, in Wells CE (ed), Dementia, 2nd ed. Philadelphia, Davis, 1977

Wells CE: Chronic brain disease: An overview. American Journal of Psychiatry 125:1, 1978

Wells CE: Pseudodementia. American Journal of Psychiatry 136(7):895, 1979

Whitehouse FW: Ten questions physicians most often ask about treating diabetic complications. Consultant 19:59, 1979

Wiener M, Pepper G, Kuhn-Weisman G, Romano J: Clinical Pharmacology and Therapeutics in Nursing. New York, McGraw-Hill, 1979

Williams TF: Diabetes mellitus in the aged, in Greenhall RB (ed), Geriatric Endocrinology: Aging, Vol. 5. New York, Raven, 1978

Wilson EA, Hadden DR, et al : Dietary management of maturity-onset diabetes. British Medical Journal 280(6228):1367, 1980

Windsor ACM: Nutrition in the elderly. Practitioner 222(1331):625, 1979

Zarit SH: Aging and Mental Disorders: Psychological Approaches to Assessment and Treatment. New York, Free Press, 1980

17

Nursing the Client Experiencing Problems of Fluids and Electrolytes

Maintenance of a healthy balance of fluids and electrolytes depends upon an adequate intake and the synergistic interaction of various body systems to ingest, process, and distribute these elements and then eliminate the products of metabolism. This chapter discusses three problems that commonly affect older people and have implications for their overall fluid and electrolyte balance. Congestive heart failure, a serious problem in older people, ultimately affects the functioning of nearly every body system and results in imbalances of both fluids and electrolytes. Pathological changes in the heart and kidney as well as certain of the client's behavior patterns have been implicated in the development of heart failure. Other problems discussed in this chapter include diverticular disease and urinary incontinence. These are prevalent problems among the elderly and have far-reaching effects not only on their patterns of elimination but on their quality of life.

Older clients who are coping with these and other chronic health problems often need to manage a complicated medication regimen in order to maintain optimal adaptation. Some must acquire new habits to meet a basic need—hygiene. To accommodate declining energy reserves, many older people must give up past behavior patterns and modify activities of daily living. This chapter discusses the nurse's role in helping older clients manage their medications safely and cope with changes in hygiene patterns and activities of daily living.

SIGNIFICANT PROBLEMS

Congestive Heart Failure

Congestive heart failure refers to a complex of adaptations that develop when the heart fails as a pump. Cardiac output may fall or it may fail to rise when the client exercises. In either case, cardiac output is not sufficient to meet the body's metabolic needs. Congestive heart failure affects the functioning of the central nervous, gastrointestinal, excretory, and musculoskeletal systems. Because the elderly have few reserves, heart failure readily disrupts the delicate balance these systems maintain. As heart failure progresses, it can threaten the older person's ability to maintain an active life-style and finally to live independently.

Stresses Associated with Heart Failure. In older people, heart failure is usually a response to multiple, diverse stresses (Kleiger, 1976). The most important underlying stress associated with heart failure is cardiac disease. Older clients with heart failure usually have at least one cardiac disease, and often have two or more. A variety of other, noncardiac health problems is usually present as well. These may precipitate heart failure in susceptible individuals or aggravate already existing failure.

The most common cardiac diseases associated with the development of heart failure in older people are ischemic heart disease and hypertensive heart disease. At least one of these was present in over

80 percent of one group of elderly clients with congestive heart failure (Pomerance, 1968). Other cardiac diseases that underlie congestive heart failure include recent myocardial infarction, mitral valve changes due to rheumatic heart disease or other factors, and aortic stenosis. Less common stresses are pericarditis, subacute bacterial endocarditis, and congenital heart defects. Senile cardiac amyloidosis (the development of detectable amyloid deposits in the heart) is recognized increasingly as a significant factor associated with the development of heart failure in elderly people, especially those over 80. Senile myocardial degeneration, or heart failure without apparent cause, is believed to be related to the normal aging process. It occurs in only a small number (2.5 percent) of cases (Kleiger, 1976).

Many noncardiac diseases precipitate or aggravate heart failure in elderly clients with little cardiac reserve. Impaired pulmonary circulation may be responsible for heart failure. For example, cor pulmonale may develop as a consequence of chronic emphysema or bronchitis. Pulmonary emboli and pulmonary infarction also precipitate heart failure. Pneumonia and other respiratory infections, thyrotoxicosis, myxedema, and diabetes mellitus are associated with heart failure. Long-standing renal failure may precipitate heart failure because it causes sodium and water retention with consequent hypertension. Advanced liver disease may cause heart failure because hypoproteinemia upsets fluid balance.

Some of the medications older people take may be responsible for heart failure. Digitalis is indicated in the treatment of heart failure but digitalis toxicity is common in the elderly and often causes arrhythmias. These reduce cardiac output and can result in heart failure. Failure to take digitalis may also stimulate heart failure. Other medications, including the corticosteroids, anabolic agents, and antiinflammatory agents such as phenylbutazone, oxyphenbutazone, and indomethacin, can cause heart failure due to sodium and water retention.

Certain behavior patterns in the elderly have been associated with the development of heart failure. These include emotional stress, excessive physical activity, or insufficient physical activity. Dietary habits can also be a factor. Excessive sodium intake can result in heart failure due to retention of water and expansion of extracellular volume.

A diet too high in calories can lead to obesity, increasing the cardiac work load. A diet inadequate in protein can result in hypoproteinemia and consequent fluid retention.

The Dynamics of Heart Failure. Several theoretical models have been proposed to explain the process by which heart failure develops and the resulting adaptations. The theories include the high output/low output failure theory, the forward failure/backward failure theory, and the left failure/right failure theory.

The high output/low output failure theory seeks to explain how various stresses alter cardiac output and stimulate the development of heart failure. *Low output failure* occurs when the stress involves cardiac muscle damage or a resistance to ventricular ejection. Both of these reduce cardiac output. The heart works harder and harder to deliver oxygen to tissues but it no longer meets the body's needs. Myocardial infarction, ischemic heart disease, hypertension, arrhythmias, and valvular heart disease are some of the conditions associated with low output failure. *High output failure,* on the other hand, occurs when the body's tissues require a larger than normal blood supply. This stress elevates the pulse rate and the cardiac output, resulting in expansion of plasma volume, increased venous return, and increased circulation. When the heart can no longer handle the increased load, cardiac output drops and does not meet the body's needs. Anemia and pulmonary emphysema increase the body's need for oxygen due to the low oxygen content of arterial blood. Hyperthyroidism, Parkinson's disease, and infection increase the body's oxygen need by increasing its metabolic requirements. Congenital defects, such as an arteriovenous fistula, increase the body's need for oxygen because they short-circuit the circulating blood, depriving large areas of an adequate blood supply. A thiamine deficiency that causes deficient tissue metabolism is the reason why beriberi increases the body's oxygen need.

Both the forward/backward theory and the left/right theory seek to explain the adaptations associated with congestive heart failure. The *backward failure theory* refers to the damming effect of blood behind the failing ventricle. Because the heart cannot pump all the blood returned to it, there is an increase in end-diastolic volume, causing venous and capillary pressures behind the ventricle to rise. When hydrostatic pressure exceeds oncotic pressure, there is transudation of fluid to the interstitial spaces. In contrast, the *forward failure theory* holds that the heart pumps an inadequate supply of blood to vital organs. Renal perfusion is reduced, activating the renin–angiotensin cycle and setting up a chain of events that culminates in sodium and water retention.

Left- and right-sided failure theories are based on the fact that the left and right sides of the heart pump blood through two distinct, but connecting systems, the systemic circulation and the pulmonary circulation. The underlying stress determines which side fails first. In *left heart failure,* less blood is pumped to the systemic circulation and pressure rises in the left atrium and pulmonary vessels. Pulmonary venous hypertension and increased stiffening of the lungs account for the adaptations associated with left heart failure. Hypertension, coronary artery disease, and mitral and aortic valve disease may precipitate left heart failure. *Right heart failure* results in less blood circulating through the pulmonary system and a build-up of pressure behind the failing right ventricle in the right atrium and venous circulation. The increasing pressure accounts for the adaptations of right heart failure, including venous congestion and edema. Right heart failure may develop late in the course of left heart failure as a consequence of any of the stresses that precipitate left heart failure. Obstructions of the pulmonary system, such as those associated with pulmonary emboli and chronic obstructive pulmonary disease, and pulmonic valve defects may precipitate right heart failure.

In fact, all three theories are somewhat artificial and simplistic because the circulatory system is a closed system and the heart is a single pump. Although heart failure may involve only one chamber initially, with the other continuing to function normally, total heart failure occurs eventually. Both of the ventricles are composed of a continuous muscle mass and share a common wall. The prolonged, excessive load on the normal ventricle eventually leads to its failure as well. Failure of only one ventricle is associated with the depletion of cardiac norepinephrine and changes in the activity of myofibrillar adenosine triphosphatase (ATPase), and these affect the functioning of all myocardial muscle, not just the portion that has failed (Coakley, 1981).

Regardless of which mechanism is involved, when the heart cannot meet the demands placed on it, the response is an increased heart rate and hypertrophy of heart muscle. The heart uses more oxygen but despite increased effort, performs less effective work. When these compensatory mechanisms fail, the client exhibits adaptations of heart failure.

An understanding of congestive heart failure is based on knowledge that there is no clear dividing line between normal cardiac function and heart failure. Consequently, the adaptations of heart failure represent a continuum ranging from absent or inconspicuous to clearly evident or catastrophic (Coakley, 1981). The onset of failure ranges from acute to slow and insidious. Stresses such as acute myocardial infarction, arrhythmias, acute respiratory infection, sudden blood loss, pulmonary infarction, thyrotoxicosis, and rapid circulatory overload may precipitate acute heart failure. It may present as pulmonary edema or cardiogenic shock. Chronic heart failure involves both the right and left sides of the heart and takes many forms. Refractory heart failure, a form of chronic failure in which cardiac decompensation continues despite appropriate treatment, is especially common in the elderly.

The Client at Risk. The incidence of congestive heart failure in the aged is significant. As a result of the aging process, the heart undergoes many changes that render it more vulnerable to the cardiac and noncardiac stresses that precipitate heart failure. Aging affects the heart muscle, valves, vessels, and conduction system. As a result, cardiac output decreases, the cardiac response to stress is less efficient and effective, peripheral vascular resistance increases, and arrhythmias develop. In addition, the incidence of cardiac conditions that are the underlying cause of heart failure is highest in the elderly. In most cases, heart failure reduces the older person's quality of life. Only rarely is it the cause of their death. Most frequently, the older client with heart failure dies from its complications, not from heart failure itself. In one study, one-third of the older subjects with heart failure died from bronchopneumonia and one-seventh from pulmonary embolism (Bedford and Caird, 1960).

Diverticular Disease

Diverticular disease is a vague term that includes several conditions. Prediverticular disease is the earliest stage of the disease process. During this phase, intestinal muscle fibers undergo prolonged spasm and shortening that result in a thickening of the circular and longitudinal layer of intestinal muscle. The thickened muscle causes segmentation of the bowel and an increase in the intraluminal pressure of each segment. A diverticulum is a small bladder or sac formed by the herniation of the mucous membrane outward through a separation in the circular muscle fibers of the intestine. It develops as a consequence of the increased intraluminal pressure. Diverticula can develop in any part of the digestive tract, but they occur most frequently in the narrowest parts of the colon on the left side, that is, the descending and sigmoid colon. They occur at the weakest points of the circular muscle, normally the areas where the segmental blood vessels penetrate the circular muscles of the bowel. Colonic diverticula are almost always multiple.

When diverticula are known to be present somewhere in the intestine but the client exhibits only a few mild adaptations or no adaptations at all, diverticulosis is said to be present. When complications develop and the client exhibits adaptations, diverticulitis is said to be present, and the client moves from Adaptation Level Three to Level Four. The lumen of the sacs can become blocked with intestinal contents, causing stasis and, finally, inflammation or infection. The mucous membrane bladders may perforate or they may erode blood vessels, causing bleeding. Most frequently, diverticulitis is a consequence of the localized perforation of a single diverticulum, with subsequent inflammation involving the area near the perforated sac or a wider area of the colon (Berman and Kirsner, 1976). About 15 percent of clients with diverticula develop diverticulitis (Goldner, 1977).

Incidence and Prevalence. Diverticular disease of the colon is a disease of middle and old age. Its incidence increases sharply with increasing age. Estimates of its incidence vary widely. According to the most conservative estimate, it afflicts 20 percent of those over age 60 (Strause, 1979). Others say that diverticular disease afflicts as many as two-thirds of those over 60, and that its incidence is

reaching epidemic proportions in the United States (Goldner, 1977). Diverticular disease is becoming more common with the passage of time. Prior to 1920, diverticular disease was almost unknown. However, within the life span of this generation of older people, it has become the most common disease of the colon in the Western world (Brocklehurst, 1978a; Snel, 1981). Diverticular disease affects women more often than men (Dymock, 1974).

Stresses. The development of colon diverticula is believed to be a consequence of multiple stresses, rather than a single event. Individuals with colon diverticula have a higher incidence of hiatus hernia and esophageal diverticula. Experts are uncertain about whether this relationship is merely coincidental or suggests some form of predisposition (Strause, 1979). Aging, with associated atrophy of the musculature of the intestinal wall, may weaken the intestine and be a factor in diverticula development. Obesity is also believed to be a factor by increasing intraluminal pressure or weakening the bowel wall (Goldner, 1977; Dymock, 1974; Strause, 1979).

Diet. A chronic lack of bulk in the diet is now believed to be one of the most important stresses responsible for the development of diverticula. In the Western world during the last century, the amount of bulk in the diet has decreased significantly. Because fiber was considered an impurity, roller milling of flour became popular. This process removes two-thirds of the fiber from flour. At the same time the intake of refined sugars doubled due to new refining processes, and the consumption of meats and fats also increased. In contrast, in those parts of the world where a high-residue diet is still the custom, diverticular disease is virtually unknown (Brocklehurst, 1978a). Fiber is composed of plant materials (polysaccharides and lignen). Because it is resistant to digestion, it adds more bulk to the sigmoid than do more easily absorbed materials. Normally, food residue moves through the colon as a consequence of the contraction and relaxation of alternate segments of the colon. As more food passes through the ileocecal valve, food residue is displaced toward the rectum as intestinal contractions continue. With increased food bulk, pressure in each segment of the colon decreases. In contrast, when there is little waste in the colon, stronger muscle contractions are required to excrete it and pressure within the affected segments rises. This high pressure is associated with muscular hypertrophy and the development of outpouchings or diverticula. Because the time required to move intestinal contents through the bowel also increases, stool becomes hard and dry, causing straining. Eventually, a vicious cycle is started.

Constipation. Constipation has also been implicated in the development of diverticular disease. The definition of constipation is elusive because bowel function is a complex and individualized phenomenon and dependent on cultural variables. Constipation refers to stools that are hard, dry, or difficult to pass or to a decrease in the frequency of the individual's normal pattern of elimination. Defecation is a normal physiological process that should not be difficult. Studies on large populations indicate that the normal pattern of defecation in 99 percent of subjects varies widely, anywhere from three times a day to three times a week. Furthermore, there does not appear to be any regular or predictable increase or decrease in the frequency of defecation with aging (Brocklehurst, 1978a). There is no evidence of any age-related structural or functional changes in the gastrointestinal tract that would induce constipation (Pollman et al., 1978). Nevertheless the incidence of constipation is greater in the old than in the young for many reasons. First, older people have a high incidence of organic diseases such as hypothyroidism, neurological diseases such as cerebrovascular accident and Parkinson's disease, hypercalcemia, strictures, and tumors that cause hard dry stools. They also have a high incidence of emotional stress, such as depression, that is associated with anorexia and subsequent constipation. The elderly also take more medications than any other age group and many of these are constipating. For example, regular use of calcium carbonate or aluminum hydroxide antacids causes constipation (Gotz and Gotz, 1978). Iron salts and minerals are binding. Anticholinergic, antihypertensive, diuretic, tranquilizer, sedative, and analgesic medications are also constipating. The frequency of laxative taking is higher in this generation of older people, perhaps because of cultural factors and lifelong habits. Overuse of laxatives is

known to cause atony of intestinal muscles, with the ultimate consequence being chronic constipation (Lofholm, 1978; Brocklehurst, 1978a). The inadequate or improper diet of older people may also be a contributing factor. Some older clients cannot chew foods such as fruits and vegetables that are high in fiber and others cannot afford them. Mental and physical impairments may prevent older people from obtaining or preparing adequate food. Their fluid intake may also be too low. With inadequate fluids, water and electrolytes are reabsorbed into the circulation rather than remaining in the intestine, resulting in stools that are hard and dry. Older people often have weak or flabby abdominal musculature, thus preventing them from increasing intraabdominal pressure and expelling feces. The increased incidence of chronic illness and hospitalization in older people, coupled with lifelong habits, make immobility a major cause of constipation in the elderly. Lack of exercise decreases peristalsis. Persons who are confused or have other mental impairments may disregard or be unaware of a distended rectum and the urge to defecate (Berman and Kirsner, 1976). In summary, constipation in older people is an adaptation to a variety of stresses. It results in a buildup of pressure in the intestine that can weaken the bowel walls. When this happens, constipation becomes a stress that contributes to the development of diverticular disease.

Precipitating Stresses. In clients with diverticulosis, certain stresses are known to precipitate diverticulitis. These include dietary indiscretions such as overeating or consumption of irritating foods or alcohol. Coughing and straining at stool may also be contributory (Strause, 1979).

Potential Stresses. Diverticulitis sometimes results in serious, even life-threatening complications. These include formation of an abscess or inflammatory mass, fistulas between the intestines and the vagina or bladder, intestinal obstruction, perforation with peritonitis, and septicemia (Snel, 1981). Massive, sudden hemorrhage may also occur in a few individuals.

Urinary Incontinence
Impairment of the functional efficiency of the lower urinary tract is an important problem in old age.

Because the normal pattern of micturition changes with age, at least 30 percent of older people complain of daytime frequency and 60 to 70 percent complain of nocturia (Brocklehurst, 1978b; George and Osborn, 1981). The elderly also have a high incidence of other urinary problems including dysuria (painful urination), scalding on micturition, and difficulty (hesitancy) in micturition (Brocklehurst, 1978b). However, incontinence is the most serious problem of micturition, not only because of its prevalence but because of its psychosocial consequences for the older person.

Urinary incontinence is characterized by the involuntary passage of urine. It is not a disease, but an adaptation that can result from many stresses. Incontinence is a problem of significant proportions among the elderly. Although estimates of its prevalence vary widely, incontinence may affect 3 percent of older men and 12 percent of older women who live in the community. It is an even more common problem among institutionalized older people, affecting as many as 40 percent of older people who are hospitalized (Brocklehurst, 1978b).

Obtaining accurate statistics about incontinence is difficult. Older people often go to great lengths to conceal their incontinence rather than seek health care. Incontinence is a source of shame and embarrassment in our society and older people may believe nothing can be done for it. For a significant number of these older people, incontinence is a catastrophe that affects not only their lives, but the lives of their families and caretakers. It is the reason why some older persons can no longer be cared for at home and are placed in institutions. In addition, it may be the only reason why hospitalized older clients are not considered for home or community placement in spite of all the other positive attributes they may have.

Normal Micturition. Continence of urine is maintained by a number of factors. The lower urinary system consists of the bladder, urethra, and internal and external sphincters. The bladder is composed of three layers of smooth muscle. The outermost layer is the detrusor muscle. The bladder is supported at its base by elastic pelvic tissues. At the bladder (vesical) neck, where the urethra meets the bladder, extensions of the smooth detrusor mus-

cle fibers are arranged to form the internal urethral sphincter, or trigonal muscle. This small triangular area is not a true sphincter, but maintains closure of the urethral opening until pressure in the bladder rises high enough to overcome its tone. Skeletal muscle at the end of the urethra forms the external urethral sphincter. The length and placement of the urethra are maintained by the pelvic perineal musculature and are essential for the maintenance of continence.

During micturition the detrusor muscle contracts and the external sphincter and pelvic muscles relax, permitting passage of urine through the urethra. Abdominal muscles also aid in urination as a result of increased intraabdominal pressure when voluntarily contracted.

Normal function of the lower urinary system requires the integrity of several elements of the nervous system:

1. Isolated inefficient neuromuscular actions of the bladder wall can autonomously contract the bladder.
2. Stretch receptors in the bladder wall sensitive to tension produced as a result of filling send impulses via the afferent fibers of the parasympathetic nervous system to the micturition center at S_2–S_4. As a result of efferent impulses from S_2–S_4, detrusor contraction and relaxation of perineal muscles and the external sphincter occur, causing micturition. At all other times, motor fibers from S_2–S_4 maintain contraction of the external sphincter. This reflex arc controls the act of voiding in infants.
3. The voiding reflex in the sacrum is subject to voluntary control from higher centers in the brainstem and the cortical center in the frontal lobe. These innervate the external urethral sphincter. Central inhibition is developed in childhood. When the urge to micturate is present, it permits postponement of urination until a socially convenient time and place are available. Central control also allows urination when the urge to void is not present.

How Aging Affects Micturition. With age, normal changes occur in the structure and function of the lower urinary system. The bladder capacity diminishes to about 250 ml from the 500 to 600 ml capacity of young adults. The kidneys are no longer able to concentrate urine well. Consequently, the healthy older person experiences an increased frequency of urination and nocturia. According to Brocklehurst (1978b), 50 to 70 percent of healthy older people experience nocturia and arise two or three times each night to empty their bladders. In many older people normal bladder filling is interrupted by uninhibited bladder contractions of the detrusor muscle, causing an urgent desire to void. After voiding, however, a significant quantity of residual urine remains because the bladder loses muscle tone. With age there is a lack of cortical neuronal function, which diminishes the central inhibitory effect over the peripheral reflex arc of micturition. This loss of inhibition also leads to nocturnal frequency and to a degree of urgency in micturition because the onset of the desire to void is late (often at the limit of bladder capacity). In contrast, young adults first have the desire to urinate at about half bladder capacity. In women the length of the urethra decreases somewhat. In both sexes, the urinary stream is slower and at a lower pressure (Brocklehurst, 1979).

Although all of these factors predispose the elderly to incontinence, they do not cause it. Incontinence is not an inevitable consequence of old age. Most healthy older clients are able to maintain continence as long as they are able to adjust their environment to meet the needs of the aging bladder. Precipitating stresses superimposed upon the predisposing factors are required to cause incontinence in older people. These may be stresses that alter the environment, depriving older people of their former control over it, or stresses that alter bladder function.

Types of Incontinence. A standard system for classifying the types of incontinence does not exist. Incontinence has been classified according to its adaptations as stress, urgency, and overflow. *Stress* incontinence is an involuntary loss of small amounts of urine because of stresses that affect the pelvic musculature or increase intraabdominal pressure. *Urge* incontinence is the precipitate loss of a large amount of urine. Clients cannot voluntarily control sphincter action and once urination starts they cannot stop it. *Overflow* incontinence is the leakage of urine from a distended bladder.

Incontinence has also been categorized according to its temporal characteristics as acute or established (Brocklehurst, 1978b). *Acute* incontinence could also be called spurious. It is a transient adaptation to a specific and temporary stress. It often develops suddenly. Acute incontinence may be due to illness, environmental factors, iatrogenic factors, or psychosocial factors. These are precipitating factors that further impair bladder function in elderly clients who are already predisposed to incontinence.

Incontinence may follow serious *illness,* such as myocardial infarction, congestive heart failure, pneumonia, acute infections, toxemias, or general surgery. Any disease condition that causes acute confusion is especially likely to be associated with acute incontinence. Constipation and fecal impaction are important reasons for acute urinary incontinence in older people of both sexes. The impaction has an obstructive effect and can result in urinary retention and overflow, dysuria and frequency (Lothian, 1977).

Any change in the *environment* may cause incontinence in older people because new environments often cause temporary confusion in the elderly. Bed rest is a particularly important reason for acute incontinence because the older client is no longer able to go independently to the toilet or commode as quickly or as often as needed. The older client may be in an environment where there are too few toilets or where the distance to the toilet is too great. This is the situation in some nursing homes. Acute incontinence also encompasses problems with mobility or manual dexterity that make it difficult for older clients to reach the toilet or arrange their garments.

Iatrogenic factors include medical treatments, especially drug therapy, that may precipitate incontinence in older people. Urinary incontinence is a common consequence of diuretic therapy. The overuse of sedatives and hypnotics may depress the client's level of awareness of bladder distention and cause incontinence. It may also be caused by antihistamines, anticholinergic agents such as the atropinelike drugs, antispasmodics, tricyclic antidepressants, antiparkinsonian agents, epinephrine, phenothiazines, muscle relaxants, quinidine, and some of the ganglionic-blocking agents. Many of these agents cause urinary retention, with resulting overflow incontinence (Brocklehurst, 1978b; 1981; Pearson and Kotthoff, 1979). Urinary incontinence has been reported with the use of L-dopa, but it subsides after the client has been on the medication for several weeks (Caird, 1974).

Psychosocial stresses have also been implicated in the development of incontinence. According to social breakdown theory, older people become incontinent because this is what society expects them to do. For example, clients who are transferred to a nursing home are often incontinent at first because they are not oriented to the setting. By the time the initial transition is over, the staff may have labeled the client as incontinent and the person reacts and behaves accordingly. Clues such as failure to toilet the client, placing the commode out of reach and diapering lead clients to believe they are not capable of controlling this function (Maney, 1976). According to another theory, incontinence is a consequence of the emotional breakdown and reversion to childhood roles that can result from institutionalization and the loss of all one's familiar habits (Brocklehurst, 1978b).

In most instances, acute incontinence can be effectively treated simply by identifying and removing the precipitating stress. Nurses play an important role in preventing or eliminating acute incontinence in older clients.

Established or central (true) incontinence is that which continues even after precipitating stresses such as acute illness, environmental, iatrogenic, and psychosocial factors have been removed. In these cases, the incontinence is believed to be a consequence of habit or further damage to some element of the urinary tract. Established incontinence may also be the only significant problem apparent in an older client who seems otherwise healthy. In these cases, incontinence often develops gradually as a consequence of slowly developing, subtle, and chronic pathological processes. Many different types of established incontinence have been identified, depending upon the nature of the precipitating stress (Fig. 1). Stresses may alter neurological control, affect the bladder and its outlet, block the urethra, or weaken the supporting muscles of the pelvis. Established incontinence is complicated in the elderly because often more than one stress is responsible for its development.

Neurological Control. Stresses that affect the nervous system are the most common reason for incontinence in the elderly (Vallarino and Sherman, 1981). Four types of neurogenic bladder conditions can occur. A fifth condition, the unstable bladder, may also be due to stresses that affect bladder enervation.

UNINHIBITED NEUROGENIC BLADDER. The uninhibited neurogenic bladder is the most frequent neurological condition responsible for dysuria and incontinence in older people (Brocklehurst, 1981). It is due to lesions in the cerebral cortex or its efferent pathways that interfere with cortical inhibition of the sacral reflex arc. Consequently the reflex arc emerges in an uninhibited fashion. The uninhibited bladder is believed to develop in many older people as a consequence of the gradual loss of cortical neurons that accompanies the aging process. It may also develop as a result of cerebrovascular accident, diffuse cerebral arteriosclerosis, Parkinson's disease, multiple sclerosis, dementia, and frontal lobe tumor. The uninhibited neurogenic bladder is characterized by a small capacity. Normal bladder filling and distention stimulate bladder contractions that result in micturition when the bladder is only partially filled. Awareness of bladder filling is absent and the sensation of the desire to void is delayed until the bladder is near capacity and contractions are large. Sensation is followed quickly by precipitate and uncontrolled bladder emptying. This explains the main adaptation of the uninhibited neurogenic bladder—urgency. Unfortunately, the uncoordinated nature of reflex bladder activity prevents the bladder from emptying properly. Consequently, the uninhibited neurogenic bladder is associated with significant residual urine, encouraging bacterial overgrowth (Lothian, 1977).

ATONIC NEUROGENIC BLADDER. Stresses that affect the posterior nerve roots or posterior horn cells (lower motor neuron lesions) and interrupt the afferent fibers of the reflex arc are associated with the atonic neurogenic bladder. Voluntary micturition is possible but reflex micturition is prevented. The bladder can be emptied effectively only when the client increases intraabdominal pressure or applies manual pressure. Because clients no longer experience the sensation of bladder distention, they often forget to urinate. The bladder becomes overdistended and eventually atonic. Bladder capacity

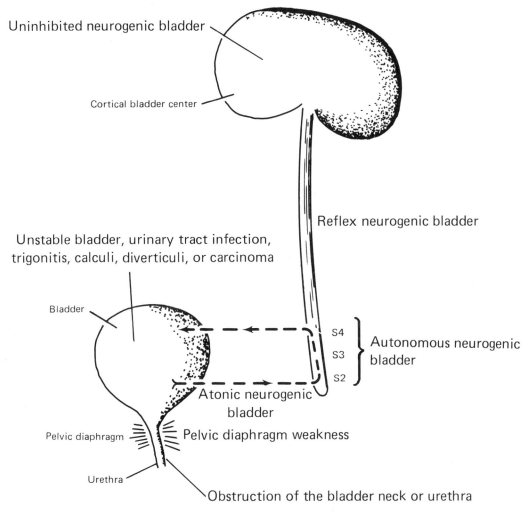

Figure 1. Stresses that precipitate established incontinence.

may increase to 1500 to 3000 ml. Chronic retention with overflow incontinence results. This type of incontinence occurs most commonly in older clients with diabetes but is also associated with tabes dorsalis (Brocklehurst, 1977).

AUTONOMOUS NEUROGENIC BLADDER. This type of incontinence develops when the sacral bladder center is destroyed and the bladder is completely cut off from the central nervous system. Normal voluntary and reflex micturition are absent. The client does not have a sensation of bladder filling or well-formed bladder contractions. The bladder empties in small quantities by weak local myoneural contractions. This type of incontinence is uncommon in the elderly. It is associated with metastatic carcinoma and infarction at the lower end of the spinal cord.

REFLEX NEUROGENIC BLADDER. In this condition, the stress (upper motor neuron lesion) affects the area between the sacral bladder center and the cortical center. Both afferent and efferent fibers are destroyed. There is no awareness of bladder distention and no ability to inhibit reflex bladder contractions. Micturition is reflex and unconscious. The bladder fills up and empties but the client has no awareness of what is happening. This type of incontinence is uncommon in old age. It is associated with paraplegia (Brocklehurst, 1979).

THE UNSTABLE BLADDER. Stresses responsible for the unstable bladder (also called detrusor instability) are uncertain. It may be associated with defective cortical control, although demonstrable pathology is not apparent. Other causes may be pelvic surgery, prostatic involvement, prostatectomy or emotional stress (Brocklehurst, 1979). The unstable bladder is characterized by the development of intrinsic contractions that result in bladder emptying. Some authors do not differentiate between unstable bladder and uninhibited bladder, but they are separate types of incontinence. In uninhibited bladder, bladder contractions develop spontaneously as the bladder fills, whereas, in unstable bladder, contractions develop in response to a provocative stimulus, such as coughing or changing position. The unstable bladder is characterized by a stimulus, a momentary delay, and then the loss of a large amount of urine (Brocklehurst, 1981).

The Bladder. The incidence of chronic urinary tract infection increases dramatically in women over age 70 and men over age 75. Chronic urinary tract infections are most prevalent in the institutionalized elderly. They have been associated with dementia and fecal contamination of the perineum. In most cases, however, chronic infections are relatively benign conditions in the elderly. They are less likely to produce incontinence in the elderly than in younger individuals (Vallarino and Sherman, 1981). On the other hand, acute urinary tract infections in older people have been associated with the development of dysuria, precipitancy, and incontinence due to the increased sensitivity of stretch receptors in the inflamed bladder.

Atrophic senile vaginitis with associated trigonitis is a common cause of acute incontinence in older women. The trigone of the bladder is related developmentally to the vagina, and like the vagina is estrogen dependent. As estrogen levels decline, these tissues atrophy and become less resistant to pathogens. As a result, inflammation and infection may develop in the areas of the vulva, vagina, and

urinary tract. The most common adaptations are urgency and frequency of urination (Brown, 1978). Other stresses that affect the bladder, such as cancer, calculi, and diverticula can also cause urinary incontinence.

The Bladder Neck and Urethra. Prostatism is a general term applied to the condition produced by obstruction at the vesical neck or compression of the urethra in men. It may be due to several stresses, including bladder neck sclerosis, nodular hyperplasia of the prostate (benign prostatic hypertrophy), and carcinoma of the prostate. Usually carcinoma does not result in obstruction until it is advanced. Benign prostatic hypertrophy is the most common cause of urinary obstruction in old age (Sourander, 1978). After age 60, 70 to 80 percent of men develop prostatic hypertrophy and half of these develop serious difficulties with micturition (deVoogt, 1981). When prostatic obstruction first occurs the detrusor muscle adapts by compensatory hypertrophy, which continues until the bladder can no longer overcome the obstruction. Then decompensation occurs and the older man develops residual urine. Whenever residual urine is present, the client is at risk for urinary tract infection. As urinary retention continues, the bladder wall thins out and becomes flabby. Finally, hydroureter, hydronephrosis, a declining glomerular filtration rate, and uremia can occur.

The adaptations that accompany benign prostatic hypertrophy range from subtle to overt. Sometimes adaptations are minimal until another stress affecting bladder function is superimposed upon the first stress. For example, the older man may use a decongestant for a common cold. A side effect is increased bladder neck tone. Or he may take anticholinergic or tranquilizer medications that decrease detrusor tone. These agents may be the stresses that precipitate painful and frightening acute urinary retention in the man with prostatic hypertrophy (Basso, 1977).

The Pelvic Diaphragm. Normally the bladder is supported on the pelvic diaphragm, principally on the pubococcygeous muscle and the levator ani. The proximal two-thirds of the urethra is above the pelvic floor and pressure on the proximal urethra exceeds that in the bladder. In addition, the pelvic muscles support the urethrovesical junction at an angle that helps maintain continence.

In many postmenopausal women, the pelvic muscles weaken and no longer provide adequate support for the bladder base, vesical neck, and proximal urethra. As the vesical neck descends, the bladder outlet is distorted and the urethrovesical angle is altered to a straight line, thus losing its mechanical advantage. When urine distends the bladder it also distends the urethrovesical segment. Consequently, whenever there is a sudden increase in intraabdominal pressure, there is an opening pull on the bladder surface and a small amount of urine escapes. Incomplete bladder emptying, residual urine, and infection can also occur. Stresses that can cause an increase in intraabdominal pressure include sneezing, coughing, laughing, bending over, stooping, sitting down, standing up, walking, getting out of bed, straining at stool, or wearing a tight girdle.

This type of incontinence is called stress incontinence. It is the most frequent reason for incontinence in postmenopausal women (Brown, 1978). Stresses that weaken the pelvic musculature in older women are not completely understood. Muscle relaxation occurs as a consequence of the atrophic changes of the aging process and the decline in estrogen levels. Traumatic deliveries and multiparity are implicated because they may stretch the pelvic floor, including the perineum, to the point where normal urethral resistance gives way under sudden strain (Butts, 1979). Stress incontinence is seen less often in virginal and nulligravid women, and when it develops it is believed to be associated in part with an intrinsic fault in tissue tone (Soule, 1976). Pelvic surgery, radiation therapy, and obesity are other stresses associated with the development of stress incontinence. Recurrent urinary tract infections that cause scarring and adhesions near the urethrovesical junction are also a factor.

Stress incontinence is usually, but not always, associated with prolapse of the anterior vaginal wall and displacement of the bladder (cystocele). Usually, there is a coexisting urethrocele as well (Soule, 1976; Brocklehurst, 1979). Stress incontinence may also be associated with uterine prolapse or prolapse of the posterior vaginal wall and displacement of the rectum (rectocele), or peritoneal tissues (enter-

ocele) through the vaginal wall (Soule, 1976). These conditions should become less common with improved obstetric management.

ASSESSING THE CLIENT'S ADAPTATIONS

Congestive Heart Failure

Classic adaptations to left-sided heart failure include breathlessness, dyspnea on exertion or at rest, cough, pulmonary congestion, rales, wheezing, extra heart sounds, and nocturia. These may vary from mild nocturnal dyspnea, vague chest tightness, and a persistent but mild cough to orthopnea that is so intense that clients struggle out of bed to open the window and spend the rest of the night in a chair. Pulmonary edema may develop secondary to left ventricular failure when left atrial pressure rises to such levels that pulmonary capillary pressure exceeds that of the oncotic pressure of plasma proteins and fluid exudes out of the capillaries into the interstitial lung tissues and finally into the alveoli, decreasing lung compliance and interfering with oxygen transport. Adaptations are severe and life threatening and include hypoxia, hypercapnea, cyanosis, frothy sputum, hemoptysis, intense dyspnea, cough, noisy respirations, diaphoresis, tachycardia, chest pain, and intense fear. Classic adaptations to right-sided heart failure include edema of the lower extremities, engorgement of veins, hepatic enlargement and tenderness, abdominal distention, anorexia, nausea, vomiting, ascites, and renal insufficiency or oliguria.

The nurse should be skilled in recognizing adaptations to heart failure. Doing so in older people is particularly difficult. Adaptations to heart failure are nonspecific and mimic many of the diseases of old age as well as the changes of old age itself. In addition, normal adaptations of aging make the assessment and interpretation of findings more difficult. The classic signs of heart failure—dyspnea, edema, rales, and cardiomegaly—are those seen in middle-aged and "young" elderly. They may be absent altogether in very old clients with heart failure. On the other hand, many older clients exhibit a combination of adaptations to both left- and right-sided failure as well as additional, nonspecific adaptations that are not seen in younger clients and may go unnoticed. The nurse who knows the older client well and views the client holistically is best able to identify the subtle cues of heart failure that differentiate it from other disease processes or the aging process. If the nurse recognizes early signs of heart failure, it is important to refer the older client to a physician to identify and treat the underlying stresses responsible for it.

The Client History. The older client's description of adaptations may provide helpful clues to recognizing congestive heart failure. On the other hand, increasing heart failure in older people often results in mental changes secondary to hypoxia and reduced cerebral blood flow. Mental status changes due to heart failure may compound existing poor memory, chronic brain syndrome, or other problems, making the history unreliable or unobtainable. If this is the case, the nurse should enlist the aid of a relative or friend of the client in order to validate the client's history and obtain an accurate picture of the client's behavior. During the history, the nurse should gather data related to the presence of congestive heart failure and the stresses that precipitate it. If the data lead the nurse to suspect the presence of an underlying stress, such as anemia, pneumonia, or a thyroid condition, the nurse should follow up with questions to determine the presence or absence of these conditions. Data should be obtained in the following categories: respiratory, cardiac and gastrointestinal systems, urinary output, integument, patterns of activity and sleep, nutrition assessment, medication history, and mentation.

Respiratory Complaints. One of the earliest signs of left heart failure in the older client is coughing. Usually, it is a mild, persistent cough that is nonproductive or productive of a frothy white or mucoid sputum (Elkowitz, 1981). These adaptations are characteristic of left-sided failure. A cough that is productive of pink-tinged sputum may indicate pulmonary emboli or pulmonary edema. The client should be referred immediately to a physician. A cough that is productive of thick or purulent sputum may indicate pneumonia. Pneumonia and heart failure often go hand in hand in the elderly; one may precipitate the other. If the client's cough is productive, the nurse should follow up to determine whether or not it might be associated with pulmonary emboli, pulmonary edema, pneumonia, or other respiratory problems.

Shortness of breath is a classic early adaptation to congestive heart failure in the elderly. In the early stages, breathlessness may occur only on exertion, but as failure progresses, it occurs at rest. Breathlessness is a consequence of insufficient oxygen being delivered to meet the metabolic demands of tissues. Breathlessness due to heart failure is easy to overlook in the elderly because it may also be associated with aging, obesity, and declining cardiopulmonary reserves. In addition, some older clients never complain of breathlessness because they voluntarily restrict their activities to avoid it. The nurse should question older clients about what activities they do and do not perform and why they do not perform certain activities until specific answers are obtained.

Gradually breathlessness progresses to dyspnea on exertion (DOE) and then dyspnea at rest. Dyspnea is another early sign of left-sided failure. It is the result of venous engorgement, which produces decreased compliance of the lungs. More effort is needed to inhale and expiration requires muscular effort rather than passive movement. The nurse should obtain information about the presence of each type of dyspnea: dyspnea at rest, dyspnea on exertion, orthopnea, and paroxysmal nocturnal dyspnea. Complaints of orthopnea by older people point strongly to heart failure. Orthopnea refers to shortness of breath in the recumbent position and occurs when blood and fluid from the lower extremities are redistributed and returned to the lungs and heart. Intrathoracic blood volume increases, reducing vital capacity and increasing pulmonary vascular pressure. As a consequence of breathlessness, the client awakens and sits upright. The change in position alters blood volume and pulmonary pressures and relieves breathlessness. As heart failure progresses, the client is unable to recline and must sit upright to breathe comfortably. Paroxysmal nocturnal dyspnea (PND) is a suffocating feeling accompanied by anxiety that occurs 1 to 2 hours after the client retires in the recumbent position. When it occurs, the client may appear pale or cyanotic. Profuse cold sweats may occur because the client becomes anxious while struggling for air. When paroxysmal nocturnal dyspnea is accompanied by wheezing it is called "cardiac asthma." The differentiation of cardiac from bronchial asthma may be difficult. Bronchial asthma is usually less frequent and accompanied by a long history of repeated attacks (Rodstein, 1979). Paroxysmal nocturnal dyspnea develops when fluid that accumulated during the day is reabsorbed, overloading the left ventricle and causing lung congestion. This condition is temporarily relieved when the client sits up. The nurse should ask clients whether they use extra pillows at night and how many or whether they make other arrangements to sleep in the semi-Fowler's position. The nurse should ask clients what happens when they sleep in the recumbent position and whether or not they have ever awakened feeling breathless or needing fresh air at night.

The nurse should also ask the client or a concerned family member about the presence of Cheyne-Stokes respirations. These are a late sign of heart failure. They may be related to a prolongation of circulation time from the lungs to the medulla, reducing the effectiveness of the feedback mechanisms that control respirations.

Cardiac Complaints.   The nurse should question the client about the presence of chest pain or tightness, which sometimes accompanies heart failure. These adaptations occur with many other conditions, including myocardial infarction. The presence of pain may be difficult to ascertain due to the increased pain threshold and memory impairments that may accompany old age. The nurse should also ask the client about palpitations. These may suggest arrhythmias or hyperthyroidism, both of which may precipitate heart failure by altering cardiac output.

Gastrointestinal Complaints.   A detailed history of gastrointestinal function is important because right-sided heart failure results in edema of abdominal organs due to venous engorgement as pressure in the capillaries rises. Edema may produce a sense of fullness in the abdomen, anorexia, nausea, vomiting, abdominal pain, or tenderness and enlargement of the liver. Interpreting these adaptations is more difficult in older clients who are taking digitalis since the adaptations may be due to digitalis toxicity. This may be the stress that precipitated the heart failure. Bowel habits should also be determined because stresses that precipitate heart failure

are associated with changes in patterns of elimination. Both hyperthyroidism and digitalis toxicity may cause diarrhea whereas hypothyroidism is associated with constipation.

Urinary Output.   Information about changes in the client's pattern of urination gives clues about the presence of heart failure. Nocturia is a frequent complaint of older clients with heart failure. At night, when the client is in the recumbent position and the cardiac work load is reduced, renal perfusion is increased and edema fluid is absorbed and then excreted. Nocturia due to heart failure must be differentiated from nocturia due to normal, age-related changes in diurnal patterns. A pattern of oliguria during the day with polyuria at night is a late and ominous adaptation to heart failure. This pattern may occur with both left- and right-sided heart failure but is more common with right-sided heart failure.

The Integument.   Dependent edema is a classic but late complaint in right-sided heart failure. The dynamics associated with the development of edema probably involve elements of both forward and backward failure theories. When a ventricle fails, the amount of blood ejected from it during systole declines, resulting in a buildup of pressure in the vessels behind the ventricle. This pressure buildup results in an increase in the hydrostatic pressure of blood. When it exceeds oncotic pressure, fluid moves from the venous system to the interstitial space. Concurrently, the reduced cardiac output associated with heart failure causes a decrease in the perfusion of the kidneys, which stimulates the synthesis of renin. Renin is converted to angiotensin I and then to angiotensin II, a potent vasoconstrictor that further reduces renal perfusion. At the same time angiotensin II stimulates aldosterone secretion by the renal cortex. Salt and water are retained, increasing the circulating blood volume and increasing the hydrostatic pressure in the arterial end of capillaries causing fluid to move to the interstitial space, aggravating edema.

The nurse should ask the client about changes in the fit of shoes, rings, and belts. If edema is present, the nurse should determine whether it is always present or subsides periodically. The client should also be questioned about weight patterns because a fluid accumulation equal to ten percent of the client's weight is needed before edema is present. Initially, the onset of dependent edema from heart failure is gradual. If the client is ambulatory, edema may subside at night. Its disappearance may be the result of shifts of fluid to other areas such as the sacrum or lungs during the night. Consequently, the client may complain not only of edema during the day but of paroxysmal nocturnal dyspnea at night. As heart failure progresses, edema persists and increases. Fluid collects in the subcutaneous tissues of dependent areas—the sacrum if the client is bedridden, the flanks, thighs, abdomen, pretibial areas, and ankles if the client is ambulatory. The peripheral edema of heart failure is bilateral and pitting. However, determining the meaning of edema in the elderly is difficult because so many conditions cause unilateral and even bilateral edema in older people. Malnutrition, varicose veins, anemia, inactivity, pelvic and intraabdominal masses, neurological conditions, renal disease, and lymphatic obstruction are among the many noncardiac causes of edema in older people.

Patterns of Activity and Sleep.   The nurse should obtain an accurate picture of the client's normal daily routine, including any recent reduction in activity level or difficulty completing activities of daily living (ADLs). Observing the client carrying out ADLs also provides useful information. Difficulties in carrying out the normal routine may be manifestations of weakness and fatigue. These two vague, nonspecific adaptations are associated with both left- and right-sided heart failure. They are due to impaired circulation, which reduces the oxygen supply to tissues and slows the removal of waste products; thus the muscles are unable to regain their strength. Weakness may be exacerbated by malnutrition, hypokalemia and depression. It may also be due to hypothyroidism, thyrotoxicosis or anemia, any of which may have precipitated the heart failure.

A detailed history of the client's sleep patterns is important. Insomnia and nocturnal wandering occur with congestive heart failure and may be a response to the adaptations of heart failure such as breathlessness, dyspnea, Cheyne-Stokes respirations, confusion, or nocturia, or to the treatment of heart failure with diuretics. The nurse must differ-

entiate between normal, age-related changes in sleep patterns and disruption of sleep or insomnia due to congestive heart failure itself, the stresses that precipitate heart failure, such as hyperthyroidism, or other health problems, such as prostatism or depression.

Diet and Medication Histories.   The nurse should obtain a detailed diet history and a medication history because the intake of both nutrients and medications can precipitate or exacerbate heart failure. The nurse should identify eating patterns including a diet high in sodium or deficient in protein. Both of these diets are associated with fluid retention. Many clients are unaware of hidden dietary sources of sodium such as those contained in some seafoods, meats and dairy products, in canned foods, condiments, and sugar substitutes. The client's prescription and nonprescription medications should be evaluated for their sodium content. Many of the nonprescription drugs that older clients frequently buy, including antacids, analgesics, and cathartics and bulk laxatives, contain appreciable quantities of sodium either as an active ingredient or part of their dosage formulation (Goldberg, 1980; Shomaker, 1980).

Mental Status Assessment.   When congestive heart failure is suspected, the nurse should include a complete mental status assessment. Irritability, restlessness, agitation, confusion, disorientation, and impairment of memory may result from heart failure. Although mental status changes do not usually occur in younger clients with uncomplicated heart failure, they are more common in the elderly. Aging changes may compromise the reserve of the brain and central nervous system, so that when hypoxia develops in response to reduced cardiac output, cerebral impairment may result. Concurrent illnesses, such as renal disease or fever, may further reduce the older client's ability to adapt to hypoxia. Cerebral impairment may be complicated by the medications used to treat heart failure. Digitalis toxicity and electrolyte imbalances due to the use of diuretics may affect mental status.

The Physical Assessment.   The physical assessment should include assessment of vital signs, cardiovascular system, respiratory system, gastrointestinal system, and integument.

Vital Signs.   Subtle changes in the vital signs may indicate heart failure. Slight increases in pulse and respiratory rates may be noted. The increase in respiratory rate is due to a fall in arterial pO_2, stimulating the carotid bodies. Tachycardia is one of the first compensatory mechanisms in heart failure. The increase in pulse rate that accompanies heart failure in the elderly is usually not as great as that in younger persons. A pulse rate of 90 in an older person may be a significant tachycardia. The character of the pulse should also be noted. Arrhythmias, especially atrial fibrillation, frequently accompany heart failure in the elderly (Coakley, 1981). Pulsus alternans, which occurs when the heart alternates one strong beat with one weak beat during sinus rhythm, may also be noted when palpating the pulse. The alternating pulse quality is due to variations in the strength of ventricular contraction that result in a smaller quantity of blood being ejected during the weaker beat.

Cardiovascular System.   The nurse should palpate the point of maximal intensity (PMI) and percuss and palpate the precordial area to determine the presence of cardiac dilatation or hypertrophy. Displacement of the PMI laterally or downward toward the diaphragm may be indicative of left ventricular hypertrophy. However, if the older client has kyphoscoliosis, chronic obstructive pulmonary disease, or other thoracic cage deformities, displacement of the PMI is an unreliable sign. Left ventricular hypertrophy is evidenced by the presence of a strong and prolonged precordial impulse. In left ventricular dilatation, the impulse feels very diffuse.

The nurse should auscultate the chest for one full minute to detect any abnormal rate or rhythm. Certain systolic and diastolic murmurs may indicate underlying valvular disease. The nurse should also auscultate over the apex of the heart to determine the presence of a gallop rhythm. Three types of gallop rhythm may occur in heart failure: S_3 (ventricular gallop), S_4 (atrial gallop), and S_3 and S_4 (summation gallop). The S_3 gallop is indicative of left ventricular failure and is caused by vibrations of the ventricular walls as the flow of blood into

the ventricles is abruptly stopped. It is heard immediately after the second heart sound (S_2). S_4, which usually accompanies ventricular hypertrophy, is caused by atrial contractions and is related to a resistance to ventricular filling. S_4 occurs toward the end of diastole, just before the first heart sound (S_1). A summation gallop is a triple rhythm that occurs during tachycardia and is caused by resistance to ventricular filling (Tanner, 1977).

The veins should be observed for distention, a sign of right-sided heart failure. Elevated venous pressure can be detected in several ways. The nurse can observe the veins of the back of the hand as the client raises the arm above the level of the heart. Normally, these veins collapse, but in heart failure they remain distended. With the client in the recumbent position, the nurse can observe for distended neck veins. Normally these collapse when the person stands or sits, but as venous pressure increases, they protrude. Venous congestion is also demonstrated by the presence of a positive hepatojugular reflux. With the client sitting at a 45 degree angle, pressure is applied over the liver for 30 to 60 seconds while the neck veins are observed for distention. Pressure over the hepatic vessels increases the amount of blood returning to the heart. The increased flow raises venous pressure in clients with right heart failure because the heart is unable to accommodate an increased blood supply. The consequence is neck vein distention.

Respiratory System.   Evaluating the findings of the respiratory assessment in the older client with heart failure is complicated when the older client cannot cooperate by taking deep breaths or has distant breath sounds due to kyphoscoliosis or chronic obstructive pulmonary disease. The nurse should auscultate the lungs to determine the presence of bilateral rales. These develop when plasma capillary pressure exceeds osmotic pressure and fluid moves from the capillaries to the alveoli. At first, the rales are fine and crepitant and heard in the bases of the lungs. They do not clear with coughing. The height of the rales indicates the extent of the edema. Percussion over the lung bases will produce a dull sound, indicating the presence of fluid. Pulmonary basilar rales occur in older people for many reasons other than heart failure, and may develop, for example, after only 24 hours on bed rest (Rodstein, 1979). The nurse should also observe the client for cough, Cheyne-Stokes respiration, or wheezing.

Gastrointestinal System. The abdomen should be inspected for signs of distention. Flabby abdominal musculature in older people may make an accurate determination of early distention difficult. If indicated, the abdominal girth should be measured and remeasured at intervals. The nurse should palpate the liver for enlargement and tenderness. These are late signs of heart failure. In congestive heart failure the liver can be palpated below the level of the ribs and feels smooth and firm. Percussion will reveal an increased expansion of the liver as well. Pain in the right hypochondrium and epigastrium is a response to stretching of Glisson's capsule as the liver enlarges due to edema (Hyams, 1978). The nurse may also note splenomegaly, especially if the client with heart failure also has anemia.

Integument. The extremities should be checked for the presence of bilateral, pitting edema. In older people, the edema of heart failure often results in cellulitis of the legs or decubiti. These may be the reason the client seeks health care (Coakley, 1981). Because edema is not noticeable until a significant amount of fluid has been retained, the client's weight should be monitored regularly. This is probably the best indicator of fluid retention in older people, and, if treatment is begun, edema may never form. The nurse should bear in mind that malnutrition in the elderly can mask weight gains due to fluid retention. Skin color should also be noted. The client may appear pale if anemia complicates the heart failure. Cyanosis of the skin and nail beds may occur. Rarely, mild jaundice may develop secondary to hepatomegaly (Hyams, 1978). The skin of the extremities may feel cool due to poor perfusion (Coakley, 1981). The skin, hair, and nails should also be evaluated for adaptations associated with hypothyroidism or hyperthyroidism that may have precipitated the heart failure.

Laboratory and Diagnostic Tests. The most useful tool for evaluating congestive heart failure is the chest radiograph, taken in full inspiration in the standing position. It detects changes in the pulmonary vessels and lung fields indicative of the earliest, as well as later, stages of heart failure. The chest x-ray also reveals cardiac dilatation, particularly of the left ventricle.

The physician makes the diagnosis of congestive heart failure based on the results of the history, physical examination, and chest x-ray. There are no laboratory tests available to confirm the diagnosis of congestive heart failure. Laboratory tests are performed to identify or rule out any stresses that may have precipitated the heart failure or to monitor the client's response to treatment. A complete blood count is done to rule out infection and anemia as precipitating causes of heart failure. The sedimentation rate, another indicator of infection, may also be ordered. Serum enzymes, including CPK, LDH, and SGOT, are measured. Increases may be associated with congestive heart failure and with certain precipitating causes, including myocardial infarction and liver disease. Blood urea nitrogen (BUN) and creatinine levels are monitored because renal disease may result in hypertension and heart failure. A urinalysis is done to rule out renal disease. In addition, if the client with congestive heart failure is experiencing oliguria, the urine specific gravity will be increased. A thyroid panel (serum T_3 and T_4) should be drawn to rule out thyroid problems as underlying causes. The ECG is obtained in order to determine abnormalities in rate and rhythm as well as the presence of cardiac hypertrophy and dilatation.

Summary. The assessment of congestive heart failure is based on the presence of a complex of adaptations apparent during the history and physical examination. The chest x-ray is the only reliable diagnostic test to confirm the presence of heart failure. Because the adaptations associated with heart failure are nonspecific, the presence of only one or two adaptations is not enough to indicate the presence of heart failure. When evaluating the data, the findings must be considered in the context of the total person.

Diverticular Disease

History and Physical Assessment. Because older people have gastrointestinal complaints so frequently, a thorough assessment must be performed to assure that the problem is accurately identified and appropriately treated. This is accomplished by ruling out the range of health problems that can alter elimination in the elderly. These vary from constipation unaccompanied by serious complications to more ominous problems, such as Crohn's disease or cancer of the colon. When taking the client's history, the nurse should assure that the client gives specific and detailed information rather than general impressions of the problem.

The nurse needs data about the client's elimination pattern and any recent changes in it. Clients with diverticular disease experience a variety of adaptations that range from mild to severe. Frequently, the client with diverticulitis experiences a sudden onset of adaptations with no previous warning. Over half the clients with diverticular disease experience some change in bowel habits. Most clients experience constipation. Less often, the client complains of diarrhea or constipation alternating with diarrhea. Stools may be pencil thin with evidence of blood. They may be black, indicating that the proximal portion of the colon is involved, or frankly bloody, indicating that the distal colon is involved (Elkowitz, 1981). Bloody stools require thorough investigation. Hemorrhoids, rectal polyps, and rectal cancer are also associated with bloody stools, especially stools streaked with bright red blood (Wheeler, 1981; Berman and Kirsner, 1976).

To validate the older client's complaint of constipation, the nurse should determine the frequency of defecation, the characteristics of the stool (color, size, consistency), the time span of the constipation (recent, chronic), its course (improving, worsening), and the client's toileting habits. Many older people may complain of constipation when there are no data to support their complaint. Today's older generation lived through a time when the theory of autointoxication from the colon was popular. Infrequent bowel movements were believed to be a cause of many serious health problems. As a result, some people developed unrealistic ideas about the nature of normal bowel habits and overconcern about defecation. They may complain of constipation because they have a mistaken idea of what it is (Brocklehurst, 1978a). On the other hand, older clients with mental impairments may complain of constipation because they forget they have moved their bowels. Constipation may present in unusual ways in some older people. Fecal incontinence is not an uncommon consequence of constipation in the elderly. It may be an overflow incontinence of formed stool or a mucus diarrhea owing to the irritation of the mucosa by fecal masses (Agate, 1979).

If the nurse establishes the presence of constipation, efforts should be made to determine the reasons for it. Constipation is one of the most important factors implicated in the development of diverticular disease, and the prevention or elimination of constipation is an important part of the treatment plan. To identify the reasons for the constipation, the nurse should gather data in the following areas:

1. *Current health status*

   Complaints, including intolerance to cold, malaise, weight changes, weakness, anorexia, nausea, vomiting, flatulence, bloating sensation, pain, tenesmus.

   Present illnesses, including hemorrhoids, anal disease, hernia, cancer, neurological disorders, thyroid problems, mental status changes, emotional problems.

   Exercise patterns.

   Nutritional assessment (including fluid intake).

   Medication history.

2. *Past health history*

   Hemorrhoids, anal disease, bowel surgery, hernia, emotional problems, cancer, neurological disorders, thyroid problems.

3. *Family history*

   Polyps, cancer of the colon.

4. *Personal and social history*

   Recent losses or life crises.

In addition to changes in bowel habits, the client with diverticular disease usually experiences abdominal tenderness or a cramplike pain in the lower left quadrant that is worse during defecation. Flatulence, nausea, vomiting, and heartburn are other frequent complaints.

The nurse should examine the abdomen and rectum. Physical assessment usually reveals tenderness in the lower left quadrant, with muscle spasm and rebound tenderness. For this reason, diverticulitis is sometimes referred to as "left-sided appendicitis." A palpable mass, reflecting an abscess, may be present in the abdomen. The rectum may be tender. Diverticula are the most frequent reason for rectal bleeding in older people (Snel,

1981). Frank, even massive, bleeding may be present. Although this is not a frequent occurrence, it is a serious one. The client should be referred for immediate medical attention. The client with diverticulitis may also have chills and mild temperature elevation.

Laboratory and Diagnostic Tests.   A variety of tests are performed to confirm the presence of diverticular disease and any of its complications and to rule out other gastrointestinal disorders. A complete blood count is done. It may show an increase in polymorphonuclear leukocytes if infection is present. This finding is less likely in older clients than in younger ones. The erythrocyte sedimentation rate may be elevated if infection is present (Anderson, 1976). A mild anemia may be present if bleeding has occurred. Serum electrolytes are assessed to rule out specific causes of constipation, such as potassium or calcium imbalances. Stool specimens should be checked for occult blood on three consecutive dates. Bleeding with diverticula is usually brisk, in contrast to the slow, insidious bleeding associated with rectal cancer.

When diverticulitis is suspected, a barium enema and sigmoidoscopy are performed to investigate the colon and rule out other disorders. The barium enema will reveal spasm, narrowing or obstruction, hypermotility, diverticula, and other changes. The sigmoidoscopy will reveal irritability and spasm but no tumors or masses. A colonoscopy may also be performed using a flexible, fiberoptic colonoscope, especially if bleeding is present. Because of its maneuverability, the colonoscope has special advantages in the elderly. The colonoscope can easily reach the descending colon, where most diverticula are located. The procedure takes 30 or 40 minutes. Clients are usually given mild sedation, such as intravenous diazepam 10 to 15 mg immediately before the procedure (Snel, 1981). The nurse should bear in mind that the bowel preps for these examinations involve a regimen of low-residue diets, enemas, and cathartics that extend over a period of several days. This regimen may be especially demanding for the elderly. The nurse should observe the older client closely for signs of fluid and electrolyte imbalance and heart failure throughout the period of the bowel prep.

Urinary Incontinence

Urinary incontinence in older people may be due to a single stress or to multiple stresses. Many of these are amenable to medical or nursing interventions. A thorough assessment is essential if all the precipitating stresses are to be uncovered—identifying and correcting only one stress may not eliminate the client's problem with incontinence.

The Health History.   Older men and women are reticent to complain of problems affecting the urinary tract. Often they do not report their symptoms until a late stage. Consequently, when taking the client's history, the nurse should ask direct questions to elicit complaints about micturition.

The Record of Incontinence.   The nurse should determine whether the onset of urinary difficulties was sudden or gradual, the duration of the problem, and whether the incontinence is continuous or episodic. Acute incontinence, whether due to illness, medication, emotional factors, or environmental factors, is often of sudden onset. Established incontinence usually has a gradual onset due to slowly worsening chronic processes. Determining the duration of incontinence provides data about the severity of the problem. Incontinence of long-standing duration can become a habit so that even when the precipitating stress is removed, the incontinence will remain (Bonner, 1974). Determining whether the incontinence is continuous or episodic provides information about the precipitating stresses. For example, neurogenic incontinence is usually continuous, while incontinence due to inflammatory or obstructive processes is often episodic.

The nurse should determine the frequency and volume of urination. Because these characteristics are highly subjective, the nurse should have the client keep a chart to make an objective determination. If clients are institutionalized or mentally impaired, the nursing staff can keep the chart. The client should be instructed to record the time, volume, place, and circumstances surrounding the urine loss. Charting these data for 1 to 2 weeks allows patterns to emerge. The chart can be used to identify diurnal and nocturnal patterns of micturition. Normal diurnal frequency is two to four times. Eight to ten times is abnormal. Increased frequency often occurs with urinary tract infection or inflammation, prostatism, and neurogenic incontinence. Frequency may also be due to systemic diseases such as diabetes mellitus. A decrease in frequency may occur with an atonic bladder. Normal nocturnal frequency is one time. Three or four times is abnormal. Determining how often the client is awakened to urinate is especially difficult. The fact that older people sleep less soundly and awake more frequently may lead them to place undue emphasis on nocturia. Nocturia may be misinterpreted as a genitourinary problem when, in fact, it is due to systemic diseases such as renal failure, diabetes mellitus, or congestive heart failure. It may also be a consequence of excessive fluid intake late in the evening or during the night. Nocturnal frequency is an adaptation to the uninhibited neurogenic bladder and prostatism. It may occur whenever the client develops overflow incontinence, as with the atonic neurogenic bladder or advanced prostatic hypertrophy.

Noting the volume of urine lost is helpful in differentiating between various types of incontinence. Clients with acute urinary tract infections and the uninhibited neurogenic bladder void small amounts of urine. Even smaller amounts are lost with stress incontinence. The client with diabetes mellitus would be likely to void large amounts of urine.

Recording the place where the client was incontinent may pinpoint environmental factors, such as distance from the toilet, that contribute to the incontinence. Noting the circumstances surrounding the urine loss helps to identify precipitating stimuli, such as coughing or sudden movements, that are associated with stress incontinence and the unstable bladder.

Various types of incontinence charts have been developed for use in institutional settings. All provide for the nurse to record every 2 or 4 hours whether the client is wet or dry, change the bed linens if necessary, and take the client to the toilet or provide a bedpan. Such a chart shows the incidence of incontinence through the 24 hours, its pattern through several days, and whether or not regular toileting is having any effect. If a considerable number of incontinent episodes are present, the observations and toileting should be done every 2 hours.

The nurse should determine whether or not the client is aware of the urge to void and the length of time between awareness of the urge and incontinence. The client with certain neurological problems, such as the atonic bladder and reflex neurogenic bladder, is not aware of bladder filling. In contrast, clients with acute urinary tract infections, inflammation, benign prostatic hypertrophy, or the uninhibited neurogenic bladder may experience urgency and an acute desire to void but be unable to control the response. After voiding, the client with benign prostatic hypertrophy often experiences a feeling of incomplete relief, so that several trips to the bathroom are needed.

Complaints of dysuria, or painful urination, should also be investigated. Dysuria may be the result of any inflammatory process of the bladder or urethra. It may be secondary to vaginal infection in women. Pain does not usually accompany benign prostatic hypertrophy, but it may be present if residual urine has caused a urinary tract infection. The nurse should bear in mind that, unlike their younger counterparts, older people with urinary tract infections do not always experience dysuria.

The nurse should gather data about the characteristics of the urinary stream. A slow, weak stream is characteristic of benign prostatic hypertrophy. The older man may also complain of hesitancy, "start-and-stop" urination, and terminal (postvoiding) dribbling. These adaptations are worse in cold weather and in the morning. Some men achieve adequate urinary flow only by abdominal straining, a habit that can cause hemorrhoids. Men often experience a gradual worsening of the urinary stream over many years and may not be aware of the extent of the problem until they are directly questioned about it.

The client should describe the characteristics of the urine. Changes in color and odor and an increase in sediment may indicate urinary tract infection. The nurse should ask about hematuria. Urologically, this adaptation is classified as initial, terminal, or total (all urine is bloody). Initial hematuria is due to lesions below the bladder neck, while terminal hematuria is due to lesions in the trigone area. Hematuria frequently accompanies prostatic hypertrophy because the veins that course over the urethra become fragile and dilated and rupture easily (Bowles, 1976; Elkowitz, 1981). Whenever the nurse notes hematuria, the client should be referred to a urologist for follow up.

The nurse should ask the client about abdominal pain or discomfort. Although clients with acute urinary retention may complain of severe pain, clients with chronic retention of as much as three liters of urine may not experience pain. Their only complaint may be that their clothes are too tight (George and Osborn, 1981). Stress incontinence is accompanied by a sensation of abdominal discomfort that worsens as the client's muscle relaxation and prolapse progress. Women may complain of a bearing-down discomfort, a feeling of "falling" pelvic organs, or a sense of weight in the pelvis. Women may also complain of a greater than normal pressure with a full bladder and almost complete relief after voiding (Soule, 1976; Butts, 1979).

A detailed history of the older client's pattern of urination is useful not only as the basis for treating incontinence but as a way of preventing incontinence. The nurse should assess the urinary patterns of every older client who is admitted to the hospital so that an appropriate schedule of elimination is set up. Doing so can prevent many older clients from developing acute incontinence.

Current Health Status.   The nurse should ask the client about any other health problems, such as neurological disorders, heart failure, renal disease, disc disease, pelvic fractures, or diabetes, that may account for the incontinence. A chronic cough or chronic obstructive pulmonary disease may be associated with the onset of stress incontinence. Clients should describe their bowel habits. Changes in bowel habits and difficulty with fecal elimination accompany rectocele and enterocele and may indicate stress incontinence. If the client has neurological disease, fecal incontinence as well as urinary incontinence may result. Fecal incontinence with subsequent contamination of the urinary tract is a frequent reason for urinary tract infections in women. Constipation, which may present as a decrease in the number of stools or as diarrhea, may be the cause of urethral obstruction and urinary incontinence.

The nurse should ask clients to describe their usual daily fluid intake. Alcohol usage should also be determined. Overuse of alcohol may precipitate urinary retention in clients with benign prostatic hypertrophy. A detailed medication history should be taken. The nurse should determine whether the client takes diuretics, sedatives, hypnotics, or drugs with anticholinergic effects.

Past Health History.   The nurse should question the client about the number of pregnancies, the spacing between them, and whether or not there is a history of difficult deliveries. A history of previous pelvic and abdominal surgery should be taken. Incontinence may occur as a consequence of surgical trauma, neurological damage, or fistula formation.

Family History.   A family history of diabetes mellitus, syphilis, cancer, calculi, and renal diseae should alert the nurse to the possibility that these conditions are responsible for the client's incontinence. The nurse should question the client about sexual functioning. In males, impotence may be secondary to diabetic neuropathy, tabes dorsalis, and neurological conditions that also cause incontinence.

Physical Assessment.   The nurse should perform a complete pelvic examination for women and genitourinary examination for men. In women, the vulva should be inspected for atrophic changes indicative of senile vaginitis and trigonitis. The urethral oriface and perineum should be inspected for inflammation. The vaginal area should be assessed and any discharge noted. A bloodstained vaginal discharge, with or without pruritis, and small red spots or excoriation in the vaginal area suggest trigonitis. During the pelvic examination, the nurse should palpate for a relaxed anterior vaginal wall or protrusion of a mass through a vaginal wall. These findings suggest stress incontinence. The nurse should also observe for uterine prolapse, noting its degree. Although first-degree prolapse is minimal, second-degree prolapse involves protrusion of the cervix into the vagina. Third-degree prolapse involves complete extrusion of the cervix. The nurse should also observe for the presence of fistulas, which can cause incontinence. If these are present, urine may be seen in the vagina.

When the client's bladder is partially full and she is in the lithotomy position, she should be asked to cough or to bear down. Leakage or projectile expulsion of urine indicates stress incontinence. If this test is negative, the client should be asked to make an expulsive effort while standing up. The nurse should observe for leakage of urine during this maneuver.

In men, the external genitalia should be observed for phimosis, meatal stenosis, and urethral trauma. Any urethral discharge should be noted. This finding may indicate urethritis, prostatitis, or venereal disease.

A complete rectal examination provides valuable information about several stresses that precipitate incontinence. The nurse should estimate the character of sphincter tone. Lax sphincter tone may indicate impaired bladder enervation. The presence of a fecal mass may indicate that impaction is the cause of incontinence. A thorough rectal examination may reveal a protrusion of the rectal wall, adding to data obtained from the vaginal examination and helping the nurse differentiate between rectocele and enterocele.

The size, contour, and consistency of the prostate gland should be estimated, although accuracy is difficult and requires judgment and experience. Only the anterior surface of the prostate is palpable through the anterior rectal wall. The normal prostate is oval or conical in shape, elastic, and weighs 20 to 25 g. Because the normal size of the gland varies, the prostate must be one and one-half to two times normal size before enlargement can be detected by rectal examination. If benign prostatic hypertrophy is present, the prostate feels firm, smooth, slightly elastic, and symmetrical. It may bulge into the rectal lumen. Irregular induration or hard nodules on the prostate gland are strongly suggestive of cancer. The nurse should bear in mind that the size of the gland does not correlate well with the severity of urinary difficulties (Anderson, 1976).

The abdomen should be palpated and percussed. A soft, flabby, very relaxed abdomen indicates poor muscle tone. This finding is common in older people, and, together with obesity, suggests stress incontinence. Palpation and percussion of the abdomen should be performed to identify or exclude a midline mass that is the distended bladder. The client with chronic urinary retention and overflow incontinence may not complain of pain or discomfort and the bladder is less easily palpated (Anderson, 1976). In these cases, findings of the rectal and vaginal examination are useful in verifying the presence of bladder distention. The older client with urinary retention may exhibit other adaptations, including restlessness, nausea, and vomiting.

The back should be percussed for signs of costovertebral angle tenderness, which may accompany acute urinary tract infection (Butts, 1979). A mild elevation in temperature may also be noted with acute urinary tract infection.

A thorough neurological examination should follow to identify any signs of central nervous system disease. The nurse should assess the client's general mobility and dexterity since these affect the client's ability to reach and use a toilet. Many older clients are unable to inhibit voiding for more than a few seconds or minutes. Slow, painful mobility or dexterity may be the only reason for their incontinence.

Throughout the examination the nurse should note the client's general appearance and mental state. In some cases, a thorough mental status assessment should be performed. Diminished awareness and confusion may impair the older client's perception of the need to urinate.

Psychosocial Assessment. The nurse should assess the environment of incontinent clients, whether they live at home or in institutions, to identify environmental stresses that may precipitate incontinence. How far are the client's bedroom and living areas from the toilet? If the client is in an institution, are there enough toilets so that clients do not have to wait? If not, are commodes provided? Can clients in wheelchairs reach the toilet easily? Does the staff in the institution respond quickly to the client's request for a bedpan or assistance to the bathroom? Is privacy provided for urination? Is the toilet seat at a comforatable height for the client? Is the bed low enough so that the client can quickly move out of bed to the toilet? Does the client's clothing have fasteners that the client can manage quickly?

The nurse should also assess the psychological adaptations of the client who is incontinent. The emotional distress, loss of dignity, and social degradation suffered by incontinent people cannot be overemphasized. Loss of self-esteem and lowered self-concept are frequent adaptations. Anxiety is another frequent response because the older client fears the embarrassment of being "caught short." Increased anxiety may make the client more aware of bladder discomfort; thus urinary frequency and urgency become self-fulfilling prophecies. Fear of wetting themselves may be so severe that clients restrict their fluid intake in a misguided effort to reduce urination. Urinary calculi and dehydration can result. Older clients may restrict their mobility, limit their social participation, and remain at home in order to avoid embarrassment. If the client lives with others, incontinence, with its attendant odors, creates an undesirable atmosphere. Consequently, family, friends, and even health care providers may reject the client.

The nurse can help the older client cope with normal aging changes in the urinary system and prevent or eliminate many types of acute incontinence and stress incontinence. Many types of established incontinence are amenable to medical or surgical treatment. Therefore, the nurse should assure that the incontinent client receives a thorough urological evaluation.

Diagnostic Data. The physician may perform a variety of diagnostic tests to make an accurate determination of the stresses responsible for the incontinence.

Laboratory Studies. If prostatic hypertrophy is suspected, blood urea nitrogen (BUN), nonprotein nitrogen (NPN), and creatinine levels are measured. These provide an index of renal function. Values are elevated in advanced prostatic hypertrophy (Tobiason, 1979). Acid phosphatase and alkaline phosphatase levels may also be determined. These are elevated in metastatic cancer of the prostate (Pearson and Kotthoff, 1979). If the history and physical assessment indicate diabetes, fasting blood glucose and postprandial blood sugar tests are done. Blood serology tests may be performed if latent or tertiary syphilis is suspected (Pearson and Kotthoff, 1979). Cytological examination of smears of the vaginal wall may be undertaken to reveal atrophic vaginitis.

The nurse should inspect the client's urine for changes in color or odor or an increase in sediment that may indicate urinary tract infection. Urine should be collected for microscopic examination and, if urge incontinence is present or acute infection is suspected, for culture and sensitivity. Proteinuria, casts, red blood cells, and white blood cells are indicative of an inflammatory process. In most cases,

infection is due to *Escherichia coli* or *B. proteus* (Brocklehurst, 1979).

The nurse should never obtain urine specimens from collection devices worn by incontinent clients because they contain large amounts of bacteria. Collecting the second voided portion of urine for microscopic examination and culture is just as satisfactory as a midstream specimen and simpler for the older client to understand and execute. If the voided specimen in women yields an ambiguous sediment or colony count, the physician may order a catheterized specimen to provide more reliable results (Elliot, 1981).

Catheterization. A postvoiding catheterization may be ordered to determine the amount of residual urine. The physician may order the procedure whenever an obstruction, such as prostatic hypertrophy, is suspected. Simply introducing the catheter helps identify the presence of urethral stricture (Hewitt et al., 1980).

Roentgenographic Studies. A flat plate of the abdomen is done first. It shows the position of the urinary tract within the abdomen and helps rule out tumors and kidney or bladder stones as reasons for incontinence. An intravenous pyelogram (IVP) may be done to determine defects in bladder filling or emptying, the presence of stones or changes in bladder contour. This test involves a series of x-rays taken after injecting an intravenous dye. These show the progress of the dye from the kidney through the urethral meatus. The final picture, taken after the client voids, estimates the degree of bladder emptying. Decreased bladder emptying may indicate neurogenic incontinence.

Endoscopic Examination. Cystoscopy is performed to inspect the bladder and urethra directly. It is useful in assessing the anatomy if stress incontinence is suspected (McCarron, 1979). It also reveals characteristic inflammatory changes associated with trigonitis or cystitis (Pearson and Kotthoff, 1979). Cystoscopy will also reveal the trabeculae that indicate the increasing intravesical pressure and bladder atonicity associated with prostatic hypertrophy. The physician can also estimate the size of the prostate by noting the relationship of landmarks within the bladder. This is a more accurate method than the rectal examination to determine the size of the prostate. Cystoscopic examination also allows visualization of other causes of incontinence, including diverticula, stones, and carcinoma (Vallarino and Sherman, 1981).

Micturating Cystogram. X-ray examination of the bladder after it is filled with a radiopaque fluid is a method of recording bladder pathology and changes in bladder and urethral flow during urination. In the elderly, this test assists in differentiating between neurogenic and nonneurogenic incontinence (Vallarino and Sherman, 1981).

Cystometrogram. The cystometrogram is performed by filling the bladder with sterile water in small amounts at specified intervals or continuously, while changes in bladder pressure are recorded. The test is completed when micturition occurs, when discomfort is severe, or when a large bladder volume is obtained. The cystometrogram gives information about residual urine, bladder capacity, intravesical pressure, the presence or absence of uninhibited bladder contractions, and the point at which the desire to void is first felt. It is useful in differentiating among the types of neurogenic incontinence.

NURSING INTERVENTIONS

Congestive Heart Failure

The treatment of congestive heart failure is directed toward two concerns: modifying the adaptations directly associated with the heart failure, and eliminating or controlling the cardiac or noncardiac stresses that precipitated the failure. Unless the underlying stresses are identified and managed adequately, relief of the heart failure will be difficult or only minimally effective (Rodstein, 1979).

The treatment plan has three goals:

1. to reduce the work load of the myocardium;
2. to reduce vascular congestion, thus preventing or controlling edema; and
3. to increase myocardial contractility.

The specific treatment for heart failure varies according to whether the heart failure is severe or mild, acute or chronic. Treatment of congestive heart failure in the elderly differs from that of younger individuals. The plan takes into consideration the smaller cardiac reserve of older people and the increased risks associated with immobility in the elderly. Once the elderly client with heart failure is stabilized, it is best to reduce and simplify the treatment regimen to the minimum required to control the failure. Although the client with acute or severe heart failure requires hospitalization, older clients with chronic heart failure manage their condition at home with a treatment regimen that includes medications, special diet, and modification of exercise patterns and activities of daily living.

Reducing the Cardiac Work Load. The provision of physical and emotional rest helps reduce the oxygen need of the myocardium and the cardiac output. The extent to which physical activity is restricted depends on several factors. Although strict bed rest may be ordered for elderly clients with severe heart failure or when myocardial infarction or complications are present, many physicians prefer to restrict activity only as much as is required to prevent discomfort. Consequently, walking may be forbidden and chair rest may be prescribed instead of bed rest. A bedside commode may be ordered in preference to a bedpan because for many clients, using a commode requires a lower expenditure of energy than does using a bedpan. The older client with congestive heart failure is at particularly high risk of developing the following stasis complications of heart failure: thrombophlebitis, pulmonary embolism, and pneumonia. If edema is present, the risk of the client developing decubiti is also increased. When the client's activity is restricted, nursing care is aimed at preventing complications and promoting comfort. The nurse should assure that the client is positioned comfortably. Usually, this means the Fowler's or semi-Fowler's position. To prevent pneumonia, decubiti, and stasis, the client's position must be changed at least every 2 hours, and the client should be taught how to avoid the Valsalva maneuver when turning. To prevent deep vein thrombosis and emboli, antiembolic elastic stockings should be worn. Passive and, later, active leg exercises should be performed several times a day. Quadriceps setting exercises, flexion and extension of the ankle, and movement of the feet and toes foster venous return. The nurse should examine the client's lower legs regularly for signs of redness and tenderness and check for positive Homan's sign. To prevent pneumonia, the nurse should help the client perform coughing and deep breathing exercises regularly.

Because emotional stress also taxes the heart, the nurse needs to assure provision of emotional as well as physical rest. As appropriate, the nurse can reassure clients about their prognosis and provide explanations about procedures and treatments. The nurse should monitor the client's emotional responses to the plan of care. Some older clients react to dependence and severe restrictions of their activity with extreme anxiety. This may result in consumption of far more energy than would permitting small amounts of carefully planned activity. If this is the case, the nurse should consult with the physician regarding modifications of the client's activity restrictions. The nurse should also discuss with family members and significant others the need to provide the client with emotional support and to avoid any emotionally stressful interactions with the client.

To control agitation and restlessness and to reduce anxiety, the physician may order small doses of mild sedatives or tranquilizers, such as diazepam 5 mg. These may be especially useful at night to assure sleep. Morphine sulfate (Kleiger, 1976) and meperidine (Rodstein, 1979) may also be ordered to promote rest. The nurse should carefully evaluate the older client's response to these drugs. Confusion and disorientation are common adaptations in older clients with heart failure. These may be a direct consequence of the heart failure or a response to sedatives or to bed rest in a bed with siderails. If medication is believed to be the reason for an older client's mental status changes, the drug should be changed or discontinued. If there is pulmonary involvement, such as pulmonary heart disease, morphine and barbiturates should not be given (Elkowitz, 1981).

To assure adequate rest at night, the nurse must also implement measures to promote sleep and, if it is present, eliminate insomnia. Interventions include limiting fluid intake in the evenings to relieve nocturia, helping the client at bedtime to carry out old habits or patterns that promote sleep, and administering ordered sedatives.

As the client's condition improves the nurse should provide education about the illness and advice about ways to avoid undue physical or emotional stress while maintaining a normal routine.

When the older client has severe heart failure or pulmonary edema, other measures may be used to reduce the cardiac work load. The administration of oxygen, particularly when the client is in pulmonary edema, is urged to reduce hypoxia (Kleiger, 1976). When chronic pulmonary disease is absent, oxygen is recommended in doses of 40 percent or more (Coakley, 1981). Arterial blood gas determinations should be made to measure the client's arterial oxygen.

Phlebotomy or rotating tourniquets may be used to reduce the circulatory volume, the right-sided return, and the blood flow to the lungs (Kleiger, 1976). Anticoagulants may be ordered to prevent worsening of the heart failure due to pulmonary emboli. The physician may order the intravenous administration of Nitroprusside to reduce blood pressure and decrease venous return to the right side of the heart. This medication unloads the left ventricle by dilating both the venous and arterial beds. It may result in a significant increase in cardiac output and a fall in left and right atrial pressures, with a dramatic clearing of refractory heart failure (Coakley, 1981; Kleiger, 1976). When Nitroprusside is administered, the client is usually transferred to the intensive care unit. The nurse carefully monitors both blood pressure and pulmonary capillary wedge pressure during Nitroprusside administration.

The decision to increase the older client's activity level is related to changes in adaptations: a decrease in breathlessness and dyspnea, a reduction in edema, a decline in venous pressure, and an improvement in mentation (Caird and Dall, 1978). As the failure begins to improve the client's activity is very slowly increased. First the client may be allowed to walk to the bathroom. Gradually, more walking is permitted. Finally, stair climbing is added. Once the adaptations have disappeared, walking should be increased so that the client is fully ambulatory in 10 to 14 days. Observing the client performing simple activities, such as rolling over in bed, and activities of daily living, such as eating or washing, provides the nurse with valuable information about the client's exercise tolerance. The nurse should monitor the client for weakness, dyspnea, tachycardia, weight gain, and paroxysmal nocturnal dyspnea to determine whether or not the client is tolerating the exercise regimen.

If the client has chronic heart failure, the nurse plays an important role in helping the client plan a daily routine that affords an appropriate mix of activity and rest. The energy costs of specific activities can be determined by consulting one of the many tables available for this purpose. These tables give data about the oxygen demands specific activities place on the body by giving the number of calories needed per minute to perform the activity. Data are available on the energy costs of most activities of daily living as well as recreational activities. The nurse needs to reevaluate and modify the activity plan on a regular basis, as warranted by the client's cardiac status. In addition to activity modification, the client with heart failure who is also obese may be asked to go on a weight reduction diet. Weight reduction further reduces the cardiac work load.

Decreasing Vascular Congestion. The underlying reason for vascular congestion in heart failure is sodium retention. Salt restriction is still considered the most valuable way to prevent or control sodium retention. Physicians vary widely in the amount of sodium they allow the client (Rodstein, 1979; Coakley, 1981). Usually, a daily intake of 2 to 3 g is permitted. The nurse's role in helping clients implement a sodium restricted diet is discussed in Chapter 16. Optimal nutrition is important in the client with heart failure. To prevent hypoproteinemia, which further increases the cardiac work load, clients who do not have kidney failure are often advised to eat a diet containing at least 70 to 90 g of protein (Rodstein, 1979; Elkowitz, 1981). Foods high in iron or iron supplements may be ordered if the client also has anemia. However, the anorexia and nausea that may accompany heart failure make the maintenance of an optimal nutritional status a challenge for the nurse and client. If the client has mild or moderate heart failure, fluid restrictions are usually unnecessary. In acute heart failure, moderate fluid restrictions may be ordered until the adaptations have subsided.

Diuretics are an essential element of a total plan to correct sodium and fluid retention and reduce venous congestion. They do not replace the sodium

restricted diet, but should be used as a supplement to it. Because of the limited reserves of older people, diuretic therapy should be tailored to the client's needs. Brisk diuresis is poorly tolerated in the elderly because their compensatory mechanisms may be sluggish.

The diuretics used most often to treat heart failure in the elderly are the thiazide diuretics and the loop diuretics. The diuretics used to treat heart failure, their actions, and the nursing implications are listed in Table 1. The thiazide diuretics are usually the physician's first choice. They are especially useful for the client with chronic heart failure. The thiazides may be used on a daily basis or prescribed intermittently, only when the client develops weight gain, edema, or other adaptations to heart failure. Some clinicians prefer intermittent therapy because the risk of side effects is minimized. Short-acting thiazide diuretics may be prescribed for clients who experience nocturia. The client takes the diuretic in the early evening and diuresis occurs before the client retires. The action of thiazide diuretics is self-limiting, that is, diuresis decreases after edema fluid is lost. Consequently, the thiazides are less likely to produce hemoconcentration, dehydration, and vascular collapse in older people.

Loop diuretics are more potent than thiazides and their diuresis is not self-limiting. Because they are available in intravenous as well as oral dose forms, they are especially convenient in acute or emergency situations.

Both thiazide and loop diuretics have many side effects in common. Because loop diuretics are more potent, side effects may appear earlier and be more severe. Hypokalemia is one of the most common adverse effects of diuretic therapy. Older clients are at special risk for hypokalemia because total body potassium decreases with aging. In addition, many older people eat inadequate diets that are insufficient in potassium and some overuse laxatives, further depleting their potassium. In order to prevent hypokalemia, the physician may order potassium-sparing diuretics, such as spironolactone, to be taken in conjunction with long-term thiazide therapy. The nurse must be particularly alert to potential side effects in older people because so many of them mimic common problems associated with old age. For example, the weakness and lethargy

TABLE 1. DIURETICS USED TO TREAT CONGESTIVE HEART FAILURE

Drug	Indications	Actions	Nursing Implications
THIAZIDES Hydrochlorothiazide (Hydrodiuril) Chlorothiazide (Diuril)	Used for maintenance therapy in chronic heart failure. Also recommended for intermittent use when sudden weight gain or edema develop.	Decrease absorption of sodium, chloride, and, to a lesser extent, potassium in proximal tubules.	Monitor client for side effects: hypokalemia, hyponatremia, hypochloremia, abnormal glucose tolerance in clients with predisposition for diabetes, hyperuricemia causing gout, and gastric irritation. Monitor client for dehydration: note increased pulse rate, orthostatic hypotension, confusion, complaints of thirst, and increased concentration of urine. Advise client to change position slowly. Monitor client with special care during the phase of intense diuresis when potassium losses are greatest. Institute daily weight and intake and output monitoring. Check blood pressure and pulse regularly. Tell client to report nausea, vomiting, or hypokalemia and to take potassium supplements in the form of medications or food. Advise client to have serum electrolytes monitored regularly. Monitor client for signs of toxicity: thrombocytopenia, agranulocytosis, pancreatitis, skin rash, photosensitivity, and intestinal ulceration. Contraindications: clients with renal or liver disease.
LOOP DIURETICS Furosemide (Lasix) Ethacrynic acid (Edecrin)	Potent diuretics, used for clients in acute or severe heart failure to mobilize refractory edema; in emergency situations such as pulmonary edema,	Short-acting drugs that act mainly by reducing reabsorption of sodium from the loop of Henle and proximal part of	Monitor carefully for side effects; they may be severe and occur quickly. Side effects include those associated with the thiazides, and, in addition, shock, uremia, pulmonary infarction, cerebral thrombosis, digitalis toxicity, and deep vein thrombosis due to hemoconcentration. To monitor client institute measures used with clients taking the thiazides.

pleural effusion or pericardial effusion that require rapid mobilization of fluid; for clients who do not respond to thiazides; and for clients with advanced renal disease.	distal tubule. Produce diuresis even in the presence of hypovolemia.	During rapid diuresis, monitor older client for circulatory collapse and oliguria. Monitor older men with prostatism for urinary retention. Monitor elderly clients for urinary incontinence. Give potassium supplements. Monitor client for toxic effects: hyperuricemia, agranulocytosis, and, rarely, ototoxicity.
POTASSIUM-SPARING DIURETICS Spironolactone (Aldactone) Triamterene (Dytac, Dyrenium)	When given alone, have only mild, slow diuretic activity. Antagonize effects of aldosterone by competition with distal tubule. When given with other diuretics, these potentiate their actions and reduce the likelihood of alkalosis and disturbed purine and glucose metabolism, while preventing loss of magnesium and potassium.	Observe clients who take these regularly for signs of hyperkalemia. Do not give potassium supplements. Advise client to have serum electrolytes monitored regularly. Contraindicated in clients with renal impairment because they may cause retention of toxic levels of potassium.

that accompany hypokalemia may be mistaken for changes due to the aging process or to heart failure. The disorientation, confusion, and weakness that accompany dehydration in older people may be easily mistaken for senility or adaptations to heart failure. To detect fluid and electrolyte imbalances, all older clients on long-term diuretic therapy should have blood urea, potassium, sodium, and chloride levels monitored regularly. Certain age-related changes make adverse effects to diuretic therapy more likely in older people. For example, due to age-related changes in the baroreceptor response and peripheral vascular system, older clients are more likely to exhibit orthostatic hypotension in response to the volume changes that accompany diuresis. The nurse should take the older client's blood pressure in both the reclining and standing positions. A difference of more than 10 mm Hg may indicate a need to reduce the dose of the diuretic. Changes in bladder enervation and musculature and the development of benign prostatic hypertrophy in older men increase the risks of urinary incontinence and retention in older people taking diuretics, especially when diuresis is brisk. Elderly clients are also more prone to develop dehydration, hyponatremia, and hyperglycemia.

When a diuretic is ordered for the hospitalized client, the nurse evaluates the therapeutic effect by monitoring several parameters. The nurse should weigh the client daily, preferably in the early morning after the client urinates. Noting changes in weight is the most valuable tool for monitoring diuresis and loss of edema. When the weight loss ceases in the client with acute heart failure, this usually means that heart failure is resolving. This finding is a sign that activity can safely be progressed. Clients who live at home should be taught to weigh themselves regularly. If the client is continent, the nurse should institute fluid intake and output recordings. These have little value if the client is incontinent. Edema is monitored by noting the frequency of any cough, checking on the ease of breathing, and, when appropriate, measuring ankle and abdominal girth.

A recent advance in the medical therapy of acute and chronic failure has been the use of systemic vasodilators, such as sublingual nitroglycerin 0.4 mg, to reduce venous congestion. Vasodilators work by dilating arteries, reducing arterial pressure and helping the left ventricle to empty more effectively, thus lowering pulmonary venous pressure (Elkowitz, 1981; Kleiger, 1976).

To reduce congestion further, especially in older clients with chronic severe failure, the physician may perform a thoracentesis. Aspiration of as little as 250 ml of fluid often provides dramatic relief of adaptations (Coakley, 1981; Rodstein, 1979). Only rarely is paracentesis indicated to relieve congestion (Rodstein, 1979).

The most important nursing problem associated with venous congestion is edema. To prevent venous congestion and edema in the hospitalized client the nurse should carefully monitor the client's daily weight, fluid intake, urine output, and sodium intake. Elevating the head of the bed helps to decrease pulmonary venous congestion. If peripheral edema is present, the extremities must be carefully washed, thoroughly dried, and examined for breaks in the skin. Edematous legs should be elevated and the client's position changed regularly. Edematous extremities must be protected from minor trauma to prevent skin breakdown. Clients who are being discharged or who live at home should be taught to use proper hygiene measures, elevate affected extremities, change position often, obtain as much exercise as possible, and avoid constricting clothing.

Increasing Myocardial Contractility. Cardiac glycosides are used in many forms of heart failure in the elderly. They increase left ventricular output by increasing the inotropic forces of contraction and slowing conduction in the atrioventricular node. Because perfusion of the kidneys is improved, the glycosides cause a mild diuresis. They also reduce the size of the heart.

The most commonly used cardiac glycosides are digitoxin and digoxin. The most desirable form for the older client is digoxin because it has a shorter half-life, which tends to diminish the duration and intensity of toxicity, should it occur. Digitalization and maintenance doses of digitalis vary, depending on the client's therapeutic response and renal function. Unlike digitoxin, which is metabolized in the liver, digoxin is excreted unchanged by the kidneys; therefore, lower maintenance doses are required for older clients with poor renal function. Recent evidence indicates that the inotropic effects of digitalis in heart failure are not sustained with prolonged treatment (Coakley, 1981). Therefore, the client's responses to the drug should be evaluated on a regular basis. The nurse assesses the therapeutic effects of digitalis in clients with heart failure by monitoring changes in the rate and rhythm of the pulse and changes in weight and urinary patterns.

Because the client with congestive heart failure is usually taking diuretics as well as digitalis, the risk of toxicity is especially high. Diuresis can deplete serum potassium and magnesium, increase serum calcium, or cause azotemia, making the heart more sensitive to the effects of digitalis. The nurse should advise clients taking digitalis and diuretics to have their serum digitalis level, serum electrolytes, and blood urea checked at regular intervals. A thorough discussion of the toxic effects of digitalis and the nurse's responsibility with clients on long-term digitalis therapy appears in Chapter 18, pages 442–443.

Two other inotropic preparations that are used for the short-term treatment of adults with heart failure are dobutamine (Dobutrex) and dopamine (Intropin). Dobutamine has shown more promising results in increasing cardiac output. It produces its inotropic effects by acting primarily on myocardial β_1 receptors, with few effects on β_2 and α receptors. It may be used with Nitroprusside for additive effects. Dopamine stimulates cardiac α receptors directly, but its use is limited by its moderate β-receptor activity (Coakley, 1981).

Providing Long-Term Support. Successful management of congestive heart failure depends upon the combined efforts of the physician, nurse, and client. Older clients who are able to cope with the changes in life-style that this diagnosis demands increase their chances of surviving and leading a full life. By educating, counseling, and supporting the client, the nurse can help the client adopt and maintain the necessary changes in life-style. Explaining why the adaptations develop may improve compliance and thus may prevent future episodes of acute heart failure. The client needs careful instructions about managing medication and diet therapy, about ways to minimize physical exertion by modifying activities of daily living, and about how to prevent undue emotional upset. The nurse should assess the client's health status regularly, particularly the parameters discussed earlier in this chapter.

Current adaptations should be compared with base line data. The nurse should also assure that the client has regular medical follow up, including laboratory determinations of digitalis levels, serum electrolytes, urinalysis, electrocardiogram, and chest x-ray. Periodically, the nurse should evaluate the older client's ability to adhere to the therapeutic regimen and make any needed adjustments. With appropriate support and follow up, older clients with heart failure can maintain a productive and satisfactory life-style.

Managing Activities of Daily Living

Activities of daily living (ADLs) include all activities necessary during an ordinary day, from waking up in the morning to going to sleep at night. They include everything one must do to take care of bodily functions and to maintain an independent household (Lawton, 1963). Functional independence is the term applied to the ability to attend to all one's own needs. "Difficulty," "limitation," and "inability" represent different levels of functional impairment or functional dependence (Filner and Williams, 1981).

Forty-five percent of the elderly are somewhat limited in one or more activities of daily living (Monthly Vital Statistics Report, 1979). Over 35 percent of older people living in the community have some degree of functional dependence (Shanas et al., 1968). Two major factors responsible for functional dependency among the elderly are physical restrictions and mental deterioration. Although some functional dependency may accompany normal aging changes, most often it is a correlate of the chronic, often debilitating, illnesses that affect older people (Filner and Williams, 1981). Eighty percent of older people have at least one chronic disease (Eisdorfer, 1976; Kovar, 1977). Other factors have also been linked with the ability of older people to perform ADLs, including mental health, economic status, life-style, motivation, tolerance for failure, attitude of significant others, and insight into limitations. External factors such as fear of crime and inadequate public transportation may adversely influence performance (Filner and Williams, 1981; Granger and Greer, 1976).

The final consequence of functional dependency for older people is institutionalization. However, increasing dependence is not inevitable. It can often be prevented, reversed, or reduced. Many chronic health problems that predispose older people to functional dependency are amenable to preventive intervention. For those who are already ill, the goals are to improve or stabilize the client's adaptation. In some cases, the goal must be more limited, that is, to reduce the rate of decline of functional independence. Even small changes in an older client's general health status may make major differences in the degree of independence and quality of life.

Assessing Activities of Daily Living.

The physician's responsibility is to collect data to determine what health problems affect the client. The nurse collects a similar data base, but uses it in different ways. One nursing responsibility is to determine how illness and other stresses influence the client's ability to perform activities of daily living. The purpose of the nurse's assessment of ADLs is to describe the client's current functional status as it reflects the client's capabilities over a 24-hour period. Unless the client's 24-hour status is considered, the assessment may be inaccurate. For example, the client may be able to dress and apply a leg brace when observed in the morning but unable to remove the leg brace at night. Because one assessment, in isolation, has little value, it is best to observe the client over a period of time.

Making an accurate assessment of a client's functional ability requires the use of a good ADL assessment tool. There is no one definitive form, and many useful forms are available for use with older clients. Nurses should select the form that provides the scope of data defined as important for the client population in their setting. Some forms are more useful for clients living at home and others for clients living in institutions. In addition, the form should be easy to use.

A good ADL assessment tool should allow objective evaluation and promote communication among health professionals. In particular, an ADL assessment tool should:

1. be client oriented, that is, consider the abilities clients need to maintain individualized life patterns;

2. objectively and precisely describe the client's functional ability at a given point in time;

3. be able to detect changes in functional ability, either deterioration or improvement;

4. consider short-term as well as long-term client goals;

5. reinforce progress to the client and those who work with the client;

6. promote comparability of clinical observations of different clients; and

7. enhance communication of information about clients among staff and health care facilities involved in client care (Donaldson et al., 1973; Jackson, 1979).

A complete ADL assessment tool does not consider the client's ability to perform certain activities in isolation. It should consider the client's particular environment, including the physical layout, furniture and appliances, and the client's use of specialized equipment and aids.

Donaldson et al. (1973) reviewed the literature and found that the following abilities may be part of the ADL assessment: dressing, ambulation, bathing, feeding, transferring, toileting, grooming, wheelchair activities, elevation, continence, bed activities, travel, communication, hand activities, writing, mentation, household activities, sensory input, and miscellaneous. In all, they reviewed 25 tools. Many ADL assessment tools confine themselves to self-care abilities, defined as dressing, bathing, grooming, feeding, and toileting. Other, more comprehensive tools are also available.

A good ADL assessment tool should rate the quality of the client's performance of the abilities it considers. Usually, a scale is developed that measures the client's degree of independence (for example, totally independent, independent but uses an assistive device, requires supervision, requires minimal assistance, requires maximum assistance, dependent). Other variables that may be noted include the length of time required to perform the activity and the presence or absence of pain during performance. Data about the quality of performance help the nurse determine the kind and amount of help the client needs.

An ADL assessment tool that provides valuable data about the functional abilities of older people has been developed by Lawton (1963). It measures the client's capacity to perform bed activities, wheelchair activities, self-care activities, ambulation, elevation (climbing), travel activities with or without mobility aids, and miscellaneous hand activities (telephoning, handling coins and eyeglasses, and the like). This tool is extremely comprehensive and is useful for older people living in the community and in institutions. It provides clear definitions of all activities and spells out just how the evaluation is to be done. Psychosocial problems are not included on this tool, however. Therefore, the nurse may wish to perform a comprehensive psychosocial assessment as well.

Another comprehensive ADL assessment tool is the Functional Life Scale (Sarno et al., 1973). It considers the interactive influence of physical, psychosocial, cultural, and economic variables on the client's functional ability. The scale includes 44 items in five categories: cognition, ADLs (self-care activities), home activities (preparing meals, housekeeping, and so on), outside activities (shopping, using public transportation, and so on), and social interaction. For each item, four qualities are noted: self-initiation, frequency, speed, and overall efficiency. This tool considers the client's behavior in the real world and is useful for clients who live in the community.

Other more limited assessment tools are available. Although they do not provide enough information for the nurse to determine if the client is able to live alone, they are useful in helping the nurse identify specific abilities of chronically ill older clients. The Katz Index of Independence in Activities of Daily Living is a simple tool that is easy to administer and score. It assesses the client's level of independence in six areas: bathing, dressing, toileting, continence, transfer, and feeding (Katz et al., 1970; Meissner, 1980).

The Barthel Index (BI) is meant for use primarily with clients with neuromuscular and musculoskeletal problems. It assesses the client's performance in ten areas: feeding, wheelchair transfers, personal grooming, toileting, bathing, walking, stair climbing, dressing, and continence of bowels and bladder. A numerical score is assigned to each area based on the time, amount of physical assistance, and special environmental changes the client re-

quires. A score of 100 points indicates the client is completely self-sufficient in these areas (Mahoney and Barthel, 1965).

The Kenny Self-Care Evaluation limits itself to purely physical activities necessary for self-care. A total self-care score is calculated based on the sum of the average score in each of six categories: bed activity, transfers, locomotion (walking, stair climbing, wheelchairs, and so on), dressing, personal hygiene, and feeding. Within each category, skills that require the same mobility and strength are grouped together. For example, because shaving, washing the face, brushing the teeth, and combing the hair all require that the hand be lifted above the head, they are placed in one subgroup under personal hygiene (Schoening and Iversen, 1968). When Donaldson et al. (1973) tested the Katz, Barthel, and Kenny scales on a group of 100 clients, they found that the Kenny Self-Care score was the most sensitive of the three and the Katz Index was the least sensitive.

When using an ADL assessment tool with older people, the nurse should bear in mind that functional abilities form a hierarchy that begins with learning feeding and continence, progresses to transferring and toileting, and moves up to bathing and dressing. These skills also have an orderly pattern of regression as part of illness or the aging process. Usually bathing and dressing abilities deteriorate first and feeding and continence last. If the older client is disabled, independence is recovered in a pattern similar to the developmental hierarchy (Meissner, 1980; Katz et al., 1970).

The nurse has many occasions to perform an ADL assessment of older clients. For example, this assessment is a valuable way to make an objective assessment of whether or not an elderly client should continue to live at home or consider moving to a more protected environment. ADL assessment tools are used routinely to evaluate the client's progress in rehabilitation programs. They can be used to determine whether or not the client is ready for discharge from an institutional setting or rehabilitation program. This functional assessment should be made in the client's home and is an excellent way of helping older clients regain confidence in their functional capacity. Hospitals and long-term care settings can easily foster dependence in older clients. A functional assessment on admission that is used to develop the client's nursing care plan can prevent dependence. As the client progresses, on-going assessment is used to update the plan of care.

Nursing Interventions.   The goal of nursing intervention is to foster independence in activities of daily living by providing support services and special environments and by teaching and counseling activities that maximize independence.

Support Services.   Support services include meals, homemakers, health services, and special transportation. Although the efficacy of these interventions has been demonstrated, they remain in short supply. The Nutrition Program for the Elderly (Title VII of the Older Americans Act) partially relieves some older people of the burden of shopping for food and cooking meals by providing meals at congregate sites and for housebound elderly. Homemaker services are vital to the optimal functioning of many older people. Unfortunately, many programs that provide homemakers are inadequately funded and clients who request a homemaker must often wait weeks or months before they are provided with one. Partially impaired older people often need someone to shop for them and provide assistance with laundry and housekeeping. Something as simple as the inability to dress oneself may be completely confining and extend the client's disability to shopping, recreational, and social spheres. Community-based health centers, including day-care and day-hospital programs for the elderly, can allow older people to retain a home and at least a modicum of independence. They also relieve the family of some of the burden of caring for an elderly member. Without transportation programs, many elderly people are unable to take advantage of health programs and other important services that may allow them to remain functionally independent. The absence of public transportation in rural areas can prevent the elderly from obtaining services they need in order to live at home. In urban areas, unsafe and inaccessible public transportation creates similar problems for the elderly. Public transportation systems should be expanded and, as mandated by the Secretary of Transportation, modified to meet "barrier-free" design regulations. Successful pilot projects have been undertaken that provide regular trans-portation between housing projects for the elderly and medical centers, senior citizen centers, and sometimes even shopping centers. In most cases, special vehicles are used that have been adapted for wheelchairs. Scheduled services may be supplemented by "on-call" door-to-door transportation services. These efforts to provide special transportation for the elderly should be expanded.

Modifying the Environment.   Modifying living units is one way to maximize the older client's functional independence. Many older people own their own homes, but they were built 40 to 50 years ago without the conveniences older people need to remain independent. Provision of ramps, handrails, adequate lighting, secured carpeting, soft surfaces, and rounded edges assures comfort and safety. Installing a flexible shower hose and a tub bench can make bathing possible. A raised toilet seat or a portable commode placed over the toilet allows the client to use the toilet in comfort. The nurse can suggest ways the client can modify clothing to make dressing and undressing possible. Zippers and Velcro fasteners can replace buttons. Garments that open in the front, not the back, should be selected. Reorganizing drawers and closets can make needed supplies and equipment more accessible. Everyday dishes, appliances, and frequently used foods should be kept on the lower shelves or the counter top.

A limited number of special housing units and apartment complexes for the elderly are available. Some have living units designed for wheelchair-bound older people. More special facilities are needed to serve our growing older population.

Some older clients who have deficits in neuromuscular or musculoskeletal function can benefit from the use of specially designed aids to perform ADLs. Kitchen and eating utensils with built-up handles make preparing and eating meals more convenient for some. Personal hygiene may be facilitated by the use of a long-handled brush to wash the back and a toothbrush with a built-up handle. Special equipment may be purchased from surgical supply houses or inexpensively made. The cost of some equipment is covered by Medicare or Medicaid when prescribed by a physician.

Teaching and Counseling.   Some older clients need help learning new ways to perform ADLs. The nurse may teach these activities or reinforce teaching done by a physiotherapist. The first step in teaching any ADL is to analyze the activity and identify each of its component motions. The client needs to practice each component motion as an exercise. Once these steps are mastered, the client practices the activity as a whole (Lawton, 1963).

Counseling elderly clients and their families is an important way of preventing unnecessary functional dependence. The nurse can support older clients as they learn to cope with chronic disability and reduced strength and endurance and learn to make appropriate adjustments in their pattern of ADLs. Counseling can assist well-meaning families who are being overprotective of their older members. Families need to understand the client's capabilities and the importance of helping the client remain as self-sufficient as possible. Families often accept the lion's share of responsibility for the functionally impaired elderly but they need support to do so.

Diverticular Disease

Treatment of clients with acute and chronic diverticular disease has three main goals: (1) to prevent or correct constipation, (2) to reduce muscle spasm, and (3) to prevent or treat infection. The specific therapeutic regimen varies according to the severity of the client's adaptations.

Acute Diverticulitis. The client with acute diverticulitis requires aggressive treatment. The goal is to put the bowel at complete rest for a period of time in order to allow the adaptations to subside. If the client is severely ill, hospitalization is indicated. Whether clients are treated at home or in the hospital they are placed on bed rest and given only oral fluids or nothing by mouth. In the latter case, intravenous therapy is initiated to maintain fluid and electrolyte balance. Gradually, the diet is progressed to low residue and finally to high residue to promote bowel regularity and keep the stool soft. If the client has lost a signficant amount of blood, blood replacement is begun. It is not unusual for the client with massive bleeding to receive five or six units of blood. The nurse administers analgesics as ordered to reduce the client's abdominal pain. Because morphine sulfate increases the intraluminal colonic pressure, meperidine is the drug of choice. Mild heat to the abdomen may also be ordered to reduce discomfort. The nurse is also responsible for administering antibiotics to control infection. Usually a broad-spectrum antibiotic, such as ampicillin, or a tetracycline is ordered. In older people with reduced renal function, tetracycline is associated with special dangers. To relax the bowel, sedatives such as phenobarbital or anticholinergic, antispasmodic agents such as probantheline bromide (Pro-Banthine) or dicyclomene HCl (Dibent, Bentyl) are ordered. Anticholinergic medications are contraindicated if the client has glaucoma, obstructive uropathy, coronary disease, or obstructive disease of the gastrointestinal tract. Once oral intake is resumed, the physician orders stool softeners, such as dioctyl sodium (Colace) to regulate the bowel and prevent constipation. About 50 percent of clients with diverticulosis experience one episode of diverticulitis and no further reoccurrence (Berman and Kirsner, 1976).

About 20 percent of clients with diverticulitis require surgical intervention (Snel, 1981). Surgery is required to correct serious complications, such as obstruction, massive hemorrhage, free perforation, generalized peritonitis, toxemia, fistula formation, or unresolved abscess (Berman and Kirsner, 1976). In most cases, the involved portion of the colon is resected and then a colostomy or end-to-end anastomosis is performed.

Chronic Diverticulosis. The treatment regimen for the older client with diverticulosis is aimed primarily at minimizing the stresses associated with the formation of diverticula. Although the treatment program usually involves several elements, changing the client's diet is the only element that has been clearly associated with an improvement in the client's condition (Strause, 1979). Other measures to relieve constipation and medications to reduce muscle spasm and prevent infection are also routinely employed.

The High-Residue Diet. Within the last decade, the high-residue diet has become the most important part of a treatment regimen for prevention of diverticular disease or the recurrence of adaptations in clients who have had diverticulitis. Dietary fiber is found in three carbohydrates plus noncarbohydrate lignen. These originate in plant cell walls and cannot be hydrolyzed in the human digestive tract. Fiber is not considered an essential nutrient and the

National Research Council has not established minimum daily requirements for fiber intake. In fact, there are no standard techniques available to measure fiber in foods. Some experts refer to dietary fiber whereas others refer to crude fiber, the residue that remains after boiling fiber with dilute acid and dilute alkali. Crude fiber measures about 50 percent of dietary fiber (Pollman et al., 1978; Battle and Hanna, 1980). The average American diet contains about 4 g crude fiber per day (McKechnie, 1976). For clients with diverticular disease, fiber has several useful effects on the gastrointestinal tract. Most important, because of its water-binding properties, fiber is a bulkating agent and stools are heavier, bulkier, and softer. Therefore, fiber helps to reduce the intracolonic pressure, relieve pain associated with defecation, and promote regular defecation. In many people, fiber also reduces the transit time through the colon, further preventing hard, dry stools. Although the high-fiber diet changes stool patterns to normal, it does not reduce the number or size of existing diverticula. Many questions remain about the long-term effects of the high-fiber diet on nutritional status. Fiber has been found to alter lipid absorption in the gastrointestinal tract, affect protein absorption, and alter the plasma concentrations of calcium, phosphate, zinc, magnesium, and other trace metals (Cummings et al., 1976; Ismail-Beigi et al., 1977; Battle and Hanna, 1980; McKechnie, 1976).

Clients with diverticular disease and other gastrointestinal problems should consult with their physician before beginning a high-fiber diet. Table 2 lists the fiber content of foods. Some clients believe that eating a high-fiber diet limits them to bran cereals and similar bland foods. On the contrary, a high-fiber diet can be varied and tasty. Fruits, vegetables, and whole grains, cooked and raw, are among the many high-fiber foods. It is best to advise clients with diverticular disease to avoid high-fiber foods that may become lodged in the diverticula. These include nuts, corn, popcorn, foods with seeds, such as tomatoes, cucumbers, figs, strawberries, and raspberries, and breads with poppy, sesame, or caraway seeds (Berk et al., 1979). Estimates of the amount of daily dietary fiber that are protective range from 20 to 60 g (Webster, 1980; Strause, 1979).

Increasing fiber in the diet may be simple for

TABLE 2. THE FIBER CONTENT OF SELECTED FOODS

Foods With No Fiber
  Meats, fish, poultry, eggs
  Fats, oils
  Dairy products
  Sugar, syrups, candy

Foods With Fiber
  Vegetables
    Fresh and frozen
    When possible, do not peel

  Dried beans, peas, legumes, nuts, seeds
  Whole grains
    Cereals
    Breads
    Crackers

  Fruits
    Dried fruits are highest
    Fresh or frozen
    When possible, do not peel
    Unstrained juices

young people but may create special problems for the elderly, especially those who are ill or frail. A diet that is very high in fiber may include more food than a client can reasonably ingest in a day. Clients who cannot eat enough fruits and vegetables to overcome constipation can be advised to add supplemental dietary fiber in the form of unprocessed or miller's bran, now widely available in supermarkets. These brans are very dry and have almost no taste. They can easily be added to cereals, soups, and homemade breads, muffins, or cookies (Berk et al., 1979). Flatulence, distention, and diarrhea have been associated with the high-fiber diet and these problems are most common in the elderly. They are believed to occur when transit time through the colon is slow, thus allowing time for the bacteria that colonize the colon to act on the fiber (Webster, 1980). Older clients with ill-fitting dentures or missing teeth may find it difficult to chew some fiber foods. Some objections have been raised about the cost of fiber foods for the elderly. However, many clients can give up costly laxatives by eating a high-fiber diet. Older clients who cannot tolerate the high-fiber diet may benefit from as little as 10 g fiber a day (Burkitt, 1976). A daily diet of 10 g fiber could be maintained by eating two slices of wholemeal bread, two bran biscuits, and two spoonfuls of bran divided over the day's meals.

The nurse should advise clients to increase the amount of fiber in the diet gradually, while the nurse monitors their responses. Taking a detailed diet history or keeping a food diary for several days before initiating a change can give the nurse data about what fiber foods the client is already eating and how the diet might be modified to include more. Once the new diet is begun, the food diary can be useful in monitoring the client's progress. Because of the water-binding properties of fiber the nurse should advise clients who increase their fiber intake to increase their fluid intake as well. Up to 3 liters fluid per day may be required to maintain fluid balance. Maintaining such a high fluid intake may be a difficult task for some elderly people; therefore they need clear explanations of why additional fluids are important. Older clients in any setting can benefit from the addition of fiber in the diet. Studies of older clients in long-term care settings demonstrate that the addition of small amounts of fiber foods and prune juice to their diet resulted in a dramatic decline in the number of laxatives they required and an improvement in bowel habits (Battle and Hanna, 1980; Basso, 1977).

Relieving Constipation. The second important element in the treatment regimen for diverticular disease includes all measures to prevent or relieve constipation. This element is closely related to dietary measures because the high-fiber diet may be one of many changes advocated for the client with constipation. To prevent constipation, clients need to maintain a high fluid intake in order to soften stool. The nurse should also assure that clients obtain as much exercise as possible. Ambulatory clients should be advised to increase daily exercise whenever possible. For bedbound clients the nurse should plan passive or active exercises within the client's tolerance. When necessary, the nurse should initiate a bowel retraining program or help clients make appropriate changes in their toileting habits. Clients should be advised to sit on the toilet for 15 to 20 minutes after breakfast. They can assist defecation by placing their body in a forward thrust with thighs flexed. Some clients benefit from elevating their feet

on a small stool to increase flexion of the thighs and raise intraabdominal pressure (Kotthoff and Pearson, 1979). Nurses working with older clients in institutionalized settings can assist them by assuring that they are provided with a regular time to move their bowels. Whenever possible, older clients should be taken to the toilet or assisted to the commode rather than placed on a bedpan. Because of the position assumed when using a bedpan, clients cannot use their abdominal muscles to help them expel stool.

Laxatives are prescribed frequently for clients with diverticular disease. Usually, bulk laxatives such as methylcellulose or stool softeners such as dioctyl sodium are used to regulate the bowel (Table 3) (Dymock, 1974; Berk et al., 1979). Bowel irritants are to be avoided in these clients. Bulk enemas should also be avoided because when diverticula are present, the risk of bowel perforation is increased. In addition, large enemas harm the intestinal mucosa. Distention may cause shock in older people. Large tap water enemas have been associated with water intoxication and electrolyte loss (Brocklehurst, 1978a; Pearson and Kotthoff, 1979).

Other therapeutic measures for the client with chronic diverticular disease are used when warranted by the client's adaptations. Iron preparations may be given if bleeding has caused anemia. Clients who are obese may be placed on a weight reduction diet. If the client experiences abdominal discomfort, sedatives and antispasmodic medications may be prescribed. In addition, some clients take antibiotics to prevent infection.

Summary. The incidence of diverticular disease is highest in the older population. Many older people do not exhibit adaptations but have already developed diverticula. All older people who have not exhibited adaptations to diverticular disease can benefit from measures to prevent their development. The nurse can provide information on measures to prevent constipation and ways to modify the diet that are useful in preventing diverticula. The nurse can help clients with diverticular disease to modify their diet, improve their elimination patterns, and cope with prescribed medications. The nurse can also teach proper dietary habits and elimination patterns to others at an early age. Doing so may be an important contribution to future generations of older

TABLE 3. TYPES OF LAXATIVES

Group	Examples	Indication	Action	Nursing Implications
Bulk-forming	Psyllium (Serutan, Metamucil) Methylcellulose (Hydrolose)	Diverticular disease; constipation.	Are composed of natural or semisynthetic polysaccharides and cellulose derivatives which dissolve and swell in water, producing an emollient gel or viscous solution that hydrates feces and promotes peristalsis and defecation. Act within 12 to 72 hours.	Advise clients to increase their fluid intake if taking these agents. Because these may cause GI obstruction if taken with insufficient liquid, do not give to an immobile, older client. Contraindicated in older clients with terminal reservoir syndrome. To relieve flatulence, increase the client's fluid intake.
Softeners	Dioctyl sodium sulfosuccinate (Colace) Dioctyl calcium sulfosuccinate (Surfak)	Diverticular disease; constipation.	Soften the stool by decreasing its surface tension and allowing fats and water to enter. Act in 24 to 48 hours.	Have few adverse effects. Large doses may cause vomiting and diarrhea.
Lubricants	Mineral oil Mineral oil and magnesium hydroxide in combination (Haley's M.O.)	Not advised for use in older people.	Soften stool by retarding reabsorption of water. Interfere with absorption of fat-soluble vitamins (A,D,E,F). May leak through anal cavity and cause soiling. May be aspirated, causing lipoid pneumonia.	Advise clients to avoid these products and suggest alternatives.

Saline cathartics/ osmotic agents	Magnesium hydroxide (Milk of Magnesia) Magnesium citrate solution, sodium phosphate and sodium biphosphate (Phosphosoda Solution)	Constipation	Include magnesium, sodium, or potassium salts, which are incompletely absorbed, causing water to be retained in the intestinal lumen. These reduce transit time and deliver stool in a semisolid state. Act within 6 hours.	Advise clients to increase their water intake since all these products may draw water from circulation. Observe clients who use these regularly for fluid and electrolyte imbalance. Use magnesium cathartics cautiously in clients with poor renal function, due to increased risk of magnesium intoxication. Avoid sodium cathartics in clients with cardiovascular disease.
Irritants/ stimulants	Anthraquinone derivatives: Senna (Fletcher's Castoria, Senokot), cascara sagrada, danthron (Dorbane, Modane) Diphenylmethane derivatives: Phenolphthalen (Feen-A-Mint, Exlax), bisacodyl (Dulcolax tablet) Castor oil: various products	Constipation	These are absorbed from the small bowel and excreted in the colon. They stimulate peristalsis by stimulating the myenteric plexus or by direct action on the smooth muscle. Time of action varies widely, from 2 to 24 hours.	All of these products may cause intestinal cramps, griping, increased mucus secretions and watery stools. Warn clients that anthraquinone products may discolor the urine. Phenolphthalens may cause allergic reactions and fluid and electrolyte imbalance.

people by preventing the development of diverticular disease and other gastrointestinal problems.

Managing Medications

Without question, medications have contributed to better health and greater longevity in this century. They are almost always a component of the therapeutic regimen of elderly clients with acute and chronic diseases. The nurse encounters older clients who require medication in the hospital, clinic, long-term care setting, and home. The nurse is often the health professional best acquainted with the client and the therapeutic regimen. The role of the nurse is to coordinate the efforts of physicians, other health care providers, and family members to develop and implement a plan of care for the older person. Consequently, the nurse plays a key role in assuring that the medication regimen is safe and effective.

Although persons over age 65 years constitute only 11 percent of the present U.S. population, they use about 25 percent of the total amount of prescribed drugs and an even larger percentage of over-the-counter drugs. This means they take about three times as many drugs as their juniors (Ethel Percy Andrus Gerontology Center, 1973). The elderly spend three times more per capita on prescription drugs alone than those under 65 (Lamy and Kitler, 1971). Because of the diversity of their health problems, older people use nearly every drug. However, the drugs most commonly prescribed for older people include sedatives, hypnotics, hypoglycemics, diuretics, and cardiac glycosides. Laxatives, vitamins, and aspirin-containing preparations are the over-the-counter drugs most commonly purchased by older people (Services Research Reports, 1977).

Multiple Drug Use in the Elderly. There are justifiable reasons for the increased reliance upon drugs among older people. Although aging is not a disease, the incidence of multiple acute and chronic diseases is highest in older people (Weg, 1978). Eighty-six percent of the elderly have one or more chronic conditions (Brotman, 1974). Many of these conditions can be relieved or controlled with appropriate use of prescription or over-the-counter drugs. In recent years, the development of new drugs has proceeded at a phenomenal rate, giving physicians and clients a vast array of choices for use to treat illness or alleviate complaints. Most of

the drugs in common use today had not been developed 30 years ago (Davison, 1978).

Unfortunately, not all the reasons for the high incidence of drug use in older people can be justified. For some busy physicians the obvious solution is the simple act of prescribing medication to solve the client's problems (Offerhaus, 1981). Some pharmaceutical companies have attempted to improve drug sales by redefining psychosocial problems as medical problems and encouraging physicians to use medications to solve these complex client problems (Olsen and Johnson, 1978). Unfortunately, drugs have only a negligible or transient impact on many of the problems most often associated with aging, including psychosocial stresses such as loneliness, depression, anxiety, and insomnia, degenerative diseases such as cancer, cardiovascular disease, and arteriosclerosis, and chronic conditions such as arthritis and hypertension. Other pressures on the physician to prescribe come from older people and their families. Through advertising by television, radio, and other media forms, older people have been told that drugs are a panacea for every problem. Thus the pressure is very high to buy over-the-counter drugs or seek prescription medications for various complaints without knowing what the drugs are or how they behave. There is a high level of expectation among older people that one of the things the physician must do during the office visit is to give them some visible evidence that they have been treated to take away with them. Physicians who dispense counseling and other forms of treatment in lieu of prescriptions are in danger of hearing the client complain, "Doctor, I don't understand why you charged me for that visit. You didn't do anything. All you did was talk to me" (Pfeiffer, 1980; Offerhaus, 1981).

Adverse Drug Reactions. Although the aged benefit when medications are used judiciously, they may also demonstrate altered or unexpected responses to medications. The incidence of drug-induced side effects and adverse reactions rises steadily with age and with the number of drugs prescribed (Hurwitz and Wade, 1969). Aged clients (70 to 79 years old) have seven times as many adverse drug reactions as clients who are 20 to 29 years old (Hollister, 1981). Some adverse reactions require admission to the hospital or prolongation of a hospital stay, thus increasing health care costs. Some reduce the quality of life or hasten or cause death. Because the implications of medication therapy can be serious the nurse needs to understand the factors that place older clients at risk for adverse drug reactions.

One risk factor is multiple drug use. In one study of prescription drug use, people over age 60 (average age 71) and living at home were taking between two and nine prescription medications (Services Research Reports, 1977). In addition to prescribed medications, older people use over-the-counter and social drugs with little knowledge of the consequences of combining these substances. Older nursing home residents take an average of five drugs per day and hospitalized elderly clients take approximately ten drugs per day (Eckardt, 1978). The more drugs taken simultaneously, the greater the chances for drug interactions or unwanted drug effects.

The problem of multiple drug use has been complicated by the trend toward specialization by physicians and the likelihood that older people will be seeing several specialists simultaneously for different problems. This practice increases the possibility that different physicians will order similar medications, increasing the risk of toxicity, or that different physicians will order medications with adverse interactions.

Other reasons for the high incidence of adverse drug reactions in older people are illness and aging. Both of these may alter one or more of the processes by which the body absorbs, distributes, transforms, and excretes drugs. These processes are called pharmacokinetics. Certain diseases that affect older clients may alter the body's capacities or functions and change the pharmacokinetics, and thus the effects, of a drug. For example, reduced peristaltic activity may impair drug absorption. Cardiovascular disease may impair systemic circulation and affect drug distribution. Peripheral vascular insufficiency may also alter drug distribution.

Aging and Pharmacokinetics. Aging affects pharmacokinetics in very specific ways. Unfortunately, knowledge about pharmacokinetics in the aged is limited. While FDA regulations require the testing of drugs prior to approval, the subjects chosen for clinical trials are usually young or middle-aged and suffering from one disease, at most. Seldom are older people included in clinical trials (Sherman and Libow, 1981). Obtaining information about the effect of aging on pharmacokinetics is made more difficult because it is not chronological age per se but biological function that influences response to drugs. Not all biological functions related to pharmacokinetics age at the same rate. In addition, there is variability from one individual to another which increases progressively as years of life increase. The relative lack of data about how drugs work in older people increases the risk of physician errors, such as overprescribing, prescribing dangerous medications, or prescribing the wrong dose or dose schedule (Eckardt, 1978). In spite of the difficulties involved in obtaining data about pharmacological changes with age, however, it is possible to make some generalizations.

Absorption. Oral medications are absorbed in the upper gastrointestinal tract. Changes in gastrointestinal function with age include changes in the active transport mechanisms, decreased acid production, decreased gastrointestinal blood flow, and, possibly, decreased gastrointestinal motility. Changes in pH may affect the ionization and solubility of some drugs as well as the speed with which they are absorbed from the stomach. Changes in motility may cause some drugs to be absorbed more completely and others less efficiently. Although one might assume that absorption of oral medication is decreased in elderly persons, this assumption is not supported by available data. Most drugs are absorbed by passive diffusion, not active transport, and their absorption is not appreciably altered by age (Hollister, 1981; Plein, 1979). Where drug absorption problems occur in older people, they are often due to drug interactions that alter gastrointestinal absorption. For example, the calcium, aluminum, and magnesium salts found in antacids and iron salts found in iron preparations are often ingested by older people. If these are taken with tetracycline or digoxin, unabsorbable complexes form and the bioavailability of these latter drugs is reduced.

Distribution. Distribution of drugs may be markedly altered in older people. Because body weight and total body water are reduced with age, the size of the reservoir in which the drug is distributed is decreased. This leads to *higher* plasma concentrations of drugs that normally dissolve in water, such as ethanol and lithium, and a consequent risk of toxicity. Because there is a proportionate decrease in lean body mass and increase in body fat with age, lipid-soluble drugs such as diazepam have a *greater* reservoir in which to be diluted. These drugs accumulate in available fat, prolonging the duration of their action. The amount of total circulating plasma albumin declines with age, thus decreasing the major source of protein binding available to drugs. This change is not of much consequence for drugs that are not highly bound. However, when drugs are bound to the extent of 90 percent or more the decrease in albumin causes a proportionate increase in the unbound, pharmacologically active drug. As the amount of free drug increases and is available to receptor sites drug action is enhanced. Side effects and toxic effects with "normal" doses may occur. Increased serum levels of meperidine, warfarin, phenytoin, tolbutamide, phenylbutazone, and other drugs have been attributed to this phenomenon. If more than one such drug is being taken, they may compete for the limited binding sites on protein. Therefore, for both drugs, more free drug is available (Anderson, 1976; Dall, 1974; Hollister, 1981). Aging also results in a decline in cardiac output, with an increase in the proportion of total blood volume to the brain and heart. These changes can delay drug distribution to target organs or organs of elimination and alter the concentration of drugs sent to the heart or brain (Mullen and Granholm, 1981; Fitzgerald, 1980).

Biotransformation. Biotransformation is the process that converts substances in the blood into a form that can be excreted readily. Most drugs undergo biotransformation in the liver. The ability of the liver to transform a drug is measured indirectly by monitoring the drug's half-life. Liver blood flow declines with age and some microsomal enzyme pathways may be affected. For those drugs whose metabolism is highly dependent on the liver, it might be expected that aging would reduce the rate of metabolism. For some drugs, as indicated by their increased half-life, biotransformation by the liver apparently proceeds at a slowed rate, thus possibly

resulting in accumulation and toxicity (Hollister, 1981). Currently, there are not sufficient data to enable definite conclusions to be made about the effects of aging on drug biotransformation (Plein, 1979; Hollister, 1981).

Excretion. The main excretory routes are through the kidney and gastrointestinal tract. With age, nephrons undergo anatomical changes, renal blood flow declines, and renal function as measured by creatinine clearance decreases. These age-related changes in renal function are universal and physiological. However, the elderly are also at high risk for additional renal impairment secondary to dehydration, congestive heart failure, hypotension, and other stresses. Because of the diminished glomerular filtration rate removal by the kidney of drugs that tend to be excreted unchanged (digoxin, Kanamycin, penicillin) is delayed, with a consequent increase in the plasma concentration, sometimes to toxic levels. If the involved drug has a small margin of safety, as is the case with Kanamycin and digoxin, the consequences of decreased renal function could be a fatal overdose when it is given in a normal dose or at normal dose intervals (Hollister, 1981).

Receptor Sensitivity. Numerous receptor sites, each responsive to different drugs, are known to exist throughout the body. Clinical data indicate that many of these receptors undergo age-related changes. In most cases, the sensitivity of receptor sites increases, rendering the older person more vulnerable to the effects of certain drugs, such as diazepam, tricyclic antidepressants, and drugs used for Parkinson's disease (Allen, 1980; Hollister, 1981; Lenhart, 1976).

Compensatory Mechanisms. With age the mechanisms responsible for integrating organ functions become less effective. One important function of these mechanisms is to help the body compensate and maintain homeodynamics when under stress. As these mechanisms become less operative, they lose the ability to compensate and correct for exaggerated pharmacodynamic effects. For example, because the baroreceptors become less active with age, older clients are more likely than younger ones to experience orthostatic hypotension as a consequence of sympatholytic drugs (Fitzgerald, 1980; Hollister, 1981).

Summary. In summary, functional changes in older people affect the fate of drugs in the body and the responses to drugs. Although drug absorption is probably not impaired, drug distribution is markedly changed. This has implications for water-soluble, lipid-soluble, and bound drugs. Some decrease in the rate of biotransformation may increase the duration of action of some drugs that pass through the liver. Serious limitations in the ability to excrete drugs by the kidney occur. Finally, although changes in receptor sites increase the older client's vulnerability to the effects of drugs, changes in reserve capacity impair the ability to adapt to those effects.

Nursing Responsibilities. The changes in pharmacokinetics brought about by illness and aging coupled with the tendency toward multiple drug use in older people mean that drugs should be used with considerable caution in older people. Because the functional changes that occur are nonuniform, drug dosage must be determined on an individual basis. If adverse drug reactions are to be minimized, every older person who is taking medications should be monitored for responses to the drugs. Because nurses usually have the most regular contact with older clients in health institutions as well as the home, they play an important monitoring role. Family members and older clients themselves share responsibility for monitoring both the benefits anticipated from taking medication and the various adverse effects that might be expected to occur. Nurses are in a key position to assist older people to monitor their own drug therapy by explaining how drugs act and cautioning clients and their families about possible adverse effects. This instruction makes it more likely that problems will be reported promptly. The nursing assessment requires knowledge of the older person's psychological and physiological functioning. Many of the adverse effects mimic characteristics of old age, such as forgetfulness, weakness, confusion, anorexia, anxiety, and tremor. These can be easily overlooked. Other common adverse effects in the aged are exaggerations of known pharmacological actions of the drug. When an older client who had been in a stable condition suddenly develops new adaptations or complaints, the nurse should first consider whether these might be due to an adverse drug reaction and not to the onset of a new illness. The nurse should also urge older clients to maintain regular appointments with their physicians, who can make determinations of the plasma concentration of certain drugs. This laboratory technique is becoming increasingly available and is particularly helpful in monitoring drugs that have small therapeutic margins, such as digoxin, theophylline, tricyclic antidepressants, and antiarrhythmic agents (Hollister, 1981).

To further minimize adverse drug reactions, the nurse also serves as an advocate for both physicians and clients. On the physician's behalf, nurses need to counsel clients regarding the limited role of medications in a therapeutic regimen, indicate their support for physicians who refuse to base their treatment of the elderly on medications alone, and, in general, debunk the notion that there is a pill to solve every problem. Nurses need to stress the importance of seeking help, other than medication, in areas that require coping, not escape. Although there is no cure for many of the diseases that affect the elderly, many older people believe they will be cured by drugs and blame the physician when this does not occur. Others deny that they will need medication for the rest of their lives to control a chronic condition and discontinue essential drugs when their adaptations subside (Brock, 1979). The nurse should also be a client advocate. Because of the availability of over-the-counter drugs and the likelihood that the client sees several physicians, older clients should be urged to keep a current list of their prescribed and over-the-counter medications at home. They can present the list to the pharmacist before they purchase a new over-the-counter drug and to their physicians at each visit. Physicians are often appalled to learn how many medications a client is really taking. As a client advocate, nurses should be alert for drug interactions and mistakes in dosage and should consult with the physician or pharmacist if a question arises. Currently, physicians who care for the elderly are being advised to undertake a regular, critical drug review with their elderly clients (Pfeiffer, 1980). The review should take place at least every 6 months. Its aim is to discontinue all medications that are not absolutely necessary (Lofholm, 1978; Davison, 1978). If physicians have not made such a review with elderly clients receiving multiple medications, the nurse should urge them to do so.

Although all older clients are vulnerable to the adverse effects of medication, several research studies have been done to pinpoint older clients at particular risk (Davison, 1978; Eckardt, 1978; Sherman and Libow, 1981). This information is useful in directing the nurse's case-finding efforts. Older people most likely to suffer adverse drug reactions have a combination of the following characteristics:

1. Multiple chronic illnesses
2. Renal failure
3. Frail
4. Small build
5. Female
6. History of previous adverse reactions
7. History of allergies
8. Seeing several physicians
9. Living alone
10. Altered mental status
11. Financial difficulties

Preventing Medication Misuse. Ninety-five percent of older Americans live in the community, and these individuals are expected to assume responsibility for taking their own medications. Self-medication refers to the self-administration of prescription drugs ordered by the physician and nonprescription drugs selected by the client. The ability of older clients to medicate themselves safely has been a concern to nurses for many years. In 1962, Schwartz et al. published a classic study that provided information about problems associated with the self-administration of medications among elderly people. The findings of this and other studies indicate that a major problem among older people is medication misuse, that is, errors in medication administration. These errors are usually, but not always, unintentional. Available data about drug behavior in our current older population indicate that drug abuse, the intentional excessive use of drugs that alter feelings, and alcohol abuse are not widespread problems (Eckardt, 1978).

The research findings suggest an urgent need

for nurses to supervise older clients who are taking medications in order to prevent misuse or identify and correct it when it has occurred. The factors responsible for medication errors appear to be complex. At the very least, errors diminish the effectiveness of medication. Errors may cause great harm. The following types of drug misuse occur with frequency among older people: omission of drugs or doses; insufficient knowledge; self-prescription; and incorrect dosage, timing, or sequencing.

Omission of a drug was the most common type of misuse identified by Schwartz et al. (1962). Since then, it has continued to be identified as a serious problem (Eckardt, 1978; Bevil, 1981). Older clients omit medications knowingly and unknowingly. Multiple drug therapy and complicated dosage schedules place older people at high risk for omission errors. Often, older clients simply forget to take their medications. Drugs may not be taken at all, or only one of several daily doses may be taken, or drugs may be taken twice because the person did not remember taking the first pill. Clients who inadvertently miss a dose may try to remedy the situation by taking two doses the next time. This practice may lead to serious transient toxicity (Hollister, 1981). One way to prevent these kinds of errors is to ask the physician to simplify the client's drug schedule if possible. The periodic drug review to eliminate nonessential medications may be helpful. Drugs supplied in one long-acting dose rather than several short-acting doses help simplify drug regimens. Authorities generally agree that older clients who take more than three medications a day run the risk of becoming confused about their drug schedule (Sherman and Libow, 1981).

If omission is due to a memory deficit, the nurse can help clients select one of the many devices available to help them remember their medications. Older clients need to be involved in the selection of a device. Otherwise the nurse runs the risk of offending clients who have not completely accepted the fact that they have a memory deficit. Pill taking can be associated with daily events, such as eating meals or brushing the teeth. The nurse should use caution when advising clients to take medications with meals because many drugs are only partially absorbed if taken with food and lose their effectiveness. Large calendars can be used, with each date subdivided into sections that represent each dose taken. Appropriate drugs and directions for taking them are affixed to each subdivision of the calendar. Alternatively, clients can be taught to set an alarm clock to go off at specified times. If appropriate, they can be advised to purchase a special device, such as the Mediset, that allows for a weekly loading of all medications and only one simple action to dispense all pills necessary for a given time. Simple plastic pill boxes that dispense a day's, week's, or month's supply of pills are also available. By counting how many pills remain in these containers at regular intervals the nurse can assess the client's level of compliance. Other errors of omission arise from communication errors. Clients may dose themselves incorrectly because they are hard-of-hearing and do not hear directions, do not understand directions, cannot remember the directions they are given, or cannot read the directions written in small print on the medication bottle. Nurses can serve as client advocates by urging pharmacists to use large print type to write directions on medication bottles. Nurses should assure that when clients receive new prescriptions they have knowledge about how to take the drugs. Nurses should also review the client's total medication regimen when they make home visits.

Sometimes clients will deliberately omit medications. A significant portion of older people are at or below the poverty level and Medicare does not have outpatient drug benefits. Some clients cannot afford to buy their own prescription medications. Financial concerns may also cause some older clients to omit doses so that the medication will last longer. Older clients may intend to take their medications, but because of fatigue, poor health, lack of transportation, bad weather, or fear, some decide not to leave their homes to have prescriptions filled or refilled when they run out. Some of these problems could be eliminated by arranging for a family member or other concerned person to assist older people to obtain their medications. Some clients prematurely discontinue prescription medications. Many reasons have been suggested for doing so: insufficient funds to refill prescriptions, development of unpleasant side effects, and fear that drugs are habit forming (Gebhardt et al., 1978). Other factors, such as unpleasant taste of medications and difficulty swallowing large pills, contribute to omission of medications. Clients should be consulted

about preferred dose form whenever possible. Clients are particularly likely to omit medication when taking it interferes with their normal living pattern. If this is the case, the nurse and client need to determine a medication schedule that does not disrupt the client's normal routine (Smith, 1976).

In two studies, it was found that child-resistant safety caps were difficult for almost 60 percent of the elderly respondents to operate (Bevil, 1981; Sherman and Libow, 1981). Difficulty opening a safety cap may cause older clients to stop taking their medications, to transfer their medications to unmarked containers, to combine several medications in one container, or to leave the container open, a practice that contributes to drug decomposition.

Insufficient knowledge has been identified as one of the most common forms of medication error among older people (Bevil, 1981; Schwartz et al., 1962). In one study (Gebhardt et al., 1978) two-thirds of elderly respondents did not believe it was important to have knowledge about their drugs. Many older people hang on to the old attitude of "The doctor will tell me what I need to know. He will take care of me." Some physicians reinforce the notion that clients should be passive and unquestioning. Attitudes are difficult to change, and nurses cannot realistically expect to change the attitudes of a lifetime. However, nurses need to make concerted efforts to help older clients assume responsibility for their own health care and make informed decisions about it. One very important element of these efforts is helping clients to understand the importance of knowing about their medication regimen.

Most older clients are sadly uninformed about the medications they take. Bevil (1981) found that 66 percent of elderly clients did not have the most basic information about the purpose of their drugs. Three percent had incorrect information. In their study, Gebhardt et al. (1978) found that half of the clients believed there were no risks associated with taking medication. Lack of information about medications can have serious consequences. For example, a physician might tell a client who is taking three medications to discontinue the heart medication. The client who does not know which is the heart medication might discontinue the diuretic instead. Older clients have been known to assume that the pill they thought most important, for example the heart medication, was the biggest or most colorful pill. The pill that was least important, the vitamin, was the smallest pill.

The nurse has a responsibility to educate older clients in three domains: cognition, psychomotor skills, and attitudes. When the nurse learns that a client has received a new prescription the nurse should first determine whether or not the client has had the prescription filled and then assure that the client has the following information about the medication:

- Name
- Purpose
- Method of administration (chew, swallow, and so on)
- Specific times of administration
- Drugs, food, and activities to avoid or use
- Pertinent adverse effects
- Procedure to follow if adverse effects develop
- Proper method of storage
- How long to use the medication
- Refill procedure

Verbal instruction should be followed up in writing. In addition, the nurse should not assume that clients can remember all the elements of their drug regimen. Instead, periodic follow-up teaching should be scheduled.

Recent concern about medication errors among the elderly has stimulated the development of many educational programs that teach principles of safe drug therapy and stress compliance (Bevil, 1981; Hecht, 1974; Donahue et al., 1981). Educational programs have used numerous approaches including individualized instruction, small group techniques, and lecture. One way of reinforcing appropriate attitudes about medication behaviors may be to use a small group approach, where older people can learn from their peers. Older clients should be encouraged to develop respect for the effects of both prescription and over-the-counter drugs.

Nurses working in the hospital setting are in a key position to assure that older clients know about their medications and can implement a drug regimen prior to discharge. It is unfortunate that nurses have not played a leadership role in implementing pre-discharge training programs in the management of

a drug schedule. In some institutions, clients are allowed to take their own medications or a prearranged schedule of placebos to validate their understanding and ability to comply (Davison, 1978; Brock, 1980; Sherman and Libow, 1981).

Self-prescription is another medication error that often occurs with older people. They may borrow or lend prescription drugs if their adaptations are similar to their friends. Spouses take each other's medications both knowingly and unknowingly (Schwartz et al., 1962). Clients may also hoard old prescription medications in case their complaint returns. Doing so, they believe, may save them expensive trips to both doctor and pharmacy (Brock, 1980).

Dosage, sequence, and timing errors are also common. These may occur because of poor eyesight and a consequent inability to read a label or syringe correctly or because of confusion about instructions. Errors in timing are significant when the client takes medication that should be taken on an empty stomach with meals.

A large number of studies have been done to identify demographic, personal, and social characteristics of clients who misuse medication (Becker and Maiman, 1975; Smith, 1976; Services Research Reports, 1977). Much of the data have been contradictory. Schwartz et al. (1962) found the following client characteristics associated with medication misuse behaviors:

- Age over 75
- Living alone
- Presence of several diseases
- Taking more than three medications
- Little formal education
- Change in marital status from married to single
- Religious affiliation (Catholics make the most errors and Jews the least.)
- Rated as "coping with difficulty" by nurse

One purpose of these studies has been to aid in the prediction and screening of populations most likely to make medication errors. However, because the data have been inconclusive and because the incidence of medication errors is so high among the elderly, a thorough assessment of each older client's medication behaviors remains the most effective way of identifying whether or not there are problems with medication use.

The Medication History. The best way to determine whether or not the older client is able to manage the medication regimen safely is to take a comprehensive medication history. It can be a useful tool in clarifying the client's medication behavior. The medication history serves the following purposes:

- To screen the medication schedule for effectiveness and safety
- To identify the client's level of compliance
- To identify any teaching needs
- To determine how much responsibility the client is able to assume

A comprehensive drug history can take many forms. A sample history is illustrated in Table 4. A good way to start the history is to ask the client to describe all the medications taken in a 24-hour period. "Tell me, beginning with the time you get up, what medication you take first. How much? How often? When? What for? Then what do you take?" If possible, the nurse learns more about the client's memory if the recall is done without the medication containers within the client's view. The 24-hour recall should include other drugs that the client may not consider to be drugs. These include over-the-counter preparations and home remedies. Some home remedies can serve valuable purposes,

---

TABLE 4. ELEMENTS OF A DRUG HISTORY

Biographic data
  Name
  Age
  Diagnosis

Twenty-four hour recall
  Prescription drugs:
    Does client understand directions—time, dose, storage method?
    Does client follow directions—time, dose, storage method?
    Does client have knowledge of drug actions and possible adverse effects?

  Over-the-counter drugs:
    What does client use these for?
      Pain, skin, respiration, eye, ear, nose, nutrition (vitamins), mental/emotional state, sleep, gastrointestinal (stomach, bowel)?
    What brands and dose does client use?
    How often does client use them?
    Does client have knowledge of the drugs— actions, possible adverse effects?

  Home remedies:
    Which ones does the client use?
    What is the purpose of each?

Ability to manage current regimen
  Does client feel there are any problems adhering to the above regimen?
  Does client currently take any other medications the doctor has not prescribed?
  Has client recently discontinued any medications the doctor prescribed with or without physician's knowledge?

Related habits
  Smoking
  Special diet
  Drinking
    Alcohol
    Caffeine

Past experiences with medications
  Any previous adverse drug reactions?
  What did client do about them?

Ability to assume responsibility for medications
  Sensory status—vision, hearing, touch
  Neuromuscular coordination
  Degree of motivation
  Intellectual function
  Memory
  Confusion

Available support systems
  Family
  Neighbor
  Volunteer
  Other

"Medicine cabinet" inspection
  Location of medications
  Current medications
  Old supplies

while others such as ginseng and sulfur may be dangerous. When obtaining information about over-the-counter drugs, the nurse should jog the client's memory by mentioning common preparations in language the client understands, "Do you take anything for your bowels? For pain? To help you sleep? For skin problems? Any eyedrops?" Many clients do not understand that over-the-counter preparations are chemicals with the potential to interact with prescription drugs; therefore, unless directly asked they may not report them. Knowing the brand of an over-the-counter drug is important because preparations vary widely in chemical composition. Knowing the dose and frequency used gives the nurse data about whether or not the client is misusing the drug.

Once the recall is completed, the nurse can probe more deeply for clues about any problems with medication management. For example, what does the client do about medications on outings to the senior citizen center or on weekend trips to visit the children? Data about whether the client has started or stopped taking any medications recently without notifying the doctor give the nurse information about compliance. There are many reasons why clients stop taking medications. They may experience side effects, they may no longer experience the adaptations for which they began taking the medication, or they may hear a news item reporting the dangers of the drug. Many older people do not know that they should notify the physician if they feel the need to discontinue a drug.

Information about the client's habits, including smoking and food and fluid intake, provide clues about potential food–drug interactions. In addition, clients on certain restricted diets may be unaware that certain over-the-counter preparations contain an element (sodium, for example) they are to avoid.

Other information in the drug history helps to determine whether the client is able to cope effectively with a medication regimen. Asking whether clients have experienced any "bad" reactions to medication in the past and what they did about them gives information about how the client would cope with future problems. Identifying sensory and neuromuscular impairments gives the nurse clues about potential problems managing medications and areas for teaching. For example, a client with severe visual impairment should be reminded to wear glasses

in order to read medication labels and safely differentiate between various medications. A client with arthritis or Parkinson's disease who cannot handle child-resistant caps may need to know that, simply by requesting them from the pharmacist, regular caps can be substituted. Clients with impairments of intellect or memory may be able to cope with a medication regimen if they use a memory jogging device or enlist some assistance from a willing neighbor or family member.

The "medicine cabinet inspection" refers to the assessment of all the medications, old and new, being kept in the household. Because this is the most sensitive part of the drug history, it is best to do it last. Most clients and their families will cooperate willingly with this review if the seriousness of the situation is explained to them. Some medications lose their potency or become toxic when out-of-date. A search of the home for all medications can reveal some surprising hoards. In one study, 49 percent of the senior citizens were keeping outdated prescription medication (Bevil, 1981).

A thorough drug history takes about one hour to complete. It serves as the basis for determining what interventions are necessary to assure safe management of the medication regimen.

Implications for the Future. The recent proliferation of newly introduced drugs has created challenges and problems for older people and the health care providers who treat them. For physicians the challenge is to keep abreast of data about new drugs and their actions in older people and to assure they are administered appropriately. Today's older generation grew up before drugs were generally available. Now they find themselves living in a society where health care has been transformed by the advent of drug therapy. If their promised benefits are to be realized, older people must learn to use drugs wisely. Helping older clients to do so is a nursing responsibility.

What about future generations of older people? For them, medication therapy is already a way of life. Some authorities have suggested that many young people of today have already developed a tolerance to medications in use today and, thus, will require increasing amounts of them in the future. Physicians are compounding the problem by creating a population dependent upon drugs. In contrast, others have suggested that as physicians learn to use drugs more wisely, their use in the future will be more selective and efficacious. Young people of today who are growing up in a drug society will learn the limitations as well as the benefits of drugs and exercise responsibility in drug use. In either case, the future will surely find an older population that is greater in number, better educated, and healthier. The hope is that they will be better informed about the safe use of medications. The nurse's roles in educating the young people of today and helping them to assume responsibility for their health is one way of assuring that hope becomes a reality.

Summary. The elderly need more drugs, receive more drugs, and suffer more adverse drug reactions than their younger counterparts. The reasons for the increase in adverse effects include the practice of multiple drug therapy, the effects of aging and multiple stresses on pharmacodynamics, and the lower reserve of older people for maintenance of homeodynamics under stress. Ninety-five percent of older Americans live in the community and must manage their own medication regimens. Nurses can assure that older clients who take medications do so safely and effectively. Nursing responsibilities include monitoring the older client's drug regimen, serving as an advocate, assessing the client's medication history, teaching safe medication behaviors, supervising the client's medication behaviors, and coordinating the client's plan of care. In a holistic approach to client care, medication therapy is viewed as just one component of a total plan of care that includes physical and psychosocial interventions as well.

Urinary Incontinence

Advanced age is no contraindication to thorough assessment and vigorous treatment of the client with incontinence. The plan of care should be the result of collaboration between the nurse and physician. The nursing assessment coupled with diagnostic data obtained by the physician should pinpoint the stresses responsible for the incontinence and the client's personal reactions to the incontinence. Treatment regimens vary widely according to the precipitating stress and the needs of the individual client.

Medical Management. Two major categories of medical intervention are drug therapy and surgery.

Drug Therapy. ANTICHOLINERGIC AGENTS. Because the underlying etiology of the uninhibited neurogenic bladder is the overexcitability of the sacral reflex arc, the rationale of drug therapy is to increase bladder capacity and diminish bladder contractions by blocking transmission of nervous impulses somewhere within the sacral reflex arc. Anticholinergic drugs are used for this purpose. A number of drugs have been used effectively, including belladonna, atropine, propantheline bromide, orphenadrine hydrochloride, imipramine, emepronium bromide, and flavoxate. These drugs are also effective in controlling the unstable bladder.

If incontinence is to be controlled, the medications should anticipate the periods of incontinence as documented by the client's incontinence record. For example, if the client is incontinent only at night, the drug should be taken before retiring and in the middle of the night when the client awakens to empty the bladder. If the client does not awaken, an alarm should be set (Brocklehurst, 1977). If incontinence is widespread, the drug should be taken at regular intervals throughout the 24 hours. Clients who are taking these drugs should be aware of their possible adverse effects, although these are rare with the dosages used to treat incontinence. Adverse effects include dry mouth, blurred vision, urinary retention, acute angle-closure glaucoma, and cardiovascular complications (Brocklehurst, 1977; Vallarino and Sherman, 1981).

CHOLINERGIC AGENTS. The treatment of incontinence associated with urinary retention and overflow (atonic and autonomous neurogenic bladders) is aimed at reducing residual urine. Cholinergic medication, such as bethanechal chloride, may be ordered to stimulate bladder contraction. In addition, the client is taught comfortable positioning for urination and how to manually compress the abdominal wall (Credé's method).

ESTROGENS. The use of estrogens allows clients to regain control when senile vaginitis is the reason for urethritis, trigonitis, and incontinence. Clients may be given oral estrogens or estrogen creams, such as Stilbestrol, for local application. Because older women may have limited mobility and dexterity, creams may be difficult for them to apply.

Creams may also cause side effects due to absorption. Oral estrogens are usually given as a 4-week course that is repeated at periodic intervals. If low dosages are used, the risk of uterine cancer and thromboemboli is low. Postmenopausal bleeding is a potential side effect.

DIURETICS. When diuretics are necessary but are also the cause of nocturnal incontinence, drugs with a rapid onset of action should be used. If these are taken early in the day the renal output at night is decreased.

ANTIBIOTICS. Acute urinary tract infections are usually treated with antibiotics such as sulfonamides, nalidixic acid, nitrofurantoin, and ampicillin. The latter two drugs are likely to cause side effects, especially skin rashes, in the elderly. When urinary tract infections are a consequence of residual urine, the stress responsible for the residual urine must be corrected if the infection and the subsequent incontinence are to be corrected (Brocklehurst, 1977).

Surgical Intervention. Surgical intervention may be indicated to correct stress incontinence and prostatism. A variety of procedures are available to correct stress incontinence. Surgery may be undertaken to elevate the bladder neck and realign it with its support surfaces and to suspend the urethra and restore the urethrovesical angle. In some cases, repair of the urethrocele completely cures this form of stress incontinence (Bowles, 1976). Other procedures that may be necessary to correct stress incontinence include anterior and posterior colporrhaphy and hysterectomy.

To correct incontinence associated with benign prostatic hypertrophy, the usual surgical intervention is enucleation, that is, the removal of the hyperplastic tissue on the inner part of the prostate. The compressed normal prostate tissue and the outer capsule are left intact. The term prostatectomy is a misnomer because the entire gland is not excised. An open or closed approach may be chosen based on the size and shape of the prostate, the client's age, physical condition, and sexual activity. Open approaches include the retropubic, suprapubic, and perineal routes. The suprapubic route is the safest and has the fewest complications. The closed approach is the transurethral route. It is recommended when the prostate gland is relatively small (Bowles, 1976; Tobiason, 1979).

The older client who is undergoing prostatectomy needs education to lessen anxiety about the consequences of the surgery. Many clients believe that the gland is essential to potency and that a prostatectomy automatically means the end of sexual functioning. Clients may not understand the anatomy of the lower urinary tract. In fact, while loss of sexual potency sometimes occurs as a consequence of perineal prostatectomy, it should not occur following the other surgical approaches. Ejaculation is diminished because of the retrograde flow of the ejaculate into the bladder and the ability to impregnate a sexual partner can therefore be diminished.

Following prostatectomy, the client may experience some transitory urge incontinence. If this occurs, the client should be taught to perform repeated exercises to hold back urine. These can help return sphincter function to normal within 3 months (Elkowitz, 1981).

Although surgical intervention remains the treatment of choice for benign prostatic hypertrophy, conservative treatments to relieve symptoms of acute obstruction may be attempted before a decision is made to operate. Temporary measures include prostatic massage per rectum combined with hot sitz baths to decrease the size of the gland and increase the urinary stream. Intermittent catheterization with slow decompression of the bladder to relieve acute retention may also be employed (Tobiason, 1979; Bowles, 1976).

Nursing Management. Nursing interventions fall into several distinct categories:

1. Treating constipation
2. Instituting pelvic floor exercises
3. Instituting bladder retraining and behavior modification programs
4. Modifying the environment
5. Supporting the client with intractable incontinence

Selection of the appropriate nursing intervention is based on the assessment and identification of the precipitating stress. Effective nursing intervention requires that the nurse be sensitive to the client's emotional reactions to incontinence, as these are sometimes devastating. Older clients may lose all hope of regaining control and believe they no longer have any reason to continue living. The nurse needs sensitivity and insight into the client's feelings, as well as patience. Efforts to help the client regain continence often require a long-term commitment; gains can be small and occur slowly.

Treatment of Constipation. If severe constipation or fecal impaction has been identified as the reason for the client's urinary incontinence, the nurse collaborates with the physician to correct the problem and prevent further constipation. The physician may order a series of enemas to clear the rectum and colon. Manual removal of the fecal mass may be necessary. The physician may also order stool softeners to prevent constipation in the future. The nurse should work with the client to develop a program of diet, fluid intake, and exercise (described earlier in this chapter) that will prevent constipation in the future.

Pelvic Floor Exercises. Stress incontinence often responds dramatically to exercises to retrain the muscles of the pelvic floor taught and supervised by the physical therapist or nurse. These exercises were first described by Kegel (1956) and are the first approach to stress incontinence. These exercises may be useful to women of any age, but the client must be able to understand the teaching if the exercises are to be effective. Improvement is gradual, so patience and persistence are necessary. Exercises need to be carried out for at least 3 months before significant improvement is noted. Clients are taught to tense the muscles of the seat, abdomen, legs, and anal sphincter as if to prevent diarrhea. Then they are to contract the muscles of the pelvic floor surrounding the urethra and vagina as if to stop the flow of urine in midstream. Last, they are to alternate these two exercises. The exercises should be increased until the client repeats them at least ten times, four to six times a day. They can be carried out with the client standing, sitting, or lying (McCarron, 1979; Mandelstam, 1977; Butts, 1979). The physician may order some form of electrotherapy such as Faradism to supplement the Kegel exercises. This treatment stimulates pelvic muscle contractions (Brocklehurst, 1978b). If Kegel exercises do not benefit older clients it is usually because the supporting tissues and muscles are too relaxed to be adequately strengthened by exercise.

Many other strategies also benefit the woman with stress incontinence. The physician may order

medications to suppress a chronic cough. If the woman is obese, she should be counseled to undergo weight reduction. Women should be advised not to wear tight girdles. The physician may insert a soft or hard ring pessary into the vagina to support the urethra and anterior vaginal wall. Soft pessaries are easier to insert and remove. The client with a pessary should have a vaginal examination and pessary change every three months (Brown, 1978).

Bladder Retraining and Behavior Modification. Bladder retraining is one of the most commonly used strategies for assisting the client with established incontinence. Its purpose is to help the client regain urinary control through a systematic habit-training program. Three factors are essential if bladder retraining is to be successfully accomplished: (1) communication among staff and between staff and client must be abundant; (2) a regular voiding habit must be established; and (3) fluid intake must be regular and sufficient.

COMMUNICATION. Before a retraining program is undertaken the client's voiding pattern during the day and night is identified using the incontinence chart described on page 382. This is used to determine a toileting schedule for the client. Once the training program is instituted, careful records must be kept of the client's voiding behaviors and all nursing actions to promote continence. Liberal verbal and written communication between nursing staff members is essential to assure consistency and continuity of care. The staff also needs to communicate with the client about the purposes of the retraining program. The notion that incontinence is an inevitable consequence of old age must be dispelled. If the training program is to be successful, the nursing staff must enlist the client's cooperation and enthusiasm.

HABIT. A time schedule of toileting is established for the client, who is then taken to the toilet or given the bedpan and encouraged to empty the bladder. The purpose is to help the client form patterns and routines of voiding. Data from the client's incontinence chart enable the staff to toilet the client at appropriate intervals just before incontinence is likely to occur. Initially it may be necessary to toilet the client every half hour. Intervals between toileting can be gradually increased as the client's bladder capacity improves. Clients should be encouraged to hold their urine until the preset voiding time but told that they can call the staff if they need to void at other times as well. An alternative voiding schedule is to establish voiding times around unvarying routines of the client. For example, the client could be taken to the toilet upon awakening, before retiring, and before and after every meal. If clients are incontinent at night, it may be necessary to awaken them and take them to the toilet.

If the client has neurogenic incontinence, anticholinergic drugs may be prescribed during the retraining program to anticipate periods of incontinence. If clients have weak sphincter muscles, instituting a program of Kegel exercises to supplement bladder retraining is also useful.

The bladder retraining program must take into account the client's environment and social circumstances. When working with a client who is living at home, the nurse must determine a schedule of voiding that is compatible with the client's lifestyle. This requires a careful preliminary assessment of the client's normal daily routine.

Effective toileting means that the nurse facilitates the client's use of the bedpan, commode, or toilet. If a bedpan is used the client should be positioned upright and slightly forward with adequate support behind the back. The thighs should be flexed and the abdominal muscles contracted to strain down. The client who has difficulty initiating the urinary stream can be taught to stimulate trigger areas by stroking the inner thigh or pulling on pubic hair. Whenever possible the client should be assisted to a commode or toilet in preference to the bedpan.

Behavior modification techniques are often used to complement bladder retraining programs. These techniques attempt to shape the behavior of the client by the use of positive reinforcement. Consequently, urinary continence is reinforced by the use of social or material rewards. Simple praise or a few minutes of conversation are effective rewards for many older people. Incontinence, undesirable behavior, is ignored; it is neither punished nor rewarded. Selection of appropriate reinforcers and consistency in their application are the keys to the success of behavior modification. These steps depend upon an accurate client assessment and cooperation among all the staff who work with the client (Field, 1979; Spiro, 1978). The results of behavior modification with elderly clients have been mixed. While some experts claim that behavior modification is not likely to benefit older clients, others claim success with

some groups of older people (Carpenter and Simon, 1960; Arie et al., 1976).

FLUID INTAKE. During the retraining program, the client must drink adequate amounts of fluid. Unless contraindicated, 2 to 3 liters per day should be consumed. Clients should be placed on a fluid schedule and given measured amounts at regular intervals. Fluid intake should be scheduled in relation to the client's voiding pattern. The nurse must be creative to prevent the intake of such large amounts of fluid from becoming monotonous and boring. The nurse can consult with the client and family about the client's fluid preferences, and assure that variety is provided. Fluids are usually withheld after a specific time in the evening (for example, 8:00 PM) and are restricted at night to prevent nocturia (Maney, 1976).

Modifying the Environment. Maintaining a therapeutic environment is an independent nursing function. Because acute incontinence is often a direct result of environmental stresses and chronic incontinence is exacerbated by environmental stresses, the nurse's role in monitoring the environment of the incontinent client is critical.

When the incontinent client lives at home, a nursing assessment should be undertaken to identify ways to reorganize the client's environment and routine to promote continence. Furniture could be rearranged to provide an unobstructed route to the bathroom. The client's bedroom could be moved to a room closer to the bathroom or to the same floor as the bathroom. A commode could be placed in the bedroom. Grab bars in the bathroom or a raised toilet seat could be installed to make toileting easier. Velcro fasteners could replace cumbersome buttons and hooks on clothing. The client's routine could be reorganized to assure that outings are brief and rest stops near toilet facilities are planned.

Other measures may be appropriate to help the client and family cope with incontinence. The nurse can suggest ways to protect the mattress and chairs from wetness. The nurse should determine whether or not the client has adequate supplies of bed linen and underclothing, access to convenient laundry facilities, and sufficient finances to cope with additional laundry expenses.

Nurses who work with clients in hospitals and long-term care settings should anticipate the confusion older clients often experience when moved to a new environment. At the time of admission, clients should be taken to the bathroom, shown exactly where it is in relation to their bed and told to go as often as they wish. If the client's mobility is restricted, the client needs to know how to call the nurse for assistance with a bedpan or commode. The nurse can use data from the admission history about the client's normal micturition pattern to work out a toileting schedule with the client that becomes part of the written nursing care plan. A frequent reason for incontinence in the elderly, bedridden client is a delay by the nurse in responding to the older client's request for a bedpan or help to the toilet. Nurses should ensure that their staff members are knowledgeable about the older client's special problems with micturition, especially precipitancy. This information may help the staff to recognize the need to respond rapidly to an older client's call for assistance. The nurse can also assure that the client receives adequate exercise and sensory stimulation. The client who is mentally alert and active is less likely to develop acute incontinence.

The Client with Intractable Incontinence. In a proportion of clients with established incontinence, especially older clients with dementia and uninhibited neurogenic bladder, intervention to control incontinence fails. Another group of clients with acute incontinence due to serious illness have a significant but temporary problem with involuntary micturition and wetness. In these cases, the nurse can use a number of means that protect incontinent clients and help them maintain a normal life. These include various kinds of absorbent pads and protective garments, body-worn collection devices, and catheters.

Not every device is suitable for every client because of anatomical differences among individuals and varying psychological responses to the devices. Although some clients feel that using an incontinence device allows them greater mobility, promotes socialization, and reduces odor, others perceive the devices as "diapers" and believe they have impaired the quality of their life (Beber, 1980). Whenever older clients are mentally able, they should be consulted about their preferences in regard to the use of an incontinence device and given choices about which devices are tried.

PROTECTIVE DEVICES. Incontinence pads to place across the bed and special undergarments consist of an absorbent body with a waterproof backing and a special facing made of smooth, porous, nonabsorbent material that enables fluid to pass through and be absorbed quickly into the body of the pad. The purpose of these devices is to separate the urine from the client and the bed or outer garments. Many different styles of pads and garments are available. All have one drawback in common: they are capable of absorbing only limited amounts of urine. If the client loses large amounts of urine, the skin is in constant contact with it. Consequently, protective devices are most useful for the client with intractable stress incontinence. Undergarments designed to protect against incontinence have special limitations. They are bulky and, if they are waterproof, they prevent the evaporation of sweat as well as urine from the skin, placing the client at risk for skin rashes. One garment that has been useful is the "gelling pad." It has the dimensions of a sanitary napkin and contains powder that, on coming in contact with urine, forms a gel. The pad can hold over 150 ml of fluid, and once the gel is formed the client experiences no wetness. When protective pads and garments are used, scrupulous skin care to prevent urine rash is essential. Protective pants require careful fitting and application. Clients who wear them should be taught to make regular and frequent trips to the bathroom to empty their bladder and cleanse their skin.

COLLECTION DEVICES. Body-worn collection devices to carry urine from the urethral meatus to a bag are available for men. No satisfactory appliance is available for women. The simplest device consists of a sheath that fits over the penis and is attached to a thin rubber tubing that leads to a bag or bottle. For more mobile clients the sheath urinal can be used with a bag attached to the leg. The sheath urinal is satisfactory for clients who are bedfast and chairfast, but it may become dislodged if the client is active. Even more satisfactory for mobile clients is the pubic pressure urinal. This has an open end that fits firmly against the pubis. The penis is extruded through the ring into the collecting system, making it difficult to dislodge. If the client leaks only small amounts of urine, a bag similar to a colostomy bag can be placed against the pubis to collect urine. Clients who are confused or restless require considerable nursing care to use a urine collector because they may not recognize the purpose of the device and pull it off. The nurse can advise mobile clients on how to adapt clothing to accommodate the collecting device. The client should be encouraged to wear normal clothing whenever possible. A zipper can be added to the trouser leg.

CATHETERS. Use of an indwelling catheter to treat acute or chronic incontinence is a measure of last resort. It should never be used as a convenience for nursing personnel caring for incontinent clients. Indwelling catheters are necessary for some elderly clients with chronic urinary retention, untreatable obstruction, and certain neurogenic bladder dysfunctions, as well as following certain urological, rectal, gynecological, and abdominal surgical procedures. Catheters are also used for clients who are comatose or seriously ill or who require careful monitoring of diuresis (deVoogt, 1981; Spiro, 1978). The physician makes the decision to use an indwelling catheter after weighing the considerable risks of the catheter against the possibility that it will improve the quality of the client's life. An indwelling catheter may be all that is required to permit an older client to go home.

The major problems with use of the indwelling catheter are infection, incrustation, and kidney stones. A urinary tract infection is inevitable when a catheter is used for more than a few days and may occur within 48 hours. A long-term catheter usually causes minimal damage in the older client who requires it for 1 or 2 years, but the nurse should remain alert for pathological changes in the kidney, especially when the catheter is used for longer periods. Encrustation of the catheter causes it to become blocked so that urine leaks alongside the catheter. Use of the catheter also predisposes the client to calculi, especially when the client is immobile, has a urinary tract infection, or an inadequate fluid intake.

If an indwelling catheter is required only a closed drainage system should be used to prevent cross contamination. Spigotting the catheter and emptying it at periodic intervals helps maintain bladder tone. The client needs scrupulous catheter care. Irrigation on a continuous or intermittent basis with an antiseptic or antibiotic, such as acetic acid or neomycin, is recommended to prevent infection and encrustation. This procedure is more manageable in a hospital than a nursing home. The catheter should be changed on a regular basis, at least every 2 weeks. A high fluid intake and acid–ash diet help to prevent complications. The indwelling catheter should drain into a bag suspended from the client's waist or attached to the leg. The bag should not be placed on the floor or attached to furniture. Doing so may publicize the client's problem or immobilize the client (Brocklehurst, 1978b; Brocklehurst, 1979; Spiro, 1978).

Summary. Whenever possible, interventions to treat acute and established incontinence are aimed at removing the stress or stresses responsible for the problem. Successful nursing management of the older client with incontinence depends upon knowledge of normal and pathological changes in the aging urinary tract and understanding of the psychosocial impact of incontinence on the older person. Although helping the older client regain control over micturition often requires a long-term commitment by the nurse and client, the rewards are great. Older people gain a greater sense of self-esteem and dignity, a profound feeling of accomplishment, and increased opportunities for socialization.

Modifying Hygiene Habits

Older clients with urinary incontinence need guidance about ways to modify their hygiene practices to prevent skin irritation. Older clients have special needs because they must consider not only the effects of urine but also the effects of normal aging on the skin. Habits of bathing are developed early in life and people practice them for years without consciously reflecting upon them, just as the businessman stands in front of the mirror and ties his necktie without giving a thought to the steps involved in the process. However, because hygiene practices are habits, clients need careful teaching and specific suggestions on ways to modify them when there are special needs.

Older people have thin, dry skin, with a decreased amount of subcutaneous fat. Their perceptions of heat and cold are diminished. As a general rule, older people should take only one or two baths or showers per week using small amounts of a superfatted soap. Water should be tepid and checked carefully before the client uses it. Skin should be patted thoroughly dry. After bathing, the client should apply an emollient lotion.

Older clients are at high risk for skin breakdown when urine comes in contact with skin. Because aging skin is dry and cracked, its protective function is diminished. When urine decomposes, an alkaline reaction occurs that causes skin irritation. Urine increases the bacterial count on the skin and the constant moisture promotes the development of a rash and skin breakdown. Because the epidermis thins with age, skin breakdown occurs more rapidly, but because the blood flow to the dermis is frequently impaired, healing occurs more slowly. If older clients wear waterproof protective garments to absorb urine, they may not be aware of the wetness and may forget to change the garment regularly. The accumulation of perspiration inside these garments adds to the wetness.

Older clients who are incontinent of large or small amounts of urine need to make regular, frequent trips to the bathroom to empty their bladder and change their undergarments and protective pants. Damp skin should be thoroughly washed, soap thoroughly rinsed away, and skin patted rather than rubbed dry before clean undergarments are applied. The client can use an emollient lotion on the buttocks and thighs. Corn starch is also useful in absorbing moisture. Clients should carefully inspect skin surfaces of the buttocks, thighs, and genitals each day for evidence of a rash. A mirror should be used to visualize all skin surfaces.

Older women may neglect perineal care or use incorrect technique. They may not understand the anatomical relationships between the urethra, vagina, and rectum. The nurse may need to educate older women about the anatomy of the perineum and teach them to cleanse and wipe the perineum from the urinary meatus to the rectum.

Odors are a major problem and are often the reason why friends, family, and nursing staff shun the incontinent client. Older clients often worry about the odor of urine and restrict their social activities. The nurse should reassure clients that careful hygiene and regular laundering can reduce the problem of unpleasant odors. Older clients may not know that the simple measure of hot water washing destroys pathogens on garments. Elderly people who do their own laundry by rinsing garments by hand should be assisted to make other arrangements for washing their clothes.

Special hygiene measures are necessary for the older client with an indwelling catheter. To prevent infection, the area around the urinary meatus and the point of entry of the catheter should be cleansed at least once a day and following contamination by feces or vaginal discharge. Cleansing should be performed by using single wiping motions away from the urinary meatus and down the catheter tubing. After cleansing, application of an antiseptic ointment around the urinary meatus helps prevent bacteria from ascending the indwelling tube into the urinary tract.

SUMMARY

Maintenance of fluid and electrolyte balance requires adequate functioning of many systems, including the gastrointestinal tract, excretory system, and circulatory system. All of these systems undergo normal aging changes that place them at risk when they are exposed to stress. This chapter focused on the nursing care of older clients with three common chronic illnesses that affect the body's fluid and electrolyte balance: congestive heart failure, diverticular disease, and incontinence.

Some clients with these ailments become acutely ill and move to Adaptation Level Four. For example, the client with diverticulosis may develop diverticulitis, the client with heart failure may decompensate and require hospitalization, and the client with incontinence may require surgical correction of the problem. However, many clients with the health problems discussed in this chapter are able to continue functioning independently for long periods of time. By assisting clients at Adaptation Level Three to manage complicated medication regimens and modify their activities of daily living and hygiene practices, the nurse can foster independence in clients who are chronically ill.

REFERENCES

Agate J: Special hazards of illness in later life, in Rossman I (ed), Clinical Geriatrics, 2nd ed. Philadelphia, Lippincott, 1979

Allen MD: Drug therapy in the elderly. American Journal of Nursing 80(8):1474, 1980

Anderson Sir F: Practical Management of the Elderly, 3rd ed. Oxford, Blackwell, 1976

Arie T, Clark M, Slattery T: Incontinence in geriatric psychiatry, in Willington FS (ed), Incontinence in the Elderly. London, Academic, 1976

Basen MM: The elderly and drugs—Problem overview and program strategy. Public Health Reports 92(1):43, 1977

Bass L: More fiber—Less constipation. American Journal of Nursing 77(2):254, 1977

Basso A: The prostate in the elderly male. Hospital Practice 12(10):117, 1977

Battle EH, Hanna CE: Evaluation of a dietary regimen for chronic constipation report of a pilot study. Journal of Gerontological Nursing 6(9):527, 1980

Bayless TM: Malabsorption in the elderly. Hospital Practice 14(8):57, 1979

Beber CR: Freedom for the incontinent. American Journal of Nursing 80(3):483, 1980

Becker MH, Maiman LA: Sociobehavioral determinants of compliance with health and medical care recommendations. Medical Care 13:10, 1975

Bedford PD, Caird FI: Valvular Disease of the Heart in Old Age. London, J. and A. Churchill, 1960.

Berk JE, Bentley PC, McHardy G: New perspectives on diverticulitis. Patient Care 13(2):152, 1979

Berman PM, Kirsner JB: Gastrointestinal problems, in Steinberg FU (ed), Cowdry's The Care of the Geriatric Patient, 5th ed. St. Louis, Mosby, 1976

Bevil, C: Medication management in an elderly community based population: A pilot project. Journal New York State Nurses' Association 12(2):19, 1981

Bonner CD: Medical Care and Rehabilitation of the Aged and Chronically Ill, 3rd ed. Boston, Little, Brown, 1974

Bowles WT: Urological surgery, in Steinberg FU (ed), Cowdry's The Care of the Geriatric Patient, 5th ed. St. Louis, Mosby, 1976

Brock AM: Self-administration of drugs in the elderly. Nursing Forum XVIII(4):340, 1979

Brock A: Self-administration of drugs in the elderly: Nursing responsibilities. Journal of Gerontological Nursing 6(7):398, 1980

Brocklehurst JC: Recent advances in incontinence, in Anderson WF, Judge TG (ed), Geriatric Medicine. London, Academic, 1974

Brocklehurst JC: The causes and management of incontinence in the elderly. Nursing Mirror 144(15)(Suppl):xi, 1977

Brocklehurst JC: The large bowel, in Brocklehurst JC (ed), Textbook of Geriatric Medicine and Gerontology, 2nd ed. Edinburgh, Churchill Livingstone, 1978a

Brocklehurst JC: The bladder, in Brocklehurst JC (ed), Textbook of Geriatric Medicine and Gerontology, 2nd ed. Edinburgh, Churchill Livingstone, 1978b

Brocklehurst JC: The urinary tract, in Rossman I (ed), Clinical Geriatrics, 2nd ed. Philadelphia, Lippincott, 1979

Brocklehurst JC: Modern developments of examination in patients with incontinence, in Folmer ANJR, Schouten J (eds), Geriatrics for the Practitioner. Amsterdam, Excerpta Medica, 1981

Brotman HB: The fastest growing minority: The aging. American Journal of Public Health 64:249, 1974

Brown ADG: Gynecological disorders in the elderly, in Brocklehurst JC (ed), Textbook of Geriatric Medicine and Gerontology, 2nd ed. Edinburgh, Churchill Livingstone, 1978

Burkitt DP: Economic development—Not all a bonus. Nutrition Today 1:6, 1976

Butts PA: Assessment of urinary incontinence in women. Nursing 79 9(3):72, 1979

Caird FI: Parkinsonism, in Anderson WF, Judge TG (eds), Geriatric Medicine. London, Academic, 1974

Caird FI, Dall JLC: The cardiovascular system, in Brocklehurst JC (ed), Textbook of Geriatric Medicine and Gerontology, 2nd ed. Edinburgh, Churchill Livingstone, 1978

Carpenter HA and Simon R: The effect of several methods of training on long-term incontinent behaviorally regressed hospitalized psychiatric patients. Nursing Research 9:17, 1960

Coakley D: Acute Geriatric Medicine. Littleton, MA, PSG, 1981

Cummings JH, Hill MJ, Jenkins DJS, et al: Changes in fecal composition and colonic function due to cereal fiber. American Journal of Clinical Nutrition 29:1468, 1976

Dall J: Advances in geriatric medicine, in Anderson WF, Judge TG (eds), Geriatric Medicine. London, Academic, 1974

Davison W: The hazards of drug treatment in old age, in Brocklehurst JC (ed), Textbook of Geriatric Medicine and Gerontology, 2nd ed. Edinburgh, Churchill Livingstone, 1978

deVoogt HJ: Problems and dangers of catheterization in the elderly, in Folmer ANJR, Schonten J (eds), Geriatrics for the Practitioner. Amsterdam, Excerpta Medica, 1981

Donahue E, Girton K, et al: A drug education program in the well elderly. Geriatric Nursing 2(2):140, 1981

Donaldson S, Wagner C, Gresham GE: A unified ADL evaluation form. Archives of Physical Medicine and Rehabilitation 54(4):175. 1973

Dymock IW: Progress in geriatric gastroenterology, in Anderson WF, Judge TG (eds), Geriatric Medicine. London, Academic , 1974

Eckardt MJ: Consequences of alcohol and other drug use in the aged, in Behnke JA, Finch CE, Moment GB (eds), The Biology of Aging. New York, Plenum, 1978

Eisdorfer C: Issues in health planning for the aged. Gerontologist 16:12, 1976

Elkowitz EB: Geriatric Medicine for the Primary Care Practitioner. New York, Springer, 1981

Elliot JS: Urologic problems of the elderly patient, in Ebaugh FG (ed), Management of Common Problems in Geriatric Medicine. Menlo Park, CA, Addison Wesley, 1981

Ethel Percy Andrus Gerontology Center. Drugs and the Elderly. Los Angeles, University of California Press, 1973

Field, MA: Urinary incontinence in the elderly: An overview. Journal of Gerontological Nursing 5(1):12, 1979

Filner B, Williams TF: Health promotion for the elderly reducing functional dependency, in Somers R, Fabian DR (eds), The Geriatric Imperative. New York, Appleton-Century-Crofts, 1981

Fitzgerald C: Physiological changes affecting psychotropic drug handling in the aged. Journal of Gerontological Nursing 6(4):207, 1980

Gebhardt MW, Governali JF, Hart EJ: Drug-related behavior, knowledge and misconceptions among a selected group of senior citizens. Journal of Drug Education 8(2):85, 1978

George NJR, Osborn DE: Acute urological problems in old age, in Coakley D (ed), Acute Geriatric Medicine. Littleton, MA, PSG, 1981

Goldberg PB: Medications that contain sodium. Geriatric Nursing 1:204, 1980

Goldner FH: Diverticular disease of the colon. Nursing Care 10(11):20, 1977

Gotz BE, Gotz VP: Drugs and the elderly. American Journal of Nursing 78(8):1347, 1978

Granger CV, Greer DS: Functional status measurement and medical rehabilitation outcomes. Archives of Physical Medicine and Rehabilitation 57(3):103, 1976

Hanna MJD, MacMillan AL: The skin, in Brocklehurst JC (ed), Textbook of Geriatric Medicine and Gerontology, 2nd ed. Edinburgh, Churchill Livingstone, 1978

Hecht AB: Improving medication compliance by teaching outpatients. Nursing Forum XIII(2):113, 1974

Hewitt AL, Lonamire WT, Page CF: Urinary incontinence—Another bane of aging. Patient Care 14(3):169, 1980

Hollister LE: Prescribing drugs for the elderly patient, in Ebaugh FG (ed), Management of Common Problems in Geriatric Medicine. Menlo Park, CA, Addison-Wesley, 1981

Hurwitz N, Wade LD: Intensive hospital monitoring of adverse reactions to drugs. British Medical Journal 1:531, 1969

Hyams DE: The liver and biliary system, in Brocklehurst JC (ed), Textbook of Geriatric Medicine and Gerontology, 2nd ed. Edinburgh, Churchill Livingstone, 1978

Ismail-Beigi F, Reinhold JG, Faraji B, et al: Effects of cellulose added to diets of low and high fiber content upon the metabolism of calcium, magnesium, zinc and phosphorus by man. Journal of Nutrition 107:510, 1977

Jackson A: Functional assessment of the aged. Allied Health and Behavioral Science 2(1):47, 1979

James O: Gastrointestinal emergencies in the elderly, in Coakley D (ed), Acute Geriatric Medicine. Littleton, MA, PSG, 1981

Janes L: Constipation. Nursing Mirror 149(13):i, 1979

Jette AM: Functional capacity evaluation: An empirical approach. Archives of Physical Medicine and Rehabilitation 61(2):85, 1980

Katz S, Downs T, Cash HR, Grotz RC: Progress in development of the index of ADL. The Gerontologist 10(1)(Part 1):20, 1970

Kegel AJ: Stress incontinence of urine in women, physiological treatment. Journal of International College of Surgeons 20:487, 1956

Kleiger R: Cardiovascular disorders, in Steinberg FU (ed), Cowdry's The Care of the Geriatric Patient, 5th ed. St. Louis, Mosby, 1976

Kovar MG: Health of the elderly and use of health services. Public Health Reports 92:9, 1977

Lamy P, Kitler MC: The geriatric patient: Age-dependent physiologic and pathologic changes. Journal of the American Gerontological Society 19:XX(871), 1971

Lawton EB: Activities of Daily Living for Physical Rehabilitation. New York, McGraw-Hill, 1963

Lenhart DG: The use of medications in the elderly population. Nursing Clinics of North America 11(1):135, 1976

Lofholm P: Self-medication by the elderly, in Kayne RC (ed), Drugs in the Elderly. Los Angeles, University of California Press, 1978

Lothian P: Frequent micturition and its significance. Nursing Times 73(46):1809, 1977

Lundin DV: Must taking medication be a dilemma for the independent elderly? Journal of Gerontological Nursing 4(3):25, 1978

Mahoney F, Barthel DW: Functional evaluation—The Barthel Index. Maryland State Medical Journal 14(2):6l, 1965

Mandelstam D: Support for the incontinent patient. Nursing Mirror 144(15)(Suppl):XIX, 1977

Maney JY: A behavioral therapy approach to bladder retraining. Nursing Clinics of North America 11(1):179, 1976

McCarron JP: How to diagnose and treat stress incontinence. Consultant 19(6):28, 1979

McKechnie JC: Diverticular disease and diet. Consultant 16(7):27, 1976

Meissner JE: Evaluate your patient's level of independence. Nursing 80 10(9):72, 1980

Monthly Vital Statistics Report. Vol. 28, No. 1, Supplement. U.S. Department of Health, Education and Welfare, Public Health Service, Health Resources Administration, National Center for Health Statistics, May 1979

Mullen EM, Granholm M: Drugs and the elderly patient. Journal of Gerontological Nursing 7(2):108, 1981

Offerhaus L: Dangers of drug therapy in the elderly, in Folmer ANJR, Schouten J, (eds), Geriatrics for the Practitioner. Amsterdam, Excerpta Medica, 1981

Olsen J, Johnson J: Drug misuse among the elderly. Journal of Gerontological Nursing 4(6):11, 1978

Pathy MA: Acute cardiac problems, in Coakley D (ed), Acute Geriatric Medicine. Littleton, MA, PSG, 1981

Pearson LJ, Kotthoff ME: Geriatric Clinical Protocols. Philadelphia, Lippincott, 1979

Pfeiffer E: Use of drugs which influence behavior in the elderly: Promises, pitfalls and perspectives, in Kayne RC (ed), Drugs and the Elderly. Los Angeles, University of California Press, 1978

Pfeiffer E: Pharmacology of aging, in Lesnoff-Caravaglia G (ed), Health Care of the Elderly: Strategies for Prevention and Intervention. New York, Human Sciences Press, 1980

Plant J: Educating the elderly in safe medication use. Hospital J.A.H.A. 51:97, 1977

Plein JB: Drug dosing for geriatric patients. Nurse Practitioner 4(2):30, 1979

Pollman JW, Morris JJ, Rose PN: Is fiber the answer to constipation problems in the elderly? A review of literature. International Journal of Nursing Studies 15(3):107, 1978

Pomerance A: Cardiac pathology in the aged. Geriatrics 23:101, 1968

Pope W, Reitz M, Patrick M: A study of oral hygiene in the geriatric patient. Nursing Digest 4(4):92, 1976

Rodstein M: Heart disease in the aged, in Rossman I (ed), Clinical Geriatrics, 2nd ed. Philadelphia, Lippincott, 1979

Rose J: Skin care in the elderly. Journal of Practical Nursing 30(4):20, 1980

Salter C de Lerma, Salter CA: Effects of an individualized activity program on elderly patients. The Gerontologist 14:404, 1975

Sarno JE, Sarno MT, Levita E: The functional life scale. Archives of Physical Medicine and Rehabilitation 54:214, 1973

Schoening HA, Iversen IA: Numerical scoring of self-care status: A study of the Kenny self-care evaluation. Archives of Physical Medicine and Rehabilitation 49(4):221, 1968

Schoening HA, Anderegg L, et al: Numerical scoring of self-care status of patients. Archives of Physical Medicine and Rehabilitation 46(10):689, 1965

Schwartz D, Wang M, Zeitz L, Goss MEW: Medication errors made by elderly, chronically ill patients. American Journal of Public Health 52(12):2018, 1962

Services Research Reports. A Study of Legal Drug Use by Older Americans. U.S. Department of Health, Education and Welfare. Public Health Service, Washington, D.C., May 1977

Shanas E, Townsend P, Wedderbum D: Old People in Three Industrial Societies. New York, Atherton, 1968

Sherman FT, Libow LS: Pharmacology and medication, in Libow LS, Sherman FT (eds), The Core of Geriatric Medicine: A Guide for Students and Practitioners. St. Louis, Mosby, 1981

Shomaker DM: Use and abuse of OTC medications by the elderly. Journal of Gerontological Nursing 6(1):21, 1980

Smith DL: Patient compliance with medication regimens. Drug Intelligence and Clinical Pharmacology 10:386, 1976

Snel P: Disorders of the large bowel in elderly people, in Folmer ANJR, Schouten J (eds), Geriatrics for the Practitioner. Amsterdam, Excerpta Medica, 1981

Soule SD: Gynecological disorders, in Steinberg FU (ed), Cowdry's The Care of the Geriatric Patient. 5th ed. St. Louis, Mosby, 1976

Sourander LB: The aging kidney, in Brocklehurst JC (ed), Textbook of Geriatric Medicine and Gerontology, 2nd ed. Edinburgh, Churchill Livingstone, 1978

Spiro LR: Bladder retraining for the incontinent patient. Journal of Gerontological Nursing 4(3):28, 1978

Steinberg FU: Rehabilitation medicine, in Steinberg FU (ed), Cowdry's The Care of the Geriatric Patient, 5th ed. St. Louis, Mosby, 1976

Strause B: Disorders of the digestive system, in Rossman I (ed), Clinical Geriatrics, 2nd ed. Philadelphia, Lippincott, 1979

Tanner G: Heart failure in the MI patient. American Journal of Nursing 77(2):230, 1977

Tobiason SJ: Benign prostatic hypertrophy. American Journal of Nursing 79(2):286, 1979

Todd B: Drugs and the elderly. What does a good drug history include? Geriatric Nursing 2(1):63, 1981

Todd B: Drugs and the elderly. When the patient is on diuretics. Geriatric Nursing 2(2):149, 1981

Vallarino R, Sherman FT: Stroke, fractured hip, amputation, pressure sores and incontinence: Principles of rehabilitation treatment, in Libow S, Sherman T (eds), The Core of Geriatric Medicine: A Guide for Students and Practitioners. St. Louis, Mosby, 1981

Webster SGP: Gastrointestinal function and absorption of nutrients, in Exton-Smith AN, Caird FI (eds), Metabolic and Nutritional Disorders in the Elderly. Chicago, Year Book, 1980

Weg RB: Drug interaction with the changing physiology of the aged: Practice and potential. Kayne RC (ed), Drugs and the Elderly. Los Angeles, University of California Press, 1978

Wheeler MH: Acute gastrointestinal bleeding, in Coakley D (ed), Acute Geriatric Medicine. Littleton, MA, PSG, 1981

V

Level Four Adaptation: The Aging Client Experiencing Acute Illness

18

Nursing the Client Experiencing Acute Oxygen Deprivation

Like so many health problems that afflict the elderly, those discussed in this chapter are chronic. They are characterized by brief periods when the client is acutely ill and longer periods when the client is able to cope with the illness and function independently. This chapter, and the ones that follow, emphasize the nursing care of elderly clients who have moved to Adaptation Level Four because of an inability to cope with the stress of illness. At this point clients require direct, ongoing nursing care as well as intervention by other members of the health team. They may be treated in hospitals, nursing homes, or rehabilitation settings. One aim of nursing care for clients at Adaptation Level Four is to help them find more successful ways of adapting so that they can return to a more independent level of functioning.

Because of their diminished reserve capacity the elderly are particularly vulnerable to the consequences of oxygen deprivation. This chapter explores the elderly client's adaptations to arteriosclerotic heart disease and occlusive cerebrovascular disease. Because the heart and brain are composed of postmitotic cells, ischemia causes far-reaching, lifelong adaptations. Nursing care often involves helping clients to find new ways to compensate for these adaptations and supporting them as they learn to cope with complex treatment regimens. Arteriosclerotic heart disease is the most common cause of death in persons over age 60 (Kleiger, 1976). It manifests itself in many ways, including two discussed here: myocardial infarction and arrhythmias. The incidence of cerebrovascular accident, also dis-

cussed in this chapter, rises at alarming rates in persons over age 50 (Report of the Joint Committee, Epidemiology, 1972).

In recent years a number of new interventions have been instituted and found to be effective even with the very old. These include treatment with potent drugs, and the use of new technology, such as pacemakers. In addition, following cardiovascular occlusion and cerebrovascular accident, the elderly can benefit from progressive exercise programs and rehabilitation.

SIGNIFICANT PROBLEMS

Myocardial Infarction

An important manifestation of cardiovascular disease in the aged is myocardial infarction. Age itself is a risk factor for myocardial infarction. Age-related changes in the blood, vessel walls, and hemodynamics are responsible for the frequent occurrence of myocardial infarction in the elderly. These include slowing of capillary blood flow, tortuosity of vessels, changes in vascular walls, increased adhesiveness of platelets, and age-related changes in cholesterol levels and serum lipids. Psychological factors play a smaller role in the development of acute infarction in the elderly. Physical overexertion and alimentary overload immediately before the onset are increasingly important in provoking myocardial infarction in the elderly (Chebotareo and Korkusko, 1979). In old age, there is approximately equal sex distribution of acute myocardial infarction, in contrast to the predominance of males in younger groups (Rodstein, 1979). The mortality of acute myocardial infarction is not easily determined in the aged because many infarctions are overlooked and misdiagnosed. Older victims of myocardial infarction have a smaller chance of surviving the first days of acute infarction than do younger victims. In addition, they are more likely to experience complications following myocardial infarction. However, there is basis for optimism in the long-term prognosis of myocardial infarction in the elderly. After the acute period of illness, the ratio of actual to expected mortality decreases from 2:3 in men aged 60 to 1:3 in men aged 90 (Caird and Dall, 1978).

Potential Stresses. Following myocardial infarction, the ultimate recovery of elderly clients depends upon several factors. Acute occlusion of the left anterior descending coronary artery is usually a greater threat to life than involvement of the right coronary artery. The presence of long-standing coronary heart disease often magnifies the adaptations to acute coronary occlusion (Pathy, 1981). In addition, the aged are at high risk for a number of potential stresses including arrhythmias, congestive heart failure, cardiogenic shock, digitalis toxicity, and cardiac rupture that may prolong recovery or threaten life.

In the elderly, serious arrhythmias occur with increasing frequency following myocardial infarction (Kleiger, 1976). Atrial fibrillation often accompanies atypical myocardial infarction in the elderly (Exton-Smith and Overstall, 1979). Sinus bradycardia, heart block, supraventricular arrhythmias, ventricular tachycardia, and premature contractions may also occur. Premature contractions are easily induced from the hypoxic area around the region of acute necrosis. Arrhythmias that develop following acute infarction are treated vigorously with potent medications or cardioversion. These interventions are discussed later in this chapter.

Congestive heart failure and cardiogenic shock are common potential stresses precipitated by acute infarction in the aged. Because impending failure may become apparent when the client begins to ambulate, the nurse must carefully evaluate the client's response to exercise progression. Cardiogenic shock is a consequence of deterioration of

contractile function of the heart and reduced cardiac output (Chebotareo and Korkusko, 1979). It is treated with the use of pressor drugs, such as isoproterenol hydrochloride. In selected clients treatment with low doses of dopamine (1 to 10 μg/kg body wt per minute IV) is also effective (Rodstein, 1979). The combination of cardiogenic shock and congestive heart failure has an especially high mortality in the aged.

Following myocardial infarction, the elderly are also at high risk for digitalis toxicity. It is easily precipitated because the myocardium in acute infarction is depleted of potassium and becomes more susceptible to the effects of digitalis.

Cardiac rupture, which accounts for about 10 percent of deaths from acute infarction, occurs most frequently in the aged. Cardiac rupture occurs more often in women over age 80 than in men. It is most common in those with hypertension but without a history of other types of coronary artery disease. Usually, activity is limited for 2 weeks in individuals believed to be at high risk for coronary rupture (Rodstein, 1979). Once ambulation begins, the client's response must be carefully observed. In addition, straining at stool, which may precipitate rupture, should be avoided. Therefore, careful assessment of the client's bowel habits and intervention to prevent constipation are important.

Abnormal Cardiac Rhythms

Abnormal cardiac rhythms are a consequence of stresses that alter impulse formation, stimulate premature beats, or disturb conduction. They are characterized by cardiac rates ranging from tachycardia to bradycardia together with either a regular or irregular rhythm. What constitutes excessive bradycardia or tachycardia and precipitates other adaptations in the elderly varies widely among older individuals and depends in part on the status of the cardiovascular system. Because excessively low heart rates limit the amount of blood pumped to vital organs, adaptations result. Usually, cerebral changes or loss of consciousness occur in the elderly. Tachycardias may also reduce cardiac output if ventricular filling is compromised. In addition, over time, they may result in failure of weak hearts.

Incidence. The incidence of arrhythmias and conduction disturbances increases with advancing age. According to Rodstein (1979), 26 to 36 percent of nursing home residents have arrhythmias associated with altered impulse formation or premature beats. Conduction disturbances occur in 10 to 20 percent of the elderly. Atrial fibrillation is the arrhythmia most frequently observed in older people (Vaidya et al., 1976). It has been documented in 3 to 5 percent of older people living at home and in from 15 to 21.6 percent of hospitalized elderly people (Caird and Dall, 1978; Exton-Smith and Overstall, 1979).

Stresses. Although the same factors that trigger arrhythmias in the young are also responsible for doing so in the elderly, some stresses trigger arrhythmias more easily and more often in the elderly. Table 1 summarizes the stresses that precipitate arrhythmias in the elderly. Aging alone seems to place people at greater risk for arrhythmias. The greater excitability and irritability of the aging myocardium place it at high risk for arrhythmias. Thickening and fat infiltration occur around the sinoatrial node. Muscle fibers undergo numerous changes. The amount of muscle declines and fibrous tissue increases around the sinoatrial node and internodal atrial tracts after age 75. These changes are believed to contribute to the increased incidence of atrial arrhythmias in the aged (Harris, 1978a).

Prescribed medication often precipitates arrhythmias in the elderly. If the medication is discontinued, the arrhythmia will cease, but this may take days or weeks. Cardiac arrhythmias, particularly premature ventricular contractions and atrioventricular block, may be the first evidence of digitalis toxicity. The injudicious use of potassium-sparing diuretics in elderly persons with impaired renal function may result in sinus node dysfunction. Tricyclic antidepressants, which are often prescribed for the elderly, may stimulate ventricular arrhythmias. Quinidine, hypokalemia-inducing diuretics and bronchodilators, theophylline derivatives, epinephrine, atropine, and sympathomimetic preparations may also precipitate arrhythmias.

In the elderly, arrhythmias are often an adaptation to a previously existing health condition that also requires intervention. For example, pneumonia and other acute infections, acute blood loss, myocardial ischemia, and a wide range of heart diseases frequently trigger arrhythmias in the elderly. Ischemia is a potent arrhythmic stress because it leads to acute potassium loss from injured cells, resulting in shortening of the action potential and refractory period and slowing of conduction. Unfortunately, in these cases, the arrhythmia may become an additional stress that further threatens the older person's level of adaptation. On the other hand, there are times when an arrhythmia is an important compensatory adaptation that assists older persons to cope with stress and maintain their level of adaptation. For example, thyrotoxicosis, emotional stress, and congestive heart failure may trigger paroxysmal atrial tachycardia, which will temporarily assist older persons to meet their oxygen needs. However, because elderly persons have diminished cardiac reserve, long-standing arrhythmias may become a stress for the client by impairing cerebral perfusion, or stimulating cardiovascular insufficiency or other life-threatening adaptations.

Cerebrovascular Accident

After age 55, the incidence of cerebrovascular accident (stroke) rises steeply (Table 2). It occurs with equal frequency in both sexes (Isaacs, 1978). Stroke victims are among the major users of health care resources, including hospitals, rehabilitation units, nursing homes, and community agencies (Coakley, 1981). Seventy-five percent of all stroke deaths occur in people over age 70. Stroke is the third cause of death among persons aged 55 to 74 and the second cause of death in persons over age 75.

A cerebrovascular accident is characterized by neurological adaptations to ischemic brain tissue that is a consequence of an occlusive or hemorrhagic process involving one or more blood vessels of the brain. Strokes may be classified according to their temporal characteristics:

1. Transient ischemic attack (TIA)
2. Reversible ischemic neurological deficit (RIND)
3. Stroke-in-evolution
4. Completed stroke

In transient ischemic attacks, adaptations last from several minutes to 24 hours and then disappear completely. The neurological adaptations associated with RINDs last 2 to 3 days before remitting. The stroke-in-evolution begins as a small neurological deficit and increases over several hours or days. The deficit

TABLE 1. STRESSES PRECIPITATING ABNORMAL CARDIAC RHYTHMS IN THE AGED

Arrhythmia	Stress

Altered Impulse Formation
    Sinus arrhythmias

Sinus bradycardia	Parasympathetic activity
	Beta-adrenergic blocking agents
	Excessive vagal tone
	Carotid sinus stimulation
Sinus tachycardia	Drugs
	Epinephrine
	Atropine
	Emotional stress
	Anxiety
	Excitement
	Infection
	Pain
	Hyperparathyroidism
	Anemia
	Heart Failure
Paroxysmal tachycardia	Coronary artery disease
	Digitalis intoxication
	Malignant diseases of pericardium or mediastinum
	Occult pulmonary emboli
	Hyperthyroidism
	Silent mitral stenosis
Ventricular tachycardia	Myocardial infarction
	Electrolyte imbalance
	Digitalis intoxication
Atrial fibrillation	All forms of heart disease, including myocardial infarction
	Infection
	Hyperthyroidism
	Trauma
	Surgery
	Vagal stimulation from abdominal distention
	Intoxication
	Medications
	Sympathomimetic bronchodilators
	Hypokalemic-inducing diuretics
	Digitalis
	Unknown stress
Atrial flutter	Significant heart disease
	Medications
Ventricular fibrillation	Myocardial ischemia
	Circulatory impairment from heart failure or hypertension
	Medications
	Digitalis intoxication
	Quinidine
	Tricyclic antidepressants
Sick sinus syndrome (sinus node dysfunction)	Degenerative changes in the node and atrium
	Arteriosclerotic heart disease
	Rheumatic heart disease

TABLE 1. **(Continued)**

Arrhythmia	Stress
Sick sinus syndrome (Continued)	Hypertension Hyperkalemia (as from potassium-sparing diuretics) Unknown stress
Premature Beats	

	Irritable foci anywhere in the heart
	Medications
	  Digitalis
	  Quinidine
	  Tricyclic antidepressants
	Toxic substances
	  Alcohol
	  Nicotine
	  Caffeine
	Hypokalemia
	Heart conditions
	  Pericarditis
	  Myocarditis
	  Myocardial infarction
	  Conditions characterized by ventricular hypertrophy or
	    congestive heart failure

Conduction Disturbances	

Atrioventricular block	Idiopathic fibrosis and sclerosis of conducting system
	Calcification of mitral or aortic valve with extension of
	    calcium to conducting system (Lev's Disease)
	Medications
	  Digitalis
	  Quinidine
	  Procainamide
	Heart disease
	  Inferior wall infarction reducing blood suppy to AV
	    node and inferior wall
	  Coronary artery disease

Sinoatrial block	Drugs, especially digitalis toxicity Arteriosclerosis Rheumatic heart disease

Bundle branch block	Heart disease
	  Coronary artery disease
	  Left ventricular failure

in completed stroke remains stable over a long period of time and does not completely regress (Hardin, 1976).

Strokes are also classified according to the involved vasculature as either carotid or vertebrobasilar. These classifications are significant because the client's adaptations are directly related to the area of occlusion.

Strokes are classified according to broad pathological types. Extensive classifications according to pathology are available in many texts, including Bonner's (1974). The most important classifications

TABLE 2. ESTIMATED INCIDENCE AND PREVALENCE OF CEREBROVASCULAR ACCIDENT ACCORDING TO AGE GROUP

Age Group	Estimated Incidence per 1000 Population (both sexes, all races)	Estimated Prevalence per 1000 Population (both sexes, all races)
10–35	—	—
35–44	0.25	—
45–54	1.00	20
55–64	3.50	35
65–74	9.00	60
75–84	20.00	95
85 and older	40.00	—

Source: Report of the Joint Committee for Stroke Facilities, Epidemiology Study Group, 1972, with permission.

are vascular occlusion from embolus or thrombus, and intracranial hemorrhage. Advances in diagnostic techniques in recent years have aided physicians in determining the pathological classification of stroke. Although cerebral thrombosis was once believed to be the most common type of stroke, new evidence demonstrates that about half of all infarctions of the internal carotid artery are a consequence of emboli dislodged from the heart (Isaacs, 1978). In spite of technological advances, diagnosis of the pathological lesion can be difficult, and autopsies have indicated that the incidence of diagnostic errors is high (Isaacs, 1978). The pathological classification of the stroke is an important determinant of the interventions.

The Client at Risk. Cerebrovascular accidents are not the result of a single stress. Many factors play a role in their development. Age itself is a risk factor. At any age, the nervous system is an indicator of stress anywhere in the body but it is particularly sensitive in the elderly. Normally, the brain is less able than other organs to withstand ischemia. This ability is reduced even further as the normal loss of cerebral cells occurs with age. Loss of cells is accelerated when ischemia occurs. Eventually, some areas of the brain may become abnormal, reducing the person's adaptability. Such individuals quickly exhibit disordered function in response to relatively slight degrees of oxygen or other metabolic deprivation. Brain metabolism is highly de-

pendent upon the efficient performance of other body systems: respiratory, cardiac, renal, hepatic, endocrine, and hematopoietic. As functioning of one or more of these systems is compromised by the aging process or chronic illness, the risk is increased that neurological adaptations will develop in response to a relatively minor stress.

Collateral safeguards of the cerebral circulation are now recognized to be more extensive and more efficient than was once supposed. Nevertheless, a number of stresses, either extrinsic or intrinsic to the blood vessels, may impair collateral circulation. If the stress is advanced, blood flow to some vessels may be cut to such precarious levels that even a slight change in the constancy or composition of the blood supply may reduce circulation or oxygenation of some parts of the brain below critical minimal levels, creating impending cerebral ischemia (Adams, 1974).

One of the most important stresses that impairs cerebral blood flow is atherosclerosis. It results in arterial kinks and narrowing and predisposes the person to thrombi and emboli. Atherosclerosis of either extracranial or intracranial arteries may impair cerebral blood flow. The elderly client with generalized atherosclerosis is also at risk for TIAs and strokes as a result of hemodynamic changes. These include postural hypotension after sudden rapid changes in movements or position. They may also be a consequence of certain medications, including diuretics, antihypertensives, tricyclic antidepressants, and phenothiazines. Resting blood pressure has been directly correlated with the incidence of cerebrovascular accident. Even mild elevations of either systolic or diastolic pressure are related to an increased risk of stroke.

Other stresses have also been found to increase the risk of stroke. In one study, over 1000 autopsies were performed on elderly persons in order to identify important risk factors in cerebral infarction in the elderly. In addition to mild hypertension, it was found that a hematocrit above 46 percent, atrial fibrillation, diabetes with fasting blood sugar levels above 111 mg/dl, serum triglyceride levels above 141 mg/dl, and serum cholesterol levels above 191 mg/dl increased the risk of cerebral infarction (Tohgi and Uchiyama, 1979).

The Client Experiencing TIAs. About one-half of all stroke victims experience transient ischemic attacks at least once before the onset of a stroke (Coakley, 1981). Transient ischemic attacks are an important warning sign of stroke, particularly in hypertensive individuals (Isaacs, 1978). The greatest risk of stroke is within the first year, especially in the first 2 months, after the initial transient ischemic attack (Coakley, 1981).

Transient ischemic attacks are a result of changes in the vasculature. The most important stress associated with TIAs is believed to be atherosclerosis of arteries, often accompanied by atheromatous ulceration of the intima. For example, microemboli may arise from atherosclerotic neck arteries and be carried to the carotid or vertebrobasilar tree, resulting in diminished blood supply and neurological adaptations. Or, atherosclerotic occlusion of the main neck arteries is complicated by another stress and the two in combination result in a dangerously diminished blood flow. Other stresses that may be involved include smoking, which exerts a vasoconstrictive effect, the use of hypotensive medications, or exaggerated neck movements, which reduce vertebral artery blood flow especially in persons with cervical spondylosis. Other stresses are prolonged standing or exertion, particularly in an elderly person who is anemic. This can produce hypovolemia leading to cerebral ischemia.

Often older persons with cardiac arrhythmias experience adaptations such as falls and hemiplegia due to focal cerebral ischemia. Although the ad-

aptations resemble those associated with TIAs, the focal stress is the heart, not the vasculature. Therefore, these are not transient ischemic attacks and the interventions required are different. These are described elsewhere in this chapter.

The Client with a Stroke. Stresses associated with stroke in the elderly differ very little from those seen at other ages. However, it is much more difficult for older people to survive massive cerebral infarction, and if they do survive, to achieve a high level of adaptation. Eighty percent of all strokes in the aged are associated with either cerebral thrombosis or embolism. Cerebral embolism, long recognized as a cause of infarction in younger clients, is now recognized as a significant cause of infarction in older clients as well. It is usually associated with lesions of the heart (Coakley, 1981).

ASSESSING THE CLIENT'S ADAPTATIONS

Myocardial Infarction

Elderly clients exhibit very different adaptations to myocardial infarction from the young. In the elderly, adaptations are highly variable and subtle. Consequently, a high percentage of myocardial infarctions in the elderly are misdiagnosed or completely overlooked.

Among the elderly, the most common initial adaptation to myocardial infarction is rapidly developing dyspnea or breathlessness. Dyspnea or another atypical adaptation may overshadow any chest pain which might be present. Dyspnea occurs in about 20 percent of elderly victims (Pathy, 1967; Caird and Dall, 1978), most of whom have preexisting coronary artery disease, cardiac hypertrophy, or heart failure. The dyspnea is probably a response to left ventricular failure. If an older person with good exercise tolerance suddenly develops dyspnea or if the dyspnea of an elderly person with heart or lung disease worsens without a clearcut reason, myocardial infarction should be suspected.

Other atypical adaptations to myocardial infarction also occur in the elderly. Sudden mental deterioration, particularly if it is confusional or irritable in nature, is frequent. Pathy (1967) found that confusion accompanied by agitation, noisiness, aggressiveness, or wandering behavior was the only adaptation in 10 percent of elderly clients. In an already disturbed older person confusion may increase. Other adaptations include dizziness, intense and prolonged weakness and fatigue, feelings of faintness, and loss of consciousness but without pain. These adaptations are attributed to reduced cerebral blood flow secondary to decreased cardiac output and aggravated by a sluggish carotid sinus reflex and cerebral arterial narrowing. Hemiplegia may occur due to cerebral infarction following hypotension or cerebral embolism. Mid- or lower-abdominal distress attributable to visceral congestion following right-sided heart failure may also occur. Other adaptations exhibited by the elderly include progressive renal failure with uremia, embolic occlusion of noncerebral arteries with ischemia or peripheral gangrene, vomiting, hiccoughs, and palpitations.

Silent myocardial infarction occurs in 31 percent of the elderly. In these cases, electrocardiographic changes are the only initial adaptation (Caird and Dall, 1978). Silent myocardial infarctions are often accompanied by cardiogenic shock and result in sudden death in the elderly (Villaverde and MacMillan, 1980). Several factors are believed to contribute to the high incidence of myocardial infarction without pain or other adaptations. These include the increased pain threshold that accompanies aging, loss of the meaning of the pain sensation, loss of memory, or a tendency to ignore any new physical problem amid the many preexisting ones (Rodstein, 1979).

Only 29 percent of elderly persons with myocardial infarction experience the "typical" initial adaptation of pain exhibited by younger persons (Caird and Dall, 1978). The pain may range from almost none to severe retrosternal pain and overwhelming anxiety. The pain may be in the anterior chest or referred to the neck, shoulder or mandible. It may occur during bed rest or after exertion. Clients with the "typical" adaptation of pain are usually not older than 80 and have a lower incidence of residual stresses such as coronary artery disease, cardiac enlargement, or congestive heart failure. In this group, pain is probably a consequence of a less well-developed collateral circulation, resulting in a more typical and extensive infarction (Rodstein, 1979).

Assessment of the elderly client with acute infarction reveals other adaptations. Profuse sweating is less likely to occur in the elderly than in the young. Auscultation may reveal the presence of an arrhythmia, a gallop rhythm, and reversed splitting of the second heart sound. The electrocardiogram usually indicates an elevated ST segment and, later, inverted T waves. However, because many elderly persons have abnormal ECG tracings because of previously existing stresses, the ECG following myocardial infarction can be difficult to interpret. Body temperature and blood reactions are less pronounced in the elderly than in the young. In the elderly, a temperature rise does not always follow myocardial infarction. The ESR may not be increased as is usually the case in younger persons. Laboratory values for SGOT, LDH, and CPK follow the same patterns seen in the young in 85 to 90 percent of the elderly.

Abnormal Cardiac Rhythms

Many young healthy people are able to tolerate arrhythmias for long periods of time without exhibiting significant adaptations. Older people, particularly those with atherosclerosis, are less likely to do so. In fact, the arrhythmia is likely to become a stress that threatens the older person's ability to function. The adaptations precipitated by an arrhythmia are a consequence of oxygen deprivation, which may compromise the cerebral circulation, produce congestive heart failure, or reduce blood pressure, eventually resulting in hypotension and shock. Arrhythmias may result in angina, emboli, thrombi, myocardial infarction, cardiovascular insufficiency, or death.

Abrupt changes in cardiac rhythm are poorly tolerated in the elderly person and may lead to syncope, falls, transient ischemic attacks, and even dementia. Arrhythmias should be suspected as the reason for a fall, especially if the fall is preceded by dizziness and not related to a change in posture. In about half such persons, the electrocardiogram is normal between falls (Exton-Smith and Overstall, 1979).

If an arrhythmia is suspected, the nurse should assess the older client for adaptations that result from a compromised circulation and oxygen deficit. Changes in mentation, personality, and behavior may indicate compromised cerebral circulation or cerebral emboli. Changes in the color of the urine may be due to microemboli of the renal artery. Complaints of abdominal discomfort may be due to microemboli of the mesenteric artery and infarcted bowel, rather than constipation. Blood pressure fluctuations, dyspnea, or pain may indicate myocardial ischemia. A variety of adaptations, including dyspnea, fluid retention, and blood pressure changes may indicate congestive heart failure.

Because less serious arrhythmias in the aged are often forerunners of more serious arrhythmias, the client with an arrhythmia must be assessed regularly. For example, atrial premature beats may be forerunners of atrial fibrillation. Ventricular premature beats may be forerunners of ventricular tachycardia.

Some arrhythmias such as sinus bradycardia, sinus tachycardia, and paroxysmal atrial tachycardia with a 2:1 or 3:1 block may not stimulate any adverse adaptations in the elderly. In most cases, however, arrhythmias do stimulate adaptations that may have dangerous consequences for older people.

Altered Impulse Formation. Adaptations to altered impulse formation vary widely and often depend upon the specific arrhythmia involved and the older client's general state of health. If an older client with ischemic heart disease develops sinus tachycardia, angina may occur. If the tachycardia continues, other adaptations may develop as well. Fortunately, sinus tachycardia usually disappears spontaneously once the precipitating stress, such as emotional stress, exertion, and the like, is eliminated.

When paroxysmal atrial or ventricular tachycardias occur in older people, the client may complain of feeling a shock in the chest followed by a fluttering sensation, weakness, nausea, or anginal pain. The client may have an unexplained cerebral ischemic attack. If the client has organic heart disease, the heart is less able to tolerate long periods of rapid ventricular rates (Van Durme, 1975). Therefore, the nurse must be alert for signs that the client's level of adaptation is threatened. Paroxysmal tachycardias are characterized by a sudden, rapid pulse rate up to or over 240 beats per minute. The ECG shows a rapid, irregular rhythm.

The most important arrhythmia among the aged is atrial fibrillation. It may begin by paroxysms and at a later stage become more permanent. If paroxysmal atrial fibrillation is precipitated by myocardial infarction or infection, it may revert spontaneously to normal sinus rhythm. Long-standing atrial fibrillation is dangerous because it alters the hemodynamics of the heart and can lead to mural thrombi, cerebral thrombosis, or microemboli. Atrial fibrillation is characterized by a pulse that is irregular in frequency and intensity. Cardiac output may fall 20 or 30 percent and result in palpitations, giddiness, syncope, angina, or acute heart failure. In the elderly, atrial fibrillation is difficult to control. Often, treatment is aimed at controlling the ventricular response to the arrhythmia rather than the atria because the atria often respond only temporarily to treatment with medication or cardioversion.

Atrial flutter is characterized by adaptations similar to atrial fibrillation. Atrial flutter may stimulate a rapid ventricular response or it may be accompanied by a regular ventricular response and pulse rate. Because atrial flutter usually indicates significant heart disease and is often accompanied by heart failure, the client requires prompt intervention.

Bradycardia in the elderly may be dangerous. Sinus bradycardia may cause the older person to faint. Bradycardia may also occur in older people who have sick sinus syndrome. Although some of these clients are asymptomatic, many develop mental confusion, fainting, dizzy spells, lightheadedness, lethargy, malaise, or angina as a consequence of the bradycardia. In sick sinus syndrome the bradycardia does not respond to exercise or drugs. Sick sinus syndrome is often accompanied by atrial arrhythmias or sinoatrial block.

Premature Beats. Elderly persons with premature beats exhibit ECG changes that include widened and premature QRS complexes. Few other adaptations occur. Persons may complain of feeling a shock in the chest or palpitations if premature beats occur frequently. During auscultation or palpation of the pulse, the examiner notes a beat that comes closer to the preceding one, followed by a longer pause. Ventricular permature beats are particularly frequent in the elderly (Villaverde and

MacMillan, 1980). When six or more per minute occur, they are considered dangerous since they foreshadow more serious ventricular arrhythmias (Elkowitz, 1981; Pathy, 1981).

Conduction Disturbances. Conduction disturbances may occur either proximal to the bundle of His, more distally, or diffusely throughout the conducting system. They may result in excessive bradycardia or in rapid escape rhythms. Atrioventricular block is the most common reason for heart block in the elderly. Atrioventricular block is of three degrees and adaptations vary depending upon the degree. First-degree block occurs normally in about 2 percent of healthy older persons. In the aging client, first-degree block may not precipitate any noticeable adaptations.

Second-degree block is significant because the failure to conduct some atrial impulses implies the possibility of development of complete AV dissociation. When there is only occasional failure of impulse conduction, the pulse is irregular. When there is a 2:1 or 3:1 block, there is irregular bradycardia.

In third-degree block, no impulses reach the ventricles, which eventually establish a fixed rhythm of their own. During the period between cessation of AV conduction and ventricular contraction, syncope and an absent or slow pulse result, constituting the Stokes–Adams syndrome. Initially the client's face is pale but becomes flushed upon recovery. Complete heart block can also result in tachyarrhythmias, depending upon ventricular activity. In cases of either bradycardia or tachycardia, however, transient weakness, dizziness, fainting, and convulsions result. Mortality is high.

Cerebrovascular Accident

The Client Experiencing TIAs. Adaptations to TIAs are highly variable and may be very subtle. Older persons may be unaware of them or may ignore them. In either case, older clients often do not report adaptations. The nurse who suspects that a client is having TIAs should communicate with individuals who have frequent contact with the client to determine if they have observed any changes in the client.

When taking the nursing history, the nurse should question the client to determine the specific adaptations that accompany the TIA. The adaptations depend upon the location of the temporary occlusion and usually occur on only one side of the body. If the carotid arteries are involved, adaptations are supratentorial. They may include paresis or paralysis of the face or extremities, aphasia, loss of vision in one eye or hemianopsia, areas of anesthesia, and mental changes, including confusion, loss of memory, or behavior changes. If the vertebrobasilar tree is involved adaptations are subtentorial. The client suddenly loses all postural tone and falls forward heavily on the knees without loss of consciousness. Other adaptations include vertigo, vomiting, dysarthria, perioral numbness, visual blurring, and diplopia. This is called the hindbrain syndrome.

Clients should also be assessed for anemia and other contextual or residual stresses, such as diabetes, hypertension, obesity, heavy smoking, sedentarism, or a fat-rich diet that may have contributed to the presence of atherosclerosis and place the client at risk for TIAs. Assessment of the client experiencing TIAs usually reveals the presence of enlarged, tortuous, and hard peripheral arteries. When auscultating the bifurcation of the carotid artery a murmur may be heard on the side opposite the neurological deficit.

The Client with a Stroke. The adaptations of the elderly client vary widely depending upon the pathological classification, location, and extent of the lesion. Cerebral thrombosis is usually associated with a gradually progressing onset. Loss of consciousness, if it occurs at all, occurs late. Cerebral embolism is usually associated with a rapid onset, brief loss of consciousness, and an early improvement. If the elderly person has generalized cerebral atherosclerosis, however, the classic pattern of onset associated with cerebral embolism may not be seen. The onset associated with intracranial hemorrhages, including subdural hematoma, subarachnoid hemorrhage, or intracerebral hemorrhage, is highly variable. The elderly person may not be aware that any problems are occurring, particularly if the right cerebral hemisphere is affected.

In general, the size of the involved artery and the adequacy of collateral circulation influence the extent of the deficit. Occlusion of the internal carotid artery or one of its branches, the middle cerebral or anterior cerebral artery, produces the carotid artery syndrome. The most frequent adaptation is contralateral hemiplegia or hemiparesis, but a wide variety of deficits in vision, sensation, communication, perception, cognition, and emotions may also occur. The most common adaptations are shown in Table 3.

When the posterior portion of the cerebral circulation is involved, the syndrome is referred to as the vertebrobasilar artery syndrome. Since these arteries nourish the midbrain, pons, medulla, ten cranial nerves, the end organs of hearing and balance, and parts of the cerebral hemisphere, occlusion can stimulate a myriad of adaptations (Table 4). These include loss of consciousness, memory loss, confusion, dizziness, ataxia, pupillary abnormalities, visual deficits, tinnitus, deafness, dysphagia, numbness, hemiplegia, or other paralysis or paresis.

Recovery from stroke is spontaneous and slow. It occurs in a predictable pattern and at a predictable pace and involves several intrinsic cerebral and circulatory mechanisms. Adaptations change with each stage of the recovery process. There are three stages in the recovery process:

1. Spontaneous resolution of cerebral edema usually occurs within 4 weeks. Edema is the most common reason for depressed consciousness during the first week after stroke and may contribute to paralysis.
2. Return of circulation to the ischemic areas occurs gradually. Eventually, areas of variable ischemia that surround the infarcted area may be brought back to a functional status by the return of circulation. This mechanism accounts for some improvement of neurological function up to 12 weeks following infarction.
3. Damaged neurons transfer some function to healthy neurons. Functions controlled by healthy brain tissue compensate for lost functions. This mechanism accounts for much of the improvement made in the first six months following infarction (Newman, 1972; Hurwitz and Adams, 1972).

It is believed that other recovery mechanisms also exist because improvements in neurological status take place for up to 2 years after stroke.

Assessment procedures and techniques for el-

TABLE 3. ADAPTATIONS AND THEIR APPROXIMATE FREQUENCY IN CAROTID ARTERY SYNDROME

Adaptation	Percent of Cases
Hemiplegia or hemiparesis	80+
Aphasia	30–60
Headache	20–50
Mental disturbance	20
Hemianesthesia or hemihypesthesia	15
Unconsciousness	15
Monoplegia or monoparesis	10–15
Visual disturbances	10–30
Paresthesias of one extremity	10
Seizures	10–20
Homonymous field defect	5–12
Optic atrophy	5–10
Homolateral loss of vision with contralateral hemiparesis	15–20

Source: Toole J, Patel AN, 1974, with permission.

derly stroke victims are generally the same as those for younger clients. Some alterations must be made to compensate for the effects of the aging process and for any chronic illnesses the aging client may have. Aging is not a factor in determining the client's adaptations to cerebrovascular occlusion. Age may be a factor in determining the meaning of these adaptations to the client and the ultimate level of functioning that can be achieved following stroke. Therefore, specialized knowledge is needed to interpret the data obtained from an elderly stroke victim.

The Initial Assessment. Immediately after the onset of the cerebrovascular accident, the client may be unconscious. Stertorous respirations or a Cheyne-Stokes rhythm may be noted. The pulse may be full. Bradycardia and an elevated blood pressure may be present. The client often has a flushed face. If paralysis of the face is present, one cheek inflates rhythmically with respiration. The swallowing reflex may be absent. The hand and eyes may be turned toward the injured side of the brain. A paralyzed extremity is indicated by complete muscular relaxation without tone. On the paralyzed side, deep reflexes may be absent; however, these should re-

TABLE 4. SELECTED ADAPTATIONS TO VERTEBROBASILAR ARTERY DISEASE

Location of Disease	Adaptations
Upper spinal cord and lower brainstem (anterior spinal artery)	Weakness or paralysis of legs or all four extremities (drop attacks) with preservation of consciousness Weakness and vertigo precipitated by head rotation or extension Ataxia Dysarthria and dysphagia Unilateral or bilateral hypalgesia
Cerebellum (posterior and anterior inferior cerebellar, and superior cerebral arteries)	Ataxia Dysmetria Dyssynergia
Labyrinth and cochlea (internal auditory artery)	Vertigo, nausea, and vomiting Tinnitus, sudden deafness
Pons and midbrain (basilar artery)	Occipital headache Lightheadedness and/or syncope Ocular palsies Stupor or coma, diplopia Unilateral or bilateral hypalgesia or weakness Peduncular hallucinosis Paroxysmal hypertension
Cerebral hemispheres, occipital lobes, and temporoparietal areas (posterior cerebral artery)	Homonymous or quadrantanopic visual field loss Visual agnosia Blindness, cortical type Temporal lobe seizures Amnestic syndrome (bilateral hemispheric involvement) Dyslexia without agraphia (dominant hemisphere) Visual agnosia

Source: Toole J, Patel AN, 1974, with permission.

turn spontaneously within days and eventually become hyperactive. The Babinski sign may be elicited. In the acute phase the nurse should also assess the status of the skin, the state of fluid and electrolyte balance, posture, and bowel and bladder function. Special attention should be given to noting signs of injury or trauma, such as a broken limb, which might have occurred at the time of the stroke. This is more likely in the elderly because their bones are more easily broken.

The Comprehensive Assessment.   Once the client's cooperation can be obtained, a comprehensive examination is undertaken. Several members of the health team including the nurse participate in various aspects of this extensive examination. Assess-

ment is a continuous process throughout the recovery and rehabilitation periods, and data are constantly updated.

Findings from the assessment process can be grouped into four general areas:

1. Adaptations directly associated with cerebral ischemia—these are neurological deficits and include confusion, incontinence, speech disturbances, and the like.

2. Adaptations that develop as a consequence of the neurological deficits—spasticity, contractures, shoulder pain, and the like.

3. Other adaptations to the focal stress—atherosclerosis, hypertensive heart disease, ischemic heart disease, and the like.

4. Adaptations to contextual and residual stresses—aging, arthritis, Parkinson's disease, an amputated limb, chronic obstructive pulmonary disease, and the like (Isaacs, 1978).

In each of these areas, some findings have a unique significance for the elderly client.

ADAPTATIONS ASSOCIATED DIRECTLY WITH THE STROKE. Neurological deficits following stroke occur in the following areas:

1. Motor function
2. Sensation and vision
3. Autonomic function
4. Communication
5. Perception, cognition, and emotional expression.

These need to be assessed on a continuous basis. If these resolve, they tend to do so at predictable rates reflecting the recovery mechanisms that follow stroke. Table 5 indicates adaptations that reflect cerebral ischemia and their significance to recovery. In general, as lapsed time increases, less and less resolution of adaptations should be expected.

1. MOTOR FUNCTION. Assessment should include passive range of motion, voluntary movement, muscle strength, cerebellar function, balance, and activities of daily living. Range of motion measurements should be as precise as possible. These give a good estimate of the impairment of joint function. Repeated measurements are valuable for gauging the ongoing impact of the stroke and the success of a treatment program. The strength of a muscle or a group of muscles can be tested in two ways. The client can perform a movement while the examiner gives resistance or the examiner can attempt to move a joint while the client resists. The client's ability to perform the following movements should also be determined: turning in bed, sitting up from a supine position, transferring to a chair, sitting unsupported, standing up from a chair, and standing.

Return of voluntary motion and reflexes is highly predictable. Initial flaccid paralysis reverts to spastic paralysis within 1 week. Spasticity always precedes the return of voluntary movement. Once a limb becomes spastic voluntary movement should follow within 1 to 2 months. If it does not, no voluntary movement should be expected (Zankel, 1971). Recovery of muscle function may begin as early as the first week and no later than the seventh week. The usual interval from onset to 80 percent final recovery is about 6 weeks (McDowell, 1976). Motor function recovery depends in part on the client's posture, position, and associated movements. Neurological recovery is usually greater in

TABLE 5. PROGNOSIS OF RECOVERY FROM CEREBROVASCULAR ACCIDENT

Prognostic Sign	Encouraging	Discouraging
Recovery from coma	Rapid	Slow
Incontinence	Clears in 2 to 3 weeks	Recovery delayed
Depression	Absent	Present
Dementia	Absent	Present
Recent memory	Good	Bad
Demeanor	Energetic	Apathetic
Language	Normal	Receptive aphasia
Positive supporting reaction	Early recovery	Delayed
Balance	Early recovery	Delayed
Posture	Well aligned	Eccentric
Walk	Rhythmical	Disorganized
Proprioception	Unaffected	Severe loss
Anosognosia	Absent	Present
Apraxia	Transient	Persistent

Source: Hurwitz LJ, Adams GF, 1972, with permission.

the affected leg than in the affected arm. Disturbances in cerebellar functions are more variable. Ataxia may improve over 1 to 2 years, but disturbances of balance may never be corrected (Hirschberg et al., 1976).

The client's ability to perform self-care activities should also be determined. Much time is spent in rehabilitation programs teaching the client to relearn these lost skills. A variety of charts have been developed, listing as many as 100 or as few as 6 self-care activities. These are used to determine whether the client can perform the activity independently, with supervision, with assistance, with adaptive devices, or not at all. No one system has been found to be ideal; however, if the assessment tool is to be useful, it must be sensitive enough to identify exactly what kinds of things clients can and cannot do for themselves. Self-care assessment tools are discussed in detail in Chapter 17.

In the elderly client, motor function may be adversely affected by untoward reactions to drugs, or by already existing cardiovascular or respiratory insufficiency. The immobility associated with bed rest may also contribute to muscle weakness (Adams, 1974). As a normal consequence of aging, control of posture and coordination deteriorate somewhat. These abilities may deteriorate further as a consequence of stroke. The ability to control posture and balance and perform coordinated activities is important to the return of optimal functioning (Rusk, 1964; Hirschberg et al., 1976).

2. SENSATION AND VISION. Sensory deficits are so subtle that they are often missed by the nursing staff and overlooked by the client. When strokes affect the nondominant side, clients are most likely to be unaware of their deficits. A complete sensory examination is important if an accurate level of recovery is to be predicted. Sensory losses are usually recovered in the first 3 months after onset (Granger et al., 1975). The persistence of multiple sensory deficits, particularly impaired vibratory sense, touch, pain, and temperature sensation, stereognosis, or proprioception prolong recovery and may prevent independent ambulation (Hurwitz and Adams, 1972; Moskowitz et al., 1972). The older client with severe motor and sensory losses has a poor prognosis due to being deprived of the sensory inputs needed to support development of compensatory behaviors (Robbins, 1976).

When tested for light touch the client may fail to perceive touch on the affected side (hemianesthesia) or may perceive the affected side when it is touched singly but not when both sides are touched simultaneously (suppression). The client's perception of a pin prick when the backs of both arms are pricked successively may be dulled. Proprioceptive loss may occur. In the stroke victim, the thumb-finding test may be used to test proprioception. While the examiner supports the affected arm, the client is asked to look at the affected thumb, grasp it, then let the thumb go. The client's eyes are then covered, the arm is moved to a different position by the examiner, and the client is asked to feel the thumb again. Proprioceptive loss is indicated by the client grasping air at the point formerly occupied by the affected thumb (Isaacs, 1978).

Hemianopsia, especially when it is accompanied by other sensory deficits, has been associated with poor recovery. If the assessment is to be accurate, the client who needs glasses must be wearing them. A simple way to differentiate hemianopsia from unilateral visual neglect is to give the client something to read. The person with hemianopsia turns the head toward the side of the deficit in order to bring the material into the visual field. The client with unilateral neglect looks straight ahead but fails to see the material on the affected side (Isaacs, 1978).

3. AUTONOMIC FUNCTION. Retention of urine and urinary incontinence frequently accompany the onset of stroke and may persist for several weeks. Urinary retention is more common in men and incontinence is more common in women. Loss of cortical control over the sacral reflex arc, reduced bladder sensation, and loss of locomotor ability seem to be the major factors in the development of incontinence in stroke victims. The incontinent client who has not been catheterized should be questioned about the presence of the urge to void, the time and frequency of urination, and any awareness of the inability to use the toilet. If possible, urethral catheterization should be avoided. For men, a condom sheath with a collecting bag is preferable in order to avoid urinary infections. If an indwelling catheter is necessary, it should be removed as early as possible, before bladder infections or catheter dependency develop. Little information is available about the effects of incontinence on the re-

covery of the elderly client with stroke. Bladder control often returns when ambulation is initiated (Tobis, 1979).

4. COMMUNICATION. Before testing the client for the presence of language skills, the client's hearing must be tested. If needed, a hearing aid should be used. The prognosis for survival of aphasic clients is poorer than that for nonaphasic clients with similar physical adaptations (Isaacs, 1978). For clients who do survive, aphasia usually does not limit the level of functional achievement (Thorpe and Coull, 1960). Even clients with global aphasia may progress to independence (Rusk, 1964). Recovery from aphasia is highly variable, but, in general, recovery is better in milder cases. The mechanisms associated with the return of language function are poorly understood, and the impact of speech therapy on the spontaneous recovery process is not known.

5. PERCEPTION, COGNITION, AND EMOTIONAL EXPRESSION. Deficits in perception, cognition, and emotional expression have the same devastating effects on the elderly as on younger clients. These can be classified in four groups:

1. *Disturbed awareness of self or space—with attitudes toward illness disordered by separation from reality:* Body image problems include anosognosia, neglect or denial of ownership of hemiplegic limbs, and disordered spatial orientation. Problems associated with disturbed body image impair successful training in self-care because clients ignore sensory input from the involved side and do not use the extremity even if they have the ability to do so. Loss of vertical and horizontal space perception jeopardizes the ability to assume an upright position and complicates gait training.

2. *Disordered integrative action:* Adaptations include impaired postural function, apraxia, agnosia, perseveration, and synkinesia.

3. *Disturbed emotional behavior:* Adaptations include emotional instability, loss of confidence, fear, depression, and unwillingness to try (Adams, 1974).

4. *Impaired learning ability:* Adaptations include clouded consciousness, aphasia, memory defects, and dementia. Dementia is the most serious deficit because it prevents the client from relearning lost skills (Hurwitz and Adams, 1972).

Deficits in these areas usually improve progressively, but timetables cannot be set. Recovery is greatest in the first 3 months and diminishes after 1 to 2 years (Report of the Joint Committee, Stroke Rehabilitation, 1972). Confusion and reduced alertness usually improve between the second and eighth week. Denial, especially when accompanied by hemianopsia, may never be rectified (Newman, 1972). Recovery from visual–spatial deficits is slow (Thorpe and Coull, 1960).

Motivation is a complex attribute that depends upon the client's cognitive and emotional status and is considered the key to successful recovery. In the elderly, motivation depends in part upon how much of the former youthful vigor remains at the time of the stroke and how strongly the client wishes to remain active and independent (Carter, 1979). Few clients appear highly motivated in the acute phase of illness. As they begin to recover and recognize gains made through rehabilitation, motivation improves. The client's premorbid personality and former work habits should also be determined. These have been found to influence the success of rehabilitation (Steinberg, 1976).

ADAPTATIONS TO THE NEUROLOGICAL DEFICITS. The initial neurological deficits exhibited by the stroke client act as a stress that may stimulate additional adaptations in the client. These should not be apparent during the initial assessment of the client. They develop later as a consequence of immobility and disuse, inappropriate care, or other multiple physiological processes. The elderly client is at risk to adapt unsuccessfully to immobility and disuse. If the elderly client with a stroke is immobile, contractures, pressure sores, pressure neuropathies, muscle atrophy, spasticity, shoulder pain, fractures, knee recurvatum, and mental deterioration may develop. With appropriate interventions, including correct positioning and exercise, many of these adaptations can be prevented. The processes by which some adaptations develop are complex and poorly understood. Consequently, adaptations such as edema in the affected limbs, joint calcification, and deep vein thrombosis may not be preventable in all clients.

There are several ways that adaptations to neurological deficits influence the client's recovery. Some, such as heel decubiti, knee contractures, and pressure neuropathies, make ambulation impossible. Others, such as shoulder pain, deep vein thrombosis, and muscle atrophy, limit the client's ability to participate fully in a rehabilitation program.

OTHER ADAPTATIONS TO THE FOCAL STRESS. In elderly stroke victims, the focal stress responsible for the neurological deficits often has many other far-reaching effects. For example, many elderly stroke victims exhibit adaptations to extensive atherosclerosis and cardiovascular disease. Nearly 13 percent of cerebrovascular accidents in the elderly are associated with myocardial infarction, and this must also be treated. In other elderly clients, the stroke is related to atrial fibrillation, endocarditis, infection causing clots of blood or pus, or drops of fat from bone fractures. Since these conditions prevent or delay the institution of a vigorous program of exercise they influence the client's recovery from stroke. In addition, elderly clients are likely to exhibit stroke risk factors, such as insufficient exercise, hypertension, diabetes, poor nutrition, and previous strokes, all of which have a negative impact on the client's ability to achieve an optimal recovery (Zankel, 1971; Anderson et al., 1974).

ADAPTATIONS TO CONTEXTUAL AND RESIDUAL STRESSES. The elderly stroke victim is more likely than a younger person to have multiple chronic illnesses. Although these are not related directly to the stroke syndrome, many have been associated with poor functional outcomes. Cardiovascular, peripheral vascular, and pulmonary disease may prevent or delay the institution of active exercise (Holderman, 1970; Isaacs, 1978). Because stroke clients use twice as much energy as nonparalyzed persons to walk, this may have adverse consequences on clients with cardiovascular and respiratory disorders (Isaacs, 1978). Deficits in hearing and vision and musculoskeletal problems such as arthritis, Parkinson's disease, or an amputation can increase the difficulty of relearning motor skills and limit the ultimate level of achievement.

The aging process itself is another important factor that influences the elderly stroke victim. Persons over age 65 demonstrate less functional improvement than those under 65 (Granger et al., 1975; Report of the Joint Committee, Stroke Rehabilitation, 1972). The aging process is associated with some loss of strength and endurance and reserve capacity. These factors are important for the client's full participation in a rehabilitation program. Con-

sequently, the elderly person may need a somewhat more protective rehabilitation program than a younger person and may make fewer gains.

NURSING INTERVENTIONS

Myocardial Infarction

The aged client with an acute myocardial infarction may be cared for at home, in the medical unit of a general hospital, or in a coronary intensive care unit. Data indicate that whether or not the aged client is admitted to a general medical unit or a coronary care unit depends in part on the individual's social circumstances and the availability of beds (Exton-Smith and Overstall, 1979). Older clients who are admitted to coronary care units do better than those admitted to general medical units (Williams et al., 1976).

If the infarction is mild and if the client has appropriate support systems, home care for the aged client is advocated. Older clients who are cared for at home seem to benefit from the familiar surroundings and do at least as well as those admitted to the hospital (Exton-Smith and Overstall, 1979).

Interventions for the elderly client with a myocardial infarction are similar to those used with younger clients. However, certain factors must be given special attention.

1. The decision to administer analgesia to the aging client depends upon the client's adaptations. If the client is experiencing pain, morphine sulfate in small doses or meperidene hydrochloride are effective ways to reduce pain, curb endogenous catecholamine levels, and decrease the cardiac work load by decreasing venous return.

2. Diazepam (5 to 10 mg) and chlordiazepoxide are often prescribed for the elderly if they experience anxiety or restlessness. If sedatives have been prescribed, the nurse must be aware that barbiturates may increase psychoses and sensory deprivation in elderly clients in coronary care units. In addition, undue sedation may result in difficulty feeding with the consequent danger of aspiration pneumonia. An acute toxic psychosis, exhibited as an agitated depression, may occur in elderly clients following myocardial infarction.

3. The amount of rest and exercise prescribed for the elderly client and the pace at which exercise

is progressed vary widely from one physician to another. In the very old, there is little need for complete bed rest. The advantages of chair rest and use of a bedside commode must be weighed against the risk of undue exertion if inadequate assistance is available for lifting the client in and out of bed. Provided that assistance is available, a deep comfortable chair may be preferable to bed rest for the older client. Short periods out of bed may ease dyspnea and prevent potential stresses such as hypostatic pneumonia, venous thrombosis, and cardiovascular deconditioning, to which the aged are particularly prone.

Although some physicians recommend mobilization as early as the second day (Pathy, 1981), others suggest that mobilization be delayed for 7 to 10 days (Caird and Dall, 1978; Villaverde and MacMillan, 1980). Mobilization should begin more cautiously if cardiac failure is present or more slowly if the client is at risk for cardiac rupture (Caird and Dall, 1978; Rodstein, 1979). Self-feeding and the use of bedside commodes or bathroom privileges rather than bedpans are also advocated for the elderly. An advantage of these approaches is that they tend to improve morale and promote a sense of optimism in clients about their condition. After discharge, most elderly clients are able to resume normal activity. Physical exertion, provided that it is moderate and does not produce angina or fatigue, is desirable to maintain the client's level of functioning and morale and promote collateral circulation.

4. Like younger clients, the aged exhibit anxiety, depression, and other emotional responses to myocardial infarction. A particular worry for the elderly, who experience repeated threats to their independence, is that this condition represents the final blow to an independent life-style. Some elderly persons believe that permanent disability and invalidism are certain consequences of acute infarction. The client's spouse also has questions and anxieties about the client's future level of functioning. The nurse must provide the client with psychological support, encouragement, and an optimistic outlook through both the acute and rehabilitative phases of the myocardial infarction. It is important to communicate that a return to previous activities is expected.

5. The nurse must be particularly observant for the development of systemic emboli, pulmonary emboli, and venous thrombosis in the elderly client. Anticoagulant therapy may not be given routinely to elderly clients unless they are at high risk for the development of emboli or thrombi. When given anticoagulant therapy, the elderly are susceptible to cerebral and intestinal bleeding and to hemopericardium.

The elderly are particularly sensitive to anticoagulants (Rodstein, 1979). If anticoagulant therapy is required, smaller doses are given to them than to the young. Since bleeding may occur even in those elderly with apparently normal prothrombin times, the nurse must observe the client carefully for indications of bleeding.

In the past, individuals who survived a coronary occlusion were discharged to their homes and told to "take it easy." Today, many medical centers have instituted cardiac rehabilitation programs that prescribe individualized progressive exercise programs for the client. Clients may visit the rehabilitation department several times each week for 3 months or more, depending on their response. They also progress their activity at home according to a prescribed plan. Principles of rehabilitation are discussed later in this chapter.

Abnormal Cardiac Rhythms

Assessment and treatment of the elderly client with an arrhythmia may necessitate hospitalization in an intensive care unit where the client can be continuously monitored. Cardiac monitoring is used to detect early cardiac arrhythmias, to diagnose specific arrhythmias and to maintain changes in rhythm that occur in response to the treatment regimen or other changes in the client's overall clinical picture. Some arrhythmias experienced by the elderly are paroxysmal, a characteristic that may result in sudden, dangerous adaptations such as syncope or falls and that makes diagnosis more difficult. If this situation is suspected ambulatory clients may be asked to wear a Holter monitor to detect the arrhythmia. The monitor records the electrocardiogram for 10- or 24-hour periods. If an arrhythmia is present intermittently, the monitor is likely to demonstrate its presence.

Several interventions are used to treat abnormal cardiac rhythms, but some are more suitable than others for the elderly client. The specific intervention depends in part on the nature of the stress that stimulated the arrhythmia. If possible, the stress is removed or modified. For example, some individuals with sinus bradycardia are very sensitive to carotid sinus stimulation. Even slight pressure on the neck, from a tight collar or certain head movements, may result in bradycardia and at times fainting. Teaching the client certain practices, such as the avoidance of specific head movements, may eliminate this problem. If the arrhythmia is due to an underlying cardiac or pulmonary condition, an infection or other health problem, that condition is treated. If the arrhythmia is due to a toxic substance, such as digitalis, other medications, alcohol, or cigarettes, the toxin is eliminated. If the arrhythmia is due to a deficiency, such as potassium, then that substance is replaced, provided the older client does not have renal problems.

The intervention also depends on the nature and severity of the adaptations that accompany the arrhythmia. An arrhythmia, such as premature beats, that is not accompanied by other adaptations, may not be treated.

Medication Therapy. A number of potent drugs are used to treat disorders of cardiac rate and rhythm. These include digitalis, atropine, ephedrine, and antiarrhythmic agents such as propranolol, quinidine, procainamide, lidocaine, and others. Mild sedatives, such as phenobarbital, may be given to clients with tachycardia if they are experiencing anxiety or palpitations. All these drugs have potent therapeutic effects and potentially hazardous untoward effects. Clients who are being maintained on these drugs need to be fully informed about them.

Digitalis. Digitalis is used for a wide variety of supraventricular and ventricular arrhythmias. By slowing conduction in the atrioventricular (AV) node, it is effective in preventing or controlling paroxysmal atrial tachycardia, paroxysmal and permanent atrial flutter, atrial fibrillation when ventricular rate is rapid, ventricular tachycardia, and ventricular extrasystoles. Digitalis is also useful for sick sinus syndrome if tachycardia occurs.

In the elderly, particular risks are associated with digitalis and with identifying what dose is safe and effective, but not toxic. Digitalis has a very small margin of safety because its therapeutic-to-toxic ratio is extremely low. Of those elderly persons who take digitalis preparations, 10 to 25 percent manifest toxicity at one time or another. Age itself is believed to be a factor in the development of toxicity (Kleiger, 1976). Requirements for dig-

italis decrease with age, and it is important that aged persons on digitalis be evaluated periodically to determine whether the drug should be continued. Regular monitoring of the serum digitalis level is helpful in preventing digitalis toxicity. Several factors predispose the elderly to digitalis intoxication. Digitalis is excreted by the kidney. With age, reduced renal function and slower excretion prolong the half-life of the drug. Changes in body composition also occur with age. Consequently, equal doses in young and old can produce twice the blood level in older persons. Control is particularly hard to achieve in the elderly with longer-acting preparations such as digitoxin. The vagus is particularly sensitive in the elderly and digitalization may result in bradycardia sufficient to cause dizziness and partial or complete heart block. Hypokalemia increases susceptibility to digitalis. Diuretic therapy or laxative abuse can induce hypokalemia and place the person at risk for digitalis toxicity even without the dosage being increased (Poe and Holloway, 1980). Advanced pulmonary disease, pulmonary emboli, and severe heart disease also increase the older client's risk of toxicity since hypoxemia increases the individual's susceptibility to the drug.

The first and only sign of digitalis toxicity in the aged may be serious or fatal abnormal cardiac rhythms, such as ectopic beats or conduction disturbances. If the PR interval becomes prolonged or if a previously long PR interval is further prolonged, digitalis toxicity should be suspected. These changes result from increased automaticity and slowing of conduction in junctional tissues. To detect arrhythmias, clients should be advised to have periodic electrocardiograms. Worsening of congestive heart failure may occur. Other early signs of digitalis toxicity seen in the elderly include central nervous system signs, such as malaise, lethargy, drowsiness, mental confusion, depression, paranoia, and delusions. Acute fatigue and muscle weakness occur frequently. Other early, but subtle, noncardiac signs of toxicity in the elderly may be an aversion to food or anorexia instead of nausea and vomiting. Clients should be asked about any changes in their eating patterns. Muddy or hazy vision, flashing lights, and white or yellow halos may be seen about bright objects instead of changes in color vision. The nurse should assess the client's vision regularly for acuity and color perception. Unilateral gynecomastia is an unusual form of digitalis toxicity seen in elderly males. The tender swelling recedes once digitalis is discontinued. Aged females on prolonged digitalis therapy may show estrogen changes in the vaginal mucosa. Both of these adaptations are due to impaired liver function, resulting in an estrogenic effect of digitalis.

The nurse must assure that the client is knowledgeable about the side effects of the medication. Clients must also be taught to take their pulse. Because many elderly clients have diminished tactile sensation, the nurse must assure that the older client is able to perceive and count the pulse accurately. Elderly clients also need to be assessed for deficits in short-term memory or confusion that might impair their ability to monitor their own cardiac status reliably on a daily basis. Older clients should be told that taking certain over-the-counter medications, such as antacids and Kaolin-pectin may result in a significant reduction in the amount of medication absorbed, thus altering the therapeutic effects of the drug (Rodstein, 1979). Clients should seek medical advice before taking any new nonprescription medication.

Atropine and Ephedrine.   Atropine and ephedrine are used for bradycardia, sinoatrial (SA) block, and AV block. Atropine is an anticholinergic agent, and, as such, produces severe side effects. Some of these can be particularly serious in the elderly. Constipation, dry skin, and blurred vision can occur. Difficulty urinating and urinary retention may develop, a particular problem for elderly men with prostatic enlargement. This drug also causes dilatation of the pupil and increased intraocular pressure. Because of the increased incidence of glaucoma in the elderly, atropine should be used with extreme caution.

Ephedrine is a sympathomimetic agent with long-lasting cardiovascular effects. It is particularly useful in preventing Stokes–Adams attacks. Ephedrine's side effects are more likely to occur in hypertensive individuals. It may interfere with sleep, or make the elderly client feel "jittery," by stimulating anxiety, restlessness, or tremor (Goodman and Gilman, 1970).

Antiarrhythmic Agents.   Quinidine and procainamide have similar cardiac actions. They depress myocardial excitability, conduction velocity, and contractility. Their indirect anticholinergic effects also result in a decreased heart rate. For this reason, they must be used cautiously in clients with congestive heart failure or hypertension. These drugs are used for atrial and ventricular arrhythmias, including tachycardia, flutter, and fibrillation. They may be given with potassium if ventricular extrasystoles occur.

Quinidine and procainamide are excreted by the kidneys, placing the client with declining kidney function at high risk for toxicity. A range of gastrointestinal complaints may indicate toxicity. In addition, procainamide has precipitated flushing, weakness, mental depression, psychosis, giddiness, joint and muscle pain, rash, and a lupuslike syndrome.

Propranolol is a beta-adrenergic blocking agent that reduces tachyarrhythmias caused by catecholamines by blocking the effects of epinephrine and norepinephrine on the heart. It is used to treat paroxysmal supraventricular tachycardia when it is due to digitalis toxicity, atrial flutter, atrial fibrillation that does not respond to digitalis, and sick sinus syndrome, hypertension, and angina.

Propranolol is given in low doses (5 to 10 mg four times daily) and with caution in the aged. Because catecholamines stimulate cardiac function, the blocking action of propranolol may result in deterioration of cardiac function, particularly in clients with an impaired heart muscle. This drug can produce diminished strength of contraction and slowing of heart rate and conduction with resultant hypotension, heart failure, and heart block. In the elderly, even small doses may cause bradycardia or severe exertional fatigue. Propranolol can also induce lifethreatening asthma in a susceptible person by blocking beta-adrenergic stimulation that is needed for dilation of bronchioles and effective air movement. In insulin-dependent diabetics hypoglycemia may be missed because propranolol masks tachycardia, an early adaptation to low blood sugar. The drug should not be used in clients with heart failure, heart block, or bradycardia. This drug should not be stopped abruptly. Doing so may cause life-threatening arrhythmias and coronary thrombosis.

Unlike the antiarrhythmic agents, lidocaine is not used for oral or long-term maintenance therapy. Lidocaine is an effective drug against ventricular extrasystoles and ventricular tachycardia. Its action develops very rapidly when given by intravenous administration and then declines when the infusion is discontinued. Usually, it is administered only to clients who are under close supervision in intensive care units. A potentially serious side effect of lidocaine is convulsions.

Pacemakers. Pacemakers are becoming more important in the treatment of elderly persons with a number of temporary or permanent abnormal cardiac rhythms. They are the treatment of choice to correct sick sinus syndrome characterized by either bradycardia or tachycardia. The pacemaker prevents the slow heart rate and concurrent drug therapy controls the tachycardia. For clients with complete heart block experiencing Stokes–Adams attacks, the pacemaker may be a lifesaving intervention. Often, the pacemaker is the only effective intervention for chronic complete heart block, particularly when most of the myocardial tissue is relatively normal (Rodstein, 1979). In these situations, medication therapy is unreliable or ineffective. If the client is too weak to undergo surgery for implantation of a permanent pacemaker, or if the arrhythmia is believed to be only temporary (as in heart block following inferior wall infarction) a temporary transvenous catheter pacemaker may be inserted. Because immune defenses are normally reduced in the elderly, the nurse must give special care to the site of pacemaker insertion to protect against infection.

Those aged persons in whom pacemaker implantation has been necessary usually adjust well to the presence of a pacemaker and demonstrate improved quality of life. Stokes–Adams attacks are prevented. Not only is exercise tolerance improved, but aged persons with pacemakers demonstrate improvements in personality and reduced irritability, depression, and hostility. Pacemaker implantation has very low morbidity and almost no mortality, even in the very old (Kleiger, 1976). For these reasons, it is never contraindicated on the grounds of age alone.

The elderly client receiving a pacemaker needs emotional support and instruction in order to accept the implantation of a mechanical device. Some elderly persons are not as familiar and comfortable with technology as the current younger generation and may perceive this intervention as too complex or dangerous. Older clients may be fearful of the surgical procedure itself or of the unknown con-

sequences of living with an electrical device implanted in the chest. One elderly client who was reluctant to have a pacemaker implanted said "I'm an old lady. At my age, why should I bother?" One strategy that has been successful in helping clients make the decision to have a pacemaker implanted is to have them talk with another elderly person who has gone through the procedure and adjusted to the pacemaker.

Once the pacemaker has been implanted, the nurse must ensure that clients know how to monitor their pulse rate and do not have impairments of sensation or memory that would limit their ability to do so accurately. They must also understand the importance of maintaining regular contacts with the health care system and what course of action to take if they note any change in the character of their pulse or their overall level of adaptation. Advances in computer science and other areas of technology now make it possible for individuals in some parts of the country to contact their medical center on their home telephone to have their pacemaker function checked.

Cardioversion. Electrical cardioversion is used to convert a number of arrhythmias to normal sinus rhythm. Cardioversion is a risky but acceptable procedure for use with young and middle-aged adults. There is general agreement that the risks of cardioversion, particularly the risk of thromboemboli, increase in elderly persons (Pathy, 1981; Caird and Dall, 1978; Villaverde and MacMillan, 1980). The risks of cardioversion increase further in the elderly if digitalis toxicity is present (Rodstein, 1979). In fact, Caird and Dall (1978) believe that in some cases the use of cardioversion in elderly clients is unjustified.

Cardioversion is effective for elderly clients with ventricular tachycardia, paroxysmal supraventricular tachycardias with a rapid ventricular rate, atrial tachycardia, atrial flutter, and atrial fibrillation when response to medication is poor. In elderly clients, the use of cardioversion to convert atrial fibrillation to normal sinus rhythm is usually successful only for a short period of time. Then the cardiac rhythm reverts back to atrial fibrillation. Because severe structural damage to the SA node is often the reason for atrial fibrillation in the elderly, cardioversion is not a long-term solution.

Because cardioversion is a potentially life-threatening intervention, the nurse assisting at the procedure must combine careful observation with the ability to institute prompt intervention.

Vagal Stimulation. Carotid sinus massage and other forms of vagal stimulation are used in the diagnosis and treatment of certain arrhythmias. These techniques must be performed carefully in the aged because they may result in cerebral insufficiency and strokelike adaptations. Nevertheless, a number of gerontologists believe that such procedures can be performed safely on elderly clients and recommend their use to diagnose sick sinus syndrome and to treat such arrhythmias as paroxysmal supraventricular tachycardias when they are not a consequence of digitalis intoxication. Gentle carotid massage or other maneuvers, such as the Valsalva maneuver, eyeball pressure, or drinking a glass of cold water, may terminate the paroxysms (Pathy, 1981; Kleiger, 1976; Caird and Dall, 1978). Kleiger (1976) believes that these procedures can be safely performed on any older person with normal carotid pulses and no bruits. When this procedure is performed in the hospital, the client's response must be carefully monitored because of the risk of cardiac arrest. Clients living at home may be taught to lie down and perform these maneuvers whenever they experience an episode of tachycardia. Since stimulating one's own vagal response without supervision may cause anxiety, carefully supervised instruction is essential to prepare the client.

Cerebrovascular Accident

The Client Experiencing TIAs. The nurse must ensure the safety of the client who experiences transient ischemic attacks. These clients require daily follow up. This may be done by arranging for a reliable family member or friend to telephone the client or by referring the client to a telephone reassurance program. Many social service agencies for the elderly have such programs which provide for daily phone calls and back-up service to visit clients who fail to answer the telephone. The nurse should also assure that the elderly client has telephone numbers for an emergency room, physician, or nurse readily available and understands that they should be used if any neurological deficits are noted.

In addition, the nurse should complete a home assessment to ensure that the environment is safe and free of hazards that might contribute to falls.

Measures to prevent hypotension should be taken. The client should be taught to avoid sudden movements and changes in position. Wearing elastic stockings is a simple, effective way of avoiding hypovolemia. The client's drug regimen should be carefully checked for the presence of medications that might contribute to hypovolemia.

Some clients, including those with cervical spondylosis, benefit from learning to restrict some head movements, including extension and full rotation of the head. Clients who smoke should be encouraged to stop. If the client exhibits any of the risk factors associated with hypertension, the nurse should assist the client to modify these. For example, the nurse should ensure that clients who have been prescribed antihypertensive medication for their hypertension are taking their medication regularly. Clients who are consuming high-fat diets can be assisted to modify their intake of fat.

Nursing interventions should also be aimed at maintaining or improving the client's hemoglobin level. This may involve helping the elderly person with a limited income plan grocery lists and meals that contain adequate amounts of iron. If clients are anemic, the nurse should assist clients to modify their exercise patterns to prevent undue fatigue.

Medical interventions for the client with transient ischemic attacks may include medication therapy or surgery. A number of medications may be used to treat elderly clients with TIAs. Anticoagulant therapy may be prescribed, particularly if the carotid artery is involved. The client taking anticoagulants needs to know which drugs potentiate the action of anticoagulants. These include aspirin, salicylates, thyroid preparations, and quinidine. Other drugs, such as barbiturates, inhibit the anticoagulant effect. Because the danger of hemorrhage is increased in the elderly, clients need to be taught to observe for signs of bleeding and should be assessed frequently by the nurse or physician.

The use of platelet antiaggregation agents, including aspirin and Persantine, is also being tried (Coakley, 1981). To ensure that clients comply with their medication regimen accurately, they must be instructed as to the purpose of these drugs.

Phenobarbital (30 mg twice daily) may be used

to minimize the brain's responses to ischemia. It has been successful in preventing falling attacks in some elderly clients. The nurse should observe the elderly client taking phenobarbital for drowsiness, disorientation, or depression. If side effects develop, phenytoin sodium (50 mg twice daily) may be prescribed instead. The nurse should be aware that this medication is associated with folate deficiency and ensuing megaloblastic anemia, particularly if the elderly person has nutritional problems (Carter, 1979).

Surgery to correct abnormalities associated with transient ischemic attacks has limited usefulness in the elderly because so many are poor surgical risks. Procedures used include endarterectomy and bypass operations. Particular success has been achieved with stenotic lesions of the internal carotid and middle cerebral vessels (Isaacs, 1978).

The Client with a Stroke. The recovery period after stroke can be divided into the following phases:

1. Acute phase, lasting 2 weeks, and concerned with basic survival.
2. Rehabilitative phase, lasting 8 to 12 weeks, and concerned with restoration of independence in activities such as standing, walking, and self-care. This phase often takes place in a specialized rehabilitation setting.
3. Final phase, lasting up to 2 years, and concerned with realization of the client's full capacity to participate in appropriate developmental tasks. This phase usually involves intervention by the health team in the client's home.

Medical Intervention. Although research for an effective treatment is ongoing, medical interventions for cerebrovascular accidents are, at best, of uncertain value. Dextran is used to reduce blood viscosity and increase capillary blood flow. Glycerol and steroids such as dexamethasone are given to reduced cerebral edema. In addition, glycerol improves cerebral metabolism. Hyperventilation and hypothermia have also been used to assist the spontaneous recovery process (Coronna and McDowell, 1976). There is no evidence, however, that these substances revitalize injured brain tissue or improve the functional ability of the stroke victim (Isaacs, 1978; Coakley, 1981). Anticoagulant therapy is used in some cases to limit the stroke-in-evolution, but

there are questions about its effectiveness (Villaverde and MacMillan, 1980). Vasodilators have limited value for the client with a cerebrovascular accident (Coakley, 1981).

Nursing Intervention. In the acute phase of stroke, nursing care is more important than any medical intervention in assisting and reinforcing spontaneous recovery. The primary goal of care is to maintain any existing function and prevent deleterious adaptations to immobility. If this can be accomplished, the elderly stroke victim is likely to achieve a higher level of functional achievement during rehabilitation (Granger et al., 1975).

The care of the elderly immobilized client is discussed in Chapter 19. A few special considerations are important for the client with a cerebrovascular accident. The spastic paralysis that accompanies cerebrovascular accident predisposes any stroke victim to contractures. The elderly, however, tend to develop contractures even more quickly than the young. If this occurs, the elderly may never develop full extension in the involved limbs, an adaptation that seriously impairs the ability to walk. Therefore, correct positioning and passive range of motion exercises are essential nursing considerations. Usually, the paralyzed extremities should be moved through passive range of motion several times daily. Proper positioning includes placing a pillow under the involved arm and hand to prevent swelling from dependency; placing sandbags lateral to the involved leg to prevent external rotation of the hip; and using a footboard to prevent plantar flexion. As soon as possible following the cerebral infarction, the client should begin a program of rehabilitation. The nurse's role in rehabilitation of the elderly is discussed below.

Rehabilitation

The elderly demonstrate the highest incidence of chronic disease of all age groups. Multiple impairments in the elderly chronically ill are common. Gradually, these impairments may reduce the person's functional status, impair the ability to perform activities of daily living, and prevent the client from living independently. Or at some point, multiple degenerative processes trigger a catastrophic event, such as myocardial infarction or cerebrovascular accident, which drastically reduces the client's ability to function. The individual who is disabled must learn again how to cope with the environment. The rehabilitation process seeks to restore or arrest further decline in functional capacity so that the client can resume a normal life in a familiar environment. Rehabilitation is essentially a learning process. It aims to teach the elderly how to modify ineffective adaptations or if this is not possible, to develop additional adaptations that compensate for ineffective ones. Emphasis is not so much on actual recovery of function but on ability to compensate for loss. This may involve learning to use adaptive devices or acquiring a new means of locomotion. Because so many older people live alone, regaining independence in mobility and activities of daily living is of paramount importance.

Rehabilitation of the elderly presents some unique problems. Often, the disabilities exhibited by the elderly are a consequence of stresses that are chronic in nature. These cannot be eliminated and will continue to have adverse effects on the client's ability to function. The coexistence of several chronic diseases is common in the elderly and unfavorably influences the client's prognosis and ability to tolerate an aggressive rehabilitation program. The aged person's ability to adapt to new situations and assimilate new techniques may be impaired. These problems hamper the learning process or the ability to cooperate and follow instructions, which is essential to effective rehabilitation (Steinberg, 1976). Most elderly persons who enter rehabilitation programs have not been physically active for some time and are out of condition. Recent illness or surgery further impairs their stamina. Reduced stamina places the client at risk for a number of stresses, including fatigue. In addition, the elderly disabled who are active are much more prone to falls, trauma, and accidents than their inactive counterparts. In spite of the difficulties, rehabilitation is the only alternative to prolonged bed rest with its consequent deleterious effects of immobility.

The Setting. Rehabilitation can be carried out anywhere provided a knowledgeable rehabilitation team is available. The setting for rehabilitation depends in part on the client's general condition and degree of disability. Rehabilitation takes place in general hospitals, convalescent hospitals, nursing homes, specialized rehabilitation facilities, outpatient facilities, or the home. The decision must be made in collaboration with the client and family and should be based on the following considerations:

1. Are specialized facilities required for an optimum rehabilitation?
2. Does the client have stresses other than the focal stress that require medical intervention or close nursing supervision?
3. Is it feasible to conduct the rehabilitation at home? Does the client have support systems to assure the environment is safe?
4. Are there financial considerations or conditions of insurance coverage that must be considered? (Hirshberg et al., 1976).

Inpatient Rehabilitation Services. Inpatient rehabilitation services are separate units specifically designed for the rehabilitation of severely disabled persons. These may be a department within a general hospital or they may exist as a separate facility. Separate rehabilitation facilities are often affiliated with a hospital, which provides diagnostic and therapeutic services to clients. Rehabilitation services may treat several types of disabilities or they may specialize in treating clients in a specific age group or with a specific disability. Many inpatient rehabilitation services also provide outpatient care or at least follow-up care for the clients they have served. Nursing homes may also provide rehabilitation services. Usually, the rehabilitation service associated with a nursing home is equipped, staffed, and operated on a limited basis and is capable of providing services to only a very small percentage of the residents. The rehabilitation of stroke clients takes place at all types of inpatient facilities. On the other hand, rehabilitation of clients with ischemic heart disease is limited to hospital departments that specialize in cardiac and vascular disease. Most clients visit these departments as outpatients for at least 3 months following hospital discharge.

Outpatient Rehabilitation Facilities. Outpatient rehabilitation is aimed at clients with limited disabilities. It allows clients to live at home or in a facility nearby and be transported to the outpatient facility for care. General hospitals, which may not have a rehabilitation service, may provide physical, occupational, and other therapies and social services through their outpatient departments. Many rehabilitation centers provide services on an outpatient basis. Some communities also have independent outpatient rehabilitation centers, which provide services for all types of disabilities.

Home Care.   For the elderly client, rehabilitation at home is an excellent alternative because the process is less unpleasant, less strenuous, and more efficient. The rate at which rehabilitation proceeds can be flexible. The older client is assured privacy and the comfort of living among familiar things and people. Independent living, an objective of rehabilitation, can be carried out best at home. The decision to rehabilitate a client at home should be based on the client's condition and a physical and psychological assessment of the client's home environment to determine whether therapeutic activities can be carried out. The client needs space and facilities that are capable of adaptation to the exercise and restorative programs needed. The assistance of family members or significant others is required to maintain each day's rehabilitation program. Most important, the psychological atmosphere of the home must be one of affection and interest on the part of relatives and others. There must be no sign of resentment or hostility.

Stroke victims who require intensive inpatient services can be successfully rehabilitated at home if all the necessary conditions are met and if the health team is willing to make the home visits. Some clients, who began the rehabilitation process in the hospital, have been found to make more significant progress at home (Tobis, 1979). However, three obstacles to successful home care have been identified: (1) It is becoming less common to find family members who have the time and desire to provide care. (2) Health insurance plans may cover care in the hospital but not at home. (3) Health team members, including physicians, nurses and therapists, are more efficient in an institutional setting. For example, they can see 10 to 15 hemiplegic clients in the time it takes to visit one hemiplegic client at home (Hirshberg et al., 1976).

The Rehabilitation Team.   Because of the complex nature of human aging, elderly clients benefit from a multidisciplinary, problem-oriented team approach to rehabilitation. In their 11-year study, Ka-

plan and Ford (1975) found that use of a coordinated team approach with clients over age 62 led to a high rate of discharge to the community. This approach is also compatible with a holistic philosophy. The team is usually composed of individuals with special skills, including the physiatrist, rehabilitation nurse, physical and occupational therapists, orthotist, and social worker. If needed, speech therapists, vocational therapists, psychologists, and others may be involved. Vocational rehabilitation is usually not necessary for the elderly. The success of a rehabilitation program depends in part on teamwork. The members of the rehabilitation team are interdependent, and the activities of several members may overlap. Each must understand the interrelationships of all the disciplines, which together meet the ever-changing needs of the client. A coordinated team effort allows physicians, nurses, therapists, family, and client to cooperate in formulating and implementing a plan of care.

Nurses work in a collaborative capacity with other members of the team to assess the client and develop and implement the plan of care. They are also in an excellent position to interpret the functions of the other team members to the client and family. It is important that the elderly client develop strong, positive relationships with the nurse and other significant members of the rehabilitation team. Efforts must be made to ensure that the team approach does not result in fragmented care. Some elderly deal poorly with a multiplicity of clinical contacts. If shuttled among several physicians, nurses, social workers and therapists, the elderly may become confused and detached from the rehabilitation process (Hirshberg et al., 1976).

The Rehabilitation Process.   To be effective, rehabilitation must be initiated as soon as the client's overall condition permits. The rehabilitation process consists of two parts: assessment and management. Success depends upon an accurate assessment. The stress that initiated the disabling adaptations must be identified, because it influences the prognosis as well as decisions about the type of rehabilitation program and when to begin it. The disabling adaptations must be precisely described. Most important, the effects of those adaptations on the individual's overall function must be determined. How do the adaptations affect the client's ability to live at home, communicate, and carry out appropriate developmental tasks? Because rehabilitation is expensive and skilled personnel and rehabilitation facilities are in short supply, the assessment process is also used to determine which clients will benefit from rehabilitation and when rehabilitative care should be discontinued. The assessment always includes a thorough history and physical assessment, but specific aspects vary according to the nature of the client's stress and disabling adaptations. For the client with a coronary occlusion, emphasis is placed on a thorough cardiovascular examination, including electrocardiograms and stress tests that may involve treadmills, stationary bicycles, and other devices. The duration of the test, the level of difficulty obtained and the presence or absence of ST-T changes is the basis for formulating the rehabilitation program. For the stroke client, and for many other persons disabled by neuromuscular and musculoskeletal disorders, a comprehensive assessment of the client's physical and mental condition, similar to the one described earlier, is the basis for setting realistic goals and designing a rehabilitation program.

The rehabilitation program designed for the client depends upon the general condition of the client and the long-term client goals. Generally, age is not a limiting factor. However, because so many of the elderly have limited cardiopulmonary reserves and have not been active for many years, the program that is prescribed may be more protective and progress at a slower rate. For the client with a coronary occlusion, a progressive exercise and activity program might include walking, jogging, swimming, game playing, and other activities. Clients are taught to monitor their own response to exercise. Reasons for stopping exercises or modifying the program include angina, leg cramps, excessive fatigue, or tachycardia.

For the stroke client, an active rehabilitation program is instituted as soon as the client's condition stabilizes. The main principles are:

1. Avoidance of flexion postures. *
2. Avoidance of overdependence on the normal side.
3. Maximum sensory and proprioceptive stimulation of the affected side.
4. Acquisition of balance before attempts are made to walk (Isaacs, 1978).

The program consists primarily of progressive increments in exercise and activities of daily living. Exercises are motions practiced for the purpose of maintaining or restoring range of joint motion, muscle strength, endurance, and skill in performing coordinated movements. When these motions are put to use in real life they are called activities of daily living (ADLs) and include self-care activities such as toileting and hygiene and miscellaneous activities such as using the telephone, manipulating a call bell, or turning on a light.

The program begins with passive exercise of involved limbs and active assistive or active exercises of the uninvolved side. It is generally recommended that if clients with an ischemic stroke are conscious, they should be placed in a chair on day 1, practice balancing exercises on day 2, and stand fully supported on day 3. Within a few days self-care skills should be taught. The nurse is usually in the best position to teach these skills while assisting the client with ADLs. An important nursing responsibility is to assure that the plan of care is implemented over the 24-hour day by providing opportunities for clients to perform all exercises and activities that are within their functional capacity. The nurse must be sure that the client uses what has been learned in the therapy sessions. This is only possible if the nurse knows what the client is doing in therapy and makes sure that those exercises and activities are reinforced on the nursing unit. Because nurses see the client during various daily activities and time cycles they are aware of the client's response to disability and rehabilitation. Therefore, nurses are expected to report problems and progress to other members of the health team.

The client needs to regain independence in the following areas:

1. Self-care—feeding, toileting, washing, dressing.
2. Domestic—cooking, washing, cleaning, sewing, doing the laundry.
3. Appliances—using slings, braces, walkers, wheelchairs, or canes.
4. Mobility—obtaining access to all rooms of the home and out of doors; stair climbing.

Because nurses spend more time with the client than any other member of the rehabilitation team, they are in a position to assess the client's psychological responses to disability and rehabilitation. As the rehabilitation process continues, the nurse must provide the client with ongoing emotional support. A temporary state of depression is a normal response to severe disability and a necessary part of the readjustment process. It should not be confused with emotional lability, loss of confidence, or a lack of motivation. The nurse should support the client throughout this period. If a stroke client fails to exhibit depression in recognition of the loss, this often reflects a serious intellectual deficit resulting from brain injury.

Nurses also play a special role in motivating clients to overcome disability. The nurse should ensure that realistic short-term goals are set for the client. By commenting on each bit of progress the client makes, encouraging the client to become independent, and maintaining an optimistic approach, the nurse can do much to improve the client's morale and motivation. Conveying hope is justified not only because many clients improve physically but because many find ways to compensate for weakness.

The nurse must also monitor the client's physiological responses to the rehabilitation plan. With age, physiological parameters that show little or no change at rest are significantly altered by stressful situations and return slowly to resting values. A particular concern is the energy expenditure of elderly clients. The hemiplegic person uses twice as much energy as a normal person to ambulate. The decrease in speed, strength, and coordination that accompanies aging further increases the energy cost of ambulation. These factors may strain the cardiovascular system of the elderly hemiplegic client. The nurse must carefully monitor the client's response to any exercise. The simplest way to do so is by monitoring the pulse. If the elderly client is in normal sinus rhythm, the severity of an exercise or activity and the oxygen consumed are directly related to the pulse rate. The maximum pulse rate with exercise for healthy persons aged 65 is about 165 beats per minute. However, for a severely disabled elderly person a resting pulse over 100 or an immediate post-ambulation pulse exceeding 120 is cause for concern. A pulse rate above 130 is indicative of excessive stress, and the elderly client should not be permitted to perform exercise pro-

ducing a pulse rate above this level (Tobis, 1979). The client should also be assessed for an irregular pulse or a blood pressure that increases excessively or drops below resting levels. These adaptations indicate a compromised circulation. The client should be observed for shortness of breath, excessive perspiration, cyanosis of lips or nail beds or complaints of dizziness or faintness. These adaptations indicate the client's exercise capacity has been overtaxed.

Every effort should be made to control the energy expenditure of elderly clients during exercise. The use of shoe lifts, braces, walkers, and canes can significantly reduce the energy expenditure of the hemiplegic person during ambulation. If the elderly client is overweight, weight reduction is indicated to reduce the energy costs of exercise. Skill in ambulation, the result of practice and careful supervision, also reduces energy expenditure.

Discharge.   Aged disabled clients are usually considered able to manage at home when they meet the following conditions:

1. Mental status is adequately clear.
2. Can walk or transfer from bed to chair with one assistant.
3. Can attend to own toileting.
4. Can manage all or part of self-care activities.

Discharge should be preceded by a final assessment of the client, particularly the ability to function in the home setting. If family members or significant others are to be involved in providing care at home, they must also be assessed and prepared for their role. The home should be assessed to determine if the client can enter and leave it, to identify what modifications might be needed in the client's bed and chair, kitchen, bathroom, stairways, and floor coverings. Permitting the client to spend a day or weekend at home before discharge is an excellent way to determine if the client is ready for discharge. Discharge planning is discussed in more detail in Chapter 20.

Once they have returned home, most stroke victims benefit from coordinated home care services, such as home health aides, Meals on Wheels, and visits from the nurse and therapist. These may be extremely helpful during the period of transition from home to hospital. The nurse should consider referring the client and relatives to a stroke club in their area. These provide a range of social and therapeutic activities as well as opportunities for the client and family members to discuss and share the difficulties of resuming a normal life.

Sixty percent of stroke victims who enter rehabilitation programs recover. Of these, about one-third achieve full independence, are intellectually clear, can ambulate with confidence and use their involved hand effectively. Two-thirds are more handicapped, perhaps with a mental barrier or a deficit in sensation or motor ability. These people will need to use an appliance, such as a walker or brace, on a permanent basis. Ten percent of stroke victims who enter rehabilitation programs die within the first 2 months after the stroke. The remaining 30 percent need continuous care as chairfast invalids (Hurwitz and Adams, 1972). Many of these individuals are ultimately institutionalized in nursing homes.

Institutionalization

Before 1930 most sick elderly people were cared for by their families or in almshouses. Today over one million older people in the United States live in institutions that provide long-term care (Butler and Lewis, 1977). About 4 percent of elderly men and 6 percent of elderly women live in institutions (Current Population Reports, 1977). The Social Security Act of 1935, the Kerr–Mills Act, and the passage of Medicare and Medicaid aided the development of long-term care institutions. As hospital care became more expensive, hospitals played a declining role in the long-term care of the chronically ill. However, as the aging population increased, the demand for long-term care beds increased. Changes in family structure and life-style meant that there was no longer a place in the home or a role in the family for older persons, many of whom did not have the physical or financial resources to live alone. This demand may reflect in part a failure to develop adequate comprehensive support systems to help the elderly remain in the community. The biggest growth occurred between 1960 and 1970 and took place in the commercial nursing home sector. After 1970, the pace of growth declined somewhat, reflecting a period of retrenchment in government-sponsored human service programs.

Types of Institutions. Institutions providing long-term care for the aged are resident facilities that provide nursing, medical, and rehabilitation care and personal services to the chronically ill and aged. Nursing homes, rest homes, homes for the aged, and convalescent homes are just some of the institutions that provide long-term care for older persons. These terms are unclear to many health professionals and members of the public. Often, the term "nursing home" is used to describe all types of long-term care institutions for the aged. In fact, nursing homes are intended to provide skilled, intensive nursing care and medical services. Although they were not intended to serve only the elderly, 92 percent of nursing home residents are over age 65 (Rossman, 1979). Intermediate types of institutions, such as convalescent homes and rest homes, provide personal and some skilled nursing care or personal care without professional nursing. Homes for the aged provide a protective environment for the elderly who are no longer able to function in the community but who do not show severe physical and mental impairment.

No two long-term care facilities are alike. Some have special programs to meet the needs of a specific group. This variability makes it more difficult to determine whether or not an institution will meet the needs of a specific individual. However, because no two individuals have identical needs, variability in the nature of services offered serves an important purpose (Friedman and Coleman, 1970).

Through Medicare and Medicaid, the federal government has established and subsidizes two categories of long-term care facilities. These are distinguished primarily by the types of services they render.

1. A skilled nursing facility (SNF) is a nursing home that has been certified as meeting federal standards within the meaning of the Social Security Act. It provides the level of care that comes closest to hospital care with 24-hour nursing services. Regular medical supervision and rehabilitation are also provided. Generally, a skilled nursing facility provides posthospital care for convalescent clients or those with long-term illnesses for a limited period of time.

2. An intermediate care facility (ICF) is also certified and meets federal standards. It provides less extensive health-related care and services.

It has regular nursing services, but not around the clock. Most ICFs carry on rehabilitation, but they emphasize personal care and social services. In general, these homes serve people who are not fully capable of living by themselves and require care above the level of room and board. However, residents are not necessarily ill enough to need 24-hour nursing care.

These two categories do not always clarify the amount and kind of service offered. Regardless of category, each home must be assessed for the actual services it renders.

Institutions for the aged fall into three categories of sponsorship: public (government), voluntary, and proprietary (commercial). Sponsorship is not necessarily related to the level of care provided or the organizational structure. However, most homes for the aged are sponsored by nonprofit, voluntary agencies and most nursing homes are commercial or public facilities. Considerable controversy surrounds the issue of the suitability of commercial nursing homes for providing high levels of care because of the inherent conflict between increasing expenditures to provide better care and cutting costs to yield higher profits. However, commercial ownership does not appear to be necessarily related to poor quality of care (Kahana and Kahana, 1976).

Financing Long-Term Care.   The cost of long-term institutionalization has risen rapidly. In 1977 the cost of maintaining a client in a long-term care facility was $1000 to $2000 a month. A number of financing mechanisms have been enacted to assist people who could not otherwise afford care. Only about 9 percent pay their own way. Ninety percent are supported by Medicaid and only 1 percent by Medicare. The percentage of persons supported by Medicare reflects that plan's "limited stay" regulations (Knopf, 1977). Many problems still exist regarding the financing of long-term care. For example, some members of the middle class may have too much income to be eligible for assistance but not enough to pay for care by themselves. Some of those who enter nursing homes turn over all their assets to the nursing home and then become eligible for Medicaid.

Standards of Care.   Individual nursing homes are required to meet minimal standards set by state or local laws and regulations and to have a state license or letter of approval to operate. Unfortunately homes that do not meet standards may be allowed to stay open "temporarily" on the grounds that their clients have no place to go. Some homes, classified as skilled, are also certified by the Joint Commission on Accreditation of Hospitals. Nursing homes may also choose to participate in Medicare and/or Medicaid programs. If they do, they are subject to the certification requirements associated with these programs as well. However, the federal government gives enforcement functions to state and local governments. The federal responsibility for Medicare, in contrast with state control and partial funding of Medicaid, has resulted in some differences between the standards set in the two programs. To qualify for Medicare, institutions must meet uniform standards for care. In contrast, Medicaid standards of care set by the states vary.

In recent years, dissatisfaction has been expressed about the survey and certification process for long-term care facilities. This process involved only a determination of whether a facility was capable of providing a specific service, not whether it had in fact delivered such service (Abdellah et al., 1979). Recently, the certification process for institutions receiving Medicare and Medicaid was modified to include a comprehensive client assessment system. This is one step that may improve the quality of care in long-term care facilities.

Although many long-term care facilities provide excellent care, others have been described as dumping grounds for the elderly. Public awareness of the deficiencies of institutions in caring for the aged has resulted in demands for greater accountability of such facilities. Standards based on client care outcomes are one of the best ways to determine whether standards of care are being met. Because of their central position as care providers in long-term care facilities, nurses are in a position to ensure that standards of care are being met and to work to improve the standards of care used to certify facilities.

Public concern about the basic rights of nursing home residents led to the passage of a Patients' Bill of Rights for Skilled Nursing Facilities participating in Medicare and Medicaid programs (Table 6). This document guarantees clients' most basic rights, including the right to manage their own personal affairs, receive sealed mail, be fully informed about their condition, use their own clothing and possessions, and conduct private visits with relatives and friends. Unfortunately, the frequent insertion of "when medically contraindicated" in the Bill of Rights provides a convenient excuse for those who wish to abuse clients' rights. All nurses who practice in long-term care settings should keep copies of the Bill of Rights at hand. It serves as a simple way to check whether or not the client's most basic rights are being protected.

Quality of Care. Many nursing homes are excellent institutions that endeavor to meet the needs of their residents within financial limits. Other homes have numerous fire and safety violations, are filthy, and do not provide even a minimum level of care. Staff at all levels may be insufficient. Nutrition may be poor. Recreational services and therapy may be nonexistent. Instances of physical and mental abuse have been documented. Public awareness of the poor quality of care in nursing homes has led to a search for those factors that influence quality (Bigot and Munnichs, 1978).

Homes that deliver high-quality care have been found to have certain characteristics in common. Those that conducted sound training programs for staff provided better care. The size of a home and the amount charged for services have also been correlated with quality of care. Resources are generally more adequate in larger and more expensive homes. Homes that served the aged poor and were troubled with low reimbursement rates have been found to deliver inferior care. Residents who had frequent visitors and had personal possessions received better care than those who did not (Gottesman, 1974; Greenwald and Linn, 1971; Anderson et al., 1969).

One reason for poor quality of care in long-term institutions may be the tendency of health professionals to use the medical model when dealing with residents. This model, which emphasizes curing the client's physical and mental problems, is not adequate when dealing with individuals faced with the progressive deterioration of their health status. Their goal is to slow further deterioration and to learn to live with their limitations. In addition, this model cannot accommodate the range of human needs that must be considered when an older person becomes a resident in an institutional setting. Interventions should emphasize the client's functional abilities and the gamut of psychosocial needs that can no longer be met in the community setting.

The apparent lack of understanding by most health professions of the nature of long-term care has resulted in a lack of prestige for this area of health care. As a result, few top professionals have been attracted to this area. The lack of physician involvement was documented in Senate Subcommittee Hearings (U.S. Senate, 1974). The large number of vacant positions for nurses in nursing homes is an indicator that many nurses find working with the chronically ill elderly unattractive (Kahana and Kahana, 1976).

Four avenues can be used to improve quality of care.

1. The formal policy system, including licensing, regulation, and self-policing. Upgrading standards and strict enforcement can improve quality of care.
2. The community service system, including community involvement in advocacy programs, and efforts to improve standards and community presence in nursing homes. This latter activity serves a watchdog function.
3. The professional system, including recruiting additional staff, improving staffing patterns and morale, increasing pay, and, as a result of these steps, reducing staff turnover.
4. The client system, including consideration of ways the family can forestall institutionalization of their elderly members and provide support once a parent is institutionalized (Kahana and Kahana, 1976).

Client Characteristics. Information about who seeks nursing home care and why they do so is used to meet current needs and plan for the future. At present, the average age of nursing home residents has risen from 75 in 1954 (Kahana and Kahana, 1976) to 83 (Miller, 1979). The institutionalized aged tend to have multiple stresses, resulting in physical and mental impairments. Women outnum-

---

TABLE 6.   PATIENTS' RIGHTS IN SKILLED NURSING FACILITIES

The governing body of the facility establishes written policies regarding the rights and responsibilities of patients and, through the administrator, is responsible for development of, and adherence to, procedures implementing such policies. These policies and procedures are made available to patients, to any guardians, next of kin, sponsoring agency(ies) or representative payee selected pursuant to section 205 (j) of the Social Security Act, and Subpart Q of Part 404 of this chapter, and to the public. The staff of the facility is trained and involved in the implementation of these policies and procedures. These patients' rights, policies and procedures ensure that, at least, each patient admitted to the facility:

1. Is fully informed, as evidenced by the patient's written acknowledgment, prior to or at the time of admission and during stay, of these rights and of all rules and regulations governing patient conduct and responsibilities;

2. Is fully informed, prior to or at the time of admission and during stay, of services available in the facility, and of related charges including any charges for services not covered under titles XVIII or XIX of the Social Security Act, or not covered by the facility's basic per diem rate;

3. Is fully informed, by a physician, of his medical condition unless medically contraindicated (as documented by a physician, in his medical record), and is afforded the opportunity to participate in the planning of his medical treatment and to refuse to participate in experimental research;

4. Is transferred or discharged only for medical reasons, or for his welfare or that of other patients, or for nonpayment for his stay (except as prohibited by titles XVIII or XIX of the Social Security Act), and is given reasonable advance notice to ensure orderly transfer or discharge, and such actions are documented in his medical record;

5. Is encouraged and assisted, throughout his period of stay, to exercise his rights as a patient and as a citizen, and to this end may voice grievances and recommend changes in policies and services to facility staff and/or to outside representatives of his choice, free from restraint, interference, coercion, discrimination or reprisal;

6. May manage his personal financial affairs, or is given at least a quarterly accounting of financial transactions made on his behalf should the facility accept his written delegation of this responsibility to the facility for any period of time in conformance with State law;

7. Is free from mental and physical abuse, and free from chemical and (except in emergencies) physical restraints except as authorized in writing by a physician for a specified and limited period of time, or when necessary to protect the patient from injury to himself or to others;

8. Is assured confidential treatment of his personal and medical records, and may approve or refuse their release to any individual outside the facility, except, in case of his transfer to another health care institution, or as required by law or third-party payment contract;

9. Is treated with consideration, respect, and full recognition of his dignity and individuality, including privacy in treatment and in care for his personal needs;

10. Is not required to perform services for the facility that are not included for therapeutic purposes in his plan of care;

11. May associate and communicate privately with persons of his choice, and send and receive his personal mail unopened, unless medically contraindicated (as documented by his physician in his medical record);

12. May meet with and participate in activities of social, religious, and community groups at his discretion, unless medically contraindicated (as documented by his physician in his medical record);

13. May retain and use his personal clothing and possessions as space permits, unless to do so would infringe upon rights of other patients, and unless medically contraindicated (as documented by his physician in his medical record); and

TABLE 6. (CONTINUED)

14. If married, is assured privacy for visits by his/her spouse; if both are inpatients in the facility, they are permitted to share a room, unless medically contraindicated (as documented by the attending physician in the medical record).

All rights and responsibilities specified in paragraphs 1 through 4 of this section—as they pertain to (a) a patient adjudicated incompetent in accordance with State law, (b) a patient who is found, by his physician, to be medically incapable of understanding these rights, or (c) a patient who exhibits a communication barrier—devolve to such patient's guardian, next of kin, sponsoring agency(ies), or representative payee (except when the facility itself is representative payee) selected pursuant to section 205 (j) of the Social Security Act and Subpart Q of Part 404 of the Federal Register, Oct. 3, 1974 (see source note).

Source: Federal Register, Social Security Administration, Dept. of Health, Education, and Welfare. Washington, D.C., vol. 39, No. 193, Part II, Oct. 3, 1974, with permission.

ber men and whites outnumber nonwhites. Most residents are less likely to have a living spouse or children and more likely to have lived alone than their counterparts in the community (Riley and Foner, 1968). Elderly clients are admitted to nursing homes from private homes, community hospitals, rehabilitation centers, psychiatric hospitals, and other nursing homes. Over half are referred by hospitals. Physicians, social agencies, and other sources also make referrals (Kahana and Kahana, 1976).

Since only a minority of all chronically ill elderly find their way to long-term care facilities, researchers have sought to learn what characteristics differentiate this group from those who remain in the community. Institutionalization is often preceded by a crisis. It is usually associated with a change in the balance between the older person's abilities and the availability of support services and not by sudden physical deterioration. For example, the needs of the client's family may change or an important community service is lost (Riley and Foner, 1968). Consequently, the client is unable to perform essential activities of daily living and admission to a nursing home ensues.

Adaptations to Institutionalization. Although some older persons welcome the move to a nursing home, many view institutionalization as the least desirable living arrangement and agree to it only as a last resort (Kahana and Kahana, 1976). Adjustment to an institutional environment varies widely among clients. By understanding what factors may contribute to an optimal adjustment, the nurse can intervene and assist the client. Studies of the institutionalized aged indicate that they exhibit many more adverse physical and psychosocial adaptations than do their counterparts in the community. Comparisons between the two groups may be unfair, since the institutionalized elderly may have a lifelong history of adaptations that are markedly different from the elderly who remain in the community. It may be that the personality, social characteristics, or physical stresses of the person, and not the experience of being institutionalized, contribute to an unsatisfactory adjustment to institutional life.

The client's psychosocial response to institutionalization may be a function of certain characteristics of the institution itself. Some studies have focused on clients in "total" institutions. These set up barriers between the residents inside and the community outside. They are characterized by tight schedules, a complex bureaucratic structure, an impersonal atmosphere, and a well-defined barrier between clients and staff, with a minimum of communication between them. These institutions do not seek to meet the individual needs of the client, and clients in these settings have been found to exhibit lowered self-esteem, loss of self-identity, detachment, and other negative personality characteristics (Coe, 1965).

Institutional neurosis is one response to living in a rigid, isolated setting. It has been exhibited by clients in nursing homes and other institutions such as hospitals and prisons. Adaptations can include overdependence, an expressionless face, automatic behavior, loss of interest in the world, and a general erosion of personality (Butler and Lewis, 1977).

High morale and a positive self-concept have been found in the residents of some nursing homes (Kahana and Kahana, 1976). These characteristics were exhibited when the setting was able to meet the client's needs in two important areas—privacy and gratification. If institutional patterns are adjusted to accommodate the client's wishes and needs, decline may be checked.

Cooperativeness and passivity are traits that have been traditionally associated with the "good" client. Studies have indicated, however, that residents who were assertive, narcissistic, and active appeared to thrive while their more pleasant, passive counterparts declined (Bigot and Munnichs, 1978). It would appear that a therapeutic approach would be to stimulate assertive, aggressive, and active behavior in the institutionalized client. Encouraging the client to participate in care, planning, and governance activities and to perform independently as many activities of daily living as possible are some ways for the nurse to do this.

It is well known that the mortality rates of the institutionalized aged are higher than those for similar groups in the community. One-third of those who enter long-term care institutions die within the first year and 90 percent of all those who enter them die there. Death rates are higher in nursing homes than in homes for the aged (Butler and Lewis, 1977). The reasons for the higher mortality rate are unclear. Death may be a response to the stress of moving from one setting to another, a response to the disease process that made the aged person seek institutionalization, or a response to the kind or quality of care in the institution. The impact of institutionalization may be related to the personal meaning of institutionalization to the individual. For some, the symbolic meaning may be family rejection, loss of independence, privacy, home, and possessions, or

death. When moved to an institution, these clients may experience anxiety, insecurity, or hopelessness, or give up the will to live (Bigot and Munnichs, 1978).

A move to a new setting always requires the acquisition of new patterns of behavior. It may be that the older client's ability to adapt, which has been impaired by aging and illness, is impaired further by a move that involves extensive changes in the environment. Numerous studies have been done to identify the consequences of transfers from home to institution or from one institution to another. Although many of these studies indicate that clients decline physically and psychologically following a move to an institution, some do not. In Bigot and Munnichs's (1978) study, clients transferred from a hospital to a nursing home improved after the transfer. It was speculated that the more homelike atmosphere of the nursing home contributed to an improvement in the client's level of adaptation.

Recently, some nursing homes have increased efforts to make rehabilitiation an integral part of their services. Although many elderly institutionalized people are not able to return to independent living in the community, the restorative potential of even very old people is being increasingly recognized. When rehabilitative efforts are intensive, some institutionalized older people have significantly improved their self-care abilities. This is one example of how long-term institutions can generate positive adaptations in clients (Gottesman, 1975).

Nursing Interventions. There are many ways that the nurse can minimize the negative consequences of institutionalization and humanize care. The admissions procedure should be flexible enough to accommodate individual needs. Some clients respond best to a quick admission while others respond best if admission is preceded by visits or overnight stays in the facility. Showing genuine interest in the client, calling the client by name and orienting the client to the setting should be components of the admission procedure. A complete health assessment should be done soon after the client is admitted. One goal of the assessment is to identify, and accommodate, as many of the client's preferences and needs as possible in order that the client can adapt more easily to a new, and strange, environment.

Even if they have participated in the decision to enter a nursing home and understand the need for change, clients will have some difficulty in adjusting. The nurse should identify what coping behaviors the client used to deal with past life crises and use these to help the client adjust to this crisis. Clients may exhibit anger or hostility, be threatening or aggressive, withdraw, or use threats or bragging in order to cope. The level of adjustment the client attains depends on the client's past experiences and satisfactions and current strengths and weaknesses. If clients deny the change in their life situation, they should be encouraged to review their current life situation at length. This often helps them to identify for themselves recent problems and conclude that nursing home care is needed (O'Reilly, 1971).

Early in admission, some clients may be temporarily disoriented to time, place, or person. In a new environment, clients have lost the important objects, habits, and other cues that helped them maintain contact with reality. During this period, the client needs to be reassured and reoriented frequently.

Fear of losing one's own identity in an impersonal institution is a problem for many clients. Interventions to help clients establish themselves as unique individuals should be instituted as part of the admission procedure. Nursing home staff tend to identify clients by their current behaviors, such as their level of orientation or the amount of assistance they require from the staff. Residents on the other hand, tend to identify themselves by their past accomplishments or social roles (Kahana and Kahana, 1976). When care is personalized, there is congruence between the way clients view themselves and the way they are viewed by their caretakers. Personal identity is also preserved when clients are encouraged to bring their own possessions, souvenirs, photos, and personal items to the home.

In order to minimize loss of independence and to ensure that clients remain active, the nurse should encourage them to take an active role in their care. This may involve participating in care planning and decision making whenever possible, performing as much of their own daily care as possible, and participating in client-governance activities. These ac-

tivities help clients feel they have maintained some control over their own lives. The nurse can bolster clients' self-esteem and sense of usefulness by encouraging them to give of themselves. This may include participating in foster grandparent programs, volunteering to organize group activities in the home, or befriending another resident.

Older people gradually establish fixed daily routines involving personal grooming, toileting, and other habits. In order to facilitate the client's adaptation, the nurse should preserve as many of these previous patterns as possible. Other routines, such as the scheduling of meals, bedtime, and visiting hours may undergo unavoidable changes as a result of the home's schedule. Staff should acknowledge that these changes are disruptive to clients and allow them to talk about it.

The nurse should also modify the environment of the nursing home to make it as homelike as possible. There are numerous ways to do so. For example, wearing street clothes rather than traditional white uniforms enhances a homelike atmosphere. Access to the telephone should be unlimited. Visiting hours should be liberal, with no restrictions on visits by children. Clients should not be segregated by sex and should be allowed freedom and privacy to perform sexual activities, including masturbation.

The Family's Reaction to Institutionalization. Institutionalization brings the family and nursing home staff in contact with one another on a long-term basis. During the admission process the family needs a great deal of support from the nursing staff. When an aged disabled parent is institutionalized, it can be assumed that the family has already experienced a major emotional crisis. Families who care are more common than those who do not. It is very difficult for families to take aged parents out of their own home and place them in an impersonal institution, especially if the decision was against the wishes of the aging parent. Family members are ambivalent, feeling a sense of relief as well as anxiety about the quality of institutional life, guilt about abandoning the parent, and anger at the circumstances responsible for their having to make this decision. The anger may be directed toward the nursing staff. Some families have religious or ethnic frameworks that engender a deep-rooted sense of obligation to attend alone to the needs of the client. At the time of admission, families may experience a grief reaction similar to that experienced when a loved one dies. The sense of loss may be so painful that the family is unable to return to visit the parent. Families must be helped to examine their feelings in order to accept the situation. The nurse can help the family think of ways to preserve the richness of their relationship with the aging parent (O'Reilly, 1971).

The family can be an excellent source of information about the client as well as a source of support to the institutionalized person. When the client is admitted, the nurse should ask the family about the client's health status, physical problems, and social and recreational interests. They may be reluctant to mention such problems as bedwetting, wandering, nighttime wakefulness, or periods of disorientation. The nurse should ask specific questions and be supportive throughout the history-taking procedure.

Because families may or may not wish to play a role in care, the nurse should identify the level of involvement the family desires. Whenever possible, the family as well as the client should be included in care planning. They should be encouraged to serve as volunteers in institutional activities, to take the client on visits home and weekend outings, to visit the client regularly, and to provide the extra amenities only a family can give. It has been demonstrated that taking clients on outings has an even greater effect on a client's morale than the number of visitors he or she receives (Gelfand, 1968). Visits from family to the nursing home serve a number of important functions. They provide a link for the client with activities in the community and they serve a watchdog function in the institution. The nursing staff has a responsibility to educate the family on a regular basis about changes in the client's condition, needs, and probable outcomes of treatment (Miller, 1979).

The Nurse as Leader. Nursing care is a major component of any nursing home. Nurses are in a strategic position to uphold standards, act as client advocates, and safeguard high-quality care. Nurses are directly or indirectly responsible for the major portion of services and care the nursing home client receives and for supervising and educating the nurs-

ing assistants who deliver much of the care. Geriatric nurse practitioners are also being used in expanded roles in nursing homes. In skilled nursing facilities they may supplement the services of the physicians, collaborate with other professionals in the institution, and improve the quality of care (Brody et al., 1976).

SUMMARY

This chapter focused on the nursing care of clients experiencing adaptations to oxygen deprivation. The oxygen deprivation associated with myocardial infarction, arrhythmias, and cerebrovascular accident is a consequence of multiple stresses, including normal aging changes, pathology, and lifelong behavior patterns. Because these stresses are chronic and usually irreversible, clients need permanent support. At times only minimal support is required. At other times, constant, direct care is required to preserve life. In both situations, the care of the older client is complex because oxygen deprivation is usually only one of many physical and psychosocial problems that must be addressed. In this chapter emphasis was placed on nursing intervention for the client who is acutely ill. Many chronically ill older clients benefit from rehabilitation programs and are able to regain their independence. Others, who need direct care or supervision, may be placed in long-term care settings.

REFERENCES

Abdellah FG, Foerst HV, Chow RK: Pace: An approach to improving the care of the elderly. American Journal of Nursing 79(6):1109, 1979

Adams GF: New views on stroke, in Anderson WF, Judge TG (eds), Geriatric Medicine. New York, Academic, 1974

Anderson TP, Baureston N, Greenberg F, Hilyard VG: Predictive factors in stroke rehabilitation. Archives of Physical Medicine and Rehabilitation 55:545, 1974

Anderson NN, Holmberg RH, Schneider RE, Stone LB: Policy issues regarding nursing homes: Findings from a Minnesota survey. Minneapolis Institution for Interdisciplinary Studies, American Rehabilitation Foundation, Minneapolis, MN, 1969

Bigot A, Munnichs JMA: Psychology of aging. Long-term illness and care of the older person, in Brocklehurst JC (ed), Textbook of Geriatric Medicine and Gerontology, 2nd ed. New York, Churchill Livingstone, 1978

Biörck G: The biology of myocardial infarction. Circulation 37(6):1071, 1968

Bonner CD: Medical Care and Rehabilitation of the Aged and Chronically Ill, 3rd ed. Boston, Little, Brown, 1974

Brickner PW: Caring for the newly admitted patient, in Brickner P (ed), Care of the Nursing Home Patient. New York, Macmillan, 1971

Brody SJ, Cole L, Storey PB, Wink NJ: The geriatric nurse practitioner: A new medical resource in the skilled nursing home. Journal of Chronic Diseases 29(8):537, 1976

Butler RN, Lewis MI: Aging and Mental Health, 2nd ed. St. Louis, Mosby, 1977

Caird FI, Dall JLC: The cardiovascular system, in Brocklehurst JC (ed), Textbook of Geriatric Medicine and Gerontology, 2nd ed. New York, Churchill Livingstone, 1978

Carter AB: The neurologic aspects of aging, in Rossman I (ed), Clinical Geriatrics, 2nd ed. Philadelphia, Lippincott, 1979

Chebotareo DF, Korkusko OV: Age associated factors predisposing to the development of ischemic heart disease and peculiarities of its clinical course in older people, in Orimo H, et al (eds), Recent Advances in Gerontology. Amsterdam, Excerpta Medica, 1979

Coakley D: Stroke and other neurological emergencies in old age, in Coakley D (ed), Acute Geriatric Medicine. Littleton, MA, PSG Publishing, 1981

Coe R: Self-conception and institutionalization, in Rose A, Peterson W (eds), Older People and their Social World. Philadelphia, Davis, 1965

Coronna J, McDowell FH: Atherosclerotic cerebral infarction: Pathophysiological aspects. Postgraduate Medicine 59:115, 1976

Current Population Reports. U. S. Department of Commerce, Bureau of the Census. Washington, D.C., U.S. Government Printing Office, 1977

Elkowitz EB: Geriatric Medicine for the Primary Care Practitioner. New York, Springer, 1981.

Exton-Smith AN, Overstall PW: Guidelines in Medicine. Volume I. Geriatrics. Baltimore, University Park Press, 1979

Friedman SL, Coleman MA: Evaluation of medical facilities in institutions for the aged, in Field M (ed), Depth and Extent of the Geriatric Problem. Springfield, IL, Charles C. Thomas, 1970

Gelfand D: Visiting patterns and social adjustment in an old age home. Gerontologist 8(4):272, 1968

Goodman LS, Gilman A: The Pharmacological Basis of Therapeutics, 4th ed. New York, MacMillan, 1970

Gottesman LE: Psychosocial intervention programs with the situational settings, in Sherwood S (ed), Long-term Care: A Handbook for Researchers, Planners and Providers. Englewood Cliffs, NJ, Prentice-Hall, 1975

Gottesman LE: Nursing home performance as related to resident traits, ownership, size and source of payment. American Journal of Public Health 64(3):269, 1974

Granger CV, Greer DS, et al: Measurement of outcomes of care for stroke patients. Stroke 6:34, 1975

Greenwald S, Linn MW: Intercorrelations of data on nursing homes. Gerontologist 11(4):337, 1971

Hardin WB: Neurological aspects, in Steinberg FU (ed), Cowdry's The Care of the Geriatric Patient, 5th ed, St. Louis, Mosby, 1976

Harris R: Ischemic heart disease, in Reichel W (ed), Clinical Aspects of Aging. Baltimore, Williams and Wilkins, 1978a

Harris R: Special problems of geriatric patients with heart disease, in Reichel W (ed), Clinical Aspects of Aging. Baltimore, Williams and Wilkins, 1978b

Hirschberg GG, Lewis L, Vaughan P: Rehabilitation: A Manual for the Disabled and Elderly, 2nd ed. Philadelphia, Lippincott, 1976

Holderman B: A Manual on Stroke. Monograph No. 2. Council and Task Forces of New Jersey Regional Medical Program: Council on Cerebrovascular Disease and Stroke, July 1970

Hurwitz LJ, Adams GF: Rehabilitation of hemiplegia: Indices of assessment and prognosis. British Medical Journal 1:94, 1972

Isaacs B: Stroke, in Brocklehurst JC, (ed), Textbook of Geriatric Medicine and Gerontology, 2nd ed. New York, Churchill Livingstone, 1978

Kahana E, Kahana B: Special aspects of geriatric care, in Steinberg FU (ed), Cowdry's The Care of the Geriatric Patient, 5th ed. St. Louis, Mosby, 1976

Kaplan J, Ford CS: Rehabilitation for the elderly: An eleven-year assessment. Gerontologist 15(5):393, 1975

Kleiger RE: Cardiovascular disorders, in Steinberg FU (ed), Cowdry's The Care of the Geriatric Patient, 5th ed. St. Louis, Mosby, 1976

Knopf O: Successful Aging. Boston, MA, G.K. Hall, 1977

Linn MW, Gurel L: Family attitude in nursing home placement. Part 1. Gerontologist 12(3):220, 1972

McDowell FH: Rehabilitating patients with stroke. Postgraduate Medicine 59:145, 1976

Miller MB: Current Issues in Clinical Geriatrics. New York, Tiresias, 1979

Moskowitz E: Complications in the rehabilitation of hemiplegic patients. Medical Clinics of North America 53:541, 1969

Moskowitz E, Lightbody FE, Freetag NS: Longterm followup of the stroke patient. Archives of Physical Medicine and Rehabilitation 53:167, 1972

Newman M: The process of recovery after hemiplegia. Stroke 3:702, 1972

O'Reilly M: Preparing the patient for his new life, in Brickner PW (ed), Care of the Nursing Home Patient. New York, Macmillan, 1971

Pathy MS: Clinical presentation of myocardial infarction in the elderly. British Heart Journal 29(2):190, 1967

Pathy MS: Acute cardiac problems, in Coakley D (ed), Acute Geriatric Medicine. Littleton, MA, PSG Publishing, 1981

Poe WD, Holloway DA: Drugs and the Aged. New York, McGraw-Hill, 1980

Report of the Joint Committee for Stroke Facilities. Epidemiology for Stroke Facilities Planning. I. Epidemiology Study Group, Reuel A. Stallones, Chairman. Stroke 3:352, 1972

Report of the Joint Committee for Stroke Facilities. Stroke Rehabilitation Study Group. Mieczyslaw Peszcynski, Chairman. Stroke 3:373, 1972

Riley M, Foner A: Aging and Society. New York, Russell Sage Foundation, 1968

Robbins S: Stroke in the geriatric patient. Hospital Practice 11(8):33, 1976

Rodstein M: The prognostic implications for risk factors for ischemic heart disease in the aged, in Orimo H, Shumado K, Iriki M, Maeda D (eds), Recent Advances in Gerontology. Amsterdam, Excerpta Medica, 1979

Rossman I: Environment of geriatric care, in Rossman I (ed), Clinical Geriatrics, 2nd ed. Philadelphia, Lippincott, 1979

Rusk HA: Rehabilitation Medicine: A Textbook on Physical Medicine and Rehabilitation, 2nd ed. St. Louis, Mosby, 1964

Steinberg FU: Rehabilitation medicine, in Steinberg FU (ed), Cowdry's The Care of the Geriatric Patient, 5th ed. St. Louis, Mosby, 1976

Thorpe ELM, Coull EG: Nursing the patient with cerebrovascular accident. Canadian Nurse 62:38, 1960

Tobis JS: Rehabilitation of the geriatric patient, in Rossman I (ed), Clinical Geriatrics, 2nd ed. Philadelphia, Lippincott, 1979

Tohgi H, Uchiyama S: Risk factors in cerebrovascular disease, in Orimo H, Shimada K, Iriki M, Maeda D (eds), Recent Advances in Gerontology. Amsterdam, Excerpta Medica, 1979

Toole JF, Patel AN: Cerebrovascular Disorders, 2nd ed. New York, McGraw-Hill, 1974

U.S. Department of Commerce, Bureau of the Census, Social Indicators, 1976. U.S. Department of Commerce, Bureau of the Census. Current Population Reports, 1977

U.S. Department of Health, Education and Welfare, Public Health Service, Office of Nursing Home Affairs, Long Term Care Facility Improvement Study. Introductory Report, Washington, D.C. U.S. Government Printing Office, 1975

U.S. Department of Health and Human Services, Health Care Financing Administration, Office of Standards and Certification, Division of Long Term Care. How to Select a Nursing Home. Baltimore, MD, 21207, 1980, HCFA 80-30043. Washington, D.C., U.S. Government Printing Office, 1980

U.S. Senate, 93rd Congress, 2nd Session. Special Committee on Aging. Special Subcommittee on Long-term Care. Nursing Home Care in the United States: Failure in Public Policy. Introductory Report. Washington, D.C., U.S. Government Printing Office, 1974

Vaidya PN, Bhosley PN, Rao DB, Luisada AA: Tachyarrhythmias in old age. Journal of the American Geriatrics Society XXIV(9):412, 1976

Van Durme JP: Tachyarrhythmias and transient cerebral ischemic attacks. American Heart Journal 89(4):538, 1975

Villaverde MM, MacMillan CW: Ailments of Aging. New York, Van Nostrand Reinhold, 1980

Williams BO, Begg TB, Semple T, McGuinness JB: The elderly in a coronary care unit. British Medical Journal 2(1033):4510, 1976

Zankel HT: Stroke Rehabilitation: A Guide to the Rehabilitation of an Adult Patient Following a Stroke. Springfield, IL, Charles C. Thomas, 1971

19

Nursing the Client Experiencing Immobility

The incidence of fractures escalates with advancing age. The reasons why older people sustain fractures as well as the sites of their fractures differ from young adults. This chapter focuses on the fracture of the upper end of the femur (hip fracture) because it is typically an illness of the elderly. When an elderly person fractures a hip, the goals and methods of treatment are adapted to meet the needs of the older person. The principles of care, however, are similar to those utilized for older people with fractures at other sites. The client with a hip fracture moves to Adaptation Level Four, requiring hospitalization and, in most cases, surgery. This chapter explores the implications of both hospitalization and surgery for the older person. Immobility has particularly deleterious consequences for older people. Therefore, the enforced immobility associated with hip fractures is kept to a minimum when treating the elderly. This chapter explores the effects of immobility on older people and discusses ways the nurse can minimize its hazards.

SIGNIFICANT PROBLEMS

Fractures
The risk of sustaining serious fractures rises steeply after age 40. Unless treatment is prompt and aggressive, the temporary loss of function caused by the fracture may progress to permanent disability and dependency in the elderly.

Precipitating Stresses. The stresses responsible for fractures in the elderly differ markedly from those in the young. Young adults usually sustain fractures as a result of severe direct trauma to the affected part, usually the shaft of a long bone. Often, fractures occur as a consequence of auto accidents or industrial injuries. As might be expected, young men are affected more often than young women. Among the elderly, however, the fracture site is usually cancellous (trabecular) bone next to the joint rather than the shaft of the bone (Exton-Smith, 1978). Fractures are eight times more common in elderly women than in elderly men (Avioli, 1976).

Because of the decrease in mineral content and mechanical strength of aging bone, especially cancellous bones, severe trauma is not necessary to cause fractures in the elderly. Bone loss is believed to be the most significant factor associated with the etiology of fractures in old age. The bone loss may be due to normal aging changes or pathological processes such as osteoporosis, osteomalacia, Paget's disease, hyperparathyroidism, and metastatic cancer. Other factors have also been implicated in the etiology of fractures. Not only are bones more fragile, but muscles, tendons, and cartilage are weakened due to loss of elasticity. Therefore, minor trauma is sufficient to cause severe fractures in the fragile bones of the elderly. Minimal force, such as bending over, a simple twist, or a minor misstep has been associated with hip fractures in the elderly. Falls, which cause only slight injury in young people, have been associated with serious injuries such as fractures and even death in the elderly.

The role of trauma, especially when associated with falls, as an immediate cause of fractures, is currently being reexamined. It is not clear whether the fall precedes the fracture or vice versa (Hielema, 1979). Questions have been raised about whether the fracture is caused by uncoordinated muscle contractions during the act of falling or by the force of the impaction. Further biomechanical research is needed to resolve these questions (Vallarino and Sherman, 1981).

Although the precise causal relationship remains unclear, it is true that the percentage of falls associated with fractures rises with age. In one study 20 to 25 percent of falls were associated with fractures in clients aged 65 to 74, while 30 to 40 percent of falls were associated with fractures in clients 75 and over (Exton-Smith, 1977).

Why Older People Fall. Normal aging changes, as well as pathology in the musculoskeletal, neurological, and cardiovascular systems, interact with psychosocial factors and place older clients at high risk for falls. Physical changes due to normal aging include diminished visual acuity, night vision, and depth perception; postural changes that alter the center of gravity; changes in gait; diminished proprioception; slowed reaction time; and decreased muscle mass, strength, and coordination.

Other physical changes occur as a result of chronic disease and place the older client at high risk for falls. Arthritis causes stiff, painful, and unstable joints. Foot deformities are common in older people and may cause an unstable gait and stumbling. Neurological problems, such as cerebrovascular accident and Parkinson's disease, cause gait changes that increase the risk of stumbling. Cataracts, glaucoma, macular degeneration, retinopathy, and other problems result in limited vision and lead to misplaced footing or the inability to avoid environmental hazards. Lightheadedness, dizziness, or vertigo can result from cerebral hypoxia, cardiac arrhythmias, postural hypotension, hypoglycemia, and vestibular disease. Loss of consciousness may occur due to arrhythmias, cerebral hypoxia, neurological disorders, and other stresses. Diminished sensation due to diabetes and peripheral neuropathy also increases the risk of falling.

Still other older people fall due to medication effects. Certain antihypertensives cause postural hypotension. The client becomes lightheaded when changing position and falls. Any drug that alters

fluid or electrolyte balance can increase the risk of falling if it results in hypovolemia or arrhythmias. Sedatives and tranquilizers decrease awareness and increase confusion, thus leading to falls. Many other drugs, such as nitroglycerin, may cause lightheadedness.

Psychosocial factors include behaviors such as improper use of walkers and canes, improper footwear and clothing (long nightgowns and robes), and environmental hazards such as poor lighting, obstructions, the lack of handrails on both sides of the staircase, and stairways and floors that are unsafe. Physical factors interact with psychosocial factors, increasing the older client's risk of falling.

Additional risk factors have been identified in elderly clients who live in nursing homes (Feist, 1978). Falls are most likely to occur in the first few weeks following admission and in the evening, when clients are likely to be fatigued and engaged in bedtime activity. Confusion and the use of tranquilizers or sedatives have also been associated with falls in nursing home residents.

Common Fracture Sites in the Elderly. The most common fracture sites in the elderly are composed of cancellous bone. These include the vertebral bodies, the upper end of the femur (hip fracture), the distal end of the radius (Colle's fracture), and the proximal end of the humerus (Wallach, 1978; Green, 1981; Charlesworth and Baker, 1978). Of all these, fractures of the upper end of the femur are the most common and potentially the most disabling (Devas, 1976). Of the 200,000 hip fractures in the United States each year, 74 percent occur in individuals over the age of 70. Elderly white women sustain hip fractures three times as often as elderly white men. Blacks are rarely affected (Wylie, 1977; Vallarino and Sherman, 1981). By the age of 90, one out of five women suffers a fractured hip (Sandler, 1978). Among females in the Medicare program, fracture of the neck of the femur was the fifth most frequent hospital discharge diagnosis in 1973 (Medicare, 1978).

The fact that osteoporosis is more marked in postmenopausal women is not the only factor associated with the incidence of hip fractures in older women. Low body weight related to body height may be associated (Hielema, 1979). In addition, the pelvis is wider in women and the angle between the neck and the shaft of the femur is sharper so that more strain is thrown on the femoral neck, increasing the risk of fracture (Bonner, 1974).

Fractures of the femur can be divided into two classes: fractures of the femoral neck and trochanteric fractures (Fig. 1). Fractures of the femoral neck are intracapsular; that is, they occur inside the tenoligamentous capsule of the hip joint. Trochanteric fractures include intertrochanteric and subtrochanteric fractures. These are extracapsular.

These two classes of fractures differ in one important respect that affects the method and, at times, the outcome of treatment. The blood supply to the femoral head runs through the femoral neck and is easily damaged by the original trauma or subsequent manipulation. Nonunion and posttraumatic degenerative joint disease secondary to avascular necrosis of the femoral head may result with fractures of the femoral neck (Woogara, 1977; Val-

larino and Sherman, 1981). Complications are especially likely with displaced fractures and less likely with impacted fractures (Todd, 1977; Vallarino and Sherman, 1981). With trochanteric fractures the blood supply to the affected area is abundant and is not damaged by the trauma. Consequently, there are fewer complications than with fractures of the femoral neck.

ASSESSING THE CLIENT'S ADAPTATIONS

Fractures

Whenever an older client is admitted to the hospital with a suspected hip fracture, a complete history and physical examination should be performed as well as certain laboratory and radiographic tests. The client's age means that there are usually coincidental stresses, such as cardiovascular, renal,

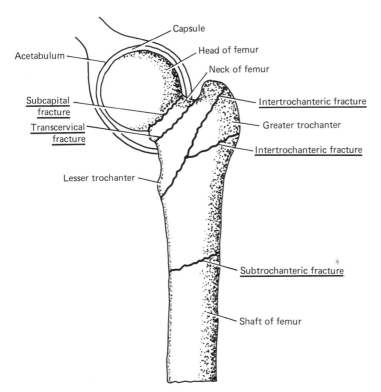

Figure 1. Four types of hip fractures. Intertrochanteric and subtrochanteric fractures are extracapsular. Subcapital and transcervical fractures are intracapsular.

or respiratory disease, diabetes, or anemia. These need to be treated, along with the musculoskeletal problem. After a musculoskeletal injury, especially one resulting from a fall, the client should be evaluated not only for the immediate injury but also for multiple musculoskeletal injuries and the reason for the fall.

The adaptations to illness exhibited by older people often vary from those of younger people, and this is true when they sustain a fractured hip. Hip fractures in the elderly are not always accompanied by acute pain, as is the case in young adults. In the elderly, the fracture site may be painless. Older clients may complain of weakness in the leg or pain in the affected knee, not the hip. Impacted fractures or those with minimal displacement often cause little pain and allow mobility, even ambulation. The only adaptation may be shortening of the leg. Older people may assume a fractured hip is a flare-up of arthritis and ignore it. Consequently, hip fractures are easily missed in older people (Anderson, 1976). Because pain is not always present in older people, the nurse should suspect a fracture whenever there is a history of possible trauma followed by a reduction or loss of function. If the fracture is pathological (due to osteoporosis or metastatic disease) the client may have experienced pain *before* the fall occurred. In this case it is the pathological fracture that causes the fall.

Observation and gentle palpation are used to assess the fracture site. The examiner should not feel for abnormal movements or crepitus. Following intracapsular fractures, the involved leg often appears shorter and displaced due to relaxation of the gluteus medius muscle, which loses its ability to abduct and rotate. Following some extracapsular fractures the affected leg may be externally rotated due to the pull of abductors and flexors of the hip or displaced posteriorly due to the pull of the gluteus maximus (Woogara, 1977).

Motor power in the affected leg should also be evaluated. It may be decreased or lost altogether. The leg may appear limp (Anderson, 1976). The client may also complain of generalized weakness.

Some older clients who live alone fall and are not found for several hours. These clients should be assessed for dehydration, hypothermia, and skin trauma. A careful mental status assessment should be made. The data should be compared with the client's preinjury mental status. An extracellular fluid volume deficit may cause the elderly client to become confused or somnolent. Unlike the younger client, the older client may neither remember the accident nor be able to give an accurate history. These clients may also exhibit hypotension and even shock. Their preinjury status will return if they are hydrated with an isotonic saline solution (Dodd, 1976; Green, 1981). Hypothermia may develop if the older client has remained on the floor without protection for several hours. If this problem is to be recognized, the client's rectal temperature should be taken on admission. The nurse should assess the client's skin for any damage predisposing to decubiti. Because their skin is fragile, older people can develop skin breakdown after lying immobile on a hard floor for only a short while (Devas, 1976).

The laboratory investigation includes the blood hemoglobin, blood type, blood urea, and serum electrolytes. X-ray examination of the anterior, posterior, and lateral pelvis is made to allow the surgeon to compare the two hips and to determine the location, extent, and severity of the fracture. Chest roentgenogram is also performed. Laboratory and radiological data are important in order to plan appropriate surgical intervention.

NURSING INTERVENTIONS

Fractures

Femoral fractures require approximately 12 weeks to heal. During this period, interventions are aimed at approximating the fragments and holding them in place. Immobilization, surgery, or a combination of these approaches can be used to accomplish this purpose.

The treatment plan for the older client with a fractured hip usually includes surgical repair followed by an aggressive period of rehabilitation. The goal of treatment is to restore the client to the prefracture level of ambulation and functioning, either unassisted or with a walker or cane. The specific treatment plan depends upon the client's overall level of adaptation as well as the type and extent of the hip fracture. Treatment of coexisting stresses is an important component of the treatment plan for every client with an orthopedic problem.

Recent advances in surgical techniques and restorative measures have revolutionized the care of older clients with hip fractures. Before these advances, the elderly were treated conservatively, with prolonged bed rest and traction. Although immobilization is a safe and effective approach for young adults with hip fractures, many elderly people cannot survive a lengthy period of immobilization. Of those who do survive, many suffer the permanent loss of ambulation, which is a major tragedy for many older people and leads to perpetual dependency. Today, surgical repair of the fractured hip is undertaken for all but a very few older clients. When the hip is repaired in this manner, early ambulation is possible. The client experiences a minimum of muscle atrophy and weakness. For elderly clients the risk associated with surgery in this instance is less than if surgery were not undertaken (Elkowitz, 1981).

Preoperative Care. The nurse integrates emotional support with all nursing care, beginning with the time of admission. Many older clients are terrified by the prospect of a broken hip. They fear they will never survive the hospitalization, and that, if they do, they will never walk again. In order to allow both the client and the surgical team sufficient time for adequate preparation, emergency surgery is usually not performed on the older client with a fractured hip. The first 24 to 48 hours after the client's admission are used to perform the assessment and prepare the client physically and emotionally for the surgery. Longer delays are usually not necessary unless the older client has an acute health problem, such as heart failure or diabetes, that should be stabilized before surgery.

Interventions prior to surgery are aimed at controlling the pain and muscle spasm associated with the fracture. The physician usually orders small amounts of meperidine, in preference to morphine, to control pain. It is important to handle the limb carefully from the time of the accident. When moving the client, the affected limb should be immobilized by wrapping the two legs together with Ace bandages or by holding both legs together. Special positioning is required prior to surgery to keep the legs in alignment and to reduce pain and muscle spasm. Some physicians may order that pillows and sandbags be used for this purpose. Others may prefer traction, especially if the pain continues. Buck's

extension traction is often used for intracapsular fractures. Russell's traction is usually preferred for extracapsular fractures. The client needs instruction about the purpose of traction and the amount of movement allowed. Before surgery, clients are usually permitted to turn only to the affected side. In order to keep movement to a minimum and promote comfort, the nurse should provide the client with a fracture pan for elimination.

The nurse should undertake preoperative teaching since careful preparation helps reduce fear of the unknown and helps the client to cooperate in the postoperative period. Clients need instruction about coughing and deep breathing and leg exercises. They should know that they will be asked to turn to the affected side after surgery. They should also be prepared if a Hemovac suction apparatus is to be used to drain off any blood, or if an indwelling catheter is to be inserted. Clients should be told that they will receive intravenous feedings instead of meals for several days after surgery. The exercise regimen and ambulation schedule clients will follow in the postoperative period should also be described and clients should practice the exercises to be performed in the postoperative period.

Surgical Intervention. Surgical intervention for the fractured hip relieves pain quickly and allows early mobilization. The choice of surgical procedure depends upon a variety of criteria, including the location and extent of the fracture (Fig. 2). Trochanteric fractures are usually repaired by internal fixation with fine pins, nails, or screws and side plates. The nails may be inserted during open surgery (open reduction) or by means of a closed method (closed reduction), their position being checked by x-ray examination. A lateral incision is made and when the wound is closed a simple occlusive adhesive dressing is applied. Because of the high incidence of complications, such as nonunion and avascular necrosis, when internal fixation is used for fractures of the femoral neck, many surgeons prefer to excise the upper fragment and replace it with a prosthesis (Devas, 1976). Some experts believe that only displaced femoral neck fractures need to be treated in this way and that slightly displaced and nondisplaced fractures can be adequately treated with internal fixation with pins after a closed reduction under radiographic control. If the upper

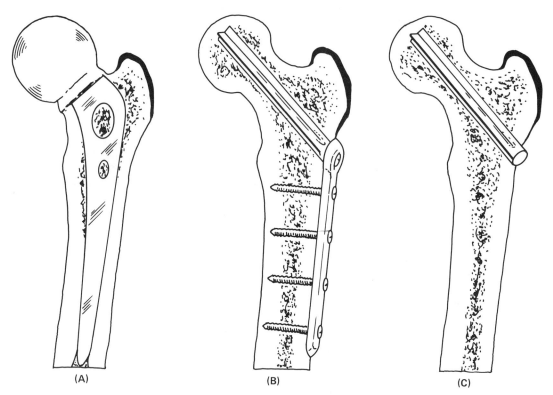

Figure 2. Common procedures used to repair fractures of the hip include the use of a prosthesis to repair a femoral fracture (A), the use of nails and a side plate for internal fixation of intertrochanteric and femoral shaft fractures (B), and the use of a nail for an intertrochanteric fracture (C).

fragment is to be replaced, several types of prostheses are available for use (Vallarino and Sherman, 1981). For example, the Thompson prosthesis is made of titanium, a very light metal. It is cemented in place to achieve firm contact with the femoral head. The Austin–Moore prosthetic device is embedded in the femur and depends in part on bone formation to hold it firmly in place (Devas, 1976). An anterolateral incision is usually made to allow access to the hip.

Postoperative Care. Nursing in the postoperative period varies according to the type of internal fixation device or prosthesis used as well as the client's general condition and ability to cooperate. In the immediate postoperative period, the nurse checks skin temperature of the affected limb. An increase in skin temperature may indicate infection or bleed-

ing. The color and pulses in the two lower limbs are assessed and compared on a regular basis. The dressing and Hemovac if present should be monitored for drainage. Elastic stockings should be applied to both lower extremities to increase circulation and prevent emboli. Thrombophlebitis and pulmonary emboli are life-threatening complications of fractures. Because decubiti prolong the rehabilitation process, meticulous skin care is essential (pp. 482–483).

Because older people are at high risk for postoperative respiratory and wound infections, the physician often orders a broad-spectrum antibiotic such as cephalothin to be administered for 1 week after surgery. In some clients, the antibiotic is begun in the preoperative period (Devas, 1976). Because anemia slows the rehabilitation of older people, the client who needs blood may be given a transfusion in the postoperative period if this was not done during the surgical procedure.

Turning and Positioning. Since physicians vary in their preferences, the nurse should obtain specific orders for turning and positioning the client. In most cases, clients with pin-and-nail repairs and prosthetic devices can be turned to the affected side. The bed acts as a splint for the affected leg and allows maintenance of alignment. During turning, the risk of displacement is highest with the Austin–Moore device. The bone is more stable when nails, pins, and the Thompson prosthesis are used. The positions the client is permitted to assume vary with each surgical procedure. The leg may be elevated to increase venous return and reduce swelling (Woogara, 1977). Often, slight hip abduction is maintained by placing pillows between the legs. Hip flexion and adduction and internal rotation are usually discouraged. Geriatric chairs and raised toilet seats are used to minimize hip flexion when sitting.

The Rehabilitation Protocol. The rehabilitation protocol is dictated in part by the surgical procedure used to correct the fracture. It may include general conditioning exercises, progressive resistive exercises, bilateral quadriceps and gluteal exercises, range of motion exercises, and progressive ambulation. The goal is early mobilization. With elderly clients, emphasis is placed on restoring safe ambulation and the ability to carry out activities of daily living. It is not necessary for elderly clients to achieve full range of motion in the joint as long as movement is sufficient to perform ADLs. Exercises are begun early in the postoperative period to increase circulation, maintain normal range of motion, strengthen muscles and prevent muscle spasm. Active and passive range of motion exercises of the feet, ankles, and knees are performed. The client is told to move the feet and ankles according to a regular schedule. Quadriceps and gluteal setting exercises are taught. The client also performs progressive resistive exercises of the upper extremities to strengthen the arms because these are needed to manage walkers and crutches. Many older people find crutches difficult to manipulate due to minor deficits in coordination, slowing of righting reflexes, and impairment of proprioception They may be more successful

with a walker. Active and progressive resistive exercises are instituted in the unaffected leg, especially if partial weight bearing must be performed. If this is the case, the unaffected leg must bear the brunt of the body's weight.

The client's weight-bearing and ambulation schedule depends upon the type of device used to repair the hip. The nurse needs specific information about the schedule to be followed for each client. The schedule may progress from non-weight-bearing ambulation (ambulation without weight on the affected limb) to full weight bearing. When a hip prosthesis is used or when special compression hip screw systems are used, clients are usually allowed partial weight bearing immediately after surgery as long as they are reasonably strong and free of pain. Full weight bearing is permitted within 1 week. When fixation pins or nails and plates are used, partial weight bearing may be delayed for several weeks or months (Vallarino and Sherman, 1981; Dunnery, 1979).

Partial weight bearing may present problems for older clients because hopping requires strength, coordination, balance, and an understanding of what is being taught. It may be difficult to hold up the affected limb. Teaching partial weight bearing or non-weight bearing to a confused elderly client may be difficult or impossible. Elderly clients are often afraid that weight bearing or ambulation will injure the hip. Consequently, the staff must have absolute confidence in the exercise program and communicate this to the client. When exercising and ambulating the client, the same routine should be used by every member of the health team. As they progress, some older clients need to understand that safe ambulation may necessitate continued use of a walker or cane because unaided ambulation may bring about another fall or another hip fracture. A few clients are able to achieve safe ambulation without an assistive device. Stair climbing should be taught if indicated.

Potential Stresses. The postoperative pain following repair of a hip fracture gradually subsides over several weeks. If it continues or increases, the physician orders a radiological examination to determine the reason. Among the many problems associated with increasing postoperative pain are separation of bone fragments, subluxation of the endoprosthesis, displacement of the fixation device, osteomyelitis, aseptic necrosis, and various types of arthritis.

Deformities of the affected limb, some of which cause serious disability, can result from both extracapsular and intracapsular fractures. Often the deformity is an external rotation of the lower limb caused by displacement of the segment or incorrect positioning after surgery that results in a contracture at the hip joint. Quadriceps palsy can develop as a consequence of injury of the femoral nerve during surgery. Foot drop can develop when splints do not fit properly and cause compression of the common peroneal nerve at the upper end of the fibula. Malunion and impaction of the fragments may lead to a difference in the length of the lower limbs. In most cases, a lift in the shoe corrects the problem.

The adaptations to immobility can also affect the elderly client with a fractured hip. These are described on pages 481 to 483. They can prolong hospitalization and the rehabilitation effort and lead to institutionalization (Vallarino and Sherman, 1981).

Prognosis. The average hospital stay for the elderly client with a fractured hip is 22.3 days (Medicare, 1978). Many older clients require long-term care before they are able to function independently. The rehabilitation process proceeds more slowly in the elderly. Advanced age (over 75 years) has been a strong predictor of unsatisfactory results following hip fracture. Impaired mental status, Parkinson's disease, and multiple chronic illnesses have also been associated with a poor prognosis (Hielema, 1979). On the other hand, fractures in clients with clinical osteoporosis tend to heal as well as those in clients without osteoporosis. There is an occasional problem of nonunion of the hip in these clients (Pont, 1981). The majority of older clients with hip fractures are eventually able to return to their home. Many are able to walk without assistive devices. Advances in surgical procedures together with early mobilization and aggressive exercise programs help to prevent complications and expedite the older client's return to the community (Vallarino and Sherman, 1981).

Management of Other Fractures. Because muscle strength and mobility are diminished in the aged, the methods used to treat most fractures in young adults are not always advisable for the elderly person. It is usually more dangerous to treat an older person with immobilization in bed than it is by surgery. Physicians who treat older people attempt to avoid immobilizing fractured limbs in plaster casts for long periods because doing so causes local osteoporosis that slows the rehabilitation process. Radial, ulnar, and Colle's fractures are usually treated with casting but early mobilization is emphasized. The cast should fit so that finger movement is not restricted. Most fractures of the tibia and femoral shaft, including those involving the knee (subcondylar fractures), are treated with internal fixation with pins or nails and plates. After the procedure, walking is permitted almost immediately. In order to allow early ambulation following fractures of the patella, the patella is usually excised. The client walks after being fitted with a special frame. Patellar cracks can be treated with nails. Many ankle fractures are treated by screwing the fractured malleolus (Devas, 1976; Elkowitz, 1981). After the fracture is repaired the elderly client needs nursing support in order to prevent immobility. Activity in the form of ambulation and exercise must be encouraged if the older client is to maintain independence.

Preventing Fractures. Nurses can help older clients prevent fractures by teaching them to remain alert for hazards in the environment and behavior patterns that promote accidents and falls. Many older clients have adjusted to their environment and do not recognize hazards and behaviors that increase the risk of falls. Much can be done to modify the client's home to prevent falls. It is essential for the nurse to obtain the client's cooperation if necessary modifications are to be made. Cost may be a limiting factor, but many alterations can be made at minimal expense. Obstacles should be removed whenever possible. Furniture should be arranged in an orderly fashion with wide traffic pathways. Extension cords should be discouraged or taped down to prevent tripping. Throw rugs should be removed, or, if the client objects, a nonskid backing should be applied. Carpets should be tacked down. Bannisters should be built on stairways. Walls and stairways should be painted different colors. Stairwells should be well lit. Grab bars and bathmats should be installed in the bathroom. The client should obtain a nightlight to assure safe passage from bedroom to bathroom.

Older clients may benefit from advice about

clothing that is safe and practical as well as attractive. Older people should wear sturdy, well-fitting shoes with substantial soles and avoid long, flowing nightgowns and robes, heelless scuffs, and thongs. Clients should be aware of other ways they can reduce the risk of falling. They should be warned not to go outside in snowy or icy weather. They should be encouraged to clean up spills and pick up fallen objects immediately. They should be discouraged from keeping their floors highly polished. To avoid environmental hazards, clients should be taught to turn their heads and use their eyes to deliberately scan the environment. Older people should also know how to check their mobility aids (walkers, canes) for any malfunctioning parts and correct problems immediately. Clients need to understand that because of the aging process, they are no longer able to correct their balance in an instant when they start to fall. They should also know that many falls are not preventable. Nurses can teach clients at high risk ways to fall, and if injuries occur, how to move across the floor to the telephone. These clients should have emergency phone numbers readily available.

Some elderly clients may be so fearful of falling that they may severely restrict their own mobility. This practice is probably more dangerous than activity because it places older clients at risk for the hazards of immobility. The nurse can refer these clients to a telephone reassurance program, in which volunteers call the client once each 24 hours. If the client does not answer, a visitor is sent to check on the condition of the client. If this system is used clients have the security of knowing they will not be left alone longer than 24 hours. Therefore, the fear of falling may not be such an overwhelming concern for them.

Supporting the Hospitalized Client

Characteristics of the Aged, Hospitalized Client. Age is a major determinant of hospital utilization. Although older people represent only 11 percent of the U.S. population they account for 34 percent of all days utilized in short-stay hospitals. Older people have at least twice as many hospital stays as their younger counterparts (Brotman, 1979), and their average length of stay per hospitalization is twice as long. The average length of stay for those aged 15 to 44 years is 5.1 days but for people over

65, it is 12.6 days (Vital Statistics, 1973). The most common reasons for the hospitalization of older people are diseases of the circulatory system, followed by diseases of the digestive and respiratory systems. The most frequent diagnoses are heart disease, hypertension, cancer, and cerebrovascular disease (Vital Statistics, 1974).

The special characteristics of elderly hospitalized clients have important implications for nursing care. When older people are hospitalized, they are more likely than younger people to be terminally ill (Kahana and Kahana, 1976). Although hospitalization constitutes a crisis situation for people of all ages, older people are the least likely to adapt to it in an optimal way because they have fewer energy reserves and their adaptive capacity has declined. Emotional reactions to hospitalization are intensified in older people. In addition, the elderly who are cerebrally impaired often fail to adapt to hospitalization and develop disturbed behaviors such as disorientation and agitation (Rossman, 1979).

Reactions to Hospitalization. Responses to hospitalization are highly individualized, depending on each person's perception and interpretation of the experience. Older people often have difficulty accurately perceiving events because of various sensory losses, especially diminished sight and hearing (Bagwell and Ludlow, 1980). Because of previous experiences as well as insufficient or inaccurate information about our modern health care system, older clients may misinterpret their experiences during hospitalization. Mental status changes and reduced reaction time reduce their abiltiy to absorb and process their new environment and the information they are given. Anxiety and depression are common responses to hospitalization and older clients who are mentally alert can be expected to react to hospitalization with heightened levels of these emotions (Rossman, 1979).

Anxiety and Fear. Most elderly clients experience significant anxiety and fear when they are hospitalized. More elderly people die in institutions than at home. Therefore, many older people view hospitals as places to die rather than places to regain their health. The enforced dependency created by hospitalization reinforces this fear. The need to be hospitalized is dramatic proof that something is wrong or that an existing disorder is worsening (Butler and

Lewis, 1977). Hospital routine may appear rational to staff members, but to older clients it may seem baffling and irrational and contribute to their anxiety. Sleep may be interrupted at an unnaturally early hour so that staff can take the client's temperature and weight. Meals may be delayed without explanation to prepare the client for tests. Uniformed attendants appear without prior warning with wheelchairs and stretchers. Nearby clients may cry out in pain or confusion. Paging systems blare forth incomprehensible phrases. In addition, procedures such as venipuncture or endoscopy have symbolic overtones that further increase anxiety. Although many diagnostic procedures are a routine part of hospital admission, older clients may interpret these tests as a sign that they may have a serious or terminal disorder (Rossman, 1979).

Helping the elderly client adjust to hospitalization begins with the admission procedure. As soon as possible, the nurse should assess the client's mental and sensory status to determine the client's ability to accurately perceive the hospital environment and process new information. To reduce anxiety, the nurse should give the client a thorough orientation to the physical setting, routines, and personnel. Because older clients absorb new information more slowly, explanations should be given at a slow pace. Unobtrusive repetition of important information is also helpful. Older clients should know the relative locations of their bed, bathroom, and day room. It is important that they know how to operate key equipment in the room, especially the bell to summon the nurse. Clients should be introduced to the personnel who will care for them. Rotations of shifts may confuse older people and disrupt their relationships with personnel. The nurse should explain who will be responsible for care on other shifts and days off. The hospital routine should also be explained. Clients need to know that certain procedures, such as vital signs, daily weights, chest x-ray, drawing blood, and so on are routine practices and do not signal deterioration in the client's condition. The times and routines for arising, retiring in the evening, morning care, and meals should also be explained. As staff members assist the client with each of these activities, they should reinforce the explanations given at the time of admission. When giving care to the client, the nurse should proceed in a calm, unhurried manner and avoid

rushing the client. Because speed of reaction declines with age, older clients can become anxious and agitated if hurried. To reduce the anxiety associated with diagnostic tests, older clients need clear explanations of their purpose, the preparation required, and how they can cooperate during the test. The nurse should also communicate regularly with clients about their progress. Whenever appropriate, the nurse should reassure older clients about their condition. Discussing and planning for returning to normal activities also helps to relieve the older person's anxiety.

The client's anxiety may be compounded by worries about the home that has been left behind. Older clients may worry about neglected pets and plants, unresolved conflicts among those living at home, or unattended mail, especially pension and social security checks. To deal with pressures at home, the nurse should involve hospital social workers or community agencies (Butler and Lewis, 1977).

The nurse should make regular assessments of the older client's anxiety level because high levels of anxiety interfere with the client's ability to perceive and interpret the experiences of hospitalization accurately. The client's expressions of anxiety and fear are highly individualized. Some clients react by making frequent requests and demands for help. These may seem unreasonable to the staff, but they are the older client's way of getting needed attention. Other older clients may respond to illness and hospitalization with regressive behaviors (Lore, 1979).

Depression. Because it is associated with so many real losses, hospitalization frequently precipitates depression or exacerbates already existing depression (Rossman, 1979). Hospitalization may precipitate the related process of grief and mourning or cause it to be reactivated from an earlier loss (Lore, 1979). Depression and grief may become stresses that contribute to or aggravate the physical condition that caused the client's hospitalization in the first place. Consequently, the nurse should be alert for signs of these responses and intervene appropriately. Older clients often express depression and grief somatically. One of the best ways to help clients resolve their feelings is to let them talk. Clients may not recognize their own feelings and may not bring them up. The nurse can initiate discussion by reflecting upon the client's mood. Touch, genuine interest, and attentive listening help older clients work through their feelings (Lore, 1979).

Reduced Self-Esteem. Hospitalization emphasizes the client's physical deterioration and loss of health, mobility, and independence. Because of illness or physician's orders, older clients may be partially or completely dependent on the staff for care. Even when they are capable of self-care, staff members may believe it is faster or easier to do things for the client, thus reinforcing the client's dependent position. These losses weaken the older client's feelings of self-confidence and sense of self-esteem.

One way of preventing dependency is to assess the client's functional capacity as soon as possible after admission. This assessment would be more meaningful if nurses could make it *before* the older person was taken from familiar surroundings to the hospital (Kemp, 1978). When the client's nursing care plan reflects the client's capacity for self-care, the client's independence and self-esteem are preserved. The room should be arranged to promote independence. The overbed table and frequently used personal items should be within easy reach. Placing an overbed trapeze above the bed of an immobile client enhances the ability to perform bed activities.

The client's self-esteem may be further damaged by the depersonalization that is associated with hospitalization. Upon admission, clients are dressed in hospital gowns. Their personal possessions and jewelry are removed. They are deprived of privacy to perform the most basic bodily functions or sustain intimate or family relationships (Kemp, 1978). If the client is placed in a ward or semiprivate room their basic territorial needs may be ignored. Some clients respond to depersonalized care by hoarding articles such as tissues or matchboxes. This behavior is a clue that clients need something that belongs to them near them to reassure them that they are still individuals (Lore, 1979). When their territory is invaded, clients may become very possessive of personal effects or certain pieces of furniture in the room.

There are many ways the nurse can personalize the client's care, beginning with admission. All older people should be greeted in a warm friendly way. The nurse should be patient and supportive when giving care and communicating with the client. When it is appropriate, older people should be encouraged to wear their own clothes and keep a treasured possession nearby. If the older client shares the room with others, the nurse should ensure that clients have furniture of their own. Clear-cut territorial boundaries reduce possessive behaviors.

Loss of Control. Hospitalized older clients experience a loss of control over their life-style. They must exchange familiar environments and routines for a bleak hospital room, institutionalized food, and incomprehensible hospital routines. Once hospitalized, the older client who is acutely ill or confined to bed may also have to cope with loss of control over bodily functions. Older clients who have urinated in bed may be so embarrassed that they claim they have spilled something in bed or perspired excessively in order to maintain some self-esteem (Lore, 1979). In order to increase their sense of control, the nurse should allow older clients to participate in decision making about their care.

Role Loss. The older client's depression is exacerbated by role loss and loss of the usual role relationships. Hospitalization may dilute or abolish the client's roles as parent or spouse. Even if older clients are functioning as homemakers in the most marginal way, they may react profoundly to the loss. The elderly spouse may be homebound and unable to visit the hospital and share the stress. Rigid visiting hours may also restrict the older client's visitors. The spouse or client may have such poor hearing that even telephone communication is impossible. It is no wonder that older clients feel isolated and lonely when hospitalized.

When family members are able to visit the hospitalized client they may experience such strain that they are unable to give the client needed emotional support. It is not unusual for adult children to act out their grief and defend themselves against rage and guilt by withdrawing their affection. Others may become overconcerned and overprotective, making decisions for the client and thus fostering psychological as well as physical dependency.

The nurse should assess the family to determine how the various members interact. When one member of a family is sick, other members also become disturbed. The nurse should consult the family about care plans and let them participate in the client's care. The nurse should also encourage families to discuss their ambivalent feelings about the older client. Elderly people often turn to their families for support when faced with hospitalization, but in order to provide support, family members also need the nurse's attention (Lore, 1979).

Mental Status Changes. Some older clients, especially those who are mentally impaired, react to hospitalization with confusion and agitation (Lore, 1979; Rossman, 1979). Any change in the environment may precipitate disorientation in the older client with organic mental syndrome. Transfer from a familiar environment causes loss of the usual visual, auditory, tactile, and olfactory cues, which help to orient the client. These losses contribute to the sensory deprivation caused when the client has impaired vision and hearing. Many pastimes, such as television and radio, that are used to reduce sensory monotony in hospitalized clients are not available to older clients with vision and hearing losses. Placing older clients in private rooms increases isolation and further aggravates sensory deprivation.

Confusion may occur immediately upon transfer to the hospital or gradually following admission. At first, clients may experience transient episodes of confusion, especially at night. Later, they forget or deny the confusion. Gradually, the confusion increases. In many cases, the confusion and disorientation disappear once the client returns to the familiar home environment.

To minimize confusion and disorientation during hospitalization clients should receive a thorough orientation to the new environment. Measures such as unrestrictive visiting hours, wearing their own clothes, keeping meaningful personal belongings nearby, and encouraging communication with family and significant others help to maintain orientation. Providing a nightlight helps to reorient forgetful older clients who awaken in an unfamiliar setting. Older clients should not be placed in a private room unless absolutely necessary. The nurse should encourage older clients to communicate with other clients on the unit. This may be accomplished in many ways, according to the client's needs. For example, the nurse can arrange for several older clients to eat their meals in the day room. If the client is deaf in one ear, the nurse can ensure that

the client is placed in a double room with the "good" ear facing the roommate's bed. Therapeutic groups can be arranged for older clients. These are often important sources of emotional support and socialization for clients, especially if they have few visitors.

More aggressive nursing measures should be undertaken if the client seems confused. For example, large clocks and calendars can be placed within the client's view, and on a frequent, regular basis, the client can be oriented to reality.

Physical Changes. As a consequence of hospitalization, older clients are also at risk for adverse physical adaptations. Their reduced immune defenses place them at high risk for the development of nosocomial infections. Mishaps such as nocturnal falls are also especially high in the elderly. The nurse has primary responsibility for ensuring that the client's environment is safe. Simple nursing measures such as scrupulous hand washing, use of low beds, side rails, and a night-light, and placing of urinal and water pitcher within reach help maintain safety.

The number of prescribed medications is highest in hospitalized older people, increasing the likelihood of adverse reactions to medications. Obtaining data about the client's physical and mental status prior to admission is useful when interpreting changes in the client's condition. The nurse should be aware that a change for the worse may not be due directly to the client's illness but to one of the medications being taken.

Summary. When the older client is hospitalized, the goal of nursing care is to help the client adapt to the experience in ways that promote personal growth. Because older people pose special problems when they are hospitalized nurses may be fearful that they are seeing their own future. Nurses must first work through these feelings in order to feel comfortable caring for hospitalized older people. The elderly respond to hospitalization with anxiety and depression. At times they may be confused. They are at high risk to develop health problems during their hospital stay. Careful assessment and thoughtful intervention can facilitate the older client's adjustment to hospitalization. Considering that hospitalization is a crisis that older people must deal with several times before they die, it is disappointing that so little nursing research has been done to document the responses of older people to hospitalization and nursing strategies that are effective in helping them cope. Helping older people cope with hospitalization is largely the nurse's responsibility. This is an area that deserves more attention on the part of nurse researchers.

Assisting the Client Who Requires Surgery

Surgical Risk in the Elderly. About 40 percent of all older people who require hospitalization undergo surgical treatment (Glenn, 1973). Surgical procedures can be especially risky in the aged, but age alone is not a contraindication to surgery. Even very old people have not necessarily reached their full life expectancy and must be considered candidates for surgical interventions to improve their quality of life. Mason et al. (1976) reviewed the literature to determine mortality data for elective and emergency surgery. They found that the risk of minor elective surgery is not significantly different from that expected in younger clients. For major elective surgical procedures, however, the mortality rate was significantly greater in the aged than their younger counterparts.

The difference in mortality rates for younger and older clients who undergo elective surgery is believed to be due to several factors. First, age-related changes in the cardiovascular, respiratory, and renal systems reduce their efficiency and reserve capacity. These systems may be well compensated under normal circumstances, but they may not be able to adapt to the stress of surgery (Mason et al., 1976). In addition, older people have the highest prevalence of certain health problems that further impair the body's ability to adapt successfully to surgery.

Older people have the highest incidence of cardiovascular disease, and this increases the risks of anesthesia and surgery. There is a mortality rate of 40 percent for surgery performed within 3 months of myocardial infarction. The greatest risk appears to be within the first 15 days after infarction. The risk gradually declines and after 2 years it is the same as for clients of the same age without heart disease. Aging clients who require nitroglycerin be-

cause of angina that occurs while they are sleeping or after slight exercise are poor surgical risks (Dodd, 1976). Acute congestive heart failure is a serious risk factor. Clients are not candidates for surgery until their cardiac status has been treated (Dodd, 1976). Another high risk group about whom there are few available data are clients with unstable arrhythmias. These should be stabilized prior to surgery. Unfortunately, digitalis is usually required to stabilize clients with heart failure or arrhythmias and the electrolyte changes that accompany surgery place the client at high risk for digitalis toxicity.

Respiratory function declines with age, and the incidence of chronic respiratory diseases increases. Older clients with chronic pulmonary diseases, including a history of respiratory failure, asthma that develops after age 50, chronic productive cough, or heavy cigarette smoking are high surgical risks. A useful preoperative test of pulmonary function is the forced expiratory volume in 1 second (FEV_1). If this is less than 1 liter, the client has a poor prognosis (Powell, 1981).

Older clients are at high risk for malnutrition, and nutritional depletion curtails their ability to withstand the risk of surgery. The decrease in gamma globulin invites infection and the reduction in plasma proteins increases the risk of shock. If the intake of protein and ascorbic acid is inadequate, wound healing can be retarded.

If the older person's hepatic or renal function is compromised, the surgical risk increases. Malfunction of either system may prolong the action of drugs used in the surgical procedure. Poor renal function, especially if cardiovascular problems also exist, places the client at risk for fluid overload during surgery (Powell, 1981). Usually, clients with severe renal disease are not considered candidates for elective surgery (Anderson, 1976).

Older people who must undergo elective surgery benefit from a thorough preoperative assessment designed to identify any functional impairments due to aging or disease. Data are used to institute measures to improve the client's adaptation before surgery and to plan for intraoperative and postoperative measures to maximize the client's adaptation to the anesthesia and surgical procedure.

In all age groups, emergency surgery carries a greater risk than planned, elective procedures. Mortality rates for emergency surgery are highest in the elderly (Powell, 1981). When emergency surgery is required, the surgical team does not have sufficient time to assess the older client and institute measures to stabilize the client's condition (Mason et al., 1976). Consequently, emergency surgery is avoided in older people whenever possible (Parkhurst, 1978). When surgery is indicated, some older clients will postpone it or refuse to have it at all, only to be admitted at a later time for emergency surgery with urgent, life-threatening complications. For this reason, when there is a good reason for older clients to have surgery, they should be advised to have it when they are "well" (Mason et al., 1976; Parkhurst, 1978).

Preoperative Care. Elderly people require a more careful assessment prior to surgery than do their younger counterparts. The preoperative assessment is a multidisciplinary responsibility. Comprehensive assessment by the nurse, surgeon, and anesthesiologist is crucial to effective care of the older client before, during, and after surgery. The assessment includes a complete history and physical examination, mental status examination, and laboratory data. Chest roentgenogram, electrocardiogram, complete blood count, urinalysis, and fasting blood sugar are routine. If indicated, the physician may order pulmonary function studies, arterial blood gases, and examination of the upper and lower gastrointestinal tract and gallbladder (Mason et al., 1976).

It is not unusual for older clients to be hospitalized several days or weeks prior to elective surgery in order to permit a comprehensive assessment and treatment of problems that increase the older client's surgical risk. During this preoperative period the nurse prepares the client for the surgery and postoperative period and uses assessment data to plan nursing interventions for the postoperative period.

Mental Status Assessment. A thorough mental status assessment is important because it is an indicator of how the client will withstand the surgical procedure. This assessment is difficult if clients have Parkinson's disease because their masklike facies do not reflect emotions accurately. Mood is important. Motivation and a will to live are believed to compensate for some physical problems. Older

clients with a desire and a reason for living are better surgical risks than clients who are depressed. These clients are interested in others, aware of current events, and sensitive to their own personal hygiene (Dodd, 1976). On the other hand, if the client is severely depressed, it may be important to postpone surgery. Older clients have many years of experience that influence their feelings about the surgery they will have. The nurse should also determine the client's usual pattern of coping with stress, previous experiences with surgery, and information about other people who have undergone similar surgery. These factors will affect the client's mood and response to surgery.

During the preoperative period the nurse should convey an enthusiastic and hopeful attitude to the client. All members of the surgical team should keep older clients informed about their condition and allow them to participate in decision making. Failure to involve older clients in their surgical care has a negative impact on their emotional status that may have damaging effects on their physical condition (Elkowitz, 1981).

The nurse should also determine the client's mental acuity and ability to learn. It is especially important to be alert for hearing problems or aphasia during the interview and then to determine whether or not the client's other faculties are still acute. The nurse uses these data to determine the preoperative teaching plan. Clients should be given as much information about the routines surrounding surgery and the postoperative period as they can comfortably assimilate. The type and amount of information must be tailored to the client's ability to comprehend. If older clients understand what is expected before and after surgery, they are more willing to cooperate.

Integumentary Assessment. A baseline assessment of the client's skin in the preoperative period is used to make comparisons postoperatively. Skin changes are often the first indicator that an allergic reaction is occurring. Systemic preoperative drugs and anesthesia given during surgery might cause skin eruptions if an allergic reaction occurs (Quinn and Ryan, 1979). The skin should be assessed for color changes, edema, ulcers, and any other signs of venous stasis. Poor venous return is common in older people and minor trauma during surgery coupled with immobility places older clients at high risk for postoperative venous stasis. In the preoperative period, the nurse should teach the older client passive and active exercises. These should be performed regularly if the client is immobile. Preoperatively, the nurse should measure the client for supportive hose.

Cardiovascular Assessment. The older client's exercise tolerance is the most useful indicator of cardiovascular function (Powell, 1981). The nurse should determine the client's usual pattern of ADLs and how easily the client tires. In addition, the nurse should assess shortness of breath, chest pain, vertigo, mental confusion, and unexpected mental changes. The aging heart reacts poorly to the tachycardia that often results from anxiety about the surgery. The nurse should be sensitive to the possibility of anxiety and through preoperative teaching attempt to reduce it.

The physician obtains an electrocardiogram in the preoperative period to use as a reference if complications develop later. A thorough drug history is also obtained. If an older client has a previous history of digitalis treatment, the physician may place the client on small amounts of digitalis (one-half to two-thirds of the digitalization dose) in order to protect the heart against arrhythmias and increase the force of cardiac contraction. If the client is taking antihypertensive medication, the anesthesiologist assesses blood pressure to determine the presence of acceptable vascular reactivity. In most cases, antihypertensive medication is not withdrawn prior to surgery (Powell, 1981). However, some antihypertensives reduce the variability in blood pressure and increase the risk of hypotension during surgery. If this is the case, the antihypertensive drug may be discontinued several weeks before surgery (Dodd, 1976).

Respiratory Assessment. Much can be done in the preoperative period to improve the respiratory function of older clients. Adequate preparation is important because respiratory complications remain the most common cause of death in elderly postoperative clients (Powell, 1981). The client's appearance and breathing pattern are clues to significant pulmonary disease. If the client maintains a relaxed position and speaks in complete sentences

without stopping to take a breath, respiratory impairment is probably minimal or well controlled. The client should be able to walk the length of the hospital corridor and climb a flight of stairs without becoming dyspneic. If the history, physical assessment, or chest roentgenogram suggests the presence of pulmonary disease, the physician may order pulmonary function tests (PFTs) and arterial blood gases. An oxygen tension of 70 to 85 mm Hg is normal for the elderly, but the carbon dioxide tension and pH should be in the normal range for the general population (Dodd, 1976).

If respiratory impairment exists, the physician may order oxygen or intermittent positive pressure breathing (IPPB) treatments with physiological saline and a bronchodilator in the preoperative period. The client may be given a broad-spectrum antibiotic to clear preexisting bronchitis or respiratory infection (Mason et al., 1976; Powell, 1981). In these cases, the nurse should begin chest physiotherapy in the preoperative period. Prior to surgery, the nurse should teach all older clients how to perform coughing and deep breathing exercises and how to use blow bottles and IPPB machines if these are to be employed in the postoperative period.

Musculoskeletal Assessment. The nurse should assess the client for postural changes, limitations in range of joint motion, or paralyzed limbs and carefully note any changes. This information is necessary to assure correct positioning during the surgical procedure.

Nutritional Assessment. A recent weight loss of more than 5 pounds may indicate malnutrition in an older person. If some of the weight is regained before surgery, the incidence of postoperative complications is decreased. The physician usually begins by ordering a high-calorie diet. This may be supplemented with tube feedings if the older client is anorexic. Hyperalimentation is used if the client cannot eat (Mason et al., 1976). Nursing strategies are aimed at assuring an optimal intake. Older clients should be consulted about food preferences and given help at mealtime, if needed.

Before the client is taken to the operating room, the nurse should assess the oral cavity. The nurse should remove dentures and make a written notation about any loose teeth. These may be dislodged during anesthesia and fall into the respiratory tract (Parkhurst, 1978).

Excretory System Assessment. The urinalysis, blood urea nitrogen, and creatinine levels are used to assess preoperative renal function. Because older people are at high risk to develop dehydration and become hypotensive when anesthetized, they are often given intravenous fluid replacement beginning the night before surgery or early on the day of surgery. Some physicians permit older clients to drink clear liquids up to 5 hours before surgery. Because urine output is an important indicator of renal function and hydration, the nurse should institute intake and output recordings.

Extracellular Fluid Volume Assessment. The physician orders the complete blood count, SMA panel, and serum electrolytes to assess the status of the extracellular fluid, Hydration is assessed by examination of tissue and tongue turgor, mucous membranes, jugular venous pressure, and the presence of any edema (Powell, 1981). Adequate hydration preoperatively is essential in the elderly because their reduced adaptive capacity leaves only a narrow margin of safety between overhydration and underhydration. Fluid, electrolyte and hemoglobin deficiencies are corrected before surgery (Anderson, 1976). A hemoglobin level of 10 g/dl is the usually accepted minimum in an older client who is to undergo an elective procedure with little blood loss. If a large blood loss is expected, transfusions may be given preoperatively rather than during surgery. Usually packed red cells are given rather than whole blood in order to prevent circulatory overload (Dodd, 1976). Older clients who have been vomiting or having diarrhea are at high risk for fluid and electrolyte disturbances. If gastric juice is lost, they are likely to develop a sodium or potassium deficit. Because gastric pH tends to be less acid with advanced age, loss of gastric juice is not as likely to produce metabolic alkalosis in the aged. Diarrhea may also cause hypokalemia. If the client has received repeated enemas to prepare for surgery or diagnostic procedures prior to surgery, there is an increased risk of dehydration.

Intraoperative Care. *Surgical Management.* The physician uses data from the preoperative assess-

ment to select the specific surgical procedure and incision. Because each operation performed has potential complications, the surgeon weighs carefully the question of performing multiple operations at once. In general, only procedures that are absolutely necessary are performed on older clients. For example, although it is likely that a surgeon will perform an appendectomy when doing a cholecystectomy on a 30-year-old client, it is unlikely that the same action would be taken on an elderly client. The surgeon weighs the client's tolerance in the preoperative period, considers standard staging approaches to problems, and selects the procedure the older client is most likely to withstand. The surgeon may avoid certain extensive procedures because older people do not tolerate them. Some operations commonly performed on younger clients may not be performed on very old clients in poor health because their risks outweigh their benefits. These include surgical intervention for varicose veins without leg ulcers, hemorrhoids, and small, asymptomatic gallstones. Instead, these problems would be treated medically. When choosing the incision to be used for the older client, the surgeon considers body build as well as ease of proper exposure. If the client is obese the surgeon may alter the incisional site to avoid deep fat because incisions in these areas carry an especially high risk of infection. If the surgical procedure causes a high risk of infection or if postoperative infection would result in serious morbidity or mortality, the surgeon begins antibiotic therapy in the preoperative period.

Anesthetic Management. Although preoperative medication and anesthesia are responsibilities of the anesthesiologist, the nurse should be aware of the principles of anesthetic management. After clients have discussed the selection of anesthesia with the anesthesiologist, they may ask the nurse many questions.

There have been no innovations in anesthetic methods related specifically to the older client (Dodd, 1976). The anesthesiologist uses data from the preoperative assessment to determine the type and amount, if any, of preoperative sedation and the method and agent(s) used for anesthesia. Preoperative narcotic and sedative drugs are used to calm clients so that they accept the strange surroundings of the operating room in a tranquil mood. The anesthesiologist uses data from the mental status assessment to determine preoperative medication as well as anesthesia. The dosage of preoperative medications is normally reduced by one-third to one-half the amount given to a young adult of the same size. Clients with chronic brain syndrome require an even lower dose of medication in order to prevent additional mental deterioration. In addition, they will require lower concentrations of anesthesia to achieve clinical anesthesia. Preoperative medication often includes a narcotic supplemented with a nonphenothiazine tranquilizer such as hydroxyzine hydrochloride (Vistaril) 25 to 50 mg or diazepam (Valium) 2.5 to 5 mg. Preanesthetic narcotics are helpful because there is discomfort associated with the hard operating table and the placement of needles for infusion and block anesthesia. Giving narcotics prior to surgery may also provide some residual analgesia during the early part of anesthesia so that lower concentrations of anesthesia are required. If older clients have asthma or multiple allergies, the anesthesiologist may order Benedryl 25 to 50 mg as a preoperative medication because it has sedative and antihistaminic actions. Some older clients are too frail to tolerate a narcotic. In these cases, the anesthesiologist may order only hydroxyzine hydrochloride or diazepam. In a few instances, no preanesthetic medication is used. Belladonna alkaloids (atropine sulfate, scopolamine hydrochloride) are not advised for older clients because they make secretions tenacious and difficult to remove. In addition, scopolamine may cause postoperative delirium in the elderly (Dodd, 1976).

The anesthesiologist's decision to use local or general anesthesia depends upon the type of surgery and the older client's condition. In either case, the anesthesiologist uses special care with older clients because veins and mucous membranes can be easily damaged by technical procedures. Local anesthesia is advantageous in the very frail or ill client. It may be used for upper extremity operations and extraperitoneal operations below the umbilicus. Premedication is essential when local anesthesia is used (Mason et al., 1976). General anesthesia administered through an endotracheal tube is preferred for intraabdominal operations. A thiobarbiturate such as thiopental sodium (Pentothal sodium) is given intravenously to induce anesthesia (Dodd, 1976). If the older client has heart disease, oxygen by mask

is given prior to and during injection. Many older people, especially those who are severely ill, have poor laryngeal reflexes. During emergency surgery when the stomach may not be empty they run a major risk of regurgitation during the induction of anesthesia (Parkhurst, 1978). Nitrous oxide in concentrations of 50 to 60 percent with oxygen is usually used as a carrier gas during maintenance of anesthesia. Halogenated hydrocarbons, such as enflurane (Ethrane), halothane (Fluothane), and methoxyflurane (Penthrane) are used with nitrous oxide. A major advantage of these gases is that the client rapidly returns to consciousness. In deep anesthesia, the major risk in older clients is hypotension. These agents have also been implicated in postoperative hepatitis (Mason et al., 1976). As an alternative to the hydrocarbons, nitrous oxide may be used in combination with narcotics to produce anesthesia. If muscle relaxants are needed, the anesthesiologist uses either succinylcholine chloride, *d*-tubocurarine chloride, or pancuronium bromide (Pavulon). Because skeletal mass in older people has decreased in size and vigor, the dosage must be reduced to prevent overdose (Dodd, 1976).

The anesthesiologist monitors blood pressure, pulse rate, and respiratory rate at regular intervals. Temperature monitoring is recommended because of the high risk of hypothermia in older clients, especially when viscera are exposed and surgery is lengthy. Heart tones and breath sounds should be monitored by precordial or esophageal stethoscope. Electrocardiographic monitoring may also be performed, especially if the client has heart disease. The use of intermittent positive pressure breathing to prevent blood gas imbalances is controversial. The lung volume at which dependent zones of the lungs cease to ventilate due to airway closure increases with age and is exacerbated by the supine and head-down positions. Consequently, hypoxemia is more common in older people and adequate ventilation and oxygen therapy during surgery are important (Powell, 1981).

Requirements for fluid replacement during surgery are similar in the elderly and young. If the older client is to receive large volumes of fluid or has limited cardiac or pulmonary reserves, the central venous pressure (CVP) should be monitored to help gauge the rate and volume of fluid replacement.

Central venous pressure is not a totally reliable indicator of fluid load. Some clients pass from a state of hypovolemia to pulmonary edema before a significant elevation in the CVP is recorded, especially if large volumes of electrolyte solutions are given. For this reason, pulmonary wedge pressure may also be measured. Via a catheter passed through the right side of the heart and into a peripheral pulmonary artery, a pulmonary wedge pressure that approximates left atrial pressure can be measured, giving early warning of impending left ventricular failure. Continuous monitoring of urinary output also provides valuable data about the client's fluid balance.

Nursing Management. It is a fallacy that older clients are more resigned to surgery than young clients and therefore less apprehensive. The strange environment of the modern operating room with all its equipment can be a frightening experience for an older person. Without their eyeglasses or hearing aid, the strange sights and sounds are especially difficult to interpret. Older people about to undergo surgery need reassurance and sympathetic care.

It is important to remember that elderly clients have a loss of subcutaneous tissues. This tissue cushions against trauma and, without it, older people are prone to decubiti. The operating room nurse must ensure that the moving and positioning of the older client on the operating room table are done with care.

Normal postural changes with age result in a posture of general flexion. The head and neck are bent forward and the dorsal spine becomes kyphotic. Therefore, when lying supine, the occiput will remain in midair unless at least one pillow is used. Consequently, the nurse should assess the older client's posture and ensure that adequate support is provided for the neck and head (Parkhurst, 1978).

Because of normal joint changes as well as osteoporosis and arthritis care must be taken to prevent trauma when positioning older clients. The body should be in normal alignment. When under the influence of anesthesia, arthritic joints should not be stretched beyond their normal range of motion. If the client has had a stroke, the paralyzed extremities must be protected when positioning for surgery. Even when care is used, older clients may complain of stiffness and discomfort after surgery because of prolonged immobilization.

The ability to regulate temperature declines with age and heat loss occurs readily in older people, especially when viscera are exposed for long periods of time or substantial quantities of blood or fluids are given in the operating room. At temperatures of 89°F, bradycardia, atrial fibrillation, and cardiac arrest may occur. The nurse should be sure that the operating room temperature is maintained at a reasonable level. In addition, when not contraindicated, warming all intravenous fluids and using a warm saline lavage of the abdominal cavity help to prevent hypothermia (Mason et al., 1976).

Immediate Postoperative Care. The period of return of consciousness is potentially a very dangerous time. Constant observation and adequate monitoring are of paramount importance. Pulse, blood pressure, temperature, skin color, and respiratory rate and depth should be monitored in every client. In addition, the knowledgeable recovery room nurse remains alert for the client who "just doesn't look right" before one of these parameters changes measurably. Electrocardiogram monitoring is recommended for elderly clients who have undergone major surgery or have cardiac disease. After major procedures, hourly urinary output monitoring with an indwelling catheter should be performed. Central venous pressure and pulmonary wedge pressure may also be monitored. The wound and any drainage tubes must be kept under observation (Mason et al., 1976; Parkhurst, 1978). If the client's condition warrants, the physician may order hemoglobin, electrolyte, blood gas, or other laboratory studies.

In older people, protective reflexes are sluggish and may return slowly. Consequently the nurse should not leave clients unattended until they are fully able to protect their airway. Unless contraindicated by arthritis or other serious disability, the client should be in the lateral or prone position until return of consciousness is complete.

Respiratory difficulties in the immediate postoperative period are common especially in older people. Usually these are due to an overdose of narcotics, inadequate reversal of muscle relaxants, continuing effects of anesthesia, or underlying pulmonary disease (Powell, 1981; Mason et al., 1976).

Postoperative pain and restrictive dressings also interfere with respiration (Parkhurst, 1978). Every older person who has had general anesthesia should receive oxygen until fully conscious, preferably by nasal cannula (Mason et al., 1976). Hypoxemia has been documented in the elderly immediately after surgery and up to 10 days postoperatively (Powell, 1981). Arterial blood gas analysis can be made to determine the client's need for oxygen. An excellent way to assess the adequacy of the client's respiratory efforts is to measure tidal and minute volume with a Wright respirometer. The nurse should leave the endotracheal tube in place until the adequacy of respiration and competence of reflexes have been confirmed. Once the client has been extubated the nurse should initiate coughing and deep breathing at frequent intervals. If the client's respiratory efforts are inadequate, intermittent positive pressure ventilation may be continued in the early postoperative period. If prolonged ventilation is needed, volume-limited respirators are preferred because they assure adequate tidal volume.

Hypotension may also occur in the immediate postoperative period due to continuous bleeding or to insufficient fluid replacement. If hypotension is due to hypovolemia, central venous pressure and pulmonary wedge pressure should reflect the problem. To correct hypotension, the physician usually orders rapid replacement of fluid and blood under careful observation rather than vasopressor agents. If hypotension is not corrected promptly, renal damage, a stroke, or myocardial infarction can occur. Shock becomes irreversible more quickly in the elderly than in the young (Metheney and Snively, 1978).

Hypothermia may develop in the postoperative period after extensive surgical procedures. It should be treated with the use of warming blankets and mattresses and warming all intravenous fluids and blood.

Anesthesia is associated with distinctive mental status changes in the elderly. Most older people may be sufficiently awake to respond in the recovery room but have no memory of any events until several hours following the surgery. Therefore, the nurse needs to repeat any reassurance and instructions given in the recovery room at a later time.

Studies of men over age 50 indicate that they need at least 7 to 9 hours to recover a minimum of 60 percent of normal mental efficiency (comparable to the level recorded after a totally sleepless night). These findings have implications for older people undergoing day surgery. The nurse should ensure that these clients are accompanied home by a responsible person and not allowed to drive for 24 hours.

If older clients do not return to consciousness as expected, the reason may be an overdose of premedication or anesthesia. Hypothermia and hypoglycemia are other reasons for delayed recovery of consciousness. Some degree of transient disorientation and restlessness is normal when older clients first emerge from anesthesia. If these persist the nurse should consider other reasons for them, including hypoxemia, drug effects, fluid and electrolyte imbalance, surgical pain, a full bladder, or infiltration of the intravenous infusion. In addition, if the client's position strains tender joints, restlessness may develop. In a few older people, cerebrovascular accident, embolism, and myocardial infarction are the reason for confusion and other mental status changes following surgery (Parkhurst, 1978). If the older client is moved from the recovery room to an intensive care unit, the possibility of postoperative delirium is increased. The problem can range from mild confusion to total psychotic disorientation due to a variety of environmental and physiological factors, including loss of the sleep cycle and an inability to keep track of time by normal changes in light. Transfer from the intensive care unit is one way to hasten recovery from delirium of this type (Mason et al., 1976).

Although it is true that older people are more tolerant of pain than younger people, they should not be expected to endure more pain for longer periods without relief. Evaluating an older client's need for pain relief requires clinical judgment. Pain medication is usually prescribed in small doses to avoid suppressing the client's cough reflex or causing hypotension and even coma in frail older people. However, clients need to receive enough pain medication so that incisional pain will not prevent deep breathing and coughing. Parkhurst (1978) recommends that older clients be given small doses of analgesics early in the postoperative period in anticipation of pain. Further small doses should be given when the client indicates awareness of discomfort.

General Postoperative Care. During the postoperative period, nursing care is directed at helping the client adapt to the stress of surgery in an optimal fashion. Emphasis is placed on preventing the postoperative complications for which the older client is at high risk. These include respiratory complications, infection, venous thrombosis, fluid and electrolyte imbalance, and renal insufficiency.

Preventing Respiratory Complications. Because pulmonary complications are especially hazardous in the elderly who have marginal pulmonary reserves, every effort should be made to prevent them. Atelectasis, pneumonia, and congestive heart failure are the most common reasons for postoperative respiratory distress in the aged. The nurse should be certain that the client performs coughing and deep breathing at regular intervals. Early ambulation should be practiced because it stimulates breathing. The upright position alone increases lung capacity up to 15 to 20 percent, thus decreasing the possibility of atelectasis. Ambulating an older person often requires the assistance of one or two people, but it is essential. Use of blow bottles and intermittent positive pressure breathing treatments also aids in preventing or correcting atelectasis. Because inhalation therapy equipment is a possible source of infection, the nurse must make sure that the client's equipment is scrupulously clean. The nurse should also observe for abdominal distention and see that abdominal dressings and binders are not overly tight, since both of these tend to force the diaphragm up and promote atelectasis. The physician may order nasogastric suction to prevent gastric distention.

Preventing Infection. For an infectious agent to invade tissue it must be present at a susceptible site and in an adequate concentration. Unlike young adults, the elderly are at risk for infection even when relatively small amounts of infectious organisms are present. The older person's ability to resist infection is compromised by the status of the defense mechanisms, poor nutrition, poor metabolic function, medication, and disease. After surgery, older clients are at risk for wound infections and infections of the urinary and respiratory tract. Urinary tract in-

fections are twice as common in the elderly as in the young and directly proportional to the need for catheterization (Mason et al., 1976). Sterile technique must be maintained whenever catheterization is necessary. Wound infections are no more common in older people than in the young. However, every effort must be made to prevent them because older people react poorly to infection. To prevent wound infections in the postoperative period the nurse needs to ensure that strict sterile technique is used during dressing changes. The physician usually removes drains as soon as useful function no longer exists, which is usually on the second or third postoperative day. Skin sutures are usually removed 1 week postoperatively unless the client is poorly nourished.

Preventing Venous Thrombosis. Venous thrombosis is a common and potentially serious postoperative complication. Although clients of all ages are at risk for this complication, the elderly are at highest risk when they are kept in bed. Venous thrombosis may occur in the superficial veins, but generally only thrombosis of the deep veins of the legs and pelvis is serious because of the potential for pulmonary emboli. Factors that place the elderly postoperative client at risk for venous thrombosis include reduction of venous circulation to the legs due to bed rest, cardiac problems, and local venous compression; injury to veins from surgery, venous catheters, or adjacent inflammatory reactions; and hypercoagulability due to injury or disease.

Preventative nursing action includes careful assessment coupled with active and passive exercise, use of antiemboli stockings, and elevating the foot of the bed (p. 483). In the postoperative client, early ambulation may be the most important measure for preventing venous thrombosis.

Preventing Fluid and Electrolyte Imbalances. Because of their reduced adaptive capacity, the elderly are at high risk for a variety of fluid and electrolyte disturbances in the postoperative period. Their degree of risk depends in part on their preoperative nutritional status and the extent of the surgical procedure. The body normally responds to injury by increasing aldosterone and antidiuretic hormone. Therefore for several days after surgery the body retains sodium and water. If the older client has reduced cardiovascular function, excessive fluid administration must be avoided in this period. The nurse monitors urine and other sources of fluid loss so that fluids can be replaced. Usually the elderly client requires 1.5 to 2.5 liters of fluid in 24 hours. Excessive amounts of fluid may be sequestered after surgery, especially if the client develops ileus. The sequestered fluid is not available for use and increases the client's fluid requirement postoperatively. Paralytic ileus is especially common in older people because of bowel edema, peritonitis, or handling of the intestines during surgery. The nurse should assess the client regularly for abdominal distention, bowel sounds, and the passing of flatus. Once any sequestered fluid is remobilized the nurse must be alert for signs of fluid overload.

In the early postoperative period when the client retains sodium, requirements for sodium are minimal. Clients should receive about 75 mEq of sodium per 24 hours to prevent hyponatremia (Mason et al., 1976). If the client has nasogastric suction or diarrhea, sodium requirements are increased. Water intoxication can develop in the aged if the client receives excessive amounts of carbohydrate and water. Adaptations include behavior changes, weight gain, headache, blurred vision, incoordination, convulsions, and coma (Metheney and Snively, 1978).

Because potassium is not retained postoperatively, older clients with adequate renal function require 40 to 60 mEq potassium per 24 hours. It is essential to maintain serum potassium levels, especially if the client is receiving digitalis. After most surgical procedures clients should receive 100 to 150 g glucose in order to minimize protein and fat catabolism. A weight loss of up to one-half pound is expected (Mason et al., 1976). Once older clients are permitted to eat the nurse must assure that they receive enough assistance to permit optimal nutrition.

Preventing Renal Insufficiency. The older client with preexisting renal disease is at high risk in the postoperative phase. Oliguric renal failure is most common but high output renal failure also occurs. Both cause azotemia with blood urea nitrogen levels over 30 mg/dl and serum creatinine levels over 3 mg/dl. Fluid and electrolyte depletion in the postoperative period is the most common reason for renal failure, but the use of nephrotoxic antibiotics

(gentamicin, Kanamycin, and colistin), the use of the anesthetic agent methoxyflurane and the prolonged use of vasopressor agents may also be responsible. The older client may be maintained on peritoneal dialysis or hemodialysis (Mason et al., 1976). In most cases, efforts are made to control the stress responsible for the renal failure. The client is placed on fluid restriction and actions are taken to control azotemia and hyperkalemia. Spontaneous diuresis occurs in 1 to 2 weeks, but months may pass before normal renal function develops.

Summary. Older people are able to adapt successfully to the stresses of anesthesia and surgery. To do so, however, they require a thorough assessment and careful management by all members of the surgical team. The nurse plays an integral role in the client's care in the preoperative, intraoperative, and postoperative phases. Extensive preoperative planning is especially important in successful management of the intraoperative and postoperative periods.

Preventing Complications in the Immobile Aged Client

Why the Elderly Are at High Risk. Many of the stresses that affect the elderly place them at high risk for physical immobility. Although exercise is being encouraged for others in our society, many older people are still being advised, "Take it easy, since you are not getting any younger." Such advice is based on the false belief that people are born with limited energy resources and should expend less and less energy as they grow old so as not to run out of it. Modern conveniences such as automobiles and elevators also promote immobility. The result is that many older people move very little. Normal aging changes in nerves, muscles, bones, and joints are magnified because the older person is out of condition. Chronic health problems that affect the elderly may also restrict mobility. Older clients with poor eyesight may restrict their mobility because they cannot maintain their balance or avoid obstacles. Pain in the joints or feet can prevent walking. Clients with angina and peripheral vascular disease may avoid even minimal exercise. Acute illness is another common reason for immobility in the aged. For example, older clients may be confined to bed at home and upon recovering may find that they are unable to stand. Older clients who are mobile may be hospitalized and during their stay become immobile. Bed rest is a necessary, but risky, intervention for many health problems that affect the elderly.

Special Hazards in the Elderly.   The hazards of immobility due to bed rest have been well documented. They affect every body system as well as the psychosocial spheres of life. For the older client, the hazards develop earlier and last longer (Gore, 1972). Although young people may be immobilized for long periods without developing irreversible adaptations, older clients, even those who are initially well, deteriorate rapidly when placed on bed rest. Special risks that face the immobile older person include contractures, osteoporosis, urinary calculi, dehydration, decubiti, thromboemboli, and pulmonary emboli. These are discussed here. Other common complications include respiratory infection (p. 480) and incontinence and constipation discussed in Chapter 17. Limiting the hazards of immobility is the nurse's responsibility. By preventing these complications the nurse also limits the length of time the client is immobilized.

Contractures.   Immobility affects joints, bones, and muscles. Contractures are fixed deformities that result when joints are held immobile. At first, contractures can be corrected by passive movement. Eventually, however, fibrosis of periarticular structures, tightening of tendons, and weakening, shortening, and atrophy of muscles take place. These changes can be corrected only by dangerous and tedious surgery and casting procedures. Older people are at high risk for contractures. They tend to flex their arms and legs when lying in bed. Clients with neuromuscular and joint diseases may develop contractures after only a few days of bed rest. The most common contractures in the elderly are at the knee and hip joints. A person affected in this way may be able to stand and walk only with great difficulty.

When the elderly client is bedridden, preventative nursing care involves frequent passive range of motion exercise to keep joints straight and active exercise to prevent muscle wasting. When positioning the client, flexion postures should be avoided.

Pillows should not be placed under the knees. The nurse needs to ensure that elderly clients who are able to sit in chairs also receive range of motion exercises. Very old people can develop ninety degree contractures at the knees and hips simply by sitting still all day and lying at night without straightening their legs.

Osteoporosis, Urinary Calculi, and Dehydration. Bed rest or immobilization in any form increases osteoporosis and complicates the osteoporosis of aging (Chapter 15). The extent to which this process is reversed when the client is remobilized is still debated by experts (Exton-Smith, 1978). The loss of calcium from bones results in increased fecal calcium excretion and urine calcium rates as high as 500 mg per day. Hypercalciuria, especially when combined with urinary stasis associated with the supine position, places the older client at high risk for stone formation.

In order to stimulate osteoblastic activity, mechanical stress is required. Weight bearing, oscillating beds, and active exercise help to minimize bone loss. The nurse also needs to assure that the immobilized client receives enough fluid to facilitate urine calcium excretion. A jug of water and a glass at the bedside are insufficient for most older clients, as they are often unable to reach or handle this equipment or unwilling to drink fluids for fear of incontinence. This problem not only increases the risk of urinary calculi but places the elderly at risk for dehydration. The nurse should look for signs of dehydration, including sunken cheeks, a dry brown tongue, increasing confusion, and an elevated blood urea nitrogen. Every immobile client should be kept on intake and output. Without this record, the nurse cannot observe for urinary problems.

Decubiti.   When immobilized, the elderly are more likely than any other age group to develop decubiti. Many have sensory deficits so that they have no warning that a problem is developing. Because of motor deficits and pain, many are unable or unwilling to change position. Other problems that place the elderly at high risk for decubiti are obesity, anemia, poor nutrition, circulatory deficiency, incontinence, and confusion.

Decubiti are the result of prolonged pressure over a bony prominence so that tissues are deprived of blood and die. Friction, shearing stresses, and traumatized, infected, and wet skin contribute to the development of decubiti. Muscle and fat layers are more vulnerable than the dermis. The areas of highest risk are the heels, greater trochanters, sacrum, elbows, scapular spines, and the dorsal spine in thin, kyphotic individuals. In very vulnerable older clients, the knees may break down due to the weight of bedcovers and the head and ears can develop sores due to contact with the pillows.

To prevent decubiti, the nurse must change the client's position at regular intervals both day and night. If clients protest about losing sleep to be turned, the nurse can explain the importance of this intervention. Skill is needed to turn and reposition clients by lifting them rather than dragging them across the sheets. Vulnerable areas must be kept clean and dry and massaged with powder. Heel protectors should be used routinely to prevent skin breakdown. Pillows, pneumatic rings, and foam supports are also useful to prevent pressure areas. A bedcradle is especially valuable for elderly clients to remove the weight of the bedcovers from the feet and knees. Many other devices such as special mattresses and beds are also available but these should never substitute for fundamental nursing care.

Venous Thrombosis. Bed rest predisposes clients of all ages, but especially the elderly, to thrombosis of superficial and deep veins. The nurse should make daily assessments of the client for adaptations to venous thrombosis. Adaptations to superficial phlebitis are usually readily apparent and include pain, tenderness, and erythema over the palpable thrombus. Adaptations to deep vein thrombosis are more difficult to assess. The client may complain of a vague ache or tightness in the leg. Fever, tachycardia, and leukocytosis may be present; however, these adaptations are common in many conditions and following surgery. The nurse should inspect and measure the girth of the legs. Swelling and possibly pitting edema in one leg may indicate thrombosis. Bilateral swelling is very widespread in the elderly and complicates the assessment. If venous thrombosis is present, a slight prominence of the venous system, slight cyanosis, or rubor may be seen. The affected leg may feel appreciably warmer. The nurse should palpate gently for tenderness and observe for calf pain produced by dorsiflexion (Homan's sign). To aid the physician in making a diagnosis of deep vein thrombosis, Doppler ultrasound equipment is available to detect abnormal venous flow patterns in the legs.

Nurses can take several measures to prevent venous thrombosis. Passive and active leg exercises are especially important for older clients, who tend to be less active in bed than younger clients. Made to measure, graduated elastic support stockings are also of value. Stockings are available in knee length, thigh length, and full leg length. The stockings should be removed for 30 minutes each shift so that air can reach the skin. Ready made elastic stockings and poorly applied elastic bandages should not be used. Frequently these are tighter proximally on the leg than distally and promote rather than prevent venous stasis. Elevating the foot of the bed is also effective in preventing venous thrombosis.

If the client develops superficial thrombosis, treatment includes rest, elevation of the feet, local heat application, and anticoagulation therapy if the process is widespread. Treatment of deep vein thrombosis is more aggressive in order to prevent long-term venous stasis and pulmonary emboli. This serious and sometimes fatal complication of deep venous thrombosis occurs most often in the elderly. Heparin administration is continued for 7 to 10 days; before it is discontinued, clients are given oral Coumadin, which is continued for several months. Bed rest is maintained until the adaptations subside and oral anticoagulants are begun. Then ambulation with elastic stockings is gradually initiated. The client is taught never to sit with the legs down (Avioli, 1976; Agate, 1979).

If the client develops venous thrombosis, the nurse observes for adaptations to pulmonary emboli. The classic adaptations of dyspnea, chest pain, hemoptysis, fever, rales, tachycardia, and reduced blood pressure may or may not be present in the elderly. If the physician is uncertain about the diagnosis, a lung scan may be ordered. However, this test is also difficult to interpret because other respiratory diseases that affect the elderly give an identical picture (Avioli, 1976).

Summary. Immobility is to be avoided in the elderly. Some older people may not understand the importance of remaining active in spite of their natural inclination to slow down as they age. Immobility may be unavoidable when the older client is ill. When bed rest is mandatory, excellent nursing care is the key to preventing the hazards of immobility in the aged.

SUMMARY

This chapter focused on the care of the elderly client with a hip fracture not only because this is one of the most common orthopedic problems among the elderly but because it is a frequent reason why older people experience immobilization, hospitalization, and surgery. However, age-related and pathological changes place the elderly at high risk for serious complications whenever they experience immobilization, hospitalization, or surgery. The nursing interventions discussed in this chapter can minimize the hazards of immobility and promote optimal adaptation during hospitalization and surgery.

REFERENCES

Agate J: Common symptoms and complaints, in Rossman I (ed), Clinical Geriatrics, 2nd ed. Philadelphia, Lippincott, 1979

Anderson F Sir: Practical Management of the Elderly, 3rd ed. Oxford, Blackwell Scientific Publications, 1976

Avioli LV: Aging, bone, and osteoporosis, in Steinberg FU (ed), Cowdry's The Care of the Geriatric Patient, 5th ed. St. Louis, Mosby, 1976

Bagwell M, Ludlow E: The elderly patient in the hospital. Supervisor Nurse 110(2):32, 1980

Boardman KD: Fractures in an elderly population in a psychiatric hospital. Nursing Mirror 144(9):52, 1977

Bonner CD: Medical Care and Rehabilitation of the Aged and Chronically Ill, 3rd ed. Boston, Little, Brown, 1974

Brotman H: Every ninth American, in Developments in Aging 1978. I. A Report of the Special Committee on Aging, United States Senate. Washington, D.C., U.S. Government Printing Office, 1979, p 20

Butler RN, Lewis MI: Aging and Mental Health, 2nd ed. St. Louis, Mosby, 1977

Charlesworth D, Baker RH: Surgery in old age, in Brocklehurst JC (ed), Textbook of Geriatric Medicine and Gerontology, 2nd ed. New York, Churchill Livingstone, 1978

Devas M: Orthopedics, in Steinberg FU (ed), Cowdry's The Care of the Geriatric Patient, 5th ed. St. Louis, Mosby, 1976

Dodd RB: Anesthesia, in Steinberg FU (ed), Cowdry's The Care of the Geriatric Patient, 5th ed. St. Louis, Mosby, 1976

Dunnery E: Fractured hip. RN 42(6):45, 1979

Elkowitz EB: Geriatric Medicine for the Primary Care Practitioner. New York, Springer, 1981

Exton-Smith AN: Clinical manifestations, in Exton-Smith AN, Evans JG (eds), Care of the Elderly: Meeting the Challenge of Dependency. London, Academic, 1977

Exton-Smith AN: Bone aging and metabolic bone disease, in Brocklehurst JC (ed), Textbook of Geriatric Medicine and Gerontology, 2nd ed. New York, Churchill Livingstone, 1978

Feist RR: A survery of accidental falls in a small home for the aged. Journal of Gerontological Nursing 4(6):15, 1978

Filner B, Williams TF: Health promotion for the elderly reducing functional dependency, in Somers AR, Fabian DR (eds), The Geriatric Imperative. New York, Appleton-Century-Crofts, 1981

Glenn F: Pre- and postoperative management of elderly surgical patients. Journal of the American Geriatrics Society 21:385, 1973

Gore I: Physical activity in old age. Nursing Mirror 142(7):48, 1976

Gore IY: Physical activity and aging—A survey of Soviet literature. Gerontologica Clinica 14:65, 1972

Green MF: Metabolic emergencies, in Coakley D (ed), Acute Geriatric Medicine. Littleton, MA, PSG Publishing, 1981

Green MF: Endocrinology in the elderly, in Anderson WF, Judge TG (ed), Geriatric Medicine. London, Academic, 1974

Hielema FJ: Epidemiology of hip fracture. Physical Therapy 59(10):1221, 1979

Johnson RE, Specht EE: The risk of hip fracture in postmenopausal females with and without estrogen drug exposure. American Journal of Public Health 71(2):138, 1981

Jones E: Immobilization syndrome in the elderly. Nursing Times 72(26):1009, 1976

Kahana E, Kahana B: Health care facilities, in Steinberg FU (ed), Cowdry's the Care of the Geriatric Patient, 5th ed. St. Louis, Mosby, 1976

Kemp J: Planning hospital care. Nursing Times 74(5):198, 1978

Kolodny AL, Klipper AR: Bone and joint diseases in the elderly. Hospital Practice 11(11):91, 1976

Kovar MG: Health and health care of the elderly. Public Health Reports 92:9, 1977

Lore A: Supporting the hospitalized elderly person. American Journal of Nursing 79(3):496, 1979

Mason JH, Gau FC, Byrne MP: General surgery, in Steinberg FU (ed), Cowdry's The Care of the Geriatric Patient, 5th ed. St. Louis, Mosby, 1976

Medicare. Inpatient Utilization of Short-Stay Hospitals by Diagnosis, 1973. Research and Statistics Note No. 5. DHEW, HCFA, Office of Policy, Planning and Research, U.S. Government Printing Office, Washington, D.C., June 1978

Metheney NA, Snively WD: Perioperative fluids and electrolytes. American Journal of Nursing 78(5):840, 1978

Marcinek MB: Stress in the surgical patient. American Journal of Nursing 17(11):1809, 1977

Parkhurst J: Anesthesia in old age, in Brocklehurst, JC (ed), Textbook of Geriatric Medicine and Gerontology, 2nd ed. New York, Churchill Livingstone, 1978

Pont A: Management of osteoporosis, in Ebaugh FG (ed), Management of Common Problems in Geriatric Medicine. Menlo Park, CA, Addison Wesley, 1981

Powell DR: Emergency anaesthesia in the elderly, in Coakley D (ed), Acute Geriatric Medicine. Littleton, MA, PSG Publishing, 1981

Quinn JL, Ryan NE: O.R. nursing assessment. AORN Journal 29(2):236, 1979

Rossman I: Environments of geriatric care, in Rossman I (ed), Clinical Geriatrics, 2nd ed. Philadelphia, Lippincott, 1979

Sandler RB: Etiology of primary osteoporosis: An hypothesis. Journal of the American Geriatrics Society 26:209, 1978

Todd R: Fractures of the femur. Nursing Mirror 144(11):62, 1977

Vallarino A, Sherman FT: Principles of rehabilitation treatment, in Libow LS, Sherman FT (eds), The Core of Geriatric Medicine: A Guide for Students and Practitioners. St. Louis, Mosby, 1981

Vital Statistics. U.S. Department of H.E.W.: Utilization of Short-Stay Hospitals, United States, 1971. July 22, 1973

Vital Statistics. U.S. Department of H.E.W.: Utilization of Short-Stay Hospitals by Diagnosis, United States, 1972. July 18, 1974

Wallach S: Management of osteoporosis. Hospital Practice 13(12):91, 1978

Williams MA, Holloway JR, et al: Nursing activities and acute confusional states in elderly hip fractured patients. Nursing Research 28(1):25, 1979

Witte NS: Why the elderly fall. American Journal of Nursing 79(11):1950, 1979

Woogara R: Sub-trochanteric fracture of femur. Nursing Times 73(51):1986, 1977

Wylie CM: Hospitalization for fractures and bone loss in adults. Public Health Reports 92(1):33, 1977

Yen PK: Nutrition: Fractures and diet—What's the relationship? Geriatric Nursing 2(6):327, 1981

20

Nursing the Client Experiencing Acute Problems of Regulation

Normal, healthy aging depends upon the synergistic interaction of complex neurological, hormonal, metabolic, and immunological mechanisms. This chapter explores two stresses that alter important regulatory functions in the elderly—cancer and cataracts.

Cancer could be considered a disease of aging. Its increasing frequency has been related directly to the extension of the human life span. Yet in some ways, normal aging changes and malignant changes are diametrically opposed. Malignancy interferes with growth regulation and leads to accelerated, uncontrolled growth. In contrast, normal cells from aging persons show slowed, reduced growth (Jarvik, 1979).

Although some diminution in neurosensory function is an unavoidable part of the aging process, severe disability need not permanently impair the older person's ability to function. Cataracts are the most common visual problem affecting the aged. They represent a disturbance in metabolic function that is not fully understood (Kornzweig, 1979).

Advanced medical and surgical interventions and combination therapies are available to treat these two problems of regulation. Despite their advanced years, older people deserve the same vigorous intervention afforded to the young. Some health professionals and family members are reluctant to consider these therapies for the elderly, believing that older people have already suffered enough or that expensive resources should not be expended on those who have already enjoyed many years of life. Alternatively, what would the future be like for the older person if treatment were withheld? Who would care for the older client if these problems were allowed to take their course? Older clients have the right to assess for themselves the impact of various treatment options and to make informed decisions about their care. The nurse can give older clients neutral information about treatment alternatives and support them while they consider their options. Many clients with problems of regulation can be completely cured. When this is not possible, interventions are available to minimize suffering, promote independence, and improve the quality of life remaining.

Because of sensory, perceptual, or social isolation, clients with cancer or cataracts are at risk for sensory deprivation. Nursing interventions to minimize this problem are discussed in this chapter. Interventions to correct problems affecting regulatory functions often involve hospitalization. When treatment is completed, older clients need help to make the transition from hospital to community. This chapter explores the nurse's role in discharge planning.

SIGNIFICANT PROBLEMS

Cancer

Cancer is not one disease, but a large group of diseases characterized by the uncontrolled growth and spread of abnormal cells. It can affect every organ and system of the body. If the spread is not checked, it results in death. Although the topic of cancer is vast, this chapter focuses on those aspects of the problem and its management that pertain specifically to the elderly.

Precipitating Stresses.   Malignancy has been seen as a phenomenon closely linked with aging itself. Although aging is not a direct cause of cancer, several possible mechanisms associated with aging may account for the relationship between aging and cancer. The relationship of malignancy to age could be due in part to accumulation of or repeated contact with chemical, physical, or biological carcinogens, to the effects of a slowly acting carcinogen over a prolonged period, to a prolonged preexposure period, or to a reduction in exposure for successive cohorts (Hodkinson, 1978). For example, the relationship between bone cancer and radioactive paint became apparent only 10 to 25 years after workers who had used such paint began to develop cancer. There may be a delay of 20 years between asbestos exposure and the development of bronchogenic carcinoma (Serpick, 1978).

Age-related changes in immune functions and a decline in immunological competence may set the stage for an increase in cancer in the elderly. The number of circulating lymphocytes declines due to a reduction in the number of T cells. B cells, which are responsible for the quick destruction of all abnormal cells in the body, suffer a decline in function and are no longer able to do so efficiently (Clifford and Bewtra, 1979). With age, the body's ability to repair itself also declines, allowing more abnormal cells to be produced. Although many cancers arise and are destroyed early by the immune system in younger people, the immune system in the elderly is less effective. A decline in certain hormones with age and the accumulation of exposure to many antigenic stimuli may contribute to the decline in host resistance in older people (Serpick, 1978). An increased incidence in autoimmune phenomena in old age has also been documented, and there is a higher incidence of malignancy in organs under immune attack (Hodkinson, 1978).

Epidemiology.   Cancer is more common in the elderly than the young. In general, both cancer incidence and cancer deaths rise with age and are highest among the oldest. Although the elderly comprise only 11 percent of the U.S. population,

over 60 percent of all malignancies occur in people over 60 years of age (Third National Cancer Survey, 1975). The longer a person lives, the more likely he or she is to develop cancer.

Incidence.   A very few sites account for most malignancies in the elderly. Skin cancer is almost exclusively a disease of older persons. An estimated 400,000 new cases occur each year (American Cancer Society, 1983). Excluding skin cancer, half of all cancers in the elderly arise in only four areas—the prostate, breast, lung, and gastrointestinal tract. In men ages 75 and older the prostate accounts for 25 percent of all cancers. At least 80 percent of men over age 85 have prostate cancer. Cancers of the stomach, large intestine, and rectum account for an additional 25 percent of cancers in men over age 75. Among women over age 75, 21 percent of all cancers occur in the breast and 28 percent in the stomach, large intestine, and rectum (Serpick, 1978).

Only a few cancers deviate from the expected age-related rise. Wilms's tumor, osteogenic sarcoma, and neuroblastoma are characteristic of childhood. Carcinoma of the testis peaks sharply and declines after age 30. Carcinoma of the cervix rises at age 30 and peaks at age 45. Cancers that peak in childhood and early adult life may be due to heightened mitotic activity in the tissue or to a brief exposure to a carcinogenic agent (Rossman, 1979).

Some cancers seem to occur almost exclusively in the elderly. As mentioned earlier, skin cancer, which affects more men than women, is predominantly a disease of older persons. Carcinoma of the prostate occurs almost exclusively in men over age 50. Nine out of ten cases are discovered in men over age 60. Carcinoma of the bladder is a relatively uncommon disease but is seen almost exclusively in older people, particularly men. Multiple myeloma is occurring with increasing frequency, but 80 percent of cases occur in people over age 50. Men are more likely to be affected than women. Although the public has the impression that leukemia is a childhood disease, it is another cancer primarily of older people. Mortality rates for groups over age 45 are higher than for those under age 15. The most common form of leukemia in older adults is chronic lymphocytic leukemia. Men have a higher death rate than women. Two types of gynecologic malignancies occur predominantly after age 60. One is carcinoma of the vulva and vagina. The other, carcinoma of the endometrium, particularly affects elderly obese women who are diabetics.

Mortality. In the United States, cancer is the leading cause of death after heart disease (Table 1).

Cancer mortality rates provide a distorted picture of the prevalence of malignancy in the elderly. The death certificate identifies the primary cause of death; however, many clients with cancer die *with* malignant disease rather than *of* it. Some other disease, such as cardiovascular or lung disease, overtakes the cancer and is responsible for the person's death.

TABLE 1. MORTALITY, TEN LEADING CAUSES OF DEATH, BY AGE GROUP AND SEX, UNITED STATES, 1978

	Ages 55–74		Ages 75+	
	Male	*Female*	*Male*	*Female*
1.	Heart diseases 191,713	Heart diseases 99,994	Heart diseases 160,793	Heart diseases 216,286
2.	Cancer 120,955	Cancer 90,016	Cancer 62,863	Cerebrovascular diseases 72,229
3.	Cerebrovascular diseases 27,169	Cerebrovascular diseases 24,543	Cerebrovascular diseases 41,076	Cancer 58,656
4.	Accidents 12,359	Diabetes 8,350	Pneumonia, influenza 17,223	Pneumonia, influenza 19,437
5.	Chronic obstructive lung diseases 11,208	Accidents 6,313	Chronic obstructive lung diseases 8,735	Arteriosclerosis 15,328
6.	Cirrhosis of liver 10,152	Pneumonia, influenza 5,315	Arteriosclerosis 8,710	Diabetes 9,789
7.	Pneumonia, influenza 9,472	Cirrhosis of liver 5,053	Accidents 7,036	Accidents 8,027
8.	Diabetes 6,843	Chronic obstructive lung diseases 4,297	Diabetes 4,954	Chronic obstructive lung diseases 3,041
9.	Emphysema 6,570	Emphysema 2,211	Emphysema 4,601	Pulmonary infarction 2,739
10.	Aortic aneurysm 5,243	Pulmonary infarction 2,101	Cirrhosis of liver 4,047	Aortic aneurysm 2,501

Source: Vital Statistics of the United States, 1978.

This phenomenon is especially true in the elderly. Nevertheless, cancer mortality rates are highest in the elderly regardless of whether the overall death rate for a particular cancer is increasing, decreasing or remaining the same.

Table 2 identifies the most common causes of cancer deaths in men and women ages 55 to 74 and over age 75. Among men over age 55, lung cancer accounts for the most cancer deaths, followed by cancer of the colon and rectum. Among women in this age group, breast cancer accounts for the most cancer deaths, followed closely by cancer of the colon and rectum.

Prognosis. A widely held opinion exists that cancers grow more slowly, are less aggressive, and less likely to metastasize in the elderly. Although this pattern is characteristic of some malignancies in the elderly, it is not true of all malignancies. In fact, the decline in metastasis noted in the elderly population may exist because the elderly are frequently afflicted by intercurrent diseases that become fatal before there is time for the development of metastatic cancer and not because the cancer is less aggressive (Rossman, 1979; Hodkinson, 1978).

One cancer that does have a better prognosis in the elderly is cancer of the breast. Although older women are more likely than younger ones to develop breast cancer, the more removed from menopause, the less aggressive the disease will be. Because of hormonal factors that are poorly understood, this tumor grows more slowly in older women. It tends to metastasize to the bone and soft tissues in the elderly, and not to the liver and lungs. Both bone and soft tissues are more amenable to palliative treatment than are the liver and lungs.

Some other malignancies are more aggressive in the aged. Papillary carcinoma of the thyroid gland is relatively benign and easily treatable in young women, but in women over 65 it is more aggressive and more likely to metastasize. One type of thyroid carcinoma, undifferentiated anaplastic carcinoma, occurs almost exclusively in women in their late 60s or older and results in early death. Malignant melanoma is more common and more aggressive in the elderly, especially in females. Evidently, hormonal factors are involved in its behavior.

Some malignancies appear to have the same prognosis in the young and old. These include cancers of the gastrointestinal tract, oral cavity, larynx, and lung (Serpick, 1978).

Cataracts

Under ideal conditions, the eye is able to function at an optimal level for over 100 years. Normal visual acuity has been reported in individuals over age 90

TABLE 2. MORTALITY, FIVE LEADING CANCER SITES, BY AGE AND SEX, UNITED STATES, 1978

	Ages 55–74		Ages 75+	
	Male	*Female*	*Male*	*Female*
1.	Lung 46,049	Breast 17,403	Lung 14,646	Colon and rectum 12,626
2.	Colon and rectum 13,717	Lung 14,463	Prostate 12,298	Breast 8,129
3.	Prostate 9,047	Colon and rectum 12,551	Colon and rectum 9,325	Lung 4,819
4.	Pancreas 6,490	Ovary 5,992	Pancreas 3,208	Pancreas 3,939
5.	Stomach 4,558	Uterus 5,480	Bladder 3,172	Uterus 2,954

Source: Vital Statistics of the United States, 1978.

(Kornzweig, 1979). Nevertheless, changes in visual ability are commonplace in old age due to normal aging changes and to local and systemic pathology.

Diabetic retinopathy, glaucoma, macular degeneration, and cataracts are the most common pathological problems affecting the aging eye. These problems cannot be corrected with glasses. Diabetic retinopathy, described in Chapter 16, is responsible for about half the blindness encountered among the aged. The prevalence of glaucoma in individuals over age 65 is from 5 to 10 percent. Glaucoma, an abnormal increase in intraocular pressure, causes loss of vision and visual field. Macular degeneration affects about 30 percent of the elderly. Individuals sustain a gradual loss of central vision while retaining peripheral vision. Clients retain the ability to move about and care for themselves, but lose the ability to read and do other close work (Kornzweig, 1977).

This chapter focuses on the most common pathological problem of the aging eye—the formation of a cataract (Anderson, 1976). Everyone who lives long enough will develop a cataract (Kornzweig, 1977). Although some degree of cataract is present in virtually every person over age 70 (Marmor, 1981), cataracts become a stress that threatens the client's adaptation in about 5 percent of the elderly population (Exton-Smith and Overstall, 1979). Despite surgical advances to remove cataracts, they remain a major cause of blindness among the elderly (Kwitko, 1978).

Definition. The term cataract refers to any opacity of the lens whether or not it interferes with vision (Kahn, 1981). The lens is located behind the pupil and iris and is fixed by a series of suspensory ligaments called zonules. It is a small disc of transparent tissue contained within a hyaline capsule much like a cellophane wrapper. The lens helps to focus images onto the retina in the back of the eye. It has no blood supply and is dependent upon the aqueous humor for its nutrition. With age, metabolic activity in the lens undergoes a normal decline (Exton-Smith and Overstall, 1979).

The Process of Cataract Formation. The stresses responsible for cataract development as well as the process of their development are poorly understood. Numerous metabolic changes have been associated with cataract formation. Three substances are present in large amounts in the normal lens—polypeptide glutathione, ascorbic acid, and riboflavin. All three have been found to be greatly reduced or absent in the cataractous lens (Kahn, 1981). Low-molecular-weight proteins, as well as sodium, potassium, calcium, and magnesium, have been found in abnormal amounts in some types of cataracts. In addition, some lens enzymes demonstrate reduced activity (Leight, 1978). Although these metabolic changes are only incompletely understood, they are believed to be responsible for changes in the molecular structure of lens proteins that cause the lens to lose its pristine transparency and gradually become opaque.

Many factors known to trigger disturbances in the normal metabolism of the lens have been associated with cataract development. These include trauma, systemic diseases such as diabetes mellitus and hyperparathyroidism, inflammation, infection, radiation, electrical shock, heat, cold, and toxic chemicals including certain drugs. Systemic and local corticosteroid preparations have been implicated in cataract formation (Elkowitz, 1981, Kahn, 1981; Smith, 1978; Kornzweig, 1979). It is well known that cataract formation is influenced by hereditary tendencies that appear to be transmitted by a dominant pattern (Kaspar, 1978).

Although cataracts sometimes develop in young people due to genetic factors, trauma, or inflammation, most cataracts occur in the elderly. These are called senile cataracts. They almost always affect both eyes but they often develop at quite different rates. Senile cataracts fall into two major categories—cortical cataracts and nuclear cataracts. In its optimal state, the lens is perfectly clear and transparent, transmitting and refracting rays of light onto the retina. As the lens ages, new fibers are constantly being produced and old fibers are compressed toward the center of the lens away from the capsule. Hence, the lens becomes larger and more rigid with age. The old lens fibers lose their transparency due to changes in their molecular structure and deposition of pigment and assume a yellow or yellow-brown color. Eventually the lens becomes totally opaque and assumes a pearly white color. This process is considered an exaggeration of normal aging and is responsible for the development of nuclear cataracts.

Cortical cataracts are due to a degenerative breakdown in lens fibers resulting in localized opacities. The majority of these occur in the periphery of the lens, forming opaque wedges or spokes. Gradually these become more diffuse until the pupil is affected. At this point, vision diminishes. Cortical cataracts may also involve the center of the lens adjacent to the posterior lens capsule or the anterior lens capsule. In this case, a very small opacity can affect visual function (Kaspar, 1978; Exton-Smith and Overstall, 1979; Smith, 1976).

ASSESSING THE CLIENT'S ADAPTATIONS

Cancer

All elderly people should be familiar with the American Cancer Society's Seven Warning Signals (Table 3). If a problem develops in one of these areas, the client should bring it to the attention of the physician or nurse. Although these signals are not definitive signs of cancer, they provide valuable clues and should be investigated. Unfortunately, many older people do not verbalize their complaints as readily or as fully as do younger people, perhaps accepting new problems as normal concomitants of aging or as an extension of a health problem already present. For the same reason, some health professionals may fail to investigate the elderly client's complaint as fully as possible.

Concurrent health problems often mask both local and systemic adaptations to cancer in older people, making it more difficult to differentiate between new adaptations to cancer and ongoing adaptations to other health problems. When an older person complains of backache, it is tempting to assume that it is due to arthritis or osteoporosis. In fact, it may be due to metastasis of breast, bladder, lung, or prostate cancer to the vertebrae. Because complaints about digestion and elimination are so common in the elderly, important cancer warning signals may go unheeded. The complaint of changes in bowel habits by an elderly person should be taken seriously. In particular, if the client has to bear down to evacuate or complains of alternating diarrhea and constipation, the nurse must consider the possibility of carcinoma of the colon. Similarly, older clients with rectal bleeding may not report it because they believe it is due to hemorrhoids, not rectal cancer.

Many systemic manifestations of cancer are easy to overlook in the elderly. Because locomotor and rheumatic diseases are so common in this age group, metabolic presentations of carcinoma, such as osteoarthropathy, peripheral neuropathy, and myopathy may be unrecognized. Anemia, whether due to occult blood loss or to marrow replacement or aplasia in carcinoma, myeloma, or leukemia, may be mistaken for nutritional iron deficiency anemia, a common problem in old age. Special difficulties in assessment are associated with malignant disease that presents with generalized, nonspecific adaptations such as weakness, anorexia, weight loss, fatigue, and malaise. These often cause failing mobility, a tendency to fall, and a general lack of interest in living in an older person that is incorrectly attributed to "senility," "old age," or some other disease the client has. Because of metabolic changes or metastasis, malignancies frequently cause confusion and other mental status changes in the elderly. Too often, these are misdiagnosed as dementia or senility by family and others.

Because data interpretation is so complex in elderly clients with multiple health problems, it is important to obtain a complete data base at frequent intervals. New findings can be meaningfully compared and correctly interpreted when complete baseline data are available and then updated at regular intervals.

Adaptations at High-Risk Sites. The nurse assessing the elderly client needs to be knowledgeable about adaptations to cancer at the high-risk sites.

Skin Cancer. Individuals with lightly pigmented skin are most likely to develop skin cancer. Because

---

TABLE 3. AMERICAN CANCER SOCIETY'S SEVEN WARNING SIGNALS

1. Change in bowel or bladder habits
2. Sore that does not heal
3. Unusual bleeding or discharge
4. Thickening or lump in breast or elsewhere
5. Indigestion or difficulty swallowing
6. Obvious change in wart or mole
7. Nagging cough or hoarseness

Source: American Cancer Society. Cancer Detection in the Physician's Office. New York, American Cancer Society, 1967.

of their heavy skin pigmentation, skin cancer is negligible among blacks. Risk factors include excessive exposure to sun or occupational exposure to coal tar, pitch, creosote, arsenic compounds, or radium. Tumors usually develop in exposed areas of the face and scalp, the nasal labial fold, the bridge of the nose, and inner canthus of the eye. The nurse should inspect and palpate the client's skin, including the scalp, palms of the hands, and soles of the feet. Basal and squamous cell skin cancers often appear as a pale, waxlike, and pearly nodule or a red, scaly, sharply outlined patch. Melanomas often start as small brown or black molelike growths that increase in size, change color, become ulcerated, and bleed easily from slight injury. If skin cancer is suspected, the nurse should refer the client to a physician who diagnoses the cancer by excisional or incisional biopsy.

Thyroid Carcinoma. Thyroid carcinoma, especially the undifferentiated anaplastic type, often presents suddenly as a large neck mass. Other adaptations are rare until late in the disease. The carcinoma may metastasize to regional lymph nodes, liver, bone, and lungs. Thyroid cancer can be diagnosed with the aid of a simple, painless diagnostic test using tracer doses of radioactive [131]I.

Lung Cancer. This is more likely to occur with advanced age. It is very difficult to assess in its early stages. Warning signs include a persistent cough, hemoptysis, chest pain, and recurring attacks of pneumonia or bronchitis. Risk factors include a history of heavy cigarette smoking or cigarette smoking for 20 years or more, and exposure to certain industrial pollutants such as asbestos. Many elderly women are at high risk for lung cancer, just as are elderly men. Many women who are elderly today were young adults during World War II when women first began working in industries that had previously been all male. They also began smoking cigarettes, a habit that had been popular for a generation in men. Diagnosis of lung cancer is aided by chest x-ray, sputum cytology, and fiberoptic bronchoscopy (Wynne, 1979).

Oral Cancer. This is most common in men over age 40, especially those who engage in heavy smoking or drinking or the use of chewing tobacco. Elderly clients may have lived for years with poorly fitting dentures that caused ulcers; therefore, they may overlook early signs of oral cancer. These include a sore that bleeds easily or does not heal, a lump or thickening, reddish or whitish patches that persist, and difficulty chewing, swallowing, or moving the jaw or tongue. Leukoplakia is considered the most significant premalignant lesion. Often, early malignancies in the mouth are not painful. All suspicious lesions should be biopsied.

Gastrointestinal Carcinomas. These may occur at any point along the gastrointestinal tract. Adaptations are often subtle and easily missed. Esophageal cancer is most common in black males between ages 60 and 65. Adaptations include dysphagia, thirst, salivation, and hiccoughs. Chronic bleeding and anemia are common. Carcinoma of the stomach has been increasing in recent decades and is most common in men over age 50. Adaptations include anorexia, epigastric pain and discomfort, anemia, and weight loss. In contrast to the mild weight loss that is a normal manifestation of aging, the weight loss may be severe. Hematemesis and melana may also occur. Pancreatic cancer shows the correlation of increasing death rates with increasing age and is more common in men. A common manifestation is jaundice. Cancer of the colon is more common in women and cancer of the rectum is more common in men (Straus, 1979). Cancers of the ascending colon may cause a dull, aching pain, while those of the lower colon and rectum are often associated with changes in bowel patterns. Blood and mucus in the stool are other common adaptations. Because of slow blood loss, anemia is frequent (Straus, 1979).

Assessing adaptations to gastrointestinal cancers is complex in the elderly because so many factors that affect gastrointestinal function may be relevant. These include food and fluid intake, medications, activity patterns, and emotions. If lesions are suspected in the upper gastrointestinal tract, the physician may order an upper gastrointestinal series, gastric analysis, endoscopy, and exfoliative studies. The physician may order barium enemas if lower gastrointestinal lesions are suspected. The colonoscope may be used to visualize the colon and biopsy suspicious tissue.

Uterine Cancer. This is most common in middle aged women and declines slightly after age 70 (Goldfarb, 1979). In its early stages, it is most often associated with bleeding. Because the bleeding is scant and transient, many older women ignore this early warning. Endometrial cancer is most common in women ages 50 to 64 (American Cancer Society, 1983). Risk factors include a failure of ovulation, prolonged estrogen therapy, late menopause and history of diabetes, infertility, obesity, or hypertension. Women at high risk for endometrial cancer should be advised to have an endometrial tissue sample taken at menopause. If endometrial cancer remains undetected, bleeding and even hemorrhage may occur in the later stages.

Cervical Cancer. This is most likely in women who had intercourse at an early age or had multiple sexual partners. A common adaptation is vaginal discharge. Because hormonal stimulation and vaginal secretions have ceased in older women, any vaginal discharge must be considered suspicious.

Ovarian Cancer. This is often called the silent malignancy because it is so difficult to identify in the early stages. Failure to identify this cancer accounts for the high death rate in women ages 55 to 74. The most significant adaptation, a palpable ovary in a postmenopausal female, is detected by careful bimanual pelvic examination. Unfortunately, too many elderly women fail to have annual pelvic examinations. Other adaptations include mild lower abdominal discomfort or persistent bloating. In suspicious cases the physician may perform culdocentesis to obtain material for cytological study (Goldfarb, 1979).

Vulvar Malignancies. These are associated with severe pruritis, especially at night. They often occur with monilial infections, particularly in diabetic women. Cancerous lesions of the vulva are white, friable, and bleed easily. They cannot be scraped off. These can be differentiated from monilial lesions which are also white and pruritic but which can be scraped away.

Breast Cancer. This is most likely to occur in women over age 50, especially those who never had children, had their first child after age 30, or have a family history of breast cancer. Adaptations to breast cancer are easier to identify in the elderly woman. Glandular tissue atrophies, leaving only fat tissue in the lower quadrants of the breasts and

supportive tissue. Consequently, when any palpable lesion develops in the breast, it must be considered malignant until proven otherwise. Other adaptations that should be investigated are thickening, swelling, dimpling, skin irritations, retraction or scaliness of the nipple, nipple discharge, pain, or tenderness. The American Cancer Society recommends that women between ages 35 and 40 receive a baseline mammogram to be used to make future comparisons. Because of recent controversy over the safety of mammography, some women may be reluctant to undergo this diagnostic procedure. New technology assures that only a few, if any, millirads of radiation are absorbed during this procedure, especially by elderly women. Because their breast tissue is less dense than that of younger women, they need lower doses of radiation to produce quality films. A few older women may be reluctant to have the test because of a sense of modesty. Personnel working in the area should assure that clients who undergo a mammogram are supplied with gowns that open in the front. These not only protect modesty but provide some warmth as well. Needle aspiration with tissue study of suspected cysts is another helpful diagnostic tool. The breast biopsy to determine whether or not the lesion is malignant is the only certain diagnostic procedure (Elkowitz, 1981).

Prostatic Cancer. This is the second leading cause of death after lung cancer in adult males. Early assessment is important because cancer of the prostate is still highly curable in its early stages. If malignancy is present, the prostate feels hard, nodular, and fixed upon rectal examination. Other adaptations similar to those with benign prostatic hypertrophy (see Chapter 17) may also be present. Diagnostic tests that may be performed if prostate cancer is suspected include needle or open biopsy, bone scan, and blood tests for prostatic acid phosphatase. This enzyme is released by the cancer once it spreads beyond the prostatic capsule.

Bladder Cancer. This is most likely to occur in men over age 50. A positive correlation exists between smoking and bladder cancer, but the reason is unclear. The earliest adaptations may be blood in the urine, prolonged cystitis, and a feeling of bladder load. Diagnosis is made by cystoscopy, biopsy, and cytology of urine (Serpick, 1978). A routine urinalysis with particular attention to the presence of red blood cells is an important mechanism for assessing bladder cancer.

Multiple Myeloma. Increasing in males over age 50, this malignant proliferation of plasma cells in the marrow often presents as bone pain, pathological fractures, or advanced osteoporosis. Anemia, thrombocytopenia, and hypercalcemia develop as bone marrow is destroyed. The accumulation of large amounts of abnormal immunoglobulin proteins can damage the kidneys. A decrease in normal immunoglobulins places the client at high risk for an infection. The excess of proteins in the blood may damage vessels in the eye and central nervous system. Spinal cord and nerve root compression may also occur. Multiple myeloma is diagnosed by demonstrating an abnormal protein in the semen or urine in the presence of plasma cell infiltration of the marrow or of multiple plasmacytomas.

Chronic Leukemia. This may be difficult to identify in older people because the client may not have adaptations for a long period of time. It may be discovered only when blood is drawn for routine examination and a high white blood cell count is noticed. Chronic lymphocytic leukemia, the most common form of the disease in the elderly, reaches its maximum incidence in the 60- to 70-year age group. It is characterized by an accumulation of immunologically incompetent small lymphocytes in the bone marrow and lymph nodes; insidious, painless swelling, often symmetrical, in lymph nodes in the neck, axillae, and inguinal areas; and enlargement of the spleen. The white blood cell count is often in the range of 100,000 to 300,000 per microliter. Antiviral and other immune defenses become impaired. The client complains of fatigue and weight loss. Anemia may not occur until after the early stages of the disease. Eventually thrombocytopenia develops. In many cases, the client dies from infection (Serpick, 1978).

Screening Programs. If cancer is identified at a localized stage, most clients of all ages can be cured of the disease. Therefore, screening programs to identify malignancies in the early stages are just as important for the elderly as for the young. The American Cancer Society advises a cancer-related

checkup every year for individuals over age 40. It should include examination for cancer of the breast, testes, prostate, mouth, gastrointestinal tract, bladder, ovaries, uterus, skin, thyroid, lungs, and lymph nodes. Specific screening techniques are available for detecting cancer of the breast, colon, rectum, uterus, lung, prostate, bladder, and oral cavity (Table 4). Unfortunately, there is still no general agreement about what screening tests should be done to detect cancer or the frequency with which they should be carried out. When assessing the health status of the elderly client it is useful to review the client's total record and identify adaptations that have persisted despite treatment. These may indicate a malignancy.

Although there are no blood tests available as initial screening tests for cancer, work is proceeding in this area. Blood tests could be a quick, painless method of screening for malignancy. The erythrocyte sedimentation rate (ESR) is useless in the elderly because it is so frequently elevated for other reasons. Knowledge that immunological phenomena are associated with malignancy is being used to develop screening tests. The carcinoembryonic antigen (CEA) was identified in 1965 and found in individuals with certain types of cancer. Identifying this antigen is a nonspecific test for cancer. Values for cancer and noncancer clients overlap considerably. At the present time this test is not used for initial screening. Other developments include the extraction of the Caspary antigen from some types of tumors and the identification of antibodies to smooth muscle fibers associated with malignancy. It remains to be seen whether these or similar tests can be developed into practical screening tools (Hodkinson, 1978).

Diagnostic Tests. When clients are elderly, difficult decisions must be made about how far to pursue diagnostic testing for cancer. Although some tests are painless and simple to perform, many others are lengthy, complex, and painful. For example, bronchoscopy and esophagoscopy procedures are taxing to any client, especially the elderly. Older clients need to be fully involved in the decision-making process about whether or not to undergo certain diagnostic tests. They need to know exactly what will be required of them in order to prepare for and cooperate with the test. Details such as

---

TABLE 4.   RECOMMENDED SCREENING TESTS FOR COMMON TYPES OF CANCER

Site	Test	Frequency
Uterine	Papanicolaou test	Once every 3 years after two initial negative tests 1 year apart[a] or Annually[b]
Breast	Self-breast exam	Monthly[a]
	Professional breast exam	Annually after age 40[a]
	Mammogram	Annually after age 40[a]
Lung	Chest x-ray	No agreement on frequency[a,b]
Prostate	Rectal exam	Annually[b]
Oral	Checkup by dentist	Regularly[a]
Colon and Rectum	Digital rectal exam	Annually after age 40[a]
	Stool, occult blood test	Annually after age 50[a]
	Proctoscopy	Every 3 to 5 years after age 50 following two annual exams with negative results[a]

[a]American Cancer Society. Cancer Facts and Figures, 1983.
[b]Serpick A, 1978.

---

positioning during the test, length of the test, pain, risks, and costs should be discussed. The decision to undergo the test should be based on an understanding of the test procedure, the reason for the test, and the treatment alternatives available if the findings are positive for cancer. Would the client be able to undergo curative surgery? Complex treatment protocols? Limited palliative measures? In each case, what treatment modalities are available? The consequences, both positive and negative, of investigating the problem and undergoing various treatment protocols should be explored and weighed against the consequences of letting the cancer take its course. Clients must be informed about all aspects of the proposed treatment, including risks, side effects, possible complications, costs, disfigurement, pain, and length of hospitalization. In some cases, treatment extends survival time but not quality of life. In others, avoiding treatment for cancer results in intolerable pain and suffering. When clients are informed they are better able to make decisions about whether or not they wish to pursue diagnostic testing. For example, it may be difficult to justify taxing barium studies for the diagnosis of gastrointestinal cancer if the client is unable to withstand surgery.

In the long run older clients' wishes should prevail. Their ability to make informed decisions depends largely on the willingness of nurses and physicians to provide them with complete and unbiased information about the benefits and risks of diagnostic tests and treatment options. Clients require a great deal of support and understanding during the decision-making process.

Elderly clients who suspect they have cancer and are undergoing diagnostic testing carry a heavy emotional burden. They may fear death, pain, and disfigurement. The fear of many elderly clients is heightened by their perception of cancer, formed decades ago, that the diagnosis inevitably consigns one to an agonizing death. Giving older clients up-to-date information about cancer is one way to alleviate some of their anxiety.

Cataracts
Visual changes of all types are so common in the elderly that routine assessment of the elderly client's eyes is essential. The visual needs of clients living

in long-term care settings are often ignored. The nurse can incorporate routine vision screening into the nursing home routine. Although nurses are not responsible for diagnosing specific pathology, they must be able to identify deviations from normal that indicate pathological conditions. Assessment of the aging eye is described in Chapter 7. When the nurse detects deviations from normal, clients must be referred to an ophthalmologist for appropriate follow-up.

Because deviations in normal visual function occur so frequently in the elderly, the nurse should not wait for the client to complain of problems. Sometimes, the changes occur so gradually that the client is not aware that vision has deteriorated. Fear of blindness is widespread among the elderly, as is the belief that failing eyesight is an inescapable concomitant of growing old. Together these factors may be the reasons many older people remain silent about changes in vision.

In the absence of specific complaints about vision, the nurse should incorporate the eye examination into the routine assessment. To reduce the client's anxiety, the nurse can explain that performing an eye examination is part of sound preventative care at any age and does not imply that something is wrong. This reassurance may open a dialogue with the client about ways the client can preserve eyesight as well as about the many effective treatments now available for various visual disabilities.

The adaptations related to cataract development are diverse. In part they depend upon the location, extent, and stage of the opacity and the presence or absence of other eye problems. In general, cataract development is characterized by a progressive, painless loss of vision. In the early stages, increasing myopia is common. When this adaptation develops in the presbyopic or hyperopic person, it often enables them to read without glasses for the first time in years. Consequently, many clients believe their vision is improving, not worsening. This phenomenon, called "second sight," is the reason why clients with early cataracts often require several changes in the prescription of their eyeglasses (Kahn, 1981; Kaspar, 1978). Clients with early cataracts may complain of a "speck" or "spot" before the eye that always remains in the same place. Clients with central cataracts may see better in dim light when the pupil is widely dilated (Exton-Smith and Overstall, 1979). The nurse may notice these individuals prefer dark rooms to sunny ones.

If the cataract is generalized the client may complain of hazy vision. Other words to describe this adaptation are "misty," "cloudy," or "smoky." The client may believe that a film or skin has formed over the eye. The client may complain that the light is not strong enough to ready by. Visual acuity declines due to dimness and distortion. Monocular diplopia or even polyopia are other complaints (Marmor, 1981).

Because of irregular refraction, bright lights are scattered as they make their way through the visual system, causing a distressing glare. Clients may complain that car lights approaching at night are "blinding" or "dazzling." They may say that they see halos or wagon-wheel spokes radiating from lights. This complaint is also associated with glaucoma and is an indication for tonometry (Kaspar, 1978). To shield the eyes from glare, clients with cataracts may wear dark glasses and use broad-brimmed hats and eyeshades when outdoors.

As vision continues to fail, the client often complains of headaches and eye fatigue. Because they must work harder to see, clients may become irritable and frustrated.

Older clients vary widely in their ability to adapt to reduced vision. Some clients with minor impairments experience a profound inability to function. Others with major visual losses tolerate the changes and continue to function at a high level. The nursing assessment considers those factors that influence the client's adaptation to visual loss:

- The state of the remaining senses
- The physical environment
- The client's preferred life-style
- The client's personality

Clients who experience loss of vision depend more heavily upon their other senses for data about the environment. When these senses are also impaired, the elderly person may react profoundly to minor visual losses. Clients may become immobile, incontinent, and confused. Their inability to adapt is believed to be due to sensory deprivation. The nurse's role in minimizing sensory deprivation is explored later in this chapter.

When vision is diminished, the client's physical environment may promote or prevent optimal adaptation. Inappropriate lighting, furniture placement, window treatments, and colors may reduce the client's ability to move about safely and remain independent.

Life-style is an important variable in determining the impact of visual loss on the elderly individual. When the client's activities of daily living require sharp vision, even minor visual losses impair the quality of life. Some elderly persons who have given up many of these activities tolerate visual losses more readily. Some of the activities that require good vision include:

- Driving a car or using public transportation
- Watching television
- Reading
- Sewing
- Playing cards
- Gardening
- Shopping and using money
- Cooking
- Housekeeping
- Dialing the telephone
- Writing letters

Declining vision may force older clients to gradually give up many desired activities, hobbies, or habits. The nurse should identify the client's current life-style, the client's satisfaction with it, recent changes in it, and the reasons for those changes.

Clients' adaptations vary according to whether or not they view their visual loss as handicapping. Some clients experience severe anxiety when vision fails and voluntarily curtail their mobility and activities of daily living. The client may rarely venture from the home. When ambulating, movements are hesitant. Other clients may attempt to maintain their life-style in as normal a fashion as possible. When visual problems become severe, they may do so only with difficulty or by jeopardizing their safety. Because reading labels is difficult, the use of medication becomes hazardous. Shopping and cooking become chores because of difficulty reading food labels and recipes. Boredom ensues because the client is forced to give up hobbies such as television, reading, and sewing that require good vision. The

inability to perceive the environment makes mobility unsafe. Eventually, because clients fear falling, they may limit social outings, with isolation resulting.

The presence of a cataract is confirmed by direct visualization of the lens opacity. In the early stages, opacities may not be visible. Later they may partially or totally obstruct the red reflex and visualization of the fundus. Nuclear cataracts may appear as milky white opacities when viewed through the pupil. Cortical cataracts appear as areas of diffuse pigmentation or as spider webs. They give off a black reflection. The pupillary light reflex should be normal (Kaspar, 1978).

When the diagnosis of cataracts is made, elderly clients react in many ways. Some are shocked. They need time to accept the fact before they are able to give serious consideration to treatment alternatives. These clients need support while they grieve their loss. Others, who suspected a problem, are relieved to learn the nature of the problem and eager to undergo surgical correction. The nurse can help them to plan realistically for surgery and its aftermath. When surgery is not possible, the nurse can assist clients to modify their life-style and environment to promote independence.

NURSING INTERVENTIONS

Cancer

Treatment Modalities.   Modern cancer treatment uses new therapies and the combined modality approach, making treatment more aggressive than was possible a decade ago. As a result, cure can be sought in many types of cancer previously thought incurable. The three basic treatment modalities are surgery, radiation, and chemotherapy. The aim of treatment is to excise or reduce the cancer by the most direct means and then to support or stimulate the client's immune system to destroy remaining cancer cells. All three modalities are used to destroy cancer in specific primary or metastatic sites. In addition, chemotherapy can be used to destroy widely disseminated cancer cells.

The purpose of cancer treatment may be cure or palliation. Although cancer cures are aggressively sought, they are not always possible due primarily to a failure to detect the cancer when it is in a stage amenable to local therapy with surgery or irradiation. Palliative measures may take many forms. For example, palliation may involve surgery to correct acute intestinal obstruction, ulceration, or pathological fractures, radiotherapy to reduce the bone pain associated with multiple myeloma, or chemotherapy to shrink tumor size or forestall the development of pleural effusion or malignant ascites. The guiding principle for palliation must be a genuine likelihood that it will relieve complications or painful adaptations of the cancer (Hodkinson, 1978).

Surgery. This may be the primary method of treatment or used in combination with other modalities. Major surgical procedures with a low cure rate can seldom be justified in the elderly unless intended to forestall complications (Hodkinson, 1978). Breast cancer is often treated with a simple, not a radical, mastectomy as the primary treatment, followed by radiation or chemotherapy (Elkowitz, 1981; Charlesworth and Baker, 1978). Partial gastrectomy may be performed in preference to total gastrectomy. There appears to be little difference in survival rates after the two procedures. Surgery in combination with both radiation and chemotherapy may be necessary for invasive carcinoma of the prostate or bladder. Extirpative surgery is the treatment of choice when cancer of the vulva, vagina, or endometrium is present. Following surgery, radiation therapy may also be used in endometrial cancer (Serpick, 1978). Careful consideration is given before performing surgical procedures that result in important disabilities, especially when the untreated prognosis is little different than the client's likely life span without the malignancy. For example, the older client may consider a colostomy a major social handicap while the likelihood of local complications without a colostomy are small.

Radiation Therapy. This may be used alone or in combination with other modalities. Both external radiation using x-rays (cobalt-60) and internal radiation using radium, cesium, iodine-131, phosphorus-32, and other agents, are used for the elderly. Surgical removal of the cancer remains the first choice for most malignancies; radiotherapy is used only when removal of the growth is impossible

and the spread of metastasis is likely (Villaverde and MacMillan, 1980). Painful bone lesions and soft tissue lesions associated with breast cancer in the elderly often respond dramatically to radiation therapy (Serpick, 1978). Local radiation of the lymph nodes of clients with chronic lymphocytic leukemia has also been highly successful in prolonging the client's survival.

Chemotherapy. No truly cancericidal drug has been found. Cytotoxic drugs kill or injure cancer cells in doses that do not kill normal cells. These drugs have been most successful against Hodgkin's disease, other lymphomas, lymphosarcomas, and leukemias. In particular, alkylating agents such as chlorambucil have improved the prognosis of clients with chronic lymphocytic leukemia (Villaverde and MacMillan, 1980). After surgery for cancer, drug therapy is frequently initiated prophylactically based on the assumption that there may be microscopic foci of the disease elsewhere. This procedure is followed for breast cancer, carcinomas of the stomach and bowel, and other tumors. Current multiple trials with adjuvant therapy employing drugs and combinations of drugs only recently available may prove to be successful in the old as well as the young (Serpick, 1978).

Chemotherapeutic agents are also used as palliative measures to shrink tumor size. For example, Adriamycin (doxorubian hydrochloride) produces regression of some thyroid carcinomas. Antineoplastic drugs such as mephalan have extended survival for elderly clients with multiple myeloma (Serpick, 1978).

Dosage of chemotherapeutic agents must be carefully adjusted in the aged. The optimal drug dose is the one that produces maximum benefit with minimum risk. The therapeutic-to-toxic range, that is, the difference between the minimum effective dose and the maximum tolerance dose, is especially narrow in the elderly. Therefore, the hazards and risks of therapy, especially combination therapy, are greater in the elderly. Safe and effective drug dosage in the elderly is determined not just by ascertaining body weight but by assessing the presence of any disabling disease and the function of the bone marrow, kidney, liver, and brain. The function of these organs affects the older client's vulnerability to the toxicity of the drugs (Villaverde and MacMillan, 1980). In clients over age 70, a dosage reduction of over 50 percent may be required in order to prevent toxicities. In frail individuals over age 80, a careful evaluation of chemotherapy is made and drug therapy may be withheld. In the elderly, the gastrointestinal tract and central nervous system are especially vulnerable to the toxic effects of chemotherapeutic agents. Laboratory examination of the bone marrow and uric acid levels are made periodically for evidence of toxicity. The nurse needs to be familiar with the adverse reactions of the specific agents being administered to the client in order to make a knowledgeable assessment of the client's response.

Steroids and hormones have been successfully used with some elderly clients. These inhibit growth of cancer cells by altering their environment. Corticoids and adrenocorticotropic hormone (ACTH) may favorably influence the course of some lymphomas and leukemias, including chronic lymphocytic leukemia. Estrogens have been used successfully in men with prostatic cancer. The general bone involvement of breast cancer can be treated with estrogens or the newer, nonmasculizing androgens (Serpick, 1978; Villaverde and MacMillan, 1980). This therapy is effective for older women with breast cancer but less debilitating than systemic cytotoxic agents.

Immunotherapy. Host reactions against tumor cells have been recognized for many years. Recent developments hold out the hope of useful immunotherapy for malignant tumors which produce tumor-specific antigens capable of evoking immune responses in the client. Because the immune system in the elderly is already compromised, immune therapy is not used in the elderly at the present time.

Treatment Decisions. Although there are significant differences among age groups with respect to the epidemiology, presentation, and course of cancer, most experts believe that the philosophy underlying cancer treatment should be similar for all age groups. No client should be denied the employment of all appropriate therapeutic modalities on the grounds of old age alone. Despite their advanced years, elderly clients should be offered the opportunity of cure or palliation of cancer.

Treatment decisions in the older client should take into consideration both length of survival and quality of life. In younger clients, malignant disease is often the only threat to life in the setting of a relatively long life expectancy for the age group. In contrast, malignant disease in the elderly may be only one of several life-threatening diseases. Frailty and disability may also be present. The prognosis of the malignancy must be viewed against the relatively short life expectancy of nonaffected clients in the same age group. For example, the average life expectancy at age 80 is 5 or 6 years and elderly people of this age with cancer often die of some other disease before the cancer advances far enough to kill them. Consequently, in the elderly it is often preferable to substitute a simple operation for radical surgery or to select a conservative form of therapy if the primary tumor is a slow-growing one.

The older client's own wishes should be given special weight. They should not be required to accept onerous treatment if they do not wish to do so. Professionals must make certain that treatment is not being given merely to salve the feelings of health care providers or relatives who feel they must "do something." For some older clients, overall survival time may not be as important as the quality of life. For other older people, on the other hand, the desire to live is so strong that they are willing to risk a great deal to do so. Health professionals must not assume that treatment will be too painful to inflict on elderly clients. Professionals may incorrectly assume that the elderly have too short a time to enjoy the benefits of treatment or that the money and effort is not worth it because the client is old. Some older clients dread the extension or recurrence of the cancer more than the difficulties of treatment. For them abandonment by the health team may be the most terrible suffering they experience.

Other variables that must be considered when planning the older client's treatment program include the type and extent of the cancer and the client's metabolic, immunological, and nutritional status. Tumors are classified according to their type, rate of growth, size, and extent. The international TNM system provides one useful method of assessing tumor characteristics. Classification of the tumor helps the health team to plan the most effective treatment regimen.

Effective cancer treatment depends on adequate functioning of the central nervous system, heart, kidneys, and liver. In the elderly, aging changes as well as chronic illness may adversely affect one or more of these organs. Assessment data are used to select treatment modalities that spare compromised organs. For example, if the client has impaired liver or renal function, certain drugs might not be selected for use.

Because immunological competence declines with age, immune functions must be assessed before instituting any treatment plan that requires immunocompetence. Treatment plans for cancers such as leukemia are often altered because the older client's immune defenses are not adequate.

It is well known that clients who are malnourished do not respond as well to chemotherapy and radiotherapy. In addition, toxicities are more likely to occur. Because the elderly are at high risk for nutritional deficiencies, a nutritional assessment is made prior to cancer therapy. High-nutrition diets or hyperalimentation are used before and during cancer therapy to maximize the client's response.

Supporting the Older Client with Cancer. The client undergoing radiotherapy or chemotherapy is at high risk for common side effects such as skin breakdown, stomatitis, nausea, vomiting, diarrhea, taste distortions, dehydration, poor nutrition, and loss of hair. There are no data that these occur more commonly or with greater severity in the elderly than in the young. Infections are frequent in cancer clients, especially elderly clients, and are attributed to their compromised immune function. Supportive measures appropriate for younger clients should be used with the elderly to provide relief. Pain is an adaptation to many but not all types of cancer. Its management was discussed in Chapter 15.

Anxiety and depression are the two most important reactions to the diagnosis of cancer. The nurse can anticipate other reactions, including anger, denial, withdrawal, regression, and even euphoria as the client's treatment plan progresses. These reactions require the nurse's sympathetic understanding.

Rehabilitation of the elderly cancer victim is an important element of the treatment plan. Rehabilitation measures may include exercise regimens, voice retraining, or fitting prostheses. Goals for the older client must be realistic and within the client's reach. The rehabilitation program often proceeds at a slower pace for the older client. Rehabilitation benefits the older client physically and psychosocially and provides clients with hope that they can resume near-normal functioning in the future.

Terminal care of clients dying with malignant disease is an important aspect of geriatric care. Over half of all cancer victims die in the impersonal atmosphere of the hospital attached to monitoring devices, respirators, or feeding tubes. A smaller percentage die at home (Hodkinson, 1978). Terminal care is discussed in Chapter 22.

Cataracts

Because the development of cataracts is poorly understood, there is no therapeutic measure available to prevent the formation or progression of cataracts or bring about their reversal. The only definitive treatment is surgical extraction.

The Client with Failing Vision. Many elderly clients with cataracts function for years with some degree of diminished vision until the time when the problem is deemed serious enough to warrant surgery. The nurse should ensure that these clients receive regular and frequent visual checkups since changes in eyeglasses may be required more frequently. If the client has central lens opacities the ophthalmologist may order mydriatic eyedrops such as homatropine. These produce some improvement in vision, at least temporarily (Leight, 1978). The nurse should ensure that the client knows how to administer eyedrops correctly. The dropper should never touch the cornea. The older client can be taught to rest the hand on the orbital rim or the bone beneath the eye to steady the hand when administering the drops. The client also needs to understand the importance of keeping the eyedrops free of contamination.

Clients with cataracts may need tinted lenses to help them cope with glare when inside as well as outside. The nurse can suggest the use of clip-on polarized lenses that can be used over regular glasses and flipped up when not needed.

The nurse can use data from the environmental assessment to help the client plan changes that promote independence in activities of daily living, mobility, and safety. Because glare is a problem, the nurse can suggest ways to reduce glare in the environment. Flat paints and window shades are recommended. Chrome and glass furniture and mirrors should be avoided. Light sources should be directed on the object the client is viewing, not on the eyes. For maximum safety, the furniture arrangement in the home may require modification to provide unobstructed safe traffic areas. To ensure independence, strong contrasting colors can be used to code cupboards, drawers, and dials. The nurse can help the client plan systematic arrangements to facilitate identification of food supplies, clothing, and other frequently used items.

Cataract Surgery. More than 400,000 persons in the United States undergo surgery for the removal of cataracts each year. Most of these people are elderly (Kwitko, 1978). In the past, cataracts were not removed until they were "ripe," but today the client need not wait that long before undergoing surgery. It is now possible to remove the lens as soon as vision has diminished to the point at which the client is handicapped in the ability to read, write, or perform other essential, or satisfying, activities of daily living. In most cases, the decision to operate is made when the client's failing vision becomes a stress that interferes with the normal life-style (Leight, 1978). This point is highly individual and depends upon the client's habits, interests, and goals. Some clients, such as those who drive or read, may need surgery for relatively minor opacities. Other clients who live in a familiar environment and do not read or watch television may not require surgery until their vision is severely impaired (20/100 to 20/200).

Cataract surgery is an elective procedure. Theoretically, most cataracts can remain on the eye throughout life with no ill effects from a physical standpoint. However, they may severely impair the elderly client's quality of life. When advised to have cataract surgery, many elderly clients are reluctant to do so at first because of misinformation about the surgery. Many elderly clients remember parents who had cataract surgery. Sandbags and bilateral eyepatches were used to immobilize the head and eyes. The postoperative period was uncomfortable, and disorientation and mental confusion due to sensory deprivation were common postoperative complaints (Smith, 1976). Many elderly clients do not understand what cataracts are. They believe they are a growth that must be removed from the eye. They believe they will require a long period of hospitalization postoperatively. By correcting misinformation and providing the elderly client with facts about modern surgical techniques the nurse can help clients to make the decision to undergo the surgical procedure.

Modern advances in surgical techniques have simplified both the surgical procedure and the postoperative period. Usually, the surgical procedure takes less than an hour and the client is discharged from the hospital in less than a week. Some cataract extractions are done on an outpatient basis (Kwitko, 1978). Usually, the lens in the most advanced state of disease is removed in the initial operation. Surgery is performed a second time to correct the other eye. New microscopes provide the surgeon with greater magnification than has ever before been possible, allowing for precision in surgical techniques (Smith, 1976). The use of fine needles and tiny sutures to close the incision has eliminated the need for sandbags and allowed the client to ambulate almost immediately after surgery. This advance minimizes postoperative bleeding into the eye as well as postoperative pulmonary and vascular complications. It also reduces the cost of surgery because the client's hospital stay is shorter (Smith, 1976).

Removal of a cataract is one of the oldest surgical procedures. It was first described over 200 years ago. Until recently, however, the cataract could not be removed until mature, since only the lenticular material was removed by extracapsular extraction. This procedure often resulted in complications.

In the past 40 years, new methods of cataract extraction have been developed using microsurgery techniques. The traditional method of cataract removal is intracapsular extraction. A wide incision is made in the cornea to remove the lens intact in its capsule. An enzyme, alpha-chymotrypsin (1/10,000 solution), may be injected into the anterior chamber underneath the iris pillars at the time of surgery. The enzyme dissolves the zonular fibers that support the lens so that the lens can be removed within the capsule with a minimum of traction or pressure (Kornzweig, 1979). The lens may be extracted with forceps, suction, or cryoprobe. Currently cryoextraction is a very popular method of cataract extraction. The probe is cooled to $-40°C$ and when the lens contacts the tip of the cryoprobe, it adheres and is removed intact. This method reduces postsurgical complications. A partial iridectomy is done to ensure that secondary glaucoma does not result should vitreous humor move forward and block the flow of aqueous from the eye.

Extracapsular cataract extraction means that the anterior capsule and lens are removed and the posterior lens capsule remains intact. If it is cloudy at the time of surgery, a capsulotomy is done to create an opening in the membrane for light to penetrate. Usually the lens material is "spooned" out. A newer method of extracapsular extraction is phacoemulsion. An ultrasonic probe is inserted into the eyeball through a tiny incision and emulsifies and aspirates the lens material apart from the posterior capsule. This method is more difficult to execute than traditional methods and requires special training. However, because it requires a tiny incision, the postoperative period is shorter (Elkowitz, 1981).

The choice of surgical approach depends upon the client's age and needs, the nature of the cataract, and the preference of the ophthalmologist. Each method has its own specific benefits. For example, there are several advantages to preserving the posterior capsule. It serves as a barrier that prevents vitreous from escaping and causing postoperative complications, including glaucoma and detached retina. It is also advantageous to leave the posterior capsule when the client is nearsighted. If opacification of the posterior capsule develops after surgery, a posterior capsulotomy can be performed on an outpatient basis. This rapid, low-risk procedure restores visual acuity (Jennings, 1976b). Phacoemulsion is more successful on immature cataracts than old, hardened ones. It is used most often on clients under age 60 (Kornzweig, 1979). While healing usually occurs most rapidly when phacoemulsion is used, the risk of postoperative complications is somewhat higher. Because of the vibration and flow of material, there is a slightly greater risk of damage to the cornea (Marmor, 1981).

Anesthesia. Clients usually have a choice about whether local or general anesthesia is used. In most cases, local anesthesia is sufficient. It is preferred for frail elderly clients who are poor surgical risks. Because it allows complete control and relaxation, general anesthesia is often preferred for older clients who are particularly anxious or restless, are deaf,

or have Parkinson's disease or any other condition that makes it difficult for them to hold their heads still (Pilgrim and Sigler, 1975; Kornzweig, 1979; Leight, 1978).

Prognosis. Apprehension due to the fear of blindness is common in the client who anticipates cataract surgery. This fear is especially likely to occur in clients who have lost vision in the eye that is not to be operated on. The nurse can help clients deal with apprehension by encouraging them to verbalize their misgivings and by thorough explanations about the benefits of surgery. Research studies indicate that even very old persons withstand cataract surgery well and have an excellent chance of recovering functional vision. In 95 percent of cases, surgical removal of the lens is performed successfully and visual acuity is improved (Kornzweig, 1977; Marmor, 1981). As a rule, if the older person is ambulatory, oriented, and desires surgery the prognosis is excellent.

The nurse can reassure the client that the risks associated with cataract surgery are few. Complications develop in less than 4 percent of cases (Kaspar, 1978). However, the procedure does put stress on the eye. If the corneal endothelial tissue is damaged during surgery or if it was in poor health before surgery, the cornea may become edematous and cloudy. Damage to the vitreous during surgery increases the risk that vitreous contraction will occur, pulling on the retina. The incidence of retinal detachment is higher in those who have had cataract surgery than in the general population. Cataract surgery can also cause transient edema within the macula. In a few cases the edema persists, adversely affecting visual acuity (Marmor, 1981). Infection and glaucoma are other possible complications (Kaspar, 1978).

Preoperative Management. Nursing care prior to cataract surgery varies according to the type of procedure planned, type of anesthesia (local or general) to be used, and the physician's preference. Despite these differences, the nurse can help every client contemplating cataract surgery to select an appropriate time for the procedure. Because this surgery is elective, clients can plan to undergo it at a time that fits comfortably into their life-style. Postoperative healing takes a minimum of 6 weeks and a maximum of 3 months, and adjustment to glasses or contact lenses requires several more weeks or months. Therefore, clients should expect that several months will be required after the operation before they are able to function at an optimal level.

The nurse needs to assess the client's expectations about the nature of vision postoperatively. Some clients have unrealistic expectations and are deeply disappointed by the outcome of surgery. Others fear permanent dependence on other people. The client's knowledge of the lens to be used to correct postoperative aphakia should also be discussed.

Several weeks before surgery, the nurse can help the client prepare for hospitalization and the return home. Although some cataract extractions are performed on an outpatient basis, most clients are hospitalized for 2 to 7 days (Leight, 1978). Clients are admitted to the hospital the day before surgery.

Before their hospital admission, clients need to plan for ways to cope with the activity restrictions required in the postoperative period. Both the nature of the restrictions and the length of time they are imposed vary according to the nature of the surgical procedure and the physician's preference. For example, when phacoemulsion is to be performed, the incision is small, shortening the postoperative period. Lifting, bending, and stooping may be partially or completely restricted for as little as 2 weeks or as long as 6 weeks (Kornzweig, 1979). Therefore, clients should rearrange the home so that frequently used items are within easy reach. Some meals can be made in advance. Arrangements can be made for friends, relatives, or a home attendant to assist with shopping, laundry, cooking, and cleaning. If hair washing is restricted in the postoperative period, clients should be told to wash their hair before coming to the hospital.

Once the client is admitted to the hospital, a complete workup is performed. Routine preoperative teaching should be completed. Antibiotic eyedrops, ointments, or eyewashes may be ordered prophylactically. Sometimes these are instituted several days before surgery. Facial scrubs to reduce pathogens may be instituted the day before surgery as well as the day of surgery. The eyelashes are clipped.

On the morning of surgery, many physicians order medications to decrease intraocular pressure. Intravenous mannitol (Osmitrol), a fast-acting diuretic, may be administered. The nurse monitors vital signs every 5 minutes and observes the client for chest pain and shortness of breath (Pilgrim and Sigler, 1975). As an alternative, oral glycerine (Glyrol) may be administered (Smith, 1978).

Maximum dilation of the pupil is essential to facilitate the surgical procedure. Drops are usually instilled several times, beginning 1 to 2 hours before surgery. Cyclopentolate HCl (Cyclogyl 1 to 2 percent) paralyzes the muscles of accommodation in addition to dilating the pupil. Phenylephrine HCl (Neosynephrine 10 percent) is a mydriatic agent and a vasoconstrictor. Other agents with similar actions include homatropine hydrobromide (Homatropine 2 percent) and tropicamide (Mydriacyl 1 percent) (Pilgrim and Sigler, 1975; Low, 1978). Prior to the cataract extraction clients also receive sedatives, narcotics and tranquilizers or narcotic potentiators to help them relax.

Postoperative Management. The goals of postoperative care are to prevent increased intraocular pressure, stress on the suture line, and hemorrhage into the eye. Specific postoperative care varies according to the surgical procedure the client underwent. In most cases the client can ambulate and sit in a chair the day of or the day after surgery. Some clients find this early activity alarming because they are afraid of damaging the eye. Careful explanations help to reassure them. Clients are usually advised not to turn to the operated side or onto their stomach because this increases pressure on the suture line. Pillows can be placed against the client's back to prevent rolling.

The operated eye is usually covered with an eyepatch for at least 24 hours. Immediately after surgery, clients can use the other eye to watch television or read. Clients are given a plastic shield to wear over the operated eye at night to prevent them from bumping or scratching it while asleep. Before they go home, clients should be taught how to tape the shield securely to the face. The shield is worn for 4 to 6 weeks postoperatively.

Postoperative pain is usually minimal. Some discomfort is normal. The eye may feel achy or itchy, as if there were sand in it or the eyeball were rubbing against the eyepatch. Mild analgesics such as aspirin or acetaminophen are usually sufficient to control any discomfort. Tearing sometimes occurs, causing the eyepatch to become damp and the nose to drip. Photophobia may also occur in the first month. Wearing dark glasses helps to prevent this problem. If the client develops excruciating pain it is a sign of increasing intraocular pressure and requires immediate medical attention.

Vomiting can cause injury to the eye by increasing the intraocular pressure. The gagging and retching associated with vomiting increase pressure on the suture line. To avoid this, the physician orders an antiemetic to be given if necessary. Because straining at stool also increases intraocular pressure, a stool softener such as dioctyl sodium (Colace) is also ordered postoperatively.

During the postoperative period, clients usually receive antibiotic eyedrops to prevent infection and steroid eyedrops to reduce inflammation. Mydriatics such as pilocarpine or atropine may also be given after phacoemulsion because they reduce the incidence of postoperative complications. Because eyedrops are continued for several weeks after surgery clients must learn how to administer them before they leave the hospital.

Before they are discharged from the hospital, clients need clear instructions about activity restrictions. In some cases bending for brief periods (for example, when putting on shoes) is permitted. In other cases, bending is strictly prohibited. Most clients are permitted to perform basic hygiene activities. However, they must use care to avoid falling in the bathtub or shower. Clients are usually advised to avoid any situation in which the eye might be bumped or they might be jostled. Allowing the client to ask specific questions about what activities are and are not permitted helps to clarify the restrictions. Clients should also be advised to telephone their ophthalmologist or nurse if they have any questions.

Before going home, clients with absorbable sutures should be warned that these start to dissolve 4 weeks postoperatively. Usually this results in decreased vision and redness of the eye. Unless clients are prepared for this process, they may believe they are developing postoperative complications.

Clients should also know how to cleanse the eyelid by applying a clean washcloth moistened with warm tap water. This can be done for 5 or 10 minutes three or four times a day. Minor crusting and discharge that adhere to the lid margin are normal for 3 to 4 weeks postoperatively.

Managing Aphakia.   Perhaps the most significant complication of cataract surgery is aphakia, the absence of a lens. Light rays enter the eye unimpeded but remain unfocused. There are three ways to correct the aphakic state: with a lens in front of the eye, a contact lens, or an intraocular lens implanted at the time of surgery. If spectacles or contact lenses are to be used, the prescription is not given until the eye is healed and the refraction has stopped changing. Usually this is two or three months postoperatively. Nursing intervention is useful in helping clients adjust to all three methods of correcting aphakia. Table 5 summarizes some of the important characteristics of these three methods.

Spectacles.   The most common way of correcting aphakia is with the use of cataract spectacles. These are the simplest, safest, and most proven device for correcting aphakia (Marmor, 1981). Cataract glasses have thick, biconvex lenses. Although advances have been made in the type of lens used, some disadvantages remain. While the client's visual acuity with spectacles may be 20/20, visual comfort may be poor and the client may have difficulty with balance and mobility. Adjustment to the lenses is often difficult. The nurse can help by giving the client encouragement and specific suggestions. Because permanent cataract lenses are prescribed so long after surgery, it is often the community health nurse who helps the client adjust successfully to them.

The client's adjustment to cataract glasses depends on whether the client has bilateral or unilateral cataracts, and the amount of vision in the unoperated eye if the client has bilateral cataracts. The cataract lens magnifies the image as much as 20 to 30 percent. Eventually the brain adapts to the enlarged image if both eyes see it (Markovits, 1978). Magnification is the main reason for difficulty adjusting to cataract spectacles when the client has a unilateral cataract. In fact, a decision may be made not to operate on a unilateral cataract. Because of the magnified image perceived by the aphakic eye and the normal sized image perceived by the unoperated eye, the client experiences diplopia. The

TABLE 5. CHARACTERISTICS OF LENSES USED TO CORRECT APHAKIA

Characteristic	Glasses	Contact Lenses	Intraocular Lenses
Image size magnification	20–33%	4–10%	1–2%
Visual field	Limited	Full	Full
Depth perception	30%	50%	85%
24-hour use	No	No—hard lenses Yes—long wear lenses	Yes
Useful for clients with reduced dexterity	Yes	Difficult	Yes
Can be worn in dusty environments	Yes	No	Yes
Cosmetic appearance	Poor	Good	Good

brain cannot fuse these disparate images. The better the vision in the unoperated eye the more the client is bothered by the distortion of the cataract glasses. Many clients adapt to seeing unequal images (aniseikonia) by ignoring the unwanted image. They use their cataract glasses for reading, seeing little with the unoperated eye, and use the unoperated eye at other times. After their first cataract extraction, clients with bilateral cataracts may receive temporary cataract glasses. These have a blank or blurred lens so that the unoperated eye is not used and the client can see out of the operated eye. When the second operation is performed, the client receives permanent cataract glasses and is able to use both eyes together. However, the impression of nearness created by the size of the objects seen through cataract lenses is confusing. It results in reduced depth perception and a lack of coordination when reaching for objects, walking, climbing stairs, and performing other movements. Chairs, eating utensils, stairs and curbs appear closer than they really are. Clients should be warned to pour hot liquids and handle fragile objects with care. To help clients to adjust to cataract glasses, the nurse can suggest the client wear the glasses at first only when sitting. Gradually, the client can practice ambulating at home on level surfaces.

Cataract glasses have a circular blind spot around the edges of the thick lenses. This reduces the visual field and distorts objects seen through the edges of the glasses, giving them a wavy or jerky appearance. In addition, the unequal thickness of the lenses gives a jack-in-the-box effect (objects appear from out of nowhere) (Markovits, 1978). Consequently, some clients complain of dizziness or nausea. The nurse can reassure clients that the more they wear the glasses, the less discomfort they will experience. Clients should be told to look through the center of the glasses and to turn their head if they want to see something on the side. When driving a car, the person must use caution when changing lanes and turn the head far to each side to check for vehicles.

Cataract lenses may be made of glass or plastic. Although plastic lenses cost about twice as much, clients who can afford to do so should be advised to purchase them. They weigh much less than the heavy glass lenses and, therefore, they are more comfortable and easier to keep in place. In addition, because they can be ground to the edge, unlike glass, they do not cause as much peripheral visual distortion as glass lenses (Boyd-Monk, 1977).

Cataract glasses should be worn constantly while the client is awake. Without them the client is nearly blind. Clients who are forgetful may need the nurse's help in finding ways to keep the glasses from being lost.

Cataract glasses are expensive. To prevent breakage, the nurse should suggest the client find a safe place to store them. Lack of cleanliness is another problem the nurse may note. Because plastic lenses scratch easily, they must always be rinsed thoroughly before being wiped with a clean soft cloth. Plastic lenses should never be laid upon the lens surface.

Clients should be advised to have their glasses

checked regularly by an optician. Should they become loose or unaligned, vision and balance can be adversely affected. Periodically, the nurse should note whether the glasses fit correctly.

The nurse also needs to assess the client's acceptance of the cataract glasses. Some clients find them unacceptable because they are cosmetically unsightly. The magnification makes the wearer's eyes look huge to others. These clients may feel free to wear the glasses only when they are alone.

Contact Lenses.   Because a contact lens rides on the cornea, it is a centimeter closer to the retina than an eyeglass lens. It magnifies the image by only 4 to 8 percent, and the brain can accept and fuse this with the image from the other eye. For this reason, individuals with unilateral cataracts are especially likely to benefit from contact lenses (Kaspar, 1978). Contact lenses also permit adequate depth perception, peripheral vision, and far less distortion.

Elderly clients should be assessed before surgery for their ability to wear a contact lens. This lens requires a degree of manual dexterity, which older people may lack. Tremor, arthritis, and muscle weakness may make placing the lens in the eye a monumental task. Until the lens is placed in the eye, the client's vision is impaired, making it difficult to locate the lens and prepare it for insertion (Kahn, 1981). Clients who have had surgery on both eyes need to have a pair of cataract glasses to wear when the contacts are not in place. These enable the client to handle the contacts when cleaning or inserting them.

Recently a number of soft contact lenses which must be removed and cleaned only once a month have been approved for extended wear. These reduce some of the problems associated with contact lenses. Contact lenses cannot be worn in a dusty environment, and clients with ocular allergies or those with glaucoma cannot wear them. Many older clients find them uncomfortable to wear. Some believe they are a nuisance to care for. There is a poor success rate with contact lenses in persons over age 70 (Marmor, 1981). Certain risks are associated with wearing contact lenses. Prolonged wear may lead to the proliferation of blood vessels in the cornea. There is also the risk of infection (Kahn, 1981).

Clients who undergo a trial with contact lenses before surgery have a better chance of adjusting to the lens. The nurse can provide assistance and support for the client who is learning to insert, remove, and care for contact lenses. Time, practice, and patience are needed if the client is to overcome the physical and psychological difficulties associated with placing an object in the eye.

Intraocular Lenses.   A client with an implanted lens is called pseudophakic. This is by far the best optical solution to aphakia because it is placed close to the position of the natural lens. It restores normal vision almost immediately following surgery. Several different styles of lenses are used for implants. After the cataractous lens is extracted, a plastic replacement lens is inserted into the anterior chamber and the flaps of the hyaline capsule are closed over it. If the capsule is removed, the lens is held in place with tiny projecting feet or sutured to the iris or the sclera (Kwitko, 1978; Jennings, 1976a).

Better methods of sterilization and different techniques of fixation have improved the outlook for lens implants. Problems with the implants do arise, however, as a result of difficulties keeping them in place, secondary infection, and immunological rejection. The complication rate is 15 to 25 percent (Kornzweig, 1977). Complications occur because intraocular lenses represent a foreign body within the eye. Inflammation is controlled with the use of steroid eye drops. If the lens becomes displaced, it can be repositioned by dilating the pupil and then maneuvering the position of the head. If this is not successful, the lens must be removed surgically (Markovits, 1978; Jennings, 1976a).

The intraocular lens is still being evaluated for surgical risk and safety. The life of the lens has not yet been fully established. It is an excellent choice for individuals over age 70 with monocular or bilateral cataracts for whom cataract spectacles or contact lenses would be uncomfortable or unsuitable. Because their long-range complications are not known, however, intraocular lenses are used with caution in younger clients. Intraocular lenses eliminate difficulties inserting, removing, cleansing, and adapting to contact lenses. They cannot be lost or misplaced and, unlike spectacles, never need to be replaced. They are a solution for older people who cannot or will not wear contact lenses or spectacles (Kwitko, 1978).

Intraocular lenses cannot be used in all elderly clients. They are unsuitable for clients with certain types of refractive errors. In addition, they are contraindicated in clients who have vision in only one eye or who have had a poor result with an implant in the fellow eye. Clients with diabetic retinopathy, corneal dystrophy, glaucoma, retinal detachment, and certain other pathological conditions are not candidates for intraocular implants (Kahn, 1981).

Intraocular lenses are designed for distance vision. Consequently, the client needs to wear appropriate glasses to compensate for reading and other near vision (Jennings, 1976a). Clients who have intraocular lenses require miotic eyedrops, such as pilocarpine hydrochloride 2 percent. Clients may need to use these for the rest of their lives. The nurse needs to teach the older client the proper technique for introducing the drops. Many clients are apprehensive about hurting the eye. Patience and reinforcement are needed for effective teaching.

Summary. It is difficult for a person with good vision to realize how devastating it is to be unable to read a letter or sign one's name. Often, a small improvement in vision results in a major change in the client's self-esteem, outlook on life, mobility, and independence. Because the improvements are so meaningful, cataract surgery is an important intervention for many elderly clients. The nurse can play a significant role in supporting clients in their decision to undergo surgery and in helping them to adapt successfully in the postoperative period.

Providing Sensory Stimulation

In the last two decades, the concept of sensory deprivation has received serious attention in the nursing literature. Numerous laboratory investigations have been undertaken to identify the adaptations that accompany sensory deprivation and the stresses responsible for it. These studies have investigated subjects who experienced acute sensory deprivation after spending only a few hours or days in isolation or a deprived environment. Many of these studies focused on young, healthy people. A few systematic nursing studies examining the effects of an alteration in the amount of sensory stimulation clients receive have been done in the clinical setting. Many of these studied clients of all ages in acute care settings, such as intensive care units, where sensory deprivation is likely to occur. There have not been any rigorous studies focusing exclusively on the consequences of long-term sensory deprivation among the elderly.

This chapter focuses on the experience of chronic sensory deprivation, a phenomenon that is probably unique to the elderly population. Acute sensory deprivation and other varieties of sensory alteration are discussed in Chapter 21. There is no proof that chronic sensory deprivation exists. However, its presence has been postulated because so many elderly people who have multiple sensory deficits or who live in deprived environments exhibit adaptations similar to those observed in subjects experiencing sensory deprivation in experimental situations. If chronic sensory deprivation in the elderly exists, it may have a gradual onset. Adaptations may go unnoticed or be mistaken for senility (Kratz, 1979; Ernst and Shaw, 1980). The community health nurse is often the one who encounters this phenomenon in elderly people living at home who have been referred to a public health agency or visiting nurse service. Nurses who practice in long-term care facilities are also in a position to observe elderly residents suffering from sensory deprivation. As nurses understand why the aging client is at high risk for sensory deprivation, they are able to intervene more effectively.

The Normal Sensory Process. Individuals orient themselves to their surroundings by receiving stimuli through the senses and organizing them in the brain. The sensory process consists of reception and perception. Reception is the biological aspect of the sensory process. It involves vision, hearing, touch, taste, and smell, by which individuals maintain contact with the environment, and proprioception and visceral sensations, which provide information about stimuli arising within the body. Perception, the psychological aspect of the sensory process, is the selection and organization of the images received by the brain into a meaningful pattern. Perception is influenced by the intensity, size, change, or repetition of stimuli, as well as by past experiences, knowledge, and attitudes (Shelby, 1978; Boore, 1977).

The exact mechanisms involved in perception are poorly understood. Nerve fibers carry the sensory information to the cortex of the brain, where it is interpreted and a response is initiated. Collateral fibers pass to the reticular activating system (RAS). There is increasing evidence that the RAS plays an important role in the efficient processing of stimuli and the resulting behavior. The RAS is composed of a dense network of neurons, the reticular formation, which extends from the medulla to the thalamus. Functionally, it controls the overall level of central nervous system activity, including the degree of wakefulness or sleep and the ability to direct attention toward specific parts of the environment. The activity of the RAS is influenced by stimuli from the senses and the cerebral cortex.

It has been theorized that the RAS monitors incoming and outgoing stimuli and becomes attuned to a certain level of activity which is projected to the cortex. The RAS functions optimally only within this specific range of stimulation, that is, it can only adapt within certain limits. This level is required for normal perception, learning, and emotion. When this regulatory system is upset by disturbances in sensory input, including increases, decreases, and distortions of stimuli, the organism is no longer able to project a normal level of activation to the cortex. It makes compensatory adjustments to regain equilibrium. If these adjustments fail, behavior becomes disorganized (Schultz, 1965).

According to Schultz (1965) the arousal state of the RAS is a general drive state, which he called "sensoristasis." The organism strives to maintain a balance in stimulus variation to the cortex as mediated by the RAS. Individuals behave in ways that maintain an optimal arousal level. Sometimes they seek to increase stimulation and sometimes they seek to reduce stimulation. There appears to be considerable variation in the amount of stimuli different individuals consider optimal. The person's response to stimuli is influenced by many variables in the environment as well as individual differences. Consequently, it is not only the quantity of stimulation that is important for cortical arousal but the quality as reflected by the degree to which it is varied and meaningful. To maintain contact with the outside world, then, the brain needs continuous, meaningful stimuli.

Definition of Terms.   Standard terminology in the field of sensory deprivation has been lacking, hampering the efforts of theorists and researchers. Ac-

cording to Brownfield (1965) at least 25 terms have been used synonymously. *Sensory deprivation* has been defined as "a situation in which the reception or perception of stimuli is altered or blocked, or in which the environmental stimuli themselves are altered or blocked." (Chodil and Williams, 1970, p. 453). Sensory deprivation implies a relative, not an absolute, loss because the individual is not divested completely of the sensory process.

In the laboratory situation, *sensory deprivation* or *restriction* has been defined in a more restrictive way as a reduction in the amount and intensity of sensory input. The overall quantity of sensory stimuli may be reduced through a variety of means such as darkness or silence. *Perceptual deprivation* or *restriction* refers to a decrease or absence in meaningful patterning of sensory stimuli. Although the quantity of stimuli is not reduced, the quality is affected and the individual is unable to make sense of the stimuli. *Perceptual monotony* means that the sensory stimuli are normally patterned but lack variety (Bolin, 1974). *Social isolation* is a critical component of the concept of deprivation and refers to a form of perceptual monotony due to an unchanging environment and restricted social contacts (Ashworth, 1979). It occurs when an individual is isolated from other people or a familiar environment. The term *sensory-perceptual deprivation* is more inclusive and is used when the normal amount, pattern, and variety of sensory input are reduced.

According to Shelby (1978), the concept of sensory deprivation involves changes in three areas:

1. Sensory underload occurs when environmental stimuli are below the level required for attention purposes. It may be due to many factors, including stimuli of inadequate intensity, poorly functioning sensory receptors, or decreased perception, as is the case when the client is highly anxious and unable to attend to stimuli perceived by the senses.

2. Relevance deprivation occurs when there is restriction of useful information due to alteration in stimuli or blockage of receptors, making it difficult to relate to the stimuli. As relevance decreases, so does the amount of meaningful information. Various physical and emotional states affect relevance.

3. Alterations of the function of the reticular activating system may also occur as a result of too

little activity or too much activity. Too little sensory stimulation can be disruptive, causing cognitive and emotional deterioration and reducing behavioral efficiency. This can result when any single factor—amount of stimuli, level of stimuli variation, or pattern and meaning of stimuli—is insufficient.

The Elderly Client at Risk. Sensory deprivation in the elderly may result from physiological, psychosocial, or environmental stresses or from the interaction of two or more of these variables. Normal aging changes as well as many of the chronic illnesses that affect the aged place the elderly person at high risk for sensory deprivation. After middle age, there begins a decline in sensory function that affects the quantity and quality of sensory input. Vision, hearing, touch, taste, and possibly smell become less acute. Most elderly persons adapt to the loss of one sense by increased use of other senses. However, when losses develop in the compensatory senses, difficulty adapting increases.

In addition to the aging process, diseases such as cataracts and glaucoma impair the visual function of many elderly people. With age, the ability of the lens to focus the image on the retina is reduced. In addition, the cells of the retina normally become less sensitive to light so that under conditions of normal illumination, the elderly person receives less visual stimulation. When lighting is reduced, as is the case at night, the elderly client is even further deprived and may experience behavioral changes such as nocturnal restlessness (Storandt, 1976). The client with glaucoma experiences a restriction of peripheral vision. The client with macular degeneration sees only a grey shadow in the center of the visual field. With these and other diseases, visual distortions may occur, causing frightening visual impressions that resemble hallucinations (Butler and Lewis, 1977). Sensory deprivation and attendant social isolation may be the most serious consequences of impaired vision. Because of poor vision, clients may restrict their mobility, thus reducing opportunities for socialization. At the same time, moreover, reading, television and other diversions are reduced or eliminated.

Significant hearing loss is believed to have the most adverse consequences of all sensory impairments experienced by the elderly. Hearing loss causes greater social isolation than blindness, since it reduces or complicates verbal communication with others. Because there is little social sympathy for the deaf, older clients with hearing deficits may be excluded from activities and thus become less and less oriented (Butler and Lewis, 1977). Hearing loss can reduce reality testing and lead to marked suspiciousness, even paranoia. If elderly people cannot accurately hear the conversations of those about them, they may impute hostile motives when none exist in reality (Storandt, 1979). According to Foley (1975), paranoia is a nearly universal response in the elderly person who is deaf.

Somatic sensations, including touch and proprioception, decline with age. Touch is believed to be especially important for physical survival. The skin is the largest of the organs and the tactile cutaneous senses are represented by a large area in the brain. The area representing the tongue, lips, and hands is disproportionately large (Ernst and Shaw, 1980). With age, the touch threshold increases slightly. A more significant diminution of touch in the elderly is due to the effects of chronic illnesses such as diabetes and cerebrovascular accident.

The importance of proprioception (the sense of kinesthesis) in the overall sensory experience was realized in 1955 when tank respirators were first used for the victims of the polio epidemic. These clients were not able to touch or move their own bodies and suffered many cognitive, perceptual, and behavioral changes recognized later as the consequences of sensory deprivation. Proprioception is normally diminished in the elderly and is further reduced by immobility in aged clients who voluntarily restrict mobility or who suffer from arthritis, cardiovascular disease, and respiratory disease. Paralysis due to cerebrovascular disease or other neurological disorders also results in an inability to move part of the body and the loss of proprioception. It has been hypothesized that a restriction in mobility with the attendant reduction in proprioception is at least as important as other sensory restrictions in the disruption of normal functioning (Zubek, 1969).

Social isolation is a major component of sensory deprivation for many elderly people. Social interaction is especially important for the elderly because their social and emotional contacts are threatened and gradually lost. Non-English-speaking elderly persons living in America may be at the highest risk, especially if they reside in a setting where very few people know their language. The chronic, long-term illnesses that affect the great majority of older people also cause social isolation in the elderly. The disability and reduced energy level associated with chronic illness reduce the elderly client's ability to carry out normal social roles (Jones, 1976). In addition, specific communication difficulties are a component of many chronic illnesses such as Parkinson's disease and cerebrovascular accident and exacerbate social isolation. The public's attitude about certain diseases or their prognosis is another factor that may increase the victim's isolation. For example, the stigma attached to cancer and difficulty facing death commonly cause relatives and significant others to avoid the client with cancer.

Unsuitable environments, particularly in long-term care settings, are a primary reason for sensory deprivation in the elderly. When most older people are placed in long-term care settings, their well-being has already been impaired by personal and social losses as well as by restrictions in the senses due to aging and disease. When these individuals are deprived of the sensory and perceptual cues of a familiar environment and familiar people, confusion, disorientation, and other signs of sensory deprivation are the consequences (Jones, 1976). Although many long-term care settings have pleasant atmospheres, for the client who lives there 24 hours a day, the carpeted hallway and lounge may have little visual variety and meaning. Institutions may have an intercom system to communicate messages irrelevant to the client, but they do not have calendars or clocks to chime the passing of the hours. Perceptual monotony and social isolation characterize these settings and are greatest for residents who are confined to their rooms all day. Food cooked for a large group of people may lack the familiar textures, tastes, and smells that arouse a healthy appetite and may be too bland to stimulate the few remaining taste buds of the elderly resident. The slowly changing atmosphere and decline in meaningful interactions that characterize life in these settings contribute to boredom. Because one hour is no different from the next, clients are at high risk for disorientation (Wiggins, 1978).

Recognizing the Client Experiencing Sensory Deprivation. Schultz (1965) made the following observations about sensory deprivation. These serve as a framework to predict the adaptations exhibited by the client experiencing sensory deprivation.

- Conditions of diminished sensory input result in measurable changes in activity level.
- Restricted variation of sensory input activates the sensoristatic drive state, which becomes increasingly intense as a function of time and amount of deprivation.
- When sensory restrictions disturb sensoristatic balance, gross disturbances occur in perception, cognition, and learning.
- When stimulus variation is restricted, the organism lowers its sensory threshold and thus becomes increasingly sensitized to stimulation in an attempt to restore balance.
- There are individual differences in the need for sensory variation.
- Reduction of the pattern or meaning of stimuli results in greater behavioral consequences than reduction in the level of stimuli.

Adaptations to Sensory Deprivation. Extensive research has documented cognitive, affective, perceptual, behavioral, and other changes in clients experiencing sensory deprivation.

Cognitive changes include confusion, disorientation, a general slowing of intellectual activity, and difficulty concentrating, abstracting, thinking coherently, and solving problems (Shelby, 1978). Clients may experience unusual, unrealistic, even bizarre, ideas (Boore, 1977).

Affective changes include anxiety, fear, depression, and rapid mood swings (Shelby, 1978). As sensory deprivation continues, clients may become increasingly irritable and lose their sense of perspective. The intensity of these emotional changes may vary from mild to severe. If the client is ill, alterations in emotional state may be more extreme because of such stresses as pain or anxiety (Boore, 1977).

Perceptual changes range from mild daydreams to illusions and hallucinations. These may be visual, auditory, kinesthetic, or somasthetic (Shelby, 1978). Hallucinations may be an attempt to pattern stimuli or increase the level of stimuli

(Chodil and Williams, 1970). Relatively simple perceptual disorders include seeing dots, colors, or shapes and hearing strange sounds. Clients have reported experiencing minor bodily sensations such as numbness or itching. More complex perceptual distortions include seeing people, animals, or landscapes, hearing voices or music, and having the sensation that one's body is rising or falling. Clients have also reported unusual perceptions of taste and smell.

Serious *behavioral changes* are a well-recognized consequence of sensory deprivation. Many clients exhibit noncompliant behavior (Shelby, 1978). This adaptation was a significant finding of the studies of clients who were required to wear bilateral eye patches following eye surgery. In addition, clients become bored and are eager for any kind of stimulation. They may be easily amused.

Other adaptations may also accompany sensory deprivation. Some individuals have complained of increasing sensitivity to bodily discomforts or pain (Downs, 1974; Shelby, 1978). The quality of sleep and dreams may change (Shelby, 1978). Physiological changes in parameters such as the galvanic skin response, catecholamine analysis, and electroencephalogram recordings have also been documented in clients experiencing sensory deprivation (Bolin, 1974).

Many of the adaptations associated with sensory deprivation are also typical of the elderly client who is "senile." These include confusion, disorientation, hallucinations, inability to abstract, and poor judgment. Therefore, to avoid mislabeling or overlooking the elderly client suffering sensory deprivation, a thorough assessment is essential.

Assessing the Client's Adaptations. The nursing approach to the elderly client experiencing sensory deprivation needs to be characterized by tact and sensitivity. Although subjects in experimental situations of sensory deprivation are usually willing, even eager, to discuss their experiences, elderly clients are unlikely to be open about them. Many clients are frightened by hallucinatory experiences. They believe their perceptions, thoughts, and feelings are signs of an underlying mental disorder. They may fear they are "going crazy." Skillful questioning may be necessary before clients reveal their experiences. They may offer cues about the experiences by using words such as "daydream" or "nightmare."

A careful assessment involves data collection in the following areas:

- Sensory status
- Level of mobility
- Preferred stimulation level
- Sensory, perceptual, and social environment
- Mental status
- Behavioral changes
- Personal resources

The assessment begins with an examination of vision, hearing, taste, smell, touch, and proprioception. The client with multiple sensory losses is at highest risk for sensory deprivation. Because the elderly client experiences gradual but continuous changes in sensory function, these assessments are most useful when performed on a regular basis. The presence of health problems such as diabetic neuropathy, cataracts, glaucoma, macular degeneration, or cerebrovascular accident should alert the nurse to the possibility of significant sensory deficits.

A musculoskeletal examination should be performed to identify any impairment of mobility. Clients should be questioned about their normal activity level. Mobility affects the sensory experience indirectly by altering sensory input or socialization.

The client's preferred stimulation level depends upon the setting and the nature of the client's problem. Every individual has a normal stimulation level that promotes optimal functioning of the reticular activating system. The range of stimulation that may be considered normal varies from person to person, as does tolerance and response to sensory deprivation. What was the baseline of sensory stimulation before the client was transferred from the home to the long-term care setting or before the client experienced significant losses of sensory function, mobility, or health? The nurse can ask relatives and significant others about the client's previous life-style or environment. These data help the nurse determine whether the client is being subjected to too much or too little stimulation.

Identifying the client's baseline level of stimulation helps the nurse to assess the client's sensory, perceptual, and social environments. Homebound clients as well as those in long-term care settings may be living in environments that are depriving them of essential sensory input. The environment should be assessed for the quantity, kind, and quality of stimuli. Are the stimuli meaningful and relevant to the elderly client?

Mental status changes, particularly disorientation to time and place, are common responses to sensory deprivation. In contrast, other clients may hallucinate but remain oriented to time, place, and person. If the elderly client has experienced a change in mental status, efforts should be made to determine if it is related to a change in sensory input. Determining the real reason for mental status changes in the elderly client experiencing chronic sensory deprivation is difficult because the mental status may change gradually over a long period of time.

Observations of behavior are especially important when clients are reluctant to share their perceptual, cognitive, or emotional experiences with the nurse. Does the client seem bored? Apathetic? Is the client's interest in life gradually fading? Does the nurse have difficulty in getting the client's attention? Is the client withdrawn? The client's sleeping patterns provide useful data. Is the client restless at night? Does the client wander at night? The client's appetite, reaction to visitors, and attention to personal hygiene provide other valuable information.

An assessment of the client's personal resources for coping is useful in pinpointing clients at high risk for sensory deprivation. Past experiences, personality, and social relationships influence how the client will respond to sensory deprivation. Clients experiencing stress due to illness or other losses are particularly vulnerable.

Elderly clients vary widely in their need for sensory stimuli and their vulnerability to sensory deprivation. Adaptations to chronic sensory deprivation have a gradual onset and may be subtle. Each client responds in an individualized way to sensory deprivation. A careful assessment of the elderly client will prevent this problem from being overlooked.

Nursing Management.   In caring for the elderly client experiencing sensory deprivation the nurse should be aware that the client's behavior is due to a combination of physiological, psychosocial, and environmental factors. In addition, the range of stimulation that is considered normal varies from one person to another. Therefore, the nurse must be attuned to individual differences and to individual needs when planning nursing interventions. Many nursing interventions have been suggested to assist the sensorially deprived client. Although these have been tested empirically, few have been substantiated by rigorous clinical research. The nurse should carefully evaluate each client situation to determine which interventions will be effective. If the client's behavior is modified by the interventions, then the assessment was correct and similar care should continue.

Nursing interventions for clients exposed to sensory deprivation are directed toward two major goals; first, to promote an optimal level of sensory input for the client, and, second, to assist the client who is experiencing cognitive, perceptual, or behavioral changes. Data from the nursing assessment are used to identify specific stresses responsible for the sensory deprivation and suggest appropriate nursing interventions.

Maximizing Remaining Sensory Function.   If sensory deprivation is believed to be due at least in part to poorly functioning sensory receptors, nursing interventions are aimed at improving function or maximizing remaining function. A client suspected of having a correctable problem such as presbyopia, cataracts, glaucoma, or a hearing loss should be referred for appropriate medical or surgical follow-up. Sometimes this very simple intervention is overlooked, especially for clients who have resided for years in a long-term care facility.

The client with reduced vision should be advised to use glasses and other low vision aids, if appropriate. These are a positive help because they not only allow the client to maintain social contacts but increase the quantity and variety of available sensory input. For example, both illuminated and nonilluminated magnifiers are available. These may allow a client to read or to look up numbers in the telephone directory. Phone dial attachments with enlarged numbers and letters allow the client to use the telephone. Reading materials with print of varying darkness and size are available. Some of the strategies to assist clients with reduced vision do not require special equipment. Simply using a night-light may prevent sensory deprivation, with its consequent restlessness and wandering, for some elderly clients. Removing the cover over the face of the clock or watch allows the client to use touch to remain aware of the time.

Fewer effective aids are available for the client with a hearing deficit. These are described in Chapter 16. Hearing aids are not effective for a large proportion of the elderly with hearing impairments and many elderly people who might benefit from a hearing aid resist wearing one (Foley, 1975). If the client does use a hearing aid, problems arise when the client is admitted to an acute or long-term care facility where staff do not know how to operate it. Nurses can provide an enormous service to clients by ensuring that members of their staff understand how to insert the hearing aid, check and change batteries, and turn it on and off.

The use of touch is an especially important intervention for elderly clients who have deficits in vision and hearing. Touch helps to orient the person, provides stimulation, and decreases social isolation by establishing interaction with the client. Touching should be used circumspectly because an older person may interpret it as an intrusion of personal space or overfamiliarity. Mutually positive results have been reported about touching between elderly clients and nurses (Ernst and Shaw, 1980). Most clients perceive the nurse who touches them as available, ready to help, liking them, and listening to them. Touching indicates caring. It is a validation of one's existence. Touch used with praise has been found to reverse adaptations of senility (Todd, 1966). Clients who are regressed may respond more readily to touch than to other stimulation techniques (Burnside, 1976). If the client lives in a long-term care setting, many everyday tasks of nursing, such as bathing, positioning, transferring, and giving backrubs offer opportunities to use touch. The nurse can plan opportunities for the client to touch. For example, when bathing the client, the nurse might ask how the bath towel or the bar of soap feels.

Encouraging Mobility.   If immobility is one of the factors contributing to the client's sensory deprivation, the nurse should encourage mobility and activities within the limits of the client's ability. Clients who live in institutions should be encouraged to do as much self-care as possible. This activity stimulates the sense of kinesthesis. Encouraging clients to walk not only affects kinesthesis but adds variation to the sensory input through eyes, ears, and nose. Stretching exercises, calisthenics, relaxation techniques, and dancing are also useful ways to stimulate the kinesthetic sense. Activities such as these are especially useful for groups of elderly clients living in long-term care facilities or the community.

Altering the Environment.   Nurses working in long-term care settings need to be especially sensitive to the quantity, patterning, and variety of stimulation provided by the environment. Methods of improving the quality of sensory input are limited only by the imagination. Elderly clients may be unable to relate to daily routines that are different from the ones they practiced at home. Clients entering long-term care facilities benefit from early, careful, and repeated explanations of routines and practices. Clients may have difficulty relating to the sensory cues in the facility. If the client had been accustomed to a late afternoon meal using china and flatware acquired when married years ago, she may be confused when meals are served at different hours and arrive on cardboard trays set with paper dishes and plastic eating utensils. Practices such as allowing clients to wear their own clothes, encouraging them to keep old photographs and mementos in view, and assisting them to maintain as many previous hygiene rituals as possible are ways to help maintain links with meaningful stimuli.

Efforts should be made to add pattern and meaning to background stimuli in long-term care facilities. Background noises may consist primarily of the random clanking of equipment as it is moved and the ringing of phones. The facility itself may lack visual variety. Painting different rooms in differing colors helps clients to identify their surroundings and increases the pattern and variety of sensory input. Clocks that chime the hour can be placed strategically to help clients remain oriented. Encouraging clients to make regular use of telephones, televisions, and radios provides additional meaningful stimuli. Not only is each day spent in a long-term care facility almost identical to the one before it, the day may lack sufficient structure for the elderly client. Clients benefit from large calendars with the correct date clearly indicated. Clients who can do so should be encouraged to read the newspaper to remain aware of the passage of time. Assisting the elderly client to establish and maintain a daily schedule of activities of daily living and various meaningful diversionary activities increases the patterning of stimuli.

If clients cannot be moved from their rooms, changing the position of their bed at intervals so they can see through a door or window improves the variety of stimuli. Hanging a mirror on the wall enlarges the client's visual field and increases visual stimulation.

The quantity and quality of opportunities for socialization take on new importance for the elderly. It is through socialization that the individual receives positive feedback and maintains self-esteem. If the client resides in a long-term care facility, staff members provide one of the few meaningful opportunities for human contact and socialization. Nurses can help their staff maintain quality in their interactions with the residents. They also need to encourage residents to form meaningful relationships with other clients. It is often helpful if the nurse explains to the client's family and significant others the reason why telephone calls, letters, and visits are so important.

Nurses who work with the elderly should be able to conduct sensory retraining groups with ease. Sensory retraining techniques consist of structured activities designed to reawaken awareness of the environment through the senses and promote socialization. They often take place in a group setting. Sensory retraining techniques are helpful for elderly clients who are mentally impaired or regressed or who are exposed to too little or too much stimuli. The term "sensory stimulation" refers to those programs intended to improve the amount, quality, patterning, or variety of stimuli for clients experiencing, or at risk of, sensory deprivation. Sensory retraining techniques utilize repetition, reinforcement, and immediate reward in a series of activities designed to maintain the function of the senses. One technique (Richman, 1969) involves stimulating each sense individually and subsequently stimulating two or more senses. To arouse attention, the client is asked to name which sensory organ is being stimulated and by what means. Thus, clients become aware of what they see, hear, taste, touch, or smell.

Naming the stimulus to each sensory organ encourages clear, precise thinking.

Scott and Crowhurst (1975) described a variety of sensory retraining exercises conducted in a small group. Activities begin with greetings and handshakes. Clients may be assisted to look in a mirror to reinforce reality. Group members may toss a "ball" made of soft materials and filled with scraps to stimulate sight, touch, and muscle coordination. The group may play simple hand instruments or clap and sing along to music. A variety of foods may be used to stimulate taste and smell and other senses as well. For example, given a variety of fruits, the group can explore their color and texture as well as their taste and smell.

Several strategies are helpful for the client who is experiencing adaptations to sensory deprivation. Because these experiences may be disturbing, providing clients with an opportunity to relate their experiences may provide great emotional relief. The elderly client can also benefit from an explanation of the reason for the adaptations and reassurance that measures can be taken to prevent them. If the client is disoriented, other measures to assist the client experiencing sensory deprivation include orienting and reorienting the client to the environment, events in the environment, and the time and date (Bolin, 1974).

Summary. The nurse who is aware of the stresses responsible for sensory deprivation can incorporate sensory stimulation techniques into nursing care. These are most effective when the client participates in efforts to enhance the quantity, patterning or variety of sensory stimuli. The result can be a more rewarding life for the client.

Discharge Planning

Posthospital discharge planning is essential for elderly clients. The vast majority of them are discharged to the community. Only 5 percent need a protective setting, such as a skilled nursing facility (SNF) or an intermediate nursing facility (INF) (Butler and Lewis, 1977). Brocklehurst (1978) reports that 93 percent of older hospitalized clients in one study went back to the same type of accommodation (private household or long-term care facility) from which they had been admitted.

Reactions to Hospital Discharge. Perhaps the most critical point of the elderly person's hospitalization is the experience of discharge. Consequently, research has been directed toward the problems that arise when elderly clients are discharged from the hospital. Many conflicting emotional and social stresses occur. Some tend to prevent discharge while others facilitate it (Brocklehurst, 1978).

Elderly people leave the hospital with very mixed feelings. Only a few are really happy to leave, and some are positively reluctant to leave. Some elderly clients are anxious to return home alone. They are motivated to overcome incredible obstacles in order to return to the community (Keywood, 1978). Other older people fear leaving the secure environment of the hospital and dread returning to the deprivation or isolation they suffered before hospitalization.

Clients who are discharged to nursing homes also have mixed feelings. During their hospitalization a few elderly clients become dependent on others and wish to continue this life-style. For them, placement in a long-term care facility may be desirable. Other older clients facing discharge from the hospital to a nursing home may feel life is no longer worth living.

Family members also have mixed feelings about the older client's postdischarge arrangements. In one study, 21 percent of families viewed the planned discharge of the elderly person back to the family setting as unwelcome. Married and unmarried children were most likely to express this attitude, whereas spouses of elderly clients were least likely. No doubt these attitudes were the result of stress and strain on the family prior to hospital admission due to physical or mental disability of the elderly member (Brocklehurst, 1978). On the other hand, when older clients plan to return alone to their own home, families feel concerned about their relatives' welfare and worry about what possible things could happen to them in the home without supervision. These stressful situations, which may be unique to elderly clients leaving the hospital, increase the need for careful discharge planning.

The Process of Discharge Planning. The goal of discharge planning is to ensure that appropriate arrangements are made to place the client following hospitalization. Both clients and their relatives or significant others should understand the plan that is made and the reasons for it. Responsibility for discharge planning rests with several professional groups. Usually, however, it is the nurse or social worker who plays a leadership role. In some hospitals, discharge planning is the direct responsibility of the social service department. In other hospitals, special discharge planning departments are set up and staffed by professional nurses. Usually, nurses with community health experience are preferred. Alternatively, the responsibility for discharge planning may be given to the staff in the utilization review department because of the obvious link between discharge planning and utilization review. Many hospitals employ nurses to staff this department. In some instances, staff nurses who provide bedside care are given direct responsibility for discharge planning. This arrangement is most likely in settings that utilize primary care nursing. The nurse is always involved in discharge planning—if not directly, then indirectly. Clients, families, physicians, social workers, and others involved in the discharge planning process depend heavily on the staff nurse's assessment when making decisions about an appropriate setting for the client following discharge.

Every hospital has a different system for determining which clients receive formal discharge planning services. Because discharge planning is time consuming and expensive, many hospitals provide discharge planning only to selected groups of clients. Because the elderly are considered a high-risk group, however, most hospitals routinely contact every elderly client who is admitted to determine whether or not there is a need for discharge planning. Other hospitals depend heavily upon referrals from staff nurses and physicians in order to meet the client's discharge planning needs.

Nurses who have direct responsibility for discharge planning need to develop information about community resources that may assist the discharge planning process. This should include data about long-term care facilities and community agencies available to assist clients who return home. Information should be gathered about the types of services offered, types of clients who would benefit, licensure, staffing, and quality of service. After a resource is used, the discharge planner should contact the agency about any problems that it might have encountered in the referral. Feedback can be used to improve the referral system (Smith et al., 1979).

Discharge planning is most effective when begun on the first day of admission. Constant assessment and reassessment of the client's adaptation is essential if discharge placement is to be appropriate. There should be weekly conferences among physicians, staff nurses, and social workers as well as the professional in charge of the discharge planning process. Conferences are more successful when professionals from community agencies are also involved. These bring hospitals and community together and allow for feedback about clients who have already been discharged. The purpose of the conference is to discuss the discharge needs of all clients, to alert those involved of upcoming discharges, and to agree on who will be responsible for taking action on decisions made (Smith et al., 1979; Brocklehurst, 1978).

Three major variables are used to determine whether the client is a candidate for a long-term care facility or able to return home:

1. The client's physical status and self-care abilities.
2. The client's mental status.
3. The client's emotional well-being.

There are many pitfalls in determining whether the client is able to handle self-care in the home. Errors are often made because many elderly clients in the hospital setting *seem* able to do little for themselves. The nursing staff may bathe, dress, and feed them. Nevertheless, this is not an indication that clients *cannot* do things for themselves. Older clients may not help themselves in the hospital because they believe it is the nurse's job to do so.

Evaluation of mental status when older clients are hospitalized may also be misleading. Hospitalization, traumatic events, a change in routine, and unfamiliar surroundings may alter the mental status of older people. When older clients leave the continuity and familiarity of their own home, they may lose self-confidence and develop feelings of insecurity. The client's comfortable routine is abruptly exchanged for a sporadic and unpredictable hospital routine. These factors, especially when coupled with illness and anxiety, may cause disorientation, agi-

tation, and other changes, often causing staff to conclude that clients will never again be able to function in their own homes.

When assessing the client's physical or mental deterioration for purposes of discharge planning, the nurse needs to determine whether the deterioration has been developing slowly over a long period of time or has been sudden and recent. Questioning the client, relatives, and significant others is the best way to obtain this information. Knowledge of the client's medical diagnosis is useful in determining whether or not it plays a role in the client's ability to function (Anderson, 1979).

An important part of the assessment is to consider the client's emotional well-being. It is valuable to listen to the client's own view on postdischarge placement. When the client's functional status is the only variable used to determine placement, the client's own emotional needs are often overlooked. Often, the client and family disagree about appropriate placement. When this is the case, the nurse should ask, "Whose needs are being met?"

Because staff nurses spend the most time with hospitalized clients, others involved in discharge planning depend upon them for an accurate, reliable assessment. Data from the assessment are used to identify realistic discharge options for the older person. The elderly have the right to decide where they want to go after they leave the hospital. Many desire to make their own decisions and are capable of doing so. The elderly client should be made aware of the available alternatives and the probable consequences of each alternative. Discharge planning can become a moral issue when clients who do not seem able to undertake self-care decide they wish to return to their own homes. Should staff accept an aged client's decision to return home when the client seems confused or in need of nursing care? If older clients are actively involved in the discharge planning process, they usually make responsible decisions regarding their postdischarge care. In addition, when older clients make their own decisions regarding postdischarge placement, their transition to the postdischarge environment is happier and healthier (Anderson, 1979).

During the discharge planning process, it is important for the nurse to give support to the family of the elderly client. Families understandably feel concerned about their relatives' welfare, but they often become overprotective. If they believe that the client is unable to make wise decisions due to age and illness, they may treat the client like a dependent child and make decisions for the client. When home care is being considered for the aging client, family participation is often crucial to a successful outcome. Therefore, their own needs and desires must be identified and respected but with care taken to avoid negating those of the older client involved.

Planning for Discharge to a Long-Term Care Facility. The transition from acute to convalescent care is a multistage process that begins with the decision to move the client from the hospital and ends when the client has made a satisfactory adjustment to the long-term care setting. This transition can be difficult because the two systems differ regarding the goals of care, length of stay, perception of quality of care provided, and prestige afforded staff. If the transition is to be successful, communication among client, family, and staff members in both settings is essential. Although staff nurses may not be directly involved in the discharge planning process, their assessment of the client is essential if a setting is to be selected that meets the client's needs and if the client is to make a successful transition to that setting.

When long-term care is contemplated, the staff nurse completes forms that identify the client's ability to perform activities of daily living, physical care needs, and special care regimens. Inadvertent omissions of care or lack of descriptive detail may lead to inappropriate placement. When attempting to find a suitable facility for an older client, what seems like routine information takes on importance in the negotiations between discharge planning personnel and staff in long-term care facilities. Information about the older client's functional potential is also important. This information helps to determine whether the client needs a setting that emphasizes custodial care or rehabilitation.

Once a long-term care facility has been selected, the staff nurse should supply the facility with additional information about the older client. An important goal of long-term care settings is to provide a living situation for the person as well as treatment for specific health problems. Personal habits may be of secondary concern in an acute care setting

because treatment of illness takes priority. In the long-term care facility, personal habits assume priority. They may provide a link to reality for elderly clients in a strange environment.

Elderly clients making the transition from acute to chronic health care facilities bring with them personal habits, personality traits, and life experiences acquired over many decades. Nurses who have been caring for the client in the hospital can provide staff in the convalescent care facility with valuable personal information about the client. Nurses can describe the client's way of coping with the limits imposed by illness, the client's understanding of the reasons for the transfer to the long-term care setting, the manner in which the client was prepared for the new facility, and the client's perception of the future implied by long-term care. As the need for more sophisticated placement decisions for older clients increases, the staff nurse's role in this area should expand (Habeeb and McLaughlin, 1979).

Planning for Discharge to the Community. Preparing the client to function at home following hospitalization begins with a thorough assessment. Data should be obtained in the following areas:

- General health status
- Ability to function in the home environment
- Availability of community resources
- Learning needs
- Adjustment to illness

Determining the client's *general health status,* particularly the presence of multiple chronic illnesses, helps to predict the client's need for medical or nursing follow up after discharge. Some clients may require regular, frequent assessment and follow up. If this is the case, transportation arrangements to health care facilities should be made prior to discharge. As an alternative, it is sometimes possible for health team members from the acute care setting, including physicians, to make home visits to provide care. When nursing follow up is required, the best solution may be a referral to the visiting nurse service.

Several variables are assessed in order to determine the client's *ability to function in the home environment.* Some clients may be able to function if they live with others, but are not able to manage at home alone. In this instance, the people with whom the client is living must be assessed for their ability and willingness to help the client. Because it has a bearing on the ease or difficulty encountered in living in the community, the physical environment of the home should be assessed. The presence of adequate bathroom and kitchen facilities should be determined. If relevant, the environment should be checked to ensure that the client's safety and mobility are not impaired by barriers such as stairways or doorsills. It is essential that the client have a telephone readily accessible in the home in case of emergencies. The need for special equipment in the home, such as a special bed or a wheelchair, should be determined so that the equipment can be obtained prior to discharge. The client's ability to perform activities of daily living should also be determined. For this purpose, the nurse can use one of the ADL assessment tools described in Chapter 17. In particular, the nurse should identify how clients intend to obtain food and medications if they are not able to leave the home. The client's ability to function in the environment helps to determine a need for a home health aide or home attendant when family and others are not available to help with the client's care.

The *availability of community resources* may determine whether or not the client, especially the client who lives alone, is able to return to the home. The availability of supermarkets and other shops should be determined. Delivery services can be invaluable in keeping the homebound client stocked with foods, medications, and other necessities. If the client cannot make private arrangements for transportation to health facilities, the accessibility of public transportation is an important factor.

The client's *teaching needs* should be ascertained and met prior to discharge. Clients returning home need information in all of the following areas:

- Nature of health problems, including their cause, signs of reoccurrence, and ways to prevent reoccurrence.
- Medications, including actions, dose, dose schedule, and possible side effects.
- Treatments, procedures, and exercises, including their purpose, how to do them, their schedule, and potential problems.
- Special supplies and equipment, including their purpose, how to use them, how to obtain repairs, and how to obtain more of them.

- Special diet, including its purpose, foods to eat, foods to avoid, and nature and amount of allowed fluids (Stone, 1979).

Data about the client's *adjustment to illness* and the future situation may indicate a need for referral to agencies that can support the client and family through the adjustment period following discharge. Among the numerous public and private agencies to which the nurse might refer to the client are an ostomy club, the Cancer Society, the Diabetes Association, a mental health agency, or a senior citizen center.

Prior to discharge, the nurse assures that the needs identified in the assessment have been met. Any special equipment should be secured and any alterations in the structure of the home should be made. Referrals to community agencies and health care facilities should be made. The client should be given an appointment for medical follow up. Education of the client and, if necessary, the family, should be completed. Once the final discharge plan is determined, the discharge planner must ensure that the client, involved family or significant others, physician, and other involved professionals know exactly what to expect.

Facilitating Return to the Community. Many elderly people who desire to return to their home following hospital discharge must overcome formidable obstacles in order to do so successfully. The health care literature identifies a number of innovative strategies that have been used to help elderly clients adapt successfully in their home environment. Unfortunately, most of these strategies are not widely used in the United States. They include:

- Self-care apartments
- Day hospitals
- After-care programs
- Trial discharge
- Home visiting

The use of *self-care apartments* has been tried in England, where some acute care hospitals house a limited number of apartments. Each apartment is a self-contained living unit with kitchen facilities. Prior to discharge, elderly clients move into the apartment, where they can be supervised and yet remain independent in activities of daily living. The client is expected to prepare light meals and keep the apartment tidy. This experience restores self-confidence to elderly clients by allowing them to see for themselves that they can manage on their own both day and night. Family members and other concerned individuals are reassured before clients leave the protective setting that they can manage safely on their own (Alcock, 1981).

Geriatric day hospitals have proven to be an important strategy for overcoming many of the problems that face older people who return home. These provide comprehensive health-related services to clients who visit the hospital for 5- to 7-hour periods each day to achieve specific therapeutic goals (Kemp, 1978). Major emphasis is on rehabilitation and teaching family members and others how to care for the client. Diagnostic and outpatient services may also be offered. Often, the day hospital and the rehabilitation unit the client visited while hospitalized are one and the same. When this is the case, elderly clients who are going home feel more secure knowing that they will be returning to the same place and the same personnel in whom they already have confidence (Brocklehurst, 1978). Day hospital care is expensive. Participation in day hospital programs is expected to be a temporary measure, ending when the client and family are able to function alone.

After-care programs provide temporary hospital services to clients for several hours several times a week. These transitional programs offer a wide range of services designed to help clients meet specific goals that will promote their ability to function in the home environment. The advantage of this approach is that the provider is able to offer a wide range of services to a group of clients, while using professional personnel efficiently. Because most after-care programs do not provide transportation between hospital and home for elderly clients, their accessibility is reduced.

Despite careful predischarge planning, many questions often remain in the minds of the client, concerned family, and staff regarding whether or not the client will be able to function in the home. Allowing the client to go home for a day or a weekend on a *trial discharge* is an excellent way to assess the client's abilities directly (Kemp, 1978). Trial discharges are a way to identify unforeseen problems in the home that can be corrected before the client is sent home permanently.

Another strategy to facilitate the elderly client's return home is *home visiting* by hospital staff nurses who personally follow up each elderly client who is discharged. This may involve a home visit before discharge so that a direct assessment can be made of necessary modifications and special equipment in the home. Following discharge, the nurse makes home visits in order to evaluate the discharge plan and to identify whether or not the client needs additional support in order to manage in the home. Fell (1979) described a home visiting project in which the client's primary nurse who planned the discharge made a home visit on selected clients to evaluate the discharge planning. If a nurse identified a need for additional follow-up visits, a public health referral was made. The project was judged beneficial for the involved clients. While home visiting by staff nurses seems to be an excellent way to follow up clients who are discharged to their homes, there are problems implementing this strategy. The hospital must identify mechanisms to adjust nurses' hours to allow for the visit or to compensate nurses for time spent making home visits. The expense of such a plan means that the hospital must have a real commitment to the project.

Summary. Today, increasing emphasis is being placed on discharge planning. Ideally, this should begin when the elderly client is admitted to the hospital. The nurse is involved directly or indirectly in discharge planning. The nursing assessment serves as the basis for decision making. Careful preplanning will shorten the client's stay in the hospital and assure the elderly client of a prepared environment, whether this is the client's own home or a long-term care facility.

SUMMARY

Clients at Adaptation Level Four are coping with adaptations that have become additional stresses for them. Because their energy reserves have been depleted, these clients are unable to carry out ADLs without assistance. Frequently, they require care in hospitals or long-term care facilities. Often, appropriate intervention by the health care team allows clients at Adaptation Level Four to return to a higher level of adaptation.

This chapter focused on cancer and cataracts, two chronic health problems that may be the reason for the move to Adaptation Level Four. Both of these health problems are associated with changes in certain of the body's regulatory mechanisms: cataracts with sensory regulation, and cancer with immunological and growth regulation.

Although older clients with cataracts may be able to function independently for years, eventually vision is so severely impaired that clients are unable to perform ADLs or do so unsafely. Because of new microsurgical techniques, most older clients with cataracts should be able to regain their former independence. The nurse's role in preparing clients for cataract surgery and subsequent chronic aphakia helps older clients to adapt optimally. The older client with cancer may function independently for long periods of time, but may move to Adaptation Level Four when the illness advances or surgery, radiation therapy, or chemotherapy is indicated. At these times, the client requires direct nursing intervention.

Normal aging changes place older clients with serious health problems at risk for sensory deprivation. Clients experiencing sensory deprivation may be found in acute care facilities, long-term care settings, or the community. In this chapter, emphasis was given to the nurse's role in assisting clients who are experiencing long-term sensory deprivation.

Because these health problems, like so many others that affect older people, require hospitalization, the need for discharge planning from acute care settings was also discussed. The nurse is always involved, directly or indirectly, in the discharge planning process, and the need for discharge planning for the elderly is universal.

REFERENCES

Alcock J: Stepping-stone to home. Nursing Times 77(10):422, 1981

American Cancer Society. Cancer Facts and Figures, 1983

Anderson CA: Home or nursing home? Let the elderly patient decide. American Journal of Nursing 79(8):1450, 1979

Anderson F Sir: Practical Management of the Elderly. Oxford, Blackwell, 1976

Anderson MEK: Color vision defects in the elderly. Journal of Gerontological Nursing 6(7):383, 1980

Ashworth P: Sensory deprivation: The acutely ill. Nursing Times 75(7):290, 1979

Baj PA, Walker D: Management actions to humanize the health care environment. Journal of Nursing Education 19(6):43, 1980

Blot WJ: Changing patterns of breast cancer among American women. American Journal of Public Health 70(8):832, 1980

Bolin, RH: Sensory deprivation: An overview. Nursing Forum XIII(3):254, 1974

Boore J: Older people and sensory deprivation. Nursing Times 73(45):1754, 1977

Botwinick J: Aging and Behavior: A Comprehensive Integration of Research Findings, 2nd ed. New York, Springer, 1978

Boyd-Monk H: Cataract surgery. Nursing 77(6):56, 1977

Brocklehurst JC: Geriatric services and the day hospital, in Brocklehurst JC (ed), Textbook of Geriatric Medicine and Gerontology, 2nd ed. New York, Churchill Livingstone, 1978

Brownfield CA: Isolation: Clinical and Experimental Approaches. New York, Random House, 1965

Burnside IM: Clocks and calendars. American Journal of Nursing 70(1):117, 1970

Burnside IM: The special senses and sensory deprivation, in Burnside IM (ed), Nursing and the Aged. New York, McGraw-Hill, 1976

Butler RN, Lewis MI: Aging and Mental Health, 2nd ed. St. Louis, Mosby, 1977

Charlesworth D, Baker RH: Surgery in old age, in Brocklehurst JC (ed), Textbook of Geriatric Medicine and Gerontology, 2nd ed. New York, Churchill Livingstone, 1978

Chodil J, Williams B: The concept of sensory deprivation. Nursing Clinics of North America 5:453, 1970

Clifford GO, Bewtra AK: Hematological problems in the elderly, in Rossman I (ed), Clinical Geriatrics, 2nd ed. Philadelphia, Lippincott, 1979

Downs FS: Bedrest and sensory disturbances. American Journal of Nursing 74(3):434, 1974

Elkowitz EB: Geriatric Medicine for the Primary Care Practitioner. New York, Springer, 1981

Ernst P, Shaw J: Touching is not taboo. Geriatric Nursing 1(5):193, 1980

Exton-Smith AN, Overstall PW: Guidelines in Medicine. Volume I. Geriatrics. Baltimore, University Park Press, 1979

Fell PE: Making the right moves in discharge planning: Home visits to evaluate planning. American Journal of Nursing 79(8):1452, 1979

Foley JM: Sensation and behavior, in Fields WS (ed), Neurological and Sensory Disorders in the Elderly. New York, Stratton, 1975

Goldfarb AF: Geriatric gynecology, in Rossman I (ed), Clinical Geriatrics, 2nd ed. Philadelphia, Lippincott, 1979

Habeeb MC, McLaughlin FE: Making the right moves in discharge planning: Including the hospital staff nurse. American Journal of Nursing 79(8):1443, 1979

Hodkinson HM: Cancer and the aged, in Brocklehurst JC (ed), Textbook of Geriatric Medicine and Gerontology, 2nd ed. New York, Churchill Livingstone, 1978

Jackson CW, Ellis R: Sensory deprivation as a field of study. Nursing Research 20(1):46, 1971

Jarvik LF: Genetic aspects of aging, in Rossman I (ed), Clinical Geriatrics, 2nd ed. Philadelphia, Lippincott, 1979

Jennings B: Intraocular lens for cataracts. AORN Journal 23(4):664, 1976a

Jennings B: Outpatient posterior capsulotomy. AORN Journal 23(2):270, 1976b

Jones JA: Deprivation and existence or stimulation and life: Our choice for the elderly. Journal of Gerontological Nursing 2(2):17, 1976

Kahn C: Visual disorders, in Lebow LS, Sherman T (eds), The Core of Geriatric Medicine. A Guide for Students and Practitioners. St. Louis, Mosby, 1981

Kaspar R: Eye problems in the aged, in Reichel W (ed), Clinical Aspects of Aging. Baltimore, Williams and Wilkins, 1978

Kemp J: Planning hospital care. Nursing Times 74(5):198, 1978

Keywood O: Preparing the elderly to return home. Part 1. Nursing Mirror 147(10):42, 1978. Part 2. Nursing Mirror 147(11):38, 1978

Knox DL: Disorders of vision: Vascular, metabolic and endocrine, in Fields WS (ed), Neurological and Sensory Disorders in the Elderly. New York, Grune and Stratton, 1975

Kornzweig AL: The eye in old age, in Rossman I (ed), Clinical Geriatrics, 2nd ed. Philadelphia, Lippincott, 1979

Kornzweig AL: Visual loss in the elderly. Hospital Practice 12(7):51, 1977

Kratz CR: Sensory deprivation in the elderly. Nursing Times 75(8):330, 1979

Kwitko ML: Artificial lens implantation. AORN Journal 28:47, 1978

Leight DH: Special senses: Aging of the eye, in Brocklehurst JC (ed), Textbook of Geriatric Medicine and Gerontology, 2nd ed. New York, Churchill Livingstone, 1978

Low CR: Outpatient cataract surgery. AORN Journal 28(1):35, 1978

Markovits AS: What to tell your patients about intraocular lenses. Consultant 18(12):87, 1978

Marmor MF: Management of elderly patients with impaired vision, in Ebaugh FG (ed), Management of Common Problems in Geriatric Medicine. Menlo Park, CA, Addison-Wesley, 1981

Mason JH, Gau FC, Byrne MP: General surgery, in Steinberg FU (ed), Cowdry's The Care of the Geriatric Patient, 5th ed. St. Louis, Mosby, 1976

Pilgrim M, Sigler B: Phaco-emulsion of cataracts. American Journal of Nursing 75(6):976, 1975

Richman L: Sensory training for geriatric patients. American Journal of Occupational Therapy 23:254, 1969

Rossman I: Mortality and morbidity overview, in Rossman I (ed), Clinical Geriatrics, 2nd ed. Philadelphia, Lippincott, 1979

Schultz D: Sensory Restriction: Effects on Behavior. New York, Academic, 1965

Scott D, Crowhurst J: Reawakening senses in the elderly. Canadian Nurse 71(10):21, 1975

Serpick AA: Cancer in the elderly. Hospital Practice 13(2):101, 1978

Shelby JP: Sensory deprivation. Image 10(2):49, 1978

Smith JA, Buckalew J, Rosales SM: Making the right moves in discharge planning: Coordinating a workable system. American Journal of Nursing 79(8):1439, 1979

Smith J: Focusing your care for the patient with an intraocular lens implant. RN 41(3):47, 1978

Smith ME: Ophthalmic aspects, in Steinberg FU (ed), Cowdry's The Care of the Geriatric Patient, 5th ed. St. Louis, Mosby, 1976

Stone M: Making the right moves in discharge planning: Discharge planning guide. American Journal of Nursing 79(8):1446, 1979

Storandt M: Psychological aspects of aging, in Rossman I (ed), Clinical Geriatrics, 2nd ed. Philadelphia, Lippincott, 1979

Straus B: Digestive organs in the aging, in Rossman I (ed), Clinical Geriatrics, 2nd ed. Philadelphia, Lippincott, 1979

Third National Cancer Survey. Incidence Data. Monograph 41, DHEW Publication 75-787. National Institutes of Health, National Cancer Institute, Bethesda, MD, 1975

Todd RL: Early treatment reverses symptoms of senility. Hospital and Community Psychiatry 17:170, 1966

Villaverde MM, MacMillan CW: Ailments of Aging. New York, Van Nostrand Reinhold, 1980

Wiggins R: The importance of sensory stimulation in caring for the elderly. Journal of Practical Nursing 28(2):24, 1978

Worrell JN: Nursing implications in the care of the patient experiencing sensory deprivation, in Kintzel KC (ed), Advance Concepts in Clinical Nursing. Philadelphia, Lippincott, 1977

Wynne JU: Pulmonary disease in the elderly, in Rossman I (ed), Clinical Geriatrics, 2nd ed. Philadelphia, Lippincott, 1979

Young JL Jr., Percy CL, et al: Cancer incidence and mortality in the United States, 1973–1977. National Cancer Institute Monograph 57. Washington, D.C., U.S. Government Printing Office, 1981

Zubek JP (ed): Sensory deprivation. Fifteen Years of Research. New York, Appleton-Century-Crofts, 1969

VI

Level Five Adaptation: the Aging Client Experiencing Terminal Illness

21

Nursing the Client Experiencing Acute Problems of Fluids and Electrolytes

Chapter 5 of this text reviewed the normal structural and functional changes in the excretory system of the aged client. Distinguishing between these normal changes and those due to concomitant disease is difficult. Renovascular disease, secondary to hypertension and discrete urinary tract infections, seems to be the leading stress resulting in renal impairment. Since there are no specific geriatric diseases of the kidney, clinical research in this area has been almost totally ignored. The epidemiology and symptomatology of renal disease in the elderly, diagnostic difficulties, and response to treatment are problems about which there is still little basic information.

SIGNIFICANT PROBLEMS

Urinary Tract Infections

Urinary tract infections, particularly pyelonephritis, is the most common renal disease in the aged. Because pyelonephritis is frequently asymptomatic in the elderly, its exact prevalence is difficult to determine. Many times, pyelonephritis is detected when the client is being treated for some other stress and routine examination suggests pyelonephritis. At other times pyelonephritis is not detected until autopsy. Although statistics vary, the incidence of pyelonephritis found at autopsy seems to be about 28 percent (Bruückel and Wineker, 1964; Sanjurjo,

1959). Pyelonephritis is more common in men, usually due to bladder neck obstruction caused by an enlarged prostate gland. Other causes of pyelonephritis may be vascular insufficiency and urinary stasis secondary to decreased muscular tension. Special characteristics of pyelonephritis in the elderly are just now being investigated. Shapiro et al. (1978) point out that it is not even certain that for the disease to be progressive, active infection by microorganisms must be continually present. There is some thought that in the later stages the disease becomes self-progressive. Autoimmune mechanisms are also believed to be a factor in progression. In the elderly, the typical adaptations of fever, dysuria, and frequency may be absent or may not be noted. Usually, a bacterial colony count is necessary to confirm pyelonephritis. Pyelonephritis is frequently responsible for acute failure in chronic renal disease. If treated, the acute failure can usually be reversed.

Renal Calculi

The formation of renal calculi is an important consideration in the elderly because it can be responsible for acute or chronic renal failure and is a frequent cause of morbidity in the elderly. Renal calculi occur under two conditions that are prevalent in many elderly clients. The first is the presence of stone-forming crystalloids, especially calcium, in concentrated amounts. Hypercalciuria occurs in situations where dissolution of the bone occurs, such as in multiple myeloma, immobilization, and senile osteoporosis. The second condition is a change in the pH of the urine resulting in aciduria, which can lead to the formation of uric acid stones. Changes in pH occur with dehydration and infection. Hyperuricemic states such as gout and polycythemia vera can also contribute to the formation of uric acid calculi. Persistent aciduria is also seen in chronic diarrheal conditions.

Renovascular Disease

Renovascular disease is an obvious cause of renal failure in the elderly. Arteriosclerosis in the kidney is the same process occurring elsewhere in the body. Vascular changes resulting in renal hypertension include the destruction of glomeruli due to ischemia as well as the narrowing of afferent arterioles (nephrosclerosis). Nephrosclerosis can be benign and is associated with essential hypertension. These clients usually have a long course of disease with only 1 percent dying in uremia. However, the renal insufficiency contributes to the overall morbidity of the elderly by becoming one more stress in a situation of limited energy sources. Malignant nephrosclerosis, associated with malignant hypertension, occurs in a small number of those with essential hypertension (about one in eight). Here the disease progresses rapidly and mortality is very high. In both situations, lowering of the renal blood pressure is essential in restoring renal function and preventing further damage. Raji et al. (1976) have noted irreversible renal failure in the elderly with minimal vascular changes. The reasons for this are not known, but, again, the concept of cumulative stresses on the body is suggested.

Other Stresses Affecting Renal Function

Renal function can be impaired by a variety of stresses common in the elderly that generally result in the adaptations of dehydration, concentrated urine, stasis of urine, and a change in pH. The concomitant problems of these adaptations have already been presented. These additional stresses requiring early detection and vigorous treatment are: inadequate fluid intake, fluid loss due to vomiting or diarrhea, hemorrhage, cardiac failure, and inappropriate use of diuretics and laxatives.

Those stresses that are prenal (dehydration/

concentration) as well as those that are postrenal (calculi) could be treated and would cause little, if any, permanent destruction in the kidney if detected early. Detection of these stresses and differential determination is difficult in the elderly, since many of the early indicators are masked by normal aging changes in kidney function. In most cases, these stresses advance and result in renal failure or end-stage renal disease.

Renal Failure

As stated above, many disorders of diverse etiology may affect the kidneys and cause renal failure. When the kidneys fail, the nitrogeneous end products of metabolism accumulate in the blood. Renal handling of sodium and water is impaired, which compromises the body's ability to adapt to variations in food and fluid intake. Volume depletion or circulatory congestion may ensue. As urine output falls, the kidneys are unable to excrete potassium and magnesium. These metabolites accumulate in the body. The metabolic disturbances associated with renal failure affect all organ systems causing an array of adaptations commonly known as uremia.

ASSESSING THE CLIENT'S ADAPTATIONS

The assessment of renal failure in the elderly client is difficult because of the variety and nonspecific nature of the adaptations, the alterations of normal findings in the aged that mask preliminary findings, and the presence of other diseases such as cardiac failure, arteriosclerosis, or diabetes. Consequently, renal disease should be suspected in all geriatric clients and routine basic assessment should be carried out.

The basic assessment of a client for renal failure has five components; client history, physical examination, blood chemistry data, urine analysis data, and radiologic findings.

Client History

Obtaining an accurate and detailed client history is a major step in the formulation of an accurate nursing diagnosis. The elderly client in renal failure presents specific problems in obtaining this accurate history. First, the stresses leading to renal failure often present nonspecific or diffuse adaptations that may or may not be noted. Second, the accumulation of nitrogenous wastes that occurs in renal failure can lead to dullness, lethargy, and confusion. Third, the loss of recent memory or the onset of chronic brain syndrome in the elderly leads to the client's inability to provide a satisfactory history. Some of this difficulty can be overcome by the nurse's use of open-ended questions, encouraging the client to elaborate wherever possible. Data received should be reviewed with the client as well as with a family member. Data should also be compared with any recorded history and the discrepancies noted.

The history should include any and all client experiences with illness, hospitalization, and health care providers. Attention should be paid to reports of fever, nausea, vomiting, or weakness since they may indicate a hidden kidney episode.

The focus of the history is to ascertain the presence of, or suggestion of, any electrolyte or metabolic disturbance. Sodium disturbance is a notable indication of kidney failure and will affect hydration status. A detailed history of food and fluid intake, urinary and bowel output, and recent changes in these activities will aid the assessment of hydration status. Probing questions need to be used to ascertain the dimensions of adaptations such as anorexia, nausea, vomiting, thirst, polyuria, oliguria, hematuria, diarrhea, or constipation. Any history of peripheral edema, pulmonary congestion, or decrease in exercise tolerance may also indicate a change in hydration status.

A history of headaches, tremors, lethargy, failing sight, or confusion can indicate accumulating levels of metabolites in the body that are affecting the central nervous system. When calcium or uric acid levels rise, renal calculi can be formed. Any previous episodes of renal calculi are suggestive of renal damage leading to renal failure. Renal calculi are not, however, always diagnosed and the nurse should be alert to other adaptations suggestive of calcium or uric acid disturbances. These include vomiting, diarrhea, skin and hair changes, tingling in the fingers, muscle weakness, and cramps. A careful notation of the client's activity level, ability to mobilize, perceived muscle strength, range of daily activities, and complaints of failing or changing ability should be made.

Physical Examination

The physical examination is also directed at discovering or confirming adaptations that are suggestive of renal failure. Some adaptations are stronger indicators than others but a pattern of generalized adaptations is also important to note.

A full neurological examination, including testing of the cranial nerves, is necessary to discover indications of central nervous system irritability or depression. Special attention should be paid to the determination of visual disturbances, particularly nystagmus, since retinal lesions are a common result of hypertension and anemia. Sensory deficits and loss of motor function are indications of neuropathy. Disturbances of function in the autonomic nervous system, including postural hypotension or incontinence, are occasionally seen.

Alteration of hydration status is a common adaptation to renal failure. This alteration is related to the disruption of fluid volume regulation and the excessive amounts of renin that are secreted by diseased kidneys. The cardiovascular system is affected by this major alteration and function of this system needs to be carefully evaluated. Hydration status can be altered in two directions, fluid overload or dehydration. In both situations, hypertension is present and blood pressure should be carefully taken and noted. Serial recordings of blood pressure are useful tools for evaluating changes in hydration status. Serial weight recordings are also useful in evaluating hydration status.

Fluid overload may be evidenced by an increased pulse rate and an accompanying increased respiratory rate. Extremities should be examined for evidence of peripheral edema. Evaluation of breath sounds generally indicates pulmonary congestion. Heart sounds may be altered in response to fluid overload. Abnormalities in cardiac rhythm are a common response to changing levels of metabolites—especially potassium and calcium. Valvular dysfunction is a rare but potential adaptation to renal failure.

Dehydration may also be seen in clients with renal failure and in the elderly this is a particularly difficult state to assess. Usual hallmarks of dehydration—thirst, loss of skin turgor, and hydration of mucous membranes are not useful in assessing the aged client. In the elderly, the sense of thirst is normally diminished and is, therefore, not a reliable indicator. The normal skin turgor of the elderly is greatly altered due to lack of subcutaneous fat and decreased circulation to the skin. Normal elderly skin is dry, lacking turgor, and subject to injury. Likewise, mucous membranes in the elderly are generally drier than in the younger population, as circulation is decreased. Dehydration itself is not an uncommon finding in many elderly clients. Differentiation can only be made after careful evaluation of fluid intake and output. Evidence of mineral deposits on the skin and pruritis are suggestive of dehydration due to renal disease.

Other changes seen in renal failure, including anorexia, osteodystrophy, anemia, and glucose intolerance, should be noted. As stated previously, however, the common adaptations of renal failure are nonspecific and can be seen in the elderly as either normal changes of aging or as adaptations to health problems commonly seen in the elderly. The history and physical examination findings are only suggestive and need to be confirmed by laboratory data.

Blood Chemistry Data

The two major blood chemistry tests for evaluating renal function are the blood urea nitrogen (BUN) and serum creatinine. The BUN reflects the ability of the body to eliminate the waste products of protein metabolism. Unfortunately, a significant rise in the blood urea nitrogen does not occur until 65 percent of renal function has been lost (Shapiro et al., 1978). Serum creatinine levels and creatinine clearance rates correlate better with renal function. In the aged, however, the normal creatinine levels and creatinine clearance rate are decreased, possibly due to muscle atrophy (Rowe et al., 1976). Additionally, the glomerular filtration rate is also decreased (Wesson, 1969). Therefore, the interpretation of renal function needs to be based on both the BUN and creatinine levels. They should rise proportionately at approximately their normal 15:1 ratio. When both the BUN and the creatinine are high, an excess of nitrogenous compounds in the blood (azotemia) is indicated. A disproportionate rise in BUN usually indicates some form of dehydration. Chapter 7 identifies normal blood chemistry values in the elderly.

Other helpful indicators are higher levels of uric acid, serum phosphorus, and low serum calcium levels. These findings in conjunction with el-

evated BUN and creatinine levels are almost certain indicators of renal disease.

Urine Analysis Data

The urine of the client should be examined for sediment, protein, and bacteria. Essential to this examination is the collection of a fresh, concentrated, uncontaminated specimen of urine. Generally, the best specimen for this purpose is the first morning voiding of urine that has been in the bladder all night. A noncontaminated specimen is difficult to obtain in the elderly, particularly in females. Moore-Smith (1974) states that 31 percent of midstream specimens collected from elderly women were frankly contaminated and an additional 17 to 28 percent were questionably contaminated. Problems arise when the client is bedridden and must use a bedpan. Noncompliance with cleansing procedures due to forgetfulness, manipulative inability, or uncooperativeness is an additional factor. Since a noncontaminated specimen is of special importance, the nurse should carefully instruct the client or cleanse the client and catch the specimen personally.

To obtain an uncontaminated urine specimen from the incontinent client, catheterization has to be considered. Since catheterization can infect the urinary tract, exquisite sterile technique must be adhered to. Another method of collecting bladder urine is suprapubic puncture and aspiration of the bladder. In younger clients this is a safe and accurate procedure. In the elderly, however, it is technically difficult since lack of abdominal muscle tone, bladder tone, and sphincter control makes identification of the bladder and retention of contents difficult. Because the success rate in the elderly is only about 65 percent, it is impractical as a routine procedure (Moore-Smith, 1974).

Once the specimen is obtained, it should be transported to the clinical laboratory without delay. Microscopic examination is done to determine the presence of leukocytes, indicators of infection or contamination, and cell casts. Casts originate in the renal tubules and suggest renal disease. Red blood cell casts suggest glomerulitis or malignant hypertension and white cell casts indicate purulent disease within the kidney. Casts containing epithelium suggest a degenerative process and waxy casts are indicative of chronic renal disease. Fat droplets also are seen in degenerative renal disease.

Protein excretion in the urine is an abnormal

finding and should not be dismissed no matter how minor. Indications of protein found in routine urinalysis should be followed up by collection of a 24-hour urine sample for analysis of protein content. Amounts of 150 mg per 24 hours are considered significantly abnormal and indicate renal disease (Rosen, 1976).

The presence of bacteria in the urine is suspected whenever leukocytes are seen upon microscopic examination. Culture of the urine is necessary to confirm the presence of bacteria, and to identify the specific organism. If positive, sensitivity studies should be performed.

Radiologic Examination

A basic x-ray of the abdomen (KUB) will visualize the presence, location, and size of the kidneys. Renal calculi are also frequently visible and no further studies need be done. An intravenous pyelogram (IVP) provides information on the size and structure of the kidney, particularly the calyceal system, and the ureters. Renal arteriograms are useful in determining the extent and severity of renal arteriosclerosis.

Renal scans utilizing isotopic mercury may not be particularly useful. Rosen (1976) found that 70 percent of clients studied demonstrated areas of decreased uptake. Decreased uptake indicates ischemic nonfunctioning areas of the kidney. He concluded that these findings are normal in the elderly population. Without earlier comparative studies, the scan may identify how much renal damage is present but will not differentiate disease from the normal aging process.

Because of the similarities in preparation for these procedures with the younger adult, the reader is referred to a basic nursing text for details.

NURSING INTERVENTIONS

Managing the Client Moving to Level Five Adaptation: Renal Failure

The inability of the kidney to excrete the metabolites produced by the body is known as renal failure. This stress has an acute and a chronic form.

Basically, acute renal failure in the aged occurs under the same conditions as in younger age groups and its management is the same. The prognosis in the elderly, however, is generally poor. Damage to the kidneys results and when combined with the aging process in the kidney, significant alterations in function occur. Chronic renal failure is the more common situation encountered in the elderly.

The client with chronic renal failure presents many adaptations that result from the inadequate control of the composition and volume of body fluids. This condition is progressive and clients eventually move to Adaptation Level Five, becoming dependent on others to meet their needs. Nursing care is initially directed at reducing the negative nitrogen balance of the body and alleviating some of the adaptations. The stress of negative nitrogen balance results in the adaptations of a rising BUN and creatinine level, gastrointestinal irritation, alteration of the central nervous system, respiratory distress, and pruritis. Thus, the goal for the client's well-being is a lower BUN and serum creatinine. In addition, other plasma and urine electrolytes should be within normal limits.

There are three initial interventions directed at achieving this goal.

Low-Protein Diet. Protein restriction alone cannot improve the prognosis of the client with chronic disease. However, it has been successful in the elderly in lowering creatinine levels. The goal of dietary therapy is to provide sufficient calories for energy utilization and sufficient amino acids to prevent protein catabolism as well as ensuring essential vitamins and minerals. The calories should be derived chiefly from complex carbohydrates. Protein intake should be regulated to provide a minimum of 0.5 g/kg body weight per day, while keeping the serum creatinine levels below 4 mg. This usually results in 20 to 30 g of protein daily (Atkins, 1971). The protein taken in should be of high biological value, the best sources being eggs and milk.

Additional dietary considerations will depend on the serum levels of sodium, potassium, and calcium. Frequently, sodium intake as well as fluid intake need to be restricted. Fluid levels, via intake and output recording, and blood pressure recordings should be carefully monitored. The goal is to provide adequate fluids while lowering the level of fluid overload that is generally present in these clients.

Calcium also frequently needs to be supplemented. Calcium depletion is a common adaptation of chronic renal failure, partly due to the inability of the kidney to convert vitamin D to an active form.

A low serum calcium stimulates parathyroid hormone secretion. An excess of this hormone draws calcium from the bones into the serum. Supplemental calcium, vitamin D, and phosphate binders can help prevent this cycle and protect bone composition.

If the client is unable to take food orally, either because of ulcerations of the mucous membrane or severe nausea and vomiting (common adaptations seen in late stages of renal failure), essential amino acids and calories can be provided by parenteral alimentation. The procedure of infusion of hypertonic solutions carries many risks and should be used very selectively.

Restriction of Physical Activity. The client with chronic renal failure is in a precarious metabolic state. Every function of the body is conducted under stress and utilizes more energy resources than it does in healthy clients. Therefore, greater energy resources are required. The calories being consumed by the client are quickly utilized in maintaining vital functions and the client presents adaptations of malnutrition including lethargy, anemia, and weakness.

One way to reduce energy demands on the body during this time is to reduce the amount of physical activity. Restricted activity decreases the possibility of protein catabolism and resultant waste products. The nurse needs to carefully restrict client activity depending on assessment of ability. When the client's kidney function is severely impaired and metabolism and vital functions are not stabilized, bed rest is indicated. Passive range of motion exercises will aid in the maintenance of mobility functions without the client expending a lot of energy. Deep breathing exercises and careful skin care are required during this period.

As the client's condition improves active range of motion exercises can be instituted. Activity can be gradually increased as tolerated. Each expenditure of energy should be planned so that many activities do not occur simultaneously. For instance, the client should not be placed in a chair immediately after eating since the energy resources being used in maintaining the muscle strength for sitting leave fewer energy resources for food digestion. Energy expenditure should be monitored by observing the client's pulse and respiratory rate as well as the client's overall response to the activity. If a variance from normal is observed, all activity should be stopped and the client allowed to rest until a normal rate is reestablished.

Careful control of activity must be balanced with the need to maintain muscle tone, strength, and joint mobility. Exercise can be increased as the client stabilizes. At some point, it is likely that the nurse will have to encourage mobility activities since the client is usually lethargic and may be moderately depressed secondary to renal failure.

Administration of Anabolic Steroids. Although many clinicians believe anabolic steroids are effective in promoting a positive nitrogen balance, they are not widely used. In the elderly, however, anabolic steroids may be a significant treatment modality and should receive serious consideration. Snyder and Brest (1966) conducted a series of studies on elderly clients and demonstrated positive results. In their studies, elderly clients, all with chronic renal failure, received 600 mg testosterone enanthate intramuscularly four times a week for 8 weeks. They averaged a 29 percent decrease of nitrogen excretion paralleled with a fall in blood urea nitrogen levels. No increase in renal function was found. Clients demonstrated clinical improvement as evidenced by an increased appetite, a decrease in fatigue and an increased sense of well-being.

Dialysis Therapy. The point at which chronic failure can no longer be treated by conservative means is not clear. More aggressive therapy is accomplished through either peritoneal dialysis or hemodialysis. Dialysis is usually instituted when the creatinine clearance falls below 5 mm/min. The goal is to initiate dialysis therapy prior to the onset of uremic complications such as severe vomiting, pericarditis, or uremic frost. These complications are, however, reversible with careful symptomatic therapy. They should be weighed against the complications of dialysis therapy which include bleeding, shock, and sepsis, as well as the time and expense involved in long-term therapy.

In the elderly, adaptations of advancing uremia may manifest themselves at higher creatinine clearance levels; thus, dialysis procedures are instituted earlier. Access to hemodialysis for all clients is still a major problem, especially outside urban areas that contain multiple facilities. The problem is somewhat alleviated with home dialysis programs. When access is a problem, the age of the client is sometimes used as a criterion for selection. However, since the aged population in this country is increasing, the incidence of elderly clients requiring dialysis has also risen. Some opponents suggest that dialysis in the elderly is too risky a procedure. The elderly present problems of access to the circulatory system, vascular disease, and hemodynamic instability, as well as the potential for severe psychological problems. Others cite significant evidence to the contrary. For instance, Walker et al. (1976) did a ten year retrospective study of dialysis clients and found no higher mortality rate in the elderly than in younger clients.

When the elderly client receiving dialysis therapy does die it is probably due to cardiovascular disease associated with uremia. The adaptations of hypertension, glucose intolerance, hyperlipidemia, and arterial calcification lead to degenerative changes in the structure and function of the cardiovascular system. For the elderly with preexisting cardiovascular disease, the stress of uremic syndrome cardiovascular changes and the stress placed on the cardiovascular system by dialysis therapy can be overwhelming and lead to an increased incidence of cardiovascular mortality.

Dialysis therapy is based on the principles of osmosis, filtration, and diffusion to remove the waste products of protein metabolism and to restore fluid and electrolyte balance. It is accomplished by the creation of a situation whereby fluids on either side of a semipermeable membrane exchange substances through these processes until the concentrations are equalized on both sides of the membrane. Continuation of the processes, as well as regulation of substances on the input side of the membrane, controls the amount and rapidity of removal of substances from the body. The membrane used can be a physiological membrane (peritoneal dialysis) or an artificial membrane (hemodialysis). Both procedures are clinically effective in removing metabolic waste products. Which procedure is chosen depends on many factors. In general, peritoneal dialysis is used for initial therapy or for clients awaiting space in a hemodialysis therapy program. Hemodialysis is used when peritoneal dialysis is not effective enough in a given time since hemo-

dialysis can return fluid values to normal rather rapidly. Many elderly clients can be maintained by a combination of conservative therapy and intermittent peritoneal dialysis every 7 to 10 days. Each method has advantages and disadvantages and should be evaluated according to a specific client's needs. Some of these considerations are noted in Table 1.

Renal Transplantation. Renal transplantation should always be considered in clients with renal failure since it is the ultimate therapy. The assessment procedure for the potential success of a transplant varies from center to center. Usually, the purpose of the assessment is to determine which treatment modality will achieve the highest level of client adaptation possible. Both physiological and psychological evaluations are done. Generally, the fewer multiple system stresses that exist the better the chance for success of a transplant.

Careful evaluation of renal function is done, not so much for the purpose of determining the severity of damage, as to determine if the natural kidneys can be left in place. Early transplant procedures included bilateral nephrectomy. While this is still indicated in the presence of infections, uncontrolled hypertension, reflux, or tumors, the preference is to retain the client's kidneys for erythropoietin production, blood pressure control, and prostaglandin production and synthesis.

Assessment also includes the ruling out of ulcer disease, since the immunological therapy required for transplant recipients can be fatal for the client with an ulcer. Other factors to be considered in the selection of transplant recipients are a normal lower urinary tract and the absence of major associated disease, such as malignancy, infection, or chronic pulmonary disease. Cardiovascular disease needs to be carefully evaluated in terms of the impending stress of the transplant process. The presence of cardiovascular disease is not necessarily a deterrent if it is controllable, not too severe, and not accompanied by stresses involving other systems.

The age of a client is not an automatic deterrent to a renal transplant. Because most agree that the highest success rates have been documented in clients under the age of forty, age is sometimes used as a factor in excluding the elderly from consideration. However, Kjellstrand et al. (1976) studied clients

TABLE 1. FACTORS TO BE CONSIDERED IN SELECTING DIALYSIS THERAPY*

	Peritoneal Dialysis	Hemodialysis
Speed of Therapy	Slow—each treatment lasts approximately 12 to 15 hours. Initial treatment may take up to 72 hours. (This can be an advantage for elderly clients who cannot tolerate rapid fluid and electrolyte changes.)	Rapid—5 to 8 hours per treatment.
Cost	Expensive—large amounts of commercially prepared dialysate solution, skilled nursing care, equipment, and hospitalization for the procedure. Can be offset with insurance coverage.	Expensive—cost of disposable filters and lines, equipment rental, skilled nursing care, and dialysis unit overhead. Home hemodialysis is somewhat less expensive. Can be offset if specific insurance coverage is obtained.
Ease of Administration	Vascular access *not* required. Abdominal catheter easy to insert. Equipment can be relatively simple for manual manipulation of solution or complex if automated pumps are used. Client cooperation essential.	Vascular access required. Heparinization required. Complex equipment requiring specifically trained personnel. Careful monitoring during dialysis necessary.
Potential Complications	1. Perforation of bladder or intestine 2. Fluid retention (hypervolemia) 3. Pain 4. Peritonitis 5. Respiratory compromise 6. Hyperglycemia 7. Protein loss 8. Abdominal adhesions 9. Hypovolemia	1. Thrombosis 2. Hemorrhage 3. Ischemia of involved extremity 4. Infection of shunt 5. Volume depletion 6. Fluid overload 7. Dialysis disequilibrium syndrome (headache, nausea, vomiting, hypertension, confusion, seizures—due to rapid lowering of blood urea levels resulting in hypertonic cerebrospinal fluid and consequent cerebral edema due to fluid shifts) 8. Hepatitis 9. Anemia 10. Cardiac arrhythmias 11. Transfusion reaction 12. Equipment failure
Contraindications	1. Recent abdominal surgery 2. Abdominal drains 3. Undiagnosed abdominal pain 4. Fever of unknown origin 5. Abdominal adhesions 6. Colostomy 7. Active peritonitis	1. Active bleeding 2. Sclerotic vessels 3. Hemodynamic instability

*Each procedure requires specific nursing skills and fastidious observations. The reader is referred to critical care texts for specifics of the details of care in these two situations.

between 50 and 71 years of age who had renal transplants because of end-stage renal failure. A five year survival rate of 80 percent for clients who received related donor kidneys and a 43 percent survival rate for clients who received cadaver kidney transplants were found. The significant factor, in this study, was the source of donor kidney, not the age of the client.

A psychological evaluation is carried out to determine the motivation, stability, and emotional maturity of the client. The ability to participate in the care, learn the information and procedures necessary to do so, and assume self-care after recovery from the transplantation procedure are important factors.

The financial status of the client is not a factor in determining acceptability into a transplant program. Medicare currently covers 80 percent of the cost of care for any client requiring a transplant. The additional costs are usually absorbed by the institution, paid for through additional insurance coverage, or covered through private donations.

Once accepted into a transplant program, the client faces two uncertainties. These uncertainties with their associated anxiety and waiting may deter some clients from choosing the transplant option.

The first problem is that of finding a suitable donor. Tissue typing is done and a human leukocyte antigen (HLA) profile is determined. This HLA profile must be matched with a donor kidney profile before a transplant can proceed. There are two sources for donor kidneys: a living donor, usually a relative; or a cadaver kidney. Nonrelative living kidneys are rarely used because the success rate is no higher than from cadaver kidneys and there is risk to the donor. If a living relative has a compatible tissue typing, and is willing to be a donor, an extensive physical and psychological evaluation, similar to the client's, is carried out on this potential donor.

If a suitable living donor cannot be found, the recipient's name is entered into the national computer listing to be tissue matched with each cadaver kidney that becomes available. The wait for a cadaver kidney is extremely long and an appropriate kidney may never be found.

The second problem, which occurs after the transplant has taken place, is the potential stress of rejection. Immunosuppressive agents are used to prevent rejection and prolong the life of the transplanted organ. The rejection process can occur at the time of surgery (hyperacute rejection) caused by preformed circulating antibodies that attack the organ violently. There is no treatment and the kidney must be removed. Acute rejection can take place anywhere from 3 to 10 days after surgery. High doses of steroids are used to decrease the rejection syndrome and are usually successful in reversing the process. Chronic rejection can occur over an indefinite period of time up to 3 to 5 years subsequent to transplant. The symptoms of chronic rejection are very subtle and difficult to detect. Renal function must be carefully monitored and the client must adhere exactly to the drug therapy prescribed until all danger of chronic rejection has passed. This means the client and family live in a state of uncertainty for a long period of time.

The care of the transplant client requires intensive and specialized nursing techniques. However, because more and more transplants are being performed with better success rates, the gerontological nurse will be in contact with increasing numbers of transplant clients and should be familiar with the general approaches to the care of this client.

Managing the Elderly Client in the Critical Care Setting

By definition, clients at Adaptation Level Five are completely dependent upon the health care system. They are in need of multiple system support and require constant observation and intense nursing care. Such clients are found in the emergency room, recovery room, coronary care unit, or intensive care unit. The increasing majority of the clients in these units are over the age of fifty and, thus, require special consideration.

In addition to the physical adaptations the client experiences, there are certain psychosocial adaptations that occur in response to the stress of the specific illness, the stress of the environment, as well as the stress of being critically ill. In the elderly client, the energy required for adaptation is less available; thus, specific assistance from the nurse is required. The ability of a client to adapt in this situation depends upon psychological health, past experience with illness, the ability to express concerns either verbally or nonverbally, and the support systems available.

The Stress of the Specific Illness. Depending upon the particular manifestations of a disease process, the nurse may observe a number of psychological adaptations in the elderly. Many disease processes have neurological, endocrine, or biochemical stresses that result in memory loss, fluctuating levels of consciousness, and cerebral anoxia. When these stresses are combined with the normal decrease in cognitive functioning in the aged individual, adaptive behaviors resembling schizophrenic psychosis can result. The behaviors frequently seen are delusions, hallucinations, withdrawal, and a lack of touch with reality. This situation is seen more frequently in postsurgical clients but is occasionally noted in clients with renal disease, severe cardiovascular impairment, or respiratory compromise.

Assessment and correction of the physiological stressors contributing to the onset of the episode (such as lowered PaO_2 levels, fever, hypoglycemia) will help to decrease the adaptations. Continued human contact (visual, auditory, and tactile) is probably the most important factor in keeping the client from total withdrawal. The nurse should talk with the client, address the client by name, explain procedures, reorient the client to reality by telling the date, time, place, what has occurred, and the identity of others present. Family members can be useful since they may be recognized and have a calming influence on the client. Restraints should not be used, although vital equipment requires protection from manipulation by the agitated or delirious client. However, restraints will only increase agitation and may cause the client further damage either directly at the area of the restraint (friction burns or fractures) or more generally, in the increased expenditure of energy.

If necessary, drugs can be given to quiet the client. Phenothiazine is the drug of choice. The elderly client may be given an initial dose of 12.5 mg intramuscularly, to be repeated every 4 hours until the metabolic situation is corrected and the psychosis clears. The dosage may need to be adapted for each individual, but should not exceed 25 mg every 4 hours. Because of the compromised metabolic response of the ill, elderly client, there is danger of slower excretion rates and the accompanying difficulty of accumulated drug levels. It is preferable to give a regular regimen of repeated small doses to stabilize the client's condition rather than larger single time doses when severe agitation results. The client receiving phenothiazine therapy

needs to be carefully observed for cardiovascular complications.

The Stress of the Environment. The environment of the intensive care unit is unfamiliar and frightening for most clients. This stress can result in a set of psychosocial adaptations, commonly called the "Intensive Care Syndrome." The specific client adaptations observed vary from unit to unit according to the specific characteristics of the unit. Typically the adaptations begin to appear 3 to 4 days after admission to the unit. Clients then begin to experience auditory and visual illusions, hallucinations, and disorientation. Clients may also exhibit combative behavior or withdrawal. These adaptations develop gradually and may appear unnoticed as the staff goes on with routine duties.

Intensive Care Syndrome was first noted in clients undergoing open heart surgery (Blachley and Starr, 1964). Egerton and Kay (1964) identified the environment as the major factor in this phenomenon. The syndrome has been noted in all types of intensive care units and can occur in any setting where the client is experiencing a level of anxiety about the unfamiliar surroundings and equipment.

The components of Intensive Care Syndrome are client anxiety, sleep deprivation, sensory alterations, and lack of territory and privacy. These components contribute to the development of the psychoticlike behaviors mentioned above. Since nurses have adapted to the environment, it is difficult for them to perceive the impact the environment is having on the client until overt behaviors appear.

Sleep Deprivation. According to Gaarder (1966), sleep has two important functions. The first is the destructuring of neurophysiological data storage that has occurred during the day. It is a "clearing out" system whereby important data are stored in the memory and unimportant data are discarded. The second function of sleep is the reinforcement of the structure of the individual's emergent character for the purpose of adapting. It is a way of reinforcing behaviors and characteristics of the personality that aid clients in coping with future stresses. When sleep does not occur, and especially when dreaming does not occur, these functions are not accomplished. The client loses the ability to adapt to stimuli, and stimuli begin to be interpreted without discrimination of importance. Lack of sleep also leads to fatigue, irritability, and increased sensitivity to pain.

When considering the elderly client in the intensive care environment, sleep deprivation becomes a critical concern. Sleep behaviors follow regular individual patterns and these behaviors are highly developed and rigid in the elderly. In addition, in times of stress the elderly may need longer intervals of sleep because the processing of data has slowed due to lower energy resources. Sleep patterns and rituals are disturbed by the general activity in the unit. Direct care, moving of the client, lights and noise, pain, and pain medication all interfere with normal sleep patterns.

Specific measures can be taken to provide prolonged periods of sleep. First, whenever possible the usual day–awake, night–asleep pattern should be maintained. At night, lights should be lowered and noise kept to a minimum. The nurse should close doors and draw curtains between clients' units to decrease visual stimulation and create an illusion of privacy. Sound indicators on monitoring equipment should be turned off (as long as alarms are left on) and, whenever possible, monitoring leads and other devices should be removed to allow for greater mobility. Direct care activities should be scheduled to allow for prolonged periods of undisturbed rest. It is helpful to interview the client or family in order to determine presleep rituals and, whenever possible, allow for them. For instance, if a client would normally brush the teeth, wind the clock, read for fifteen minutes before turning out the lights, and then lie on the right side when falling asleep, the nurse can provide for this. After communicating the intent to aid the client in preparation for sleep, the nurse assists with mouth care. The client's own clock can be brought into the unit and, if able, the client can wind it and place it on the bedside. If the client is unable to do this independently than the nurse can assist while involving the client mentally in this activity. Reading is an activity that may be allowed depending upon the client's status. The client can be positioned on the right side. The lights are then lowered, noise reduced, and the client told that a period of undisturbed time has been set aside for sleep.

If sleep deprivation becomes severe, clients begin to withdraw and react exclusively to their own internal cues. Bodily sensations become distorted and add additional anxiety. Depersonalization experiences are common—feelings of floating, body deadness, or detached self-observation. Clients begin to associate falling asleep with death. They fear that if they should fall asleep they may never awaken. Consequently, they begin to fight the thing most needed—sleep (Luby et al., 1969). The nurse can help by understanding the client's fear, reinforcing reality, and orienting the client to reality. Frequently, if clients can have a member of the family with them it will help them to "trust themselves" to fall asleep.

As more is learned about the need for sleep and dreaming, encouraging sleep for the critically ill client takes a higher priority in the provision of quality care. The control of environmental factors that interfere with sleep as well as intervening in the presence of anxiety are areas for professional nursing care.

Sensory Alterations.   A second consideration is the effect of the environment on the client's sensory input. Behavior is based upon the input received by all of our senses—touch, sight, hearing, taste, and smell. Sensory input helps individuals adapt to their environment and alerts them to changes in the environment through the processes of perception and reception. Perception reflects the psychological interpretation of the input. Reception involves the physiological reaction functions. Individual stimuli can be ignored or received, relegated to minor or major status, acted upon or forgotten. If the system becomes overloaded either by too many stimuli occurring too rapidly or by a totally new environment, adaptation to these situations may not occur. The adaptation to sensory input requires time, energy, and familiarity (Lindsley, 1965).

Critical care clients suffer from many varieties of sensory alteration. Generally they simultaneously experience sensory overload, sensory monotony, sensory distortion, and sensory deprivation.

SENSORY OVERLOAD. Sensory overload is a multisensory experience wherein two or more senses receive stimuli of greater than normal intensity, either suddenly or in rapid succession. This rapid, multifocused assault on the receptive activities in the brain can lead to behavior immobility (confusion). Each stimulus is not fully interpreted in terms of reality, so that the client's behavior relates to his or her own interpretation of reality. Since the client is unable to alter the environment, the only alternative is to attempt to adapt to it. Behaviors are then structured to cope with this altered sense of reality. The nurse observes these behaviors in terms of external reality and in that context they are not appropriate, thus, the client is considered "confused."

Generally, sensory overload can be handled by anticipating its occurrence and by attempting to limit or at least slow down the rapidity of inputs. As each stimulus is introduced, it is helpful for the nurse to explain what it is the client is feeling or seeing or hearing. Sometimes, the use of familiar analogies helps the client to interpret the input since it relates to something familiar. This can, however, also add to the confusion. It is better if the client can suggest an analogy and the nurse correct and clarify. At least once a day, or more often if indicated, the nurse should sit quietly with the client and ask what is seen, heard, smelled, and so on, and aid in interpreting sensory input in a calm, controlled atmosphere. This may require reinforcement each day as new input continues to distort reality. For instance, the client may sense monitoring wires and hear the beeping of each cardiac impulse on the monitor. The client might interpret this as being tied down by the wires and the beeping as the literal sound of the heart beat. Consequently, the client will not move and becomes outraged when the nurse turns down the monitor to allow for sleep. The nurse should explain the difference between the monitor recording and the client's own heart beat, and encourage the individual to learn how much movement is safe without disturbing the monitor. The next day when another nurse routinely changes the monitor leads, the client may interpret this as having disturbed the leads by the movement and may become immobile again.

SENSORY MONOTONY. Sensory monotony refers to a continuous sensory input along with the reduction of other stimuli. It occurs as the client begins to adapt to the environment. Usually, the sense most affected is that of hearing. As clients begin to become aware of a respirator in the next unit or a monitor beeping at regular intervals or other steady noise, they begin to learn that this sound does not refer to them and begin to accept it

as part of the environment. This type of continuous nonthreatening sound can then become either annoying or hypnotic. The danger is that adaptation to the continuous input may prevent clients from perceiving important sensory input. Elderly clients with hearing losses can also suffer from sensory monotony as they cannot distinguish sound well, and sounds tend to blend together in their perception. Stimuli must be very loud, or lower pitched, or accompanied by another sensory stimulation, such as touch, in order for perception to occur.

SENSORY DISTORTION. Sensory distortion occurs as the client's sensory system becomes overloaded or because of sleep deprivation. Sensory distortion experiences are also called *illusions,* or misperceptions of sensory stimuli. For instance, clients may only perceive a sheet on part of the body and feel exposed when, in fact, they are totally covered. Or they may state that they smell flowers when it may be a medication they have been given. The client may see people in the room who are not there; the client, nevertheless, hears and recognizes their voices. Sensory distortion is also a common adaptation of the elderly client who, through the aging process, is developing organic brain syndrome. It is important for the nurse to recognize the differences between illusions, or sensory distortion, and hallucinations, which are vivid sensory experiences *without* sensory stimulation. The nurse should also differentiate disorientation and faulty judgment from confusion. The client suffering sensory distortion in the critical care environment can usually identify the troublesome stimuli. Control of the environment and provision of sleep should eliminate this adaptation.

SENSORY DEPRIVATION. Sensory overload, monotony, and distortion are easy to understand when it is remembered that the capacity of the elderly to process stimuli is reduced in the critical care situation. Almost exactly for that reason, as well as the lack of a caring touch, clients can also suffer from sensory deprivation. Clients suffering from sensory overload and sensory deprivation exhibit the same behavior since these two stresses are really the opposite sides of the same coin (Chodil and Williams, 1970). Sensory deprivation may be easier to understand if referred to as emotional–touch deprivation (Roberts, 1976).

The experience of sensory deprivation is situational. It occurs when clients are confined in a stressful environment and interpersonal interactions are reduced. It is a reduction in the quality of sensory input. Sensory deprivation can involve one sense, but more generally the three major senses—visual, auditory, and touch—are involved. Clients are in an unfamiliar setting, separated from those they know, and cut off from their usual activities.

Each day, people engage in a number of activities that are sensory pleasing, or at least understandable to them. Normal stimuli might be combing our hair, looking at our children, stubbing a toe, walking, sitting in the sun, feeling a cool breeze, and so on. For the client in the critical care environment all of these normal stimuli are absent. The result is that while the client is still being bombarded with stimuli, the stimuli are almost all new and need to be interpreted and processed for the first time. The client is deprived of receiving normal, familiar stimuli.

At the same time, the client is socially isolated. The family is allowed to visit for only brief periods. Their fear and grief frequently interfere with the interpersonal interaction, or the client may be unable to communicate. They are afraid to touch the client. Their fear of "disturbing the machines" combined with a subconscious fear of illness may prevent them from approaching the client.

Sensory deprivation in the elderly is intensified when the nurse removes the client's eyeglasses, hearing aid, and dentures. Removal of these sensory aids, coupled with the normal decrease in sensory input with aging, puts the elderly at particular risk.

When sensory stimulation is reduced, behavioral changes result. Usually the nurse observes client boredom, inactivity, and sleep. Reaction to familiar stimuli excites the reticular activating system and its response projects upon the cortex where perception, learning, and emotional control take place. When familiar sensory input is reduced, a void is created, with a vigorous striving taking place to stimulate this system. Sleep is an acceptable way for the client to withdraw from the environment and it helps to pass the time. Sleep also offers its own stimulation to the reticular activating system through dreaming (Chodil and Williams, 1970).

It is important for the nurse to recognize when sleep is occurring in longer than desirable periods (excluding recovery from a sleep deprivation situation). If this seems to be the case, then meaningful sensory stimulation should be provided.

ASSESSING SENSORY ALTERATIONS. As stated previously, the assessment of sensory alterations is difficult. An assessment guide to aid the nurse in maintaining awareness of the environmental impact may be helpful. The assessment should begin with a history of previous cognitive ability, sensory aids used by client, and previous hospital experience. The nurse should assess the client's immediate environment for noise or other noxious stimuli. Clients should be asked to state their understanding of what is happening and the purpose of various pieces of equipment so the nurse has clues as to their perception of events. Meaningful and concrete interactions with nursing staff and family, as well as continued reorientation to events, should aid in minimizing sensory alteration.

Lack of Territory and Privacy. Critically ill clients live in a space no larger, and frequently smaller, than a hospital bed. The area around the bed is filled with equipment and people, over which the client has no control. When the equipment also takes up bed space, the physical space, or territory, of the client is invaded. Territory is associated with status and protection. Generally territory is delineated by physical barriers of some sort. The critically ill client cannot set up a barrier, and cannot even put out the typical environmental props that delineate territory in a controlled environment. Environmental props include such things as toilet articles in the bathroom, pictures of family on the bedside table, or clothes in a closet. The critically ill client is assigned to a bed and that bed is shared with IV equipment, monitoring leads, hypothermia blankets, and so on. People set things on the bed or sit on the bed while working, put side rails up and down, and raise and lower the bed, as appropriate. The client's territory is invaded, reinforcing the feelings of vulnerability and low status. The client's reaction to this can be expressed as anger, hostility, or withdrawal.

Privacy is essential in order to preserve personal autonomy. Privacy is the right of the individual to decide what information, under what conditions, and to whom, information about self should be shared. Privacy allows the individual to integrate experiences into a meaningful pattern and exert individuality onto events. It also enables the individual to avoid manipulation and domination and provides psychological distance and selective communication experiences.

In the critical care environment, the client is frequently physically and physiologically exposed. Because of the illness, intimate contact is made by strangers. Physiological information is obtained and shared with health care providers, often to the exclusion of the individual. Others dictate the content and pattern of communication. It is most difficult for the client to refuse to communicate, or to communicate selectively. Establishing trust and confidentiality is difficult when the client visually perceives people moving in and out of the area. These intrusions and lack of privacy for maintenance of personal autonomy lead to increased levels of stress, anxiety, and fatigue.

Attention to the components of the Intensive Care Syndrome—anxiety, sleep deprivation, sensory alterations, lack of privacy and territory—can diminish untoward reactions to this specialized environment. Lazarus and Hagens (1968) demonstrated that modifications in the environment did produce a lower incidence of delirium in open-heart surgery clients. Heller et al. (1970) documented that changes in the open-heart recovery room, such as describing the environment and procedures in detail to the client, providing sleep cycles, and moving equipment out of the client's visual field all contributed to a decrease in the occurrence of psychotic disturbances.

The nurse is the vital link in altering the client's environment. With appropriate assessment and intervention, the environment can become less stressful for the elderly client, resulting in the preservation of energy resources.

The Stress of Being Critically Ill. The critically ill elderly client is an individual involved in a series of losses and faced with the prospect of death. Any critically ill client is faced with the possibility of death, but this is an intense reality in the elderly. As the client becomes more aware of the critical nature of the situation, a number of reactions may occur.

Loneliness. The client may feel lonely despite being surrounded by health care providers. In this environment, the client is the center of attention of many people but is rarely encounterd as a unique personality. The feeling of loneliness, especially in the elderly, is not an unusual experience. Loneliness is the recognition of being alone, of being separated from meaningful and comforting interaction. The feeling of loneliness is sometimes communicated as dread, desperation, or restlessness. Loneliness helps individuals look at themselves and examine the meaning of their existence. If this is done, loneliness can be a positive experience. In the situation of the client at Adaptation Level Five, there is the reality of loneliness. The client, alone, is experiencing the pain, fear, and threat of the illness. This aspect cannot be shared, only acknowledged.

Loneliness is resolved when the client overcomes anxiety and believes that the future has meaning. The nurse can reassure the client that a future does exist, and support meaningful interactions with family, friends, and others. In the elderly, loneliness is intensified by the perception of loss, adding to the series of losses already experienced. The nurse needs to be careful not to offer meaningless reassurances but to engage in realistic considerations of the future of the client.

Hopelessness. Another reaction may be the expression of hopelessness. Hopelessness arouses the feeling of entrapment, a sense of the impossible, of things being beyond one's capabilities. There is no energy available for wishing, hoping, or anticipating. When the ability to function is impaired, and clients are separated from supportive loved ones, they can become overwhelmed with despair and lose the motivation to recover. The introduction of additional treatment or medication intensifies the perception of hopelessness. Generally, these clients see no future for themselves or they see a radically altered future. They believe that because of their illness, control of the future has been lost.

There are times when the nurse perceives the client's situation as hopeless. This sense of hopelessness is easily communicated to the client despite whatever verbal encouragement the nurse might offer. It is not unusual for a nurse to feel this way about an elderly client with a catastrophic illness. When nurses communicate a sense of hopelessness either overtly or covertly to the client and/or family, the client's sense of hopelessness is intensified. If such feelings are communicated, the client may reach a level of emotional standstill and his or her health status can quickly deteriorate. On the other hand, when indications of hope are communicated by the nurse, the client will cling to these. If these indications of hope are supported by the client's perception of events, the hopelessness will be diffused. It is important for the nurse to validate the client's perception of the illness and assure that the reality of the situation is understood. False reassurances are nontherapeutic and will interfere with any meaningful communication.

The nurse can foster hopefulness by discussing other clients who have survived similar situations. The sense of "if others have done it so can I" helps clients to understand that they are not the only ones who have experienced this illness. It is also extremely helpful if a client who has had a similar experience can visit the client. They can share common experiences and feelings and the client who is more advanced in the recovery stage offers real encouragement, acting almost as a role model. The nurse can also be of prime importance. The client can draw from the nurse's strength, calmness, knowledge, and ability. If the nurse and client develop a trusting relationship, the client begins to believe the nurse has knowledge and experience in this situation. Consequently, the client will believe the actions and words as indications of hope. The nurse motivates the client toward hopefulness by altering the internal and external resources available to the client. The nurse acts as a catalyst in removing the threats and reinforces reality and support from health care providers, family, and friends. The nurse sets goals that the client can attain and reinforces the attainment of these goals as indicators of progress. Each goal attained increases motivation and decreases hopelessness.

Powerlessness. Still another reaction is powerlessness. Powerlessness is a perceived lack of personal control of events in a given situation. Loss of control begins with the illness itself. Illness makes certain physiological and psychological demands on the individual. The person has to respond to pain, dyspnea, bleeding, and the like. A loss of power over body functions forces the individual to seek aid from others. Feared loss of power in an illness frequently prevents individuals from seeking help early in the situation. It is when they acknowledge

their powerlessness that they seek and can accept aid. In accepting help from a physician or a nurse, a client relinquishes power and control.

When the client is hospitalized, more control is given up. Activities are carried on according to a hospital schedule. Diagnostic procedures and treatments that the client does not fully understand are carried out and permission is rarely asked. In a critical care area, clients cannot control information about themselves, as tests and monitoring reveal information clients do not know. Clients have no control over the environment, the people who will care for them, or the activities of daily living.

The ultimate loss of power comes about when decisions about treatment are made. Frequently, decisions about therapy are based on standardized protocols and continue on a tightly scheduled sequence. When a decision needs to be made, it is usually the physician, in consultation with other health care providers, who makes it. Sometimes, the family, instead of the client, may be consulted. When clients are consulted, they may lack a full understanding of the reality of the situation and serious decision making cannot occur. A sense of the client's wishes regarding treatment may be communicated and fed into the process, but the client often does not make the full decision.

Clients may feel guilty about this loss of control. If an individual's normal daily activities include controlling activities, for example, a manager or administrator or other such occupation, a psychological adjustment to loss of control has to be made. The sense of having others assume responsibility for care can make this individual feel guilty for not being responsible. Someone else has been burdened with the "job" of caring.

There are some clients who are relieved by this lack of control. The client is overwhelmed by the events that are occurring and does not want to be responsible for the outcome. Control and responsibility is gladly given to others. The client does not then have to worry about making correct decisions in a foreign environment and under threatening conditions. Focus of attention can be fully on survival and recovery.

Most clients, however, feel that passivity and dependency have been forced upon them and they feel frustrated by their lack of control. The sense of losing part of their uniqueness and being is intensified when control is lost. The frustration usually results in angry attempts to control the situation. For instance, they may refuse to be turned, or they may lash out at someone who moves the bedside table. As the frustration increases, the angry, hostile behavior will increase. Clients will attempt to force their uniqueness onto any situation they can. A struggle for power between the client and the system can result, and the client, who has not been provided with full knowledge of the situation, is bound to lose. This loss can lead to severe depression and feelings of helplessness. In the critical care situation, the acuteness of care needs does not allow time for teaching, and permits only minimal explanation. The client's anxiety, illness, and frustration can block or distort any knowledge that is shared. Additionally, because nurses naturally use professional language or jargon, the message may not be recognized by the client. This lack of knowledge is a critical element in the client's real and perceived lack of power.

If the nurse keeps in mind the readiness of the client and provides information that has meaning to the client, the recovery process will be aided. As the client assimilates each item of information, additional areas can be addressed and explained. The nurse needs to be truthful, answer questions as fully as possible, respond at a level that the client will understand, and validate the information received by the client. As the client's knowledge expands, intellectual control over the situation will increase.

Control and power can be restored in other ways. The reinforcement of positive physical changes should be made explicitly to the client. For instance, if a client is on a respirator and the blood gas values have been stabilized, the client should be told that while the respirator will remain in place, improvement is seen. Any knowledge of physiological improvement will aid a client in believing that he or she is reestablishing somatic control. The client's role in any improvement should also be emphasized. For instance, if turning and positioning have kept the client's lungs free from congestion, this connection should be made and the client praised for being cooperative.

Psychological control can be restored by allowing the client to participate in the care and/or make choices about the care. The nurse needs to be alert to the client's readiness to take on simple care activities without compromising energy resources.

Any time a choice is to be made, the client should make the choice, or at least be included in the discussion.

As control is reestablished, the client becomes less angry, more cooperative, more relaxed, and recovery progresses. The level of control should continue to be increased as recovery occurs.

Other Reactions to Critical Illness. The client in the critical care setting can, of course, experience a wide variety of reactions that have not been discussed here. The reaction to the situation will depend somewhat on the basic personality structure of the client and how that personality reacts to stress. Other sections of this text explore personality themes in detail.

At some point, the client and the family in the critical care situation will be confronted with the possibility or the reality of impending death. It is important to recognize that if a terminal prognosis is determined, the client and family should be fully informed so that energy can be focused on dealing with the dying process rather than expending energy on reacting to the environment and the illness. Discussion of the dying process and the nurse's role is found in Chapter 22 of this text.

The Nurse and the Critically Ill Client

Level Five clients present an extreme challenge to the professional nurse. Their total dependence—physical, psychological, and social—requires acute and astute observation and creative interventions. Occasionally, it can result in the nurse taking on a full recovery role. The Level Five client is most frequently found in a critical care unit, but can be encountered anywhere, even in a nursing home facility. Usually, Level Five is rather temporary with the client recovering or dying. Occasionally, a client remains at a totally dependent stage and requires long-term care. Long-term care of the Level Five client requires high energy nursing care, which is difficult to achieve.

Caring for a Level Five client makes several demands on the nurse. The nurse takes in a huge amount of stimuli, needs to process stimuli rapidly, functions as a technical expert, participates in a range of human interactions at a variety of intellectual and intimacy levels, absorbs anxiety from a variety of sources, and acts as teacher, comforter, caretaker, resource person, and colleague. The demands on the nurse's own resources are enormous. In this situation, the nurse needs to develop an individual coping mechanism that allows for these functions, provides support, and restores energy. Support may come from coworkers, friends, or family. Energy restoration comes from rest and diversional activities. The nurse's physical and psychological health needs to be preserved by following basic good health practices. The nurse should take advantage of support groups, stress workshops, or personal counseling whenever offered. Professional health care should be considered when indicators of stress are noted.

REFERENCES

Adler ML: Kidney transplantation and coping mechanisms. Psychosomatics 13:337, 1972

Atkins CR: Renal transplantation, in Kenner C, Guzzetta C, Dossey B (eds), Critical Care Nursing Body-Mind-Spirit. Boston, Little, Brown, 1981

Atkins RC, Leonard CD, Scribner BB: Management of chronic renal failure. Disease of the Month, March, 1971

Baehler RW, Gallas JH: Conservative management of chronic renal failure. Geriatrics 31(9):46, 1976

Benoliel JQ, VandeVelde S: As the patient views the intensive care unit and the coronary care unit. Heart and Lung 4:260, 1975

Blachley PH, Starr A: Post-cardiotomy delirium. American Journal of Psychiatry 121:371, 1964

Bolin RH: Sensory deprivation: An overview. Nursing Forum 13(3):240, 1974

Brückel RW, Wincker HJ: Clinical aspects of urinary tract infections in geriatrics. Age With A Future: Proceedings of the Sixth Annual International Congress of Gerontology. Philadelphia, Davis, 1964

Chambers JK: Assessing the dialysis patient at home. American Journal of Nursing 81(4):750, 1981

Chodil J, Williams B: The concept of sensory deprivation. Nursing Clinics of North America 5(3):453, 1970

Cianci J, Lamb J, Ryan R: Renal transplantation. American Journal of Nursing 81(2):354, 1981

Egerton N, Kay JH: Psychological disturbances associated with open heart surgery. British Journal of Psychiatry 110:433, 1964

Engel GL: Sudden and rapid death during psychological stress: Folklore or folk wisdom? Annals of Internal Medicine 74:771, 1971

Gaarder K: A conceptual model of sleep. Archives of General Psychiatry 14:253, 1966

Gutman RA: Physical activity and employment status of patients on maintenance dialysis. New England Journal of Medicine 304:309, 1981

Hackett TP: Management of the disruptive patient in the intensive care setting. Cardiovascular Nursing 11:45, 1975

Heller S, Frank KA, Malm JR: Psychiatric complications of open-heart surgery: A re-examination. New England Journal of Medicine 283:1015, 1970

Kjellstrand CM, Shideman JR, et al: Kidney transplantation in patients over 50. Geriatrics 31(9):65, 1976

Kornfield DS: The hospital environment: Its impact on the patient, in Moos RH (ed), Coping With Physical Illness. New York, Plenum, 1977

Kotchen T, Ernst C: Detecting and treating arteriosclerotic renovascular hypertension. Geriatrics 31(8):83, 1976

Lazarus RH, Hagens JH: Prevention of psychosis following open-heart surgery. American Journal of Psychiatry 125:715, 1968

Lindsley D: Common factors in sensory deprivation, sensory distortion, and sensory overload. Sensory Deprivation. Cambridge, MA, Harvard University Press, 1965

Luby E, Frohman CE, et al: Sleep deprivation: Effects on behavior, thinking, motor performance and biological transfer systems. Psychosomatic Medicine 22:182, 1960

Merail JP: The Treatment of Renal Failure, 2nd ed. New York, Grune and Stratton, 1965

Moore-Smith B: The treatment of urinary tract infections in elderly women. Modern Geriatrics 4:122, 1974

Moorthy AV, Zimmerman SW: Renal disease in the elderly: Clinicopathologic analysis of renal disease in 115 elderly patients. Clinical Nephrology 14(5):223, 1980

Raji L, Keane WF, Leonard A, Shapiro F: Irreversible acute renal failure in nephrotic syndrome. American Journal of Medicine 61:207, 1976

Roberts S: Behavioral Concepts and the Critically Ill Client. Englewood Cliffs, NJ, Prentice-Hall, 1976

Rosen H: Renal diseases in the elderly. Medical Clinics of North America 60(6):1105, 1976

Rowe JW, Andres R, et al: The effect of age on creatinine clearance in men. Journal of Gerontology 31(2):155, 1976

Sanjurjo LA: The problems of chronic pyelonephritis. Medical Clinics of North America 43(6):1601, 1959

Shapiro W, Porush J, Kahn A: Medical renal diseases in the aged, in Reichel W (ed), Clinical Aspects of Aging. Baltimore, Williams and Wilkins, 1978

Snyder A, Brest AN: Chronic renal insufficiency treated

with anabolic steroids; Effects on acid–base balance, protein metabolism and hematopoiesis. Journal of the American Geriatrics Society 14(1):21, 1966

Vertes V, Bloomfield DK, Patel R, Gary M: Peritoneal dialysis in the geriatric patient. Journal of the American Geriatrics Society 15(11):1019, 1967

Walker PJ, Ginn AE, et al: Long term hemodialysis for patients over 50. Geriatrics 31(9):55, 1976

Wesson LG: Physiology of the Human Kidney. New York, Grune and Stratton, 1969

Woods NF, Falk SA: Nurse stimuli in the acute care area. Nursing Research 23:144, 1974

22

Death—The Last Developmental Stage

Death is a natural consequence of living, and acceptance of the inevitability of one's own death is the final stage of growth. Like any period of growth and change there are accompanying fears and crises. The pain associated with the experience of accepting death can be great because the perception of potential loss is great. Unlike many other growth situations, there is no control over whether or not death will occur. Only the experience of how the separation occurs is in our control. Preparing for one's own death can result in the investment of oneself in supporting and loving relationships and positive experiences.

Erikson indicates the final stage of life is the achievement of integrity. Integrity is the acknowledgement that one's life has value and purpose (Erikson, 1959). Other psychologists have similar ideas about the completion of life. The attainment of this stage results in the acceptance of one's own ultimate death. Although developmental stages are dictated by circumstances, rather than chronological age, it can be assumed that accepting death is a major developmental task of the elderly.

This section of the text will discuss death and the dying process from this perspective. Death of the elderly client can be a fulfilling experience for all participants in the event. The professional nurse can play an important role in assisting the client and the client's family through the process.

SIGNIFICANT PROBLEMS

The Meaning of Death for the Aged Client

Growing old in the United States is difficult. This society worships youth and is youth oriented. Acknowledgement of aging is taboo. The elderly are ignored or hidden away. Aging is feared and misconceptions about the elderly abound. The elderly receive little support in coming to grips with dying. Despite some recent advances in death education, discussion of death with the elderly is avoided. Wass and Scott (1977) point out that even the experts in the field of gerontology avoid the subject of death. Frequently, the discussion of death with the elderly is avoided so as not to upset the older person or to avoid some sort of embarrassment. However, a survey done in 1968 found that the majority of the elderly think and talk about death, and do so, generally, in a positive way (Riley, 1968). Matse (1975) showed that staff of nursing homes tended to avoid talking of death with the residents, but that death was a frequently discussed topic among the residents themselves.

Fear of Death. Facing up to death or denying it is closely related to one's fear of death. Old people, while by no means a homogeneous group, do have certain characteristics in common; most important among them is the fact that they are in their final stage of life and death is approaching. There is no single attitude concerning death among the elderly, but several studies have indicated that, as a group, the elderly have less fear of death than younger groups (Kastenbaum, 1969; Kalish and Reynolds, 1976).

Fear of death is not a simple or single reaction. There is some suggestion, however, that the elderly may fear the process of dying more than death itself. Marshall (1975) identifies four components of death fear: (1) fear of dying and the pain, dependency, loss of control, and loss of functions involved; (2) fear of nonbeing; (3) fear of the consequences of death—afterlife, judgment, survivors; and (4) fear of separation and loss of loved ones. The degree and intensity of fear vary greatly from person to person due to both personality and environmental factors.

Grieving.   The reaction to the fear of death is termed *grieving*. Grieving occurs as a reaction to a real or perceived loss. Since the elderly experience losses at an increasing rate and intensity with limited time for adaptation and reintegration, they frequently experience the phenomenon of "bereavement overload." Bereavement overload refers to the absence of sufficient time to successfully work through the grieving of one loss before another occurs (Kastenbaum, 1969). For instance, an elderly individual may have lost a job through mandatory retirement, resulting in the loss of social contacts as well as the loss of disposable income for entertainment. Then a friend dies, a spouse dies, and the individual moves. The client experiences loss after loss after loss. Grief can occur at any age, but in the elderly a series of losses accompanied by a perception of their own impending death may lead to insomnia, depression, loss of appetite, and other consequences of grief. These are serious outcomes for a person who lacks the energy reserves of youth. The nurse's sensitivity to the burden of grief borne by the elderly reduces the possibility that these problems will be dismissed as inevitable consequences of advanced age.

In summary, death is a realistic concern of the elderly. It is not morbid or unhealthy to talk of one's own death. The older person has concerns about the distribution of personal possessions, arranging burial, and saying "goodbye" in a personal and meaningful way. Some people fear that the older person will become "obsessed" with death. Obsession is more likely to occur when there is no one to listen to a little "death talk" (Kastenbaum, 1977). A sensitivity to and acceptance of death is an indication of healthy achievement of the final stage of growth. The elderly need acceptance and support in their striving toward this stage.

Definitions of Death

In discussing the topic of death it might be assumed that it is relatively easy to define death. In actuality, death is extremely difficult to define. In the past, definitions of death were clear and commonly accepted by everyone. Death was frequently described by indicating the signs and characteristics that involved the entire body, such as paleness, frigidity, immobility, closed eyes, dropped jaw, and apnea. Contemporary definitions of death are more complex when one considers the varying approaches of different disciplines, especially medicine, philosophy, and the law.

Medical Definitions.   Medicine defines death by either the circulatory or neurological changes that occur. Details of changes that occur in the cardiovascular system during the dying process have been noted by Gavey (1952), Walker (1973), and others. Systemic biological changes have also been documented (Kirk, 1968). Many neurologists have indicated that bioelectrical changes in the electroencephalogram are significant in the death process (Toole, 1971). These studies have led to a fuller understanding of the physiological events that occur when a person dies.

Recently, the concept of "brain death" as the indicator of death has been developed. This concept is based on the hypothesis that the brain is the locus of control of physiological functioning. The concept of "brain death" refers to the whole brain including the cerebellum, medulla, and brain stem. It specifically includes unconsciousness and higher reflex mechanisms. Criteria for brain death have been developed in order to accurately predict and document irreversible loss of brain activity. These criteria were developed by the Ad Hoc Committee to Examine the Definition of Brain Death of Harvard Medical School (1968). The criteria they developed, commonly called the "Harvard Criteria," are widely recognized and accepted in this country. The American Bar Association has recommended these criteria as the legal definition of death. The criteria are:

1. Unreceptivity or unresponsiveness
2. No movements or breathing
3. No reflexes
4. Flat electroencephalogram

An initial documentation of these four findings followed in 24 hours by a repetition of these findings confirms brain death. The "Harvard Criteria" stand as a landmark in decision making in this difficult area.

Additional studies have noted the limitations of the criteria. For instance, in cases of extreme hypothermia the criteria are not valid until the body has warmed to a normal temperature. Also, the presence of central nervous system depressants may temporarily affect responses, so the criteria cannot be used until drug levels are lowered (Mellerio, 1971). Toole (1971) agrees that brain death is significant, but suggests that the "Harvard Criteria" are too conservative. He feels that metabolic criteria, such as measurements of metabolic products in the cerebral spinal fluid and oxygen consumption, should also be included. Others suggest additional criteria. Alexandre adds the lack of spontaneous respirations and falling blood pressure; Revillard suggests angiography to demonstrate loss of circulation to the brain (Walstenholme and O'Connor, 1966). Other suggestions for the demonstration of lack of brain circulation include radioisotopes or sonar techniques (Hadjidimos et al., 1969).

Philosophical Definitions. Another attempt to define death is to define it in philosophical or theological terms. The philosophical definition of death is related to the meaning of life, which may look to the body for clues but is not dependent upon scientific measures. This definition of death will depend upon how one evaluates the meaning of life. There are four approaches to, or definitions of, death that are based on a meaning of life.

The first of these is the cessation of the flow of vital body fluids—blood and breath. According to this view, death occurs when there is an irreversible loss of the flow of these vital fluids. This is a naturalistic approach, and is reflected in the Jewish theological phrase "breath of life."

A second definition includes the concept of the soul. Greek philosophy speaks of the soul as the significant factor in human life. It represents the essence of man, which is independent of the chemical and electrical forces that account for bodily functioning. This idea is also seen in the philosophies of gnosticism, Pauline Christianity, and later Western theologies. Death occurs when the soul leaves the body. The leaving of the soul is sometimes equated with the stoppage of body fluids. The important thought here, however, is that fluids stop flowing when the soul leaves the body and they stop because the soul is no longer present. It is the leaving of the soul, not the loss of fluids, that is death.

The third view focuses on the nature of man. The essence of man is defined as the ability to reason and think rationally. The significant abilities of man lie in two general areas: first, an ability to integrate one's internal bodily environment and second, a capacity for integrating one's self with the external environment on a conscious level. It is intellect, intuition, rationality, and the ability to control that makes man unique. Thus, when these abilities are lost, man is dead. In this view, it is not simply a loss of consciousness, but the irreversible consequences of a permanent loss of consciousness that identify death.

The fourth view is closely related to the third but includes the loss of the capacity for social interaction. Here man's uniqueness is defined by the ability to express emotion, to remember, and to care or love. If the capacity for these social interactions is lost, then the essential character of humanness is lost and, according to this definition, death has occurred. These last two views of life—consciousness and the capacity for social interaction—are viewed by some as synonymous and by others as separate and distinct.

In considering these views, most philosophers emphasize that concepts of the essence of humanity do not imply that individuals must be valued by others in order to be human. It is not a qualitative or quantitative judgment. The essence of humanness, whatever it is believed to be, is what is significant to the nature of human beings, and without it the human being is dead. It is essentially an exclusive quality—it exists or does not exist.

Legal Definitions. Legal definitions are an attempt to avoid precipitous or immoral declarations of death and have arisen because of the ability of technological devices to prolong bodily functions. As stated above, the "Harvard Criteria" serve as the basis for a legal definition. It is likely that as the philosophical definitions of death are further explored, and technological devices are further developed, legal definitions will become more significant in this society and will need further refinement.

Death can be defined in many ways, for many purposes. These definitions are somewhat interactive, since an acceptance of a measurable definition of brain death as a definition of death infers a philosophical statement that the essence of man has also died.

The Meaning of Death in America

Response to death is determined, in part, by the social norms and behavior accepted by the culture with which an individual identifies. The range of differences among cultural groups is enormous. In America, there are a rich variety of groups, each with their own ethnic, cultural, and religious practices and rituals concerning death. There is also a dominant American attitude toward death that influences all cultural practices.

There are three sociocultural responses to death. They are death-accepting, death-defying, and death-denying. Generally speaking, primitive, nontechnological societies are *death-accepting,* viewing death as natural and inevitable. The acknowledgement of a dying member is a part of the everyday pattern of life. *Death-defying* societies refuse to believe that death takes anything away or diminishes life in any way. The early Egyptian societies are good examples, illustrated by the burying of servants and possessions with the dead. In *death-denying* cultures, there is a refusal to acknowledge death and a belief that death is not a natural part of existence; rather, it is seen as something to be overcome. The United States, along with most Western advanced societies, is a death-denying culture.

Aires (1981) points out that the denial of death

in the United States has intensified since World War II. He points out that from the Middle Ages up until the mid-forties, death was noted and noticeable. Notices of bereavement were posted on doors, or drapery was hung, shutters were closed, and periods of mourning lasting a year or more were observed, with mourning clothes being worn by the bereaved. Death was a social and public fact. In only one generation, this position was virtually reversed. Mourning observances are now shortened and black is rarely worn. The dying person is frequently hospitalized or otherwise removed and isolated from the home. Discussion of death is disapproved. Children are "protected" from death by not allowing them to participate in death rituals.

Feifel (1971) suggests some reasons for the reluctance of Americans to accept death. He points out that family cohesiveness has declined along with primary group interactions. In addition, there has been an upsurge in technology resulting in alienation, isolation, and depersonalization. These losses alter our sense of continuity; thus, death is now feared as a loss of identity rather than, in the old view, a continuation into a new life.

Lifton (1968) comes to similar conclusions in his study of the survivors of Hiroshima. He identified six variables that have led American culture to its difficulty in dealing with death. The variables he suggests are increasing urbanization separating individuals from the life/death cycle of nature, separation of the aged and persons who are dying in nursing homes and hospitals, absence of an extended family, loss of religious influences, advances in medical technology, which have increased man's control over the dying process, and the threat of mass death or decreased sensitivity to an individual death in many situations such as war or nuclear attack.

American culture separates the dead by placing them in "viewing rooms," uses euphemisms such as "pass on," "at rest," or "gone to their reward," rather than the word "dead," and hides death from children, thus perpetuating the denial.

In recognizing this unnatural approach to death, sociologists and psychologists have recently taken death "out of the closet" so to speak. Unfortunately, the media—printed, verbal, and televised—seem recently to be almost morbidly preoccupied with death as entertainment. Dumont and Foss (1972) point out that death has entered the entertainment media in ways that are almost pornographic—violent, fantastic, and romanticized death is presented as entertainment. This is also a form of denial of the reality of death. Some of the recent work among health care professionals, sensitizing them to their own view of death, may be the beginning of putting death in its natural perspective in this country. Understanding the death-denying aspects of American culture will help the nurse to understand and assist the client who is dying.

The Process of Dying

It is important to distinguish death from dying. Death is the condition of being dead, having died, no longer being alive. Dying refers to a process that results in death. In this society, the words are sometimes used, inappropriately, as synonyms. It seems obvious, but nurses often consider those dying as "all-but-dead" or "as-good-as-dead." To prevent this unconscious slip, nurses need to be careful to distinguish dying persons from those who are already dead and treat them accordingly.

Phases in the Process of Dying. The process of dying can be divided into four phases: social death, psychological death, biological death, and physiological death. These phases may occur together or one at a time, generally in the following order.

- *Social Death:* Social death occurs when the individual ceases normal social interactions. Social death occurs appropriately as the terminal phase nears and the environment is contracted by the client's being bedridden or hospitalized. Social death can occur prematurely when the client is isolated in a nursing home or socially deserted long before any other indications of dying are identified.
- *Psychological Death:* Psychological death occurs when the client experiences alterations in personality. As death becomes more imminent, the dying individual withdraws from life. As a result, individuality is lost. Occasionally, personality distortions occur because of a disease process.
- *Biological Death:* Biological death occurs when consciousness and self-sustaining mechanisms are lost. Artificial support may keep certain organs alive but the person no longer exists.

- *Physiological Death:* Physiological death occurs when all organs cease to function. It generally occurs close to the time of biological death in a predictable sequence of events. It can be prolonged through the use of artificial support devices.

These four phases of dying lead to a number of adaptations that are discussed in the next section.

ASSESSING THE CLIENT'S ADAPTATIONS

Psychosocial Adaptations

The Dying Trajectory. The process of dying occurs over time. The course of the dying process has been termed the dying trajectory by Glaser and Strauss (1968). The trajectory helps to identify the length, shape, and course of the last phase of life, and serves as a useful guide for health care professionals to plan their interactions. They suggest four major types of trajectory:

1. Certain death at a known time—generally infers a rapid course and a known cause such as trauma or fatal disease.
2. Certain death but at an unknown time—typical of most chronic illnesses or advanced age.
3. Uncertain death, but resolved at a known time. This occurs when a specific threat to life is presented, such as surgery, and is resolved within a specific time frame—the individual either survives the surgery or dies.
4. Death at an unknown time. This is the situation in which most of us find ourselves. No specific threat to life exists, but it becomes more noted as the person advances in age.

It is useful to keep the trajectory in mind as reactions to dying are explored, since they too are time related. At some point, people become aware that they are dying, either because they were told so or they anticipate it because of advancing age or failing health. The knowledge that life is limited presents the individual with a crisis situation that demands accommodation and reorientation. The acknowledgement of impending death is not a fundamentally new thought for the individual but it alters the individual's perception of the remainder of life. Confrontation with the meaning of life cannot be avoided.

Death as Crisis. In a sense, dying is the most stressful crisis because it cannot be avoided. It is beyond the usual problem-solving methods. This crisis situation awakens unresolved key problems from the past so that an individual is faced with the immediate dying process as well as unresolved feelings and inevitable conflicts.

There are three commonalities that have been identified during the crisis period of dying. These are the feeling of limitation or being trapped, the feeling of loss due to the recognition that all that is presently known will be lost, and the feeling related to change from independency to dependency. Generally, these aspects of dying, rather than the knowledge of death set up the fear and accompanying crisis behaviors. Dealing with the crisis of dying is difficult because the individual has had no previous experience with personal death. Also, adaptation to a crisis is facilitated by the expectation of pleasurable results in the future; the person facing death generally does not anticipate pleasure. In addition, the ability of the elderly person to cope with this crisis may be altered by decreasing energy levels necessary to maintain appropriate defense and coping mechanisms.

Anxiety and Fear. There are some specific psychosocial adaptations that occur during the dying process. The first is anxiety. Anxiety is a natural reaction in people contemplating their own death, even if that death is not presumed to be imminent. The thought of nonbeing is anxiety provoking. Almost every client will experience some level of anxiety. While anxiety is nonspecific, it encompasses a number of fears. Each person will have specific fears about death that may be unique to him or her. In addition to specific fears, there are the four common fears among the elderly identified earlier (Marshall, 1975). They are fear of the dying process including discomfort and pain; fear of nonbeing; fear of the consequences of death; and fear of separation; and the loss of loved ones. Pattison (1977) has also identified a group of fears associated with death that are more specific than

those listed above. Pattison's list includes: fear of the unknown; fear of loneliness as isolation and withdrawal occur; fear of the loss of family or friends; fear of loss of self-control; fear of loss of body or disability; fear of suffering and pain; fear of loss of identity; fear of sorrow; fear of regression; fear of mutilation and decompensation; and fear of premature burial.

Some of these fears can be coped with if they are known to the individual and others. Interventions can be planned to assist the client should a situation arise that relates to the person's fear. With support, clients can use their capacities to deal with the realization that death is an unknown. Clients can then focus on their specific fears connected with the dying process. As each fear is identified, plans can be made to cope with it. For instance, if the client fears the loss of friends and family, plans can be made to continue these interactions as long as possible. The client can be assisted to acknowledge that they will be lost, and can be allowed to control the loss (one at a time), mourn the loss, and adapt to it.

Anticipatory Grief. Another psychosocial adaptation that occurs is anticipatory grief. This is a natural reaction to the perception of imminent loss. Anticipatory grieving can be a facilitator to prepare the person for the reality of death (Weisman, 1977). Unlike reactive grieving, anticipatory (or preparatory) grief acknowledges that there are times when it is most therapeutic to dwell on and contemplate these impending losses. These losses need to be worked through to the extent possible. This is facilitated by allowing dying persons to grieve and express their sorrow verbally, by crying, by periods of withdrawal, and any other way that is helpful. A dying person's day should not be filled with grief but grief should be expressed when it occurs.

Anger and Hostility. A third psychosocial adaptation, which again is normal, is anger accompanied by hostility. Anger is understandable; the person is being deprived of a future. The anger may be focused at "God" ("Why is He punishing me?"). These feelings of anger may also be displaced on anyone or anything available. Generally, the anger is covering up the more painful fears of loss. Anger is generally apparent near the time the person has become aware of impending death. It may be extremely intense and difficult to deal with. Expressions of anger should be encouraged as (usually) this will decrease the intensity and duration of this reaction.

Guilt. The fourth psychosocial adaptation of the dying person is guilt. Guilt develops when one is not living up to one's self-image. It is not unusual for persons who are terminally ill to believe that they are being punished for some past behavior. They feel guilty for the past offense and frequently feel shame for their current situation. Guilt may also develop over their expressions of anger to those close to them or to a caretaker. Or they may feel guilty for "losing control" by expressing their grief. When guilt develops it can be dealt with quickly by reinforcing the reality of the situation and the naturalness of associated feelings.

Defense Mechanisms. As clients struggle to deal with these adaptations to the dying process they may use a variety of defense mechanisms. Defense mechanisms used in the dying process are generally therapeutic as they assist the individual in coping with the stress. When used appropriately, these defense mechanisms serve an adaptive function. They are crucial in helping clients to live with the threat of their imminent demise.

Verwoerdt (1966) suggests that the defense mechanisms used by the dying person fall into one of three groups associated with the death crisis. The first group of defense mechanisms are those aimed at retreating from the threat and conserving energy. These include regression and dependence. The second group are those defenses aimed at excluding the threat or its significance from awareness. The specific defenses here are repression, suppression, denial, rationalization, depersonalization, and intellectualization. The last category are defenses aimed at mastering the threat: obsessive–compulsive behaviors, counterphalic mechanisms, and sublimation. Verwoerdt's framework seeks to explain the underlying reason for the use of the defense mechanism. Identification of the defense mechanism may be the first step in assisting the client to identify particular fears and cope with the dying process.

Stage Theory. Another way to look at personal and social adaptations to the dying process is stage theory, popularized by Elizabeth Kübler-Ross (1969). Stages delineate the various adaptations a person experiences while dying. There are, however, some problems with stage theory. The stages are usually seen as consecutive and inflexible. Nurses who pigeonhole clients into a stage may fail to recognize the full range of reactions clients are experiencing at any given time. Stage theory tends to neglect the individual aspects of each person.

Still, staging can be a useful tool in understanding the client's behavior. Engle (1962) did some of the initial work in stages of death, added to by Kübler-Ross, and then by Gullo et al. (1974). Their stages of grieving are listed below:

Engle	*Kübler-Ross*
1. Shock and disbelief	1. Denial
2. Developing awareness of loss	2. Anger
	3. Bargaining
3. Restitution	4. Depression
	5. Acceptance

Gullo et al.
1. Shock
2. Anger
3. Grief
4. Bargaining
5. Uncertainty
6. Renewal and rebuilding
7. Integration of experience

One of the additional things that Gullo found is that an individual has a specific response style and will go through each stage according to this style.

Further research into stage theory needs to study the interaction between coping styles and staging. Research on staging also needs to address the acutely dying client, since most work in staging has been done with the chronically dying individual. The application of stages in a shorter dying trajectory is questionable. There is also the basic question of whether staging is a universal phenomenon. Currently, evidence does not exist to suggest that the staging experience occurs in non-Western cultures. At this time, stage theory may be used as an attempt to understand reactions of the dying person as long as the stages are not applied too rigidly and the limitations of this theory are recognized.

Resolution of the Crisis. Resolution of the crisis of dying is the acceptance of one's own death. Struggling and psychic pain have stopped and the person acknowledges that death will occur. With acceptance can come peace of mind and tranquility. Also with acceptance of death can come control. Facing death requires exploration of who we really are, and of becoming joined with nature to overcome terror. If death is accepted as necessity rather than striving to demote it to the level of accident, energies that have been used in attempting to deny death will then be available for the more constructive aspects of continued life. It is not unusual for those who have accepted their impending death to become very creative and prolific in their expressions of life, love, and death. Real acceptance of death is positive and active. It is not simply passive resignation, dull reaction, or fatalism. The person achieves an intensity of meaning in existence, a unity or oneness with the world and other humans.

One of the difficulties in the process of dying is the pain of loneliness. Accounts of persons who have reached a level of acceptance indicate that they have reached a level of acceptance through interpersonal relationships with family, friends, and staff who care and who see their lives as being enriched by the person who is dying.

Acceptance of death is dependent upon the development and ratification of a philosophy of life. This is difficult to achieve because of the seeming contradiction between the attraction of understanding and the repulsion of death and dying. To incorporate death into personal philosophy demands interpretations that not only satisfy theoretically (why there is death or the need for death), but also give inner sustenance in meeting the crisis of suffering and death. This is a difficult task that requires exploration, discussion, and argument until the individual is satisfied. There is real danger of the person intellectualizing his or her own death at this point, a defense mechanism that may not be therapeutic in attempting to reach this goal.

Structural Adaptations in the Dying Process

Structural adaptations of dying occur at every age and are progressive. This statement is both obvious and surprising. Dying is often viewed as a fixed event, usually associated with the determination of

a terminal illness, and a prognosis made as to the length of survival. In reality, most diseases are long-term and may be based on hereditary factors (as in diabetes, epilepsy) or life-style (obesity, smoking, stress leading to cardiovascular disease). Nevertheless, the current medical-biological model of disease includes the premise that a medical disease "overtakes" individuals and either threatens to take or, in fact, does take their lives.

A more realistic view of the dying process might be one recognizing that with any disease process is a concurrent aging process. Aging is usually the more significant factor leading to death. There is, of course, much individual variation in the rate of aging, but most agree that after the age of 30 there is loss in functional capacity, which occurs in a linear fashion, each year of life.

There is also an impression that medical science and technology have increased the life span. It is true that life expectancy has changed. That is, more people are surviving diseases that, in the past, would have caused an early death. Thus, more people are living longer than previously. However, the overall span of life has not changed significantly during recorded history and seems to remain at about 70 years on the average. In fact, the 1980 figures, reported by the Statistical Bureau of the Metropolitan Life Insurance Company indicate a life expectancy decrease by 0.2 years, the first such decline since 1968. The current life expectancy at birth for males is 70 years, and for females, 77.6 years (1981). So, while advances in medical care have assisted individuals in living to an older age the overall span of life is still about the traditional "three score and ten."

Biological theories of aging have previously been presented in this text. Whether death occurs from a disease process, from normal aging, or a combination of both, it is not a singular discrete event. It is a series of complex interrelated changes that occur at the cellular level. It is when these changes alter the functioning of somatic systems that the death process is recognized. The death process is characterized by three basic physiological responses: failure of the brain to supply information vital for the functioning of the respiratory and cardiovascular systems, inadequate gas exchange, and inadequate circulation. Without the aid of technology, these three mechanisms generally occur in concert and death results. Technology has been used to intervene and support these systems when there has been reason to believe that the underlying stress can be corrected. To explore these mechanisms in more detail each will be discussed separately.

Central Nervous System Failure. The central nervous system (CNS) is made up of the brain and the spinal cord. This system provides regulatory control of the vital functions of the body as well as sensory and intellectual functions. A variety of stresses in the brain can result in alterations of the CNS's ability to function. Common stresses are encephalitis, meningitis, strokes, and tumors. In addition, stresses in other areas of the body, such as kidney or liver disease, can create lowered glucose levels, imbalances of electrolytes, or alterations in hormone levels leading to CNS decompensation.

There are classic adaptations seen in CNS decompensation. They occur in stages and indicate progessive decompensation. Severe *confusion* or *disorientation* occurs first. This continues to a stage of *lethargy*. At this stage, reflexes may become sluggish and cognitive functioning becomes difficult. The next stage of *stupor* indicates no wakefulness and no spontaneous movements; reflexes can only be elicited by visual, auditory, or touch stimuli and are generally very slow. Decorticate positioning may be seen at this level. The next stage is *semicoma*. In this stage, movement occurs only in response to deep pain, decerebrate posturing can occur, and generally pupils do not react. Changes in vital signs generally occur with semicoma. Blood pressure increases, pulse pressure widens, arrhythmias occur, and respirations become shallow. The final stage is *coma*, in which there are no movements and no reflexes. This stage is considered terminal and is accompanied by falling pulse and blood pressure, and shallow, irregular respirations.

Pulmonary Failure. The second mechanism is pulmonary failure, the inability to provide an adequate exchange of gases. This can occur from a variety of stresses, including an interruption of vascular supply, a depression in the lower medullary portion of the brain, the presence of congestive or emphysemic processes, or a decrease in the muscular activities of the chest. The initial adaptive response is *hypoxia,* with the accompanying adaptations of confusion, irritability, and anxiety. There are also the responses generally seen in *hypercarbia,* which quickly follows. These alterations in oxygen and carbon dioxide levels continue until breathing becomes extremely and severely impaired and may need to be assisted.

Circulatory Failure. The third mechanism in the death process is inadequate circulation to the vital organs: the brain, heart, lungs, and kidneys. Adequate circulation is dependent upon both the efficient pumping of the heart and response of the vessels to changing conditions. Stresses in this system include arrhythmias, loss of blood volume, atherosclerosis, myocardial infarction, or prolonged shock. The common adaptive response is a decreased blood supply to any or all of the vital structures. Generally, the initial response is *vasoconstriction* in the nonvital tissues including the skin, accompanied by tachycardia and decreasing blood pressure. Eventually, prolonged vasoconstriction leads to *cellular hypoxia, necrosis,* and eventual tissue and organ death.

These three mechanisms occur at varying rates of speed depending upon the circumstances surrounding the dying process. They can occur suddenly and in combination, quickly, one at a time, or over a long period of progressive deterioration. Although not totally exempt, the elderly do not usually experience sudden and unexpected deaths. Death is more apt to occur from degenerative aging or chronic disease processes.

Adaptations of Impending Death. The exact death trajectory varies from individual to individual, depending on the stress and the individual's ability to adapt. Certain adaptations usually indicate the dying process is ending and death is close at hand.

1. Temperature: Vasoconstriction causes the skin to become cold to the touch and damp. Color changes, also due to severe vasoconstriction, result in an overall pallor and cyanosis of the extremities. As the heat regulation system fails, the person's body temperature will fall. Generally the person is not aware of this drop and is not conscious of being cold.
2. Pulse: Just prior to death the pulse rate becomes extremely irregular in both rate and intensity.

The pulse may become extremely rapid and then slow, be very strong and then weak, regular and then irregular. Peripheral pulses generally fade before the apical pulse does. The apical pulse becomes softer and softer and becomes inaudible even when an electrocardiogram still indicates cardiac activity.

3. Gastrointestinal changes: As changes in consciousness occur, the person becomes less able to swallow sufficient liquids, and accompanying indications of dehydration may occur. The loss of the swallowing reflex generally indicates an irreversible loss of consciousness. Also at this level of consciousness, fecal and urinary incontinence occur. These changes by themselves do not necessarily indicate impending death, but they always are present when death is imminent.

4. Respiration: As the gas exchange becomes altered, breathing becomes labored and irregular. Respirations may increase initially to 30 to 40 per minute and then revert to Cheyne-Stokes respirations with increasingly longer periods of apnea.

5. Central nervous system: The interval of unconsciousness may range from a few seconds to several days, so this alone is not a good indicator of impending death. With loss of consciousness, movement, sensation, and reflexes are also lost. Electroencephalograms indicate that consciousness is maintained longer than seems apparent based on responses. They have also indicated that hearing is maintained longer than other senses and it is difficult to determine when, precisely, it is lost.

There is no simple way to know definitely when an individual's death will occur. These signs can be used to prepare the dying individual and the family for the closeness of the event.

NURSING INTERVENTIONS

The Nurse's Role

Caring for the person who is dying can be both stressful and rewarding for the professional nurse. Whenever a client is defined as dying, the burden of care shifts from the medical staff to the nursing staff. Care for dying clients consists of two types of activity: physical and interpersonal. The provision of physical nursing care is rewarding since it allows the nurse direct one-to-one access to the client that is frequently prevented through institutional or technological barriers. This one-to-one contact allows a trusting relationship to develop. Caring for the dying client is difficult, however, because the nurse does not derive as much satisfaction from the experience as from caring for a client who recovers. In addition, it is difficult because health care facilities are generally cure oriented and the dying client does not easily fit the orientation of most institutions.

Benoliel (1976) suggests that nursing the dying client is fundamentally an interpersonal activity with two important functions: nurses provide continuity of experience for the person who is dying; they also offer personal care and direct assistance when individuals cannot provide for themselves. The nurse is concerned with the physical, personal, and social experiences that together comprise the individual's process of dying. The nurse aids the client through the utilization of self, the health care facility, family, friends, community, and social agencies. In order to derive satisfaction from this challenging role, nurses need to accept the notion of their personal mortality. While the process of self-acknowledgement will never be complete, nurses need to come to grips with the knowledge that they will die at some time and need to develop personal philosophies that accept death as part of, or a consequence of, living.

Confirming Personal Feelings. It is not easy for healthy persons to think seriously of their own death. In doing so, nurses confront their own deep-seated feelings and fears about death. If nurses refuse to admit their own feelings, then they will not be able to assist clients to deal with theirs. Nurses, of course, are not required to confront their own death immediately; thus, they have the luxury of time to confront this problem from a variety of situations or approaches. Epstein (1975) has suggested a series of exercises in which nurses can engage in order to develop self-awareness of their own mortality. These exercises can be done privately or in a group teaching/sensitivity session. Some of the exercises she suggests are the following:

1. Ask yourself a series of questions related to where you stand about your own death:

How do you want other people to react to your death?

What type of funeral/burial do you want?

What level of grief is appropriate?

2. Write a description of the way you want your loved ones to react upon hearing about your impending death. Then compare that "wished for" reaction with a real situation. Is the wished for reaction a realistic expectation? Are you happy with the reality expectation?

3. Talk about your own death in a small group setting. Express your *feelings,* not expected behaviors.

4. Discuss a client who is dying and how you feel about that client's behavior.

Other questionnaires and sensitivity exercises have been developed and are generally included in most death education courses.

Nurses need to develop an understanding of the dying experience along with a sense of the holistic response inherent in the process. This experience of the client, as well as the holistic adaptations, were discussed earlier. More research continues to be developed to further our understanding of this process.

It is important that in caring for the dying nurses realize their own personal limitations. The nurse may need to leave the death scene or the client may need to retreat. Death is the client's crisis and the nurse can only support, not take over for the client.

Stresses Experienced by the Nurse. There are some unique stresses for the nurse who works with the dying. Working with dying clients requires that the nurse be involved in the grieving process of the client as well as the family. This grief can become cumulative and overwhelming for the nurse. It is also difficult for the nurse to measure success. The client does not "recover" in the usual sense of the word. It can be extremely frustrating for the nurse who does everything "right" when the client does not respond, or chooses a direction other than that which the nurse might have chosen.

It is openly acknowledged that involvement in another person's dying is difficult. The establishment of a social and professional network can replenish the nurse's emotional bank and decrease vulnerability to this professional stress. At the same time, involvement with the dying offers a unique opportunity for sharing the experience of living at a depth not usually found in the professional nurse–client relationship.

Ethical and Legal Issues in Death

In caring for the dying client, the nurse is presented with many ethical and legal concerns. The nurse is frequently in a critical position of contact with the client and family and, thus, will be confronted with situations that can produce conflict between the client's needs and the needs of others, or society.

Ethical Concerns. Ethics is the philosophical approach to what is "right." It is concerned with general values as well as specific moral choices made by an individual. Ethical questions do not generally have a universal answer. Instead, ethics provide a framework for discussion and reflection in order to prevent reactive decision making. The nurse needs to develop a personal value system that is congruent with professional ethical values so that questions can be dealt with when the choices are equally unattractive. It is important for nurses to make rational choices for and with the individual, and not impose their own answers. Issues requiring ethical decisions involve questions of the right to reject treatment, prolongation of life, euthanasia, and suicide.

Legal Concerns. Legal considerations involve acting within the "rules" as decided by the courts. Frequently, legal decisions have grown out of difficult ethical dilemmas. For instance, the "Natural Death Act" in California (and similar acts in other states) offers a solution to the dilemma of the right to die without artificial supports. Legal issues have also developed over the "rights" of the dead person vis-à-vis the survivors. The law has spelled out procedural and substantive rights, through the use of wills and estate planning, that allow the living to determine and control their possessions and exert influence over the survivors. These two considerations, ethical and legal, are frequently intertwined. While a particular decision may be legal, it may not necessarily be ethical. For instance, it is legal for an individual to have a will. But when confronted with a family who is pressuring the dying individual to make a will the nurse may have difficulty with the "rightness" of this decision at this time. Unfortunately, many issues such as "telling clients they are dying" have no legal basis.

Decision Making. A useful place for nurses to start in the making of an ethical decision is the *ANA Code for Nurses with Interpretive Statements*. In order to set up parameters for action, nurses can also use the Nurse Practice Act of the particular state where they are licensed. These, along with a personal philosophy of clients' rights and the meaning of life, will serve as the base for decision making in conflict situations.

In dealing with these issues, the nurse can interact in a variety of ways. Veatch (1972) suggests four basic relationships between the nurse and the client regarding decision making. She suggests the way in which the nurse relates is usually congruent with the nurse's ethical philosophy, which may be either covert or overt. In evaluating client care, the type of relationship needs to be evaluated in order to assure that it enhances the nursing care goals for the client. These relationships are as follows:

1. *The engineer.* This is a relationship in which the nurse presents all the facts to the client, allowing the client to make the decisions regarding care. The nurse carries out the client's wishes with no consideration of the nurse's own personal values. This has the potential for placing the nurse in a morally outrageous situation. This type of relationship can be implied when the nurse agrees to act as a client advocate without indicating limits to the client's right to make decisions.

2. *The priestly relationship.* This relationship is at the other end of the decision-making continuum. In this situation, the nurse decides what is in the client's best interest and a maternalistic controlling relationship is established. Obviously, this type of relationship threatens the client's autonomy.

3. *The collegial relationship.* In this relationship the client and nurse share common goals. Decisions are reached through discussion and mutual consent. The underlying assumption is that the client enjoys equal status with the nurse. This is probably an unrealistic assumption in these days of bureaucratized health care systems that exclude the client from the decision-making process.

4. *The contractual relationship.* Here, the nurse and the client acknowledge that their values may differ but the basic framework for decision making is the client's values. The care plan is negotiated, allowing the client as much control as possible, or wanted, within parameters that do not offend the moral positions of the nurse or the health care system. The contract can only be modified after discussion and agreement by all concerned. This is the model that is used in many hospice facilities.

The "Right to Die." The care of the dying client presents the potential for a range of ethical dilemmas that may or may not have a legal component. One issue that pertains particularly to the elderly is the "Right to Die." This issue is encountered partly because so many deaths take place in the hospital. Hospitals are acute care facilities designed to care for clients through an episode of illness or surgery and return them to society. In this context, a dying individual is an inappropriate client. Feelings of frustration arise in the attempt to care for this client since the client cannot respond to the usual therapies. This frustration can lead to the aggressive use of technological devices to support life systems in the vain search for cure. Decisions to stop aggressive treatment and substitute supportive care for the dying client are made, of course, every day. They are difficult decisions and the conflicts inherent in them precipitate discussions of active (killing) and passive (letting die) euthanasia. Despite the fact that the outcome is the same (death of the individual), active and passive euthanasia are distinct actions involving a variety of arguments pro and con.

It is possible to argue that passive euthanasia is defensible on the grounds of caring and kindness and that active euthanasia is indefensible on the same grounds. There are those who argue that active euthanasia at the client's request is the ultimate act of caring. Most supporters of passive euthanasia include the control of pain, despite the probability of depressing respiratory or cardiac activity as a crucial argument.

Conflicts in caring for the dying typically arise when the decision whether to continue treatment or not is made unilaterally. When the "no-code" order is written, it is nurses who carry out this order despite their own values or decisions. Realizing that someone must make a decision, and this generally is the physician, it is not unreasonable for the nurse to expect to have been consulted or, at the very least, been given the rationale for the decision. One model for making this difficult decision is the Optimum Care Committee as established at Massachusetts General Hospital. The committee serves in an advisory capacity and the mandatory discussion about the decision helps clarify the client's prognosis, treatment goals, and wishes of the client and family. In each situation, the decision not to resuscitate is based solely on the clinical interest of the client.

It is in this difficult area of decision making that more clients are assuming greater responsibility and have sought legal sanctions for their actions. This responsibility is seen in the natural death acts and in living wills that appear in many states. On the whole this has been a welcome development since it shifts the burden of decision away from the physician. The significance of living wills lies in the stimulation of discussion of treatment with the client and family. A living will focuses attention on the impending death. The prognosis is stated and shared and the dying process is eased by open and honest communication. Many states already have Right-To-Die laws and legislation is now pending in others.

One of the difficulties that arises in these situations is when the wishes of family members do not agree with the position stated by the client, and when the family members disagree among themselves as to the best course of action. This problem becomes more acute when the client is elderly and the question of competency arises. The living will, unlike the natural death acts, is not legally binding but will generally be upheld on moral grounds unless the courts intervene. The nurse can aid the family in exploring the motivation for their objections (frequently it is guilt) and support them in their grieving. The potential for family schism over this issue is substantial, and there are financial and psychological implications as well as legal ones.

Assisting the Dying Client

Communicating with the Dying Client. Communication with the dying client is the most important nursing activity and should be directed toward three types of understanding: (1) the meaning of the illness and its adaptations for the client, (2) the client's awareness of and reaction to the illness,

and (3) the fears and anxieties that the client experiences (Verwoerdt, 1966). The attending skills of the nurse (attentive body language, eye contact, active listening) will facilitate communication. It is important not to force the communication but to allow the client to lead the discussion. Willingness to listen, being there, and allowing flexibility will create a climate of trust and acceptance.

Generally, when the client is conscious, communication is verbal. The nurse also needs to be alert to the additional nonverbal communication the client expresses. A clenched fist or a look of anxiety should not be ignored. Crying or a relaxation of tension should be recognized as an important comment. The nurse also can use nonverbal methods of communication. A touch, direct eye contact, sitting by the client, or physical care can all express care and understanding.

There are some situations that present communication problems, for example, a client with a tracheostomy, or a client who is aphasic. The nurse then needs to use a large repertoire of communication approaches. Symbolic language can be developed; signs and sign language are also useful. Verbal language accompanied by appropriate body language is usually very successful in conveying meaning. Occasionally, for the aphasic client, communication in a native language might be successful. Music is also a method of communication that can be used to convey caring and emotions.

Some useful skills for the nurse to possess are the ability to listen, to interpret verbal and nonverbal behaviors, to respond appropriately, and to communicate caring to the client and the family.

Sharing the Crisis. It is the goal of nursing to assist the elderly client in attaining as positive a dying experience with the most control possible. Pattison (1977) describes this as aiding the client toward an "appropriate death." The dying elderly client has to be approached as a human being who requires continued human contact and assistance through the crisis. It cannot be assumed that the elderly are all at peace with their coming death. Some are, some are not. The elderly do think about death and understand its inevitability. Their willingness to acknowledge this does not preclude the normal difficulty inherent in facing one's own death. Interventions are planned to assist the aged person to facilitate this "appropriate death." The nurse aids in the process by sharing the crisis of dying, so that clients are helped in dealing with the first impact of the realization of their impending death. Through continued contact, the nurse helps the client clarify and define the realities of day-to-day existence as well as the potential dying trajectory. The client generally requires assistance in separating anticipatory grief from the real losses of friends, body image, and self-control. Aid in retaining communication and family relationships may also be required. Interventions that reflect an understanding of the client's individuality greatly enhance the nurse's effectiveness.

Facilitating the Grieving Process.   Kalish (1970) points out that clients react in a variety of ways when advised of their impending death. They may accept or deny the information or vacillate between acceptance or denial. They may intellectually acknowledge it and emotionally deny it. They might react in their usual manner or experience a temporary diversion from their usual response pattern. Eventually, the client assimilates the knowledge in some manner and enters the grieving process. At the same time that clients are trying to cope with the knowledge of impending death, they are confronted with a variety of other tasks. These can include getting the will in order, checking on insurance, arranging work matters, paying bills, and so on. Clients must cope with the idea of the loss of loved ones and one's self, decide about current and future medical care—including a decision about continuation of treatment—anticipate future pain and loss of abilities, and come to grips with feelings about the meaning of death or life after death.

For the individual, the dying process is, in reality, a process of grieving—grieving for the loss of loved ones, the loss of all that is held important, and, ultimately, the loss of oneself. There are "allowable" manifestations of grief in this society. Unfortunately, most of the manifestations of self-grief are not well tolerated. Expressions of self-grief are frequently seen as "self-pity" and are viewed as indulgent behavior by most people. A frequent response of health care professionals is to distance themselves from individuals engaged in self-grief and leave them to their own devices. For instance, the nurse moves to a more receptive client to provide care. By leaving, the nurse avoids observing an intense human sorrow that may make the nurse uncomfortable. This response generally results in the client's grieving in private. Privacy does allow the client to preserve dignity and a sense of self-control. In some situations, private grieving may be appropriate. Nurses, however, should be sure that private expressions of grief have not been forced on the dying individual because of society's expectations.

One situation that denies the client's expression of grief occurs when clients have been lied to or when the family is engaged in a pretense pattern. Pretense isolates the client who is grieving. The client is forced to suffer this loneliness at a time when consolation is needed. The client can observe the grief of the family—the reddened eyes, the forced cheerfulness, and the empty reassurances—and is left to grieve alone.

The nurse can be helpful by acknowledging the client's grief and allowing expressions of grief by whatever means chosen. Grieving can take forms other than the stereotyped presentation of sadness, withdrawal, or crying. Other behaviors include fainting, laughing, anorexia, screaming, leaving the area, threatening suicide, hysteria, insomnia, tight-lipped silence, and repetitive rocking motions. Expressions of grief should be allowed and the client should not be quieted or sedated unless a real threat to self occurs. It is also important that the nurse not judge this behavior. The client's grief will decrease in intensity as time passes, diversion is provided, and acceptance is attained.

The elderly client's need for a Life Review (Butler, 1963) is closely related to this need to grieve. Life Review is the remembrance of accomplishments and failures in life. The Life Review generally takes time and occurs gradually. It is supported by allowing clients to talk about themselves. It is sometimes prompted by a seemingly superficial discussion about every-day events. As the elderly recall past events, they may need assistance in summing up these events and integrating them into a meaning of life. Their self-esteem is centrally involved. The nurse's empathetic manner and encouragement can help the elderly in this case.

One goal of the dying client is frequently to maintain as much control as possible over the dying process. To that purpose, clients need to have complete and honest information so they may make choices regarding treatment. Elderly clients must not be perceived as dependent beings solely because of their advancing age, physical weakness, or minimal energy levels. The nurse assists the client by allowing and encouraging statements of preference regarding care and the environment, and carrying out those decisions with or for the client.

Providing Physical Comfort. At some point (variable according to the death trajectory, general health of the client, and cause of dying), the dying client requires interventions directed toward the structural adaptations mentioned earlier. The goal of nursing intervention is, in this situation, to enhance the client's comfort. Such interventions require basic nursing skills. Some particular considerations are mentioned below.

1. *Changes in appetite and taste*. Zinc levels in the elderly may be lowered, resulting in a decreased sense of taste. Supplements are indicated when lack of taste brings about inadequate intake. Adequate fluid intake for the maintenance of appropriate hydration is, of course, essential. The diet is planned to provide for essential energy needs. It should be palatable and attractive to the client. If nausea is present, antiemetics may be indicated.

2. *Incontinence*. Urinary incontinence is a frequently encountered adaptation in the dying client and is most distressing as an indication of loss of control. Incontinence can range from stress incontinence to dribbling to total incontinence. Inflammatory diseases of the bladder, if present, are treated with drugs. Otherwise, discussion with the client of how to handle the problem is indicated. The use of incontinence pads or disposable diapers can be utilized, but may be so distressing to the client that a catheter may be advisable. Chapter 17 discusses nursing interventions for the incontinent client in more detail.

3. *Constipation*. Decreased food and fluid intake along with decreased activity may lead to constipation. Frequency of bowel movements are observed and recorded. Dietary adjustments of increasing fiber, roughage, and fluid intake can be considered. Laxatives and enemas should be used only when necessary.

4. *Pain*. The perception of pain varies from individual to individual and seems to be affected by culture, personality, and the symbolic meaning of the pain. Pain relief methods include exercise

and positioning. Hypnosis, biofeedback, focused attention, and acupuncture can also be considered. Pharmacologic agents available for pain relief include antianxiety, antidepressant, and psychadelic agents, in addition to narcotic and nonnarcotic analgesics.

Adequate pain relief is the most common problem of the terminally ill. Anticipation of pain adds to the distress of pain, as do rigid and specified dosages and timing of pain medication. Hospice units have experimented with allowing clients to have medication available and to administer it themselves. This cuts down on the waiting time for medication and allows the client to adjust the dosage within an acceptable range, taking less or more as the need requires. Control of pain is essential in order that clients can participate in other aspects of their care. The body's reaction to pain is total and, therefore, interferes with all other activities.

5. *Skin Care*. As weight loss, decreased activity, and poor nutritional status develop, the integrity of the skin is in jeopardy. Vasoconstriction places an additional burden on the skin by decreasing the oxygen supply to the skin. Skin breakdown can be avoided by using a variety of nursing techniques: exercise, massage, padding, and positioning.

6. *Respiratory Support*. As the dying process continues, respiratory efforts may become labored. Positioning in a supported elevated position generally alleviates discomfort. The client experiencing air hunger and associated anxiety may be relieved with the administration of oxygen.

Hospice Care

An alternative approach to care for the dying client is a change in setting. The elderly client dying in the hospital is frequently placed in a degrading and isolated situation in the acute care setting. Care frequently deteriorates to the most basic physical care as other clients take a higher priority. This type of care can increase the isolation, loneliness, and confusion of the dying elderly client. An alternative to this is placement in a hospice unit. Hospice is a concept of care whereby the quality of life is maximized when life cannot be extended. Hospice care is appropriate when all other treatments have failed to reverse the dying process. A client's life is not ended prematurely in a hospice setting, although "extraordinary measures" are not used. Decisions about care are made by the client in consultation with the health care team and family.

Types of Programs.   Hospice care can take many forms. It largely depends on the services that are needed in a community, the services already existing, and the type of resources available. A *hospital based program* can consist of a special unit or individual clients scattered throughout the institution cared for by the hospice team. Clients generally retain their own physicians who work cooperatively with the hospice team, or the client's care can become the total responsibility of the hospice staff. There is an attempt to make the client's environment as comfortable and as homelike as possible by obtaining favorite objects of the clients, such as a rocking chair, family photos, or a favorite blanket. Family and friends, including children and pets, are able to visit as freely as desired. The client is encouraged to be as independent as possible. Hospital based programs frequently provide outpatient services such as bereavement clinics for the client or support groups for the family. Home care might also be an extension of a hospital based program. Generally, in this type of program, the client is returned to the home setting as quickly as possible and receives the necessary supports there, being readmitted to the inpatient setting only when necessary. The hospice team is responsible for the care in all three settings; the inpatient, outpatient, and home setting. This is the most flexible and, generally, best coordinated approach to hospice care.

A *home health agency based hospice* focuses on outpatient care. If the client needs to be hospitalized, the hospice workers stay in contact with the client and the client's family, but are not directly involved with the provision of in-hospital care. Care in the home is provided by hospice workers, volunteers, or visiting nurses. The hospice agency coordinates this care. A major focus of home health agency hospice care is family support with extended support during the funeral period, mourning, and grieving periods.

The third type of hospice is the *independent hospice*. This is a facility designed specifically for the care of the dying. This is the least common type of hospice in the United States, mainly because of the high start-up costs and associated financial problems. One of the best known of the independent

hospice programs is the Connecticut Hospice Inc. in Branford, Connecticut. The Connecticut Hospice is unique in that it is licensed by the state to serve the entire population of Connecticut at its specially designed inpatient facility. The hospice also provides outpatient services for the residents of the New Haven area.

Financing Hospice Care.   The major challenge confronting the hospice movement today is economic. Most hospice services are covered by health insurance when care is provided by licensed hospitals, nursing homes, or home health agencies. Complications arise when hospice services are not offered through the traditional channels—as when care is provided by an independent hospice organization. Further, some insurers balk at paying for bereavement counseling and other supportive services for family members. There are some demonstration projects currently in progress whose goal is to learn how to provide quality hospice care with an appropriate and effective financing model.

Licensure and Accreditation.   Licensure and accreditation are also issues that need to be fully resolved. In most states, hospice programs are not licensed. In 1982 only Connecticut, Florida, New York, Nevada, and Virginia licensed such facilities. A number of other states are considering licensing laws that would define what a hospice is, set standards for care, and help establish reasonable rates. An associated issue is the possibility of further fragmentation of services by the establishment of separate hospice facilities. Additionally, the construction of new inpatient hospice facilities is opposed by some who cite the surplus of hospital beds that exist in many areas.

There is also the danger of the exploitation of vulnerable clients and families by unscrupulous providers, a sad lesson learned through the nursing home experience. Model voluntary accreditation standards were developed several years ago by the National Hospice Organization. The resources do not exist, at this time, for a national accreditation program. Thus, an institution can choose to meet the standards or not. Programs are not currently accredited. The Joint Commission on Accreditation of Hospitals has developed standards for hospice care in hospital based programs and it is possible that in the future this group may involve itself in the accreditation of independent facilities.

The Nurse's Role. The overwhelming majority of people, when faced with the need to care for terminally ill family members, generally look to a hospital or a nursing home. In increasing numbers, this is an inappropriate approach to care. In a great many cases, hospice care is the more appropriate choice. The hospice idea has begun to take hold in this country, but it is still a new concept. Much work still needs to be done in the area of education and legislation.

Nurses may find themselves in the position of explaining the hospice concept to clients and their families. Nurses can aid the family in clearly understanding the purpose and limitations of a hospice facility. This requires being familiar with the hospice philosophy as well as the available resources in the area. One source of education for nurses and other health care providers is the Hospice Institute for Education, Training, and Research, Inc. in New Haven, Connecticut. The Institute is involved in educational programs for care-givers as well as conducting research on the hospice concept and philosophy. It offers a range of courses and seminars for a wide variety of caretakers at a nominal cost. Additional information can be obtained from the National Hospice Organization in McLean, Virginia.

Assisting the Family

The family of the dying individual has an important effect on the client. The death of the individual will also greatly influence the family. In the past, the family was not considered in the care plan for the individual. By including the family, however, the psychosocial support available to the dying person can be increased. With the family members nearby, previously unstated emotional issues (regrets, expressions of affection, resentments, goodbyes) can be expressed among family members. In addition, involvement of the family in the care of the dying relative decreases the fragmentation and disorganization of the family unit that is frequently associated with a death in the family. It also assuages some of the guilt that often accompanies the grief process.

In order to understand the impact of death on

the family, an awareness of the interrelationships, interdependencies, and reciprocity of roles in the family is needed. The family unit is a basic system of society and has, therefore, certain characteristics. The family system is a composite of both individual members' behaviors and their complex and multiple interactions with one another. Anything that affects the family as a whole affects each individual member. For instance, inflation affects the family as a unit, influencing buying power. Inflation also has an effect on each individual in the family—such as the mother who may have to work and a child who may have to take over the home care chores. Likewise, any change in one member of the family unit affects all other members individually as well as collectively. If a member of a family leaves, changes a role, or undergoes a personal crisis, other members of the family are forced to change also.

The family can be conceptualized at three levels. The *nuclear family* generally refers to that stable group of individuals who live together. For elderly clients, this may include a spouse, siblings, or children and grandchildren; however, the elderly may not have a nuclear family by virtue of their living alone. If a person resides in a nursing home, the term nuclear family does not extend to other residents of the home, although the client may identify a close friend as a member of the nuclear family in the absence of others. The *extended family* generally refers to the relationship of the nuclear family to the family of origin of both the husband and wife. Thus, the extended family includes all blood relatives and relatives by marriage. In some families, the extended family can be quite large, with some members closer physically and emotionally than other members. The third level, the *social network,* refers to friends, neighbors, coworkers, and other significant individuals. There is an implication that clients should and do receive the greatest degree of support from their nuclear family. For a variety of reasons this may not be true. The nurse needs to be alert to potential sources of comfort and conflict in the family at all levels.

The effects of the dying process on family members vary as a function of innumerable factors: the nature of the terminal condition, personality of all involved persons, prior history of family relationships, the importance of the dying individual to each member, the ability of all concerned to establish the kind of communication that is most satisfactory to everyone, and the rapidity with which death occurs. The death of an elderly family member may have been somewhat anticipated, so the family may not have to deal with shock or denial as they might when a younger member dies. Nevertheless, they will still grieve and be affected by the loss of this member.

The Grief Reaction.   Grief has been mentioned before in the context of the dying individual. It is considered again, here, in the context of grieving for another's death. Grief is a normal reaction to a significant loss. It is an expected response when the death of a family member occurs. Under these conditions, grief is generally a self-healing response and will eventually be resolved. Lindemann (1944) defined the characteristic adaptations of the grief syndrome: somatic distress, preoccupation with the image of the deceased, guilt, hostile reactions, and loss of patterns of conduct. The process of resolving grief is termed "grief work." It requires both physical and emotional energy and is no less demanding than heavy manual labor. "Grief work" encompasses three tasks: emancipation from the dead, readjustment to life without the deceased, and formation of new relationships. Grief of the family cannot be adequately described by stage theory, which applies to the individual who is dying. The accomplishment of "grief work" does not mean the deceased is forgotten or not loved. Rather, the emotional energy a family member had invested in the deceased is modified so that new relationships can be established and the survivor is not bound emotionally to an individual who is no longer alive. The process starts with the acknowledgement of loss, and the person grieving goes through a series of reactions, commonly called phases. All grief theories acknowledge at least three broad categories of immediate reactions. In *avoidance,* the bereaved experiences shock, denial, and disbelief. In an anticipated death, this phase may be shorter and less pronounced than when the death is unexpected. *Confrontation* is a highly emotional phase where grief is most pronounced and the loss is felt intensely. *Reestablishment* is the phase when grief gradually declines and the bereaved begins a social and personal reentry to the everyday world.

This description delineates normal grief. There are some variations that occur. A common variation the nurse might see is anticipatory grief. Anticipatory grief is the presentation of adaptations to grief before the actual loss has occurred. The grief that family members display while a member is actively dying is anticipatory grieving and is appropriate. Anticipatory grieving may create a problem when the family completes a detachment from the dying individual and thus does not offer the support the person needs.

Another variation is delayed grieving. In this situation, a family member may display only minimal adaptations of grief at the time of the loss. Normal grieving may be delayed for an extended period of time. Then, usually quite unexpectedly, some event will trigger the grief response and a full grieving response will occur.

Grieving may also take exaggerated or abbreviated forms and usually is related to the level of attachment the family member had to the individual who has died.

Nursing Goals.   The nursing goals for care of the family of the dying individual include:

1. *Establishing a relationship with the family.* The nurse should meet with the family whenever possible to communicate the nurse's role and the kind of support staff can offer them as a unit and as individuals. The short-term and long-range needs of the family should be assessed.

2. *Reducing the family's fear of the unknown.* The family should be oriented to the environment, institutional policies, and names of those involved in the care of the dying person. The nurse should clearly communicate all information about the client, the prognosis, and the anticipated trajectory.

3. *Involving the family in the physical care of the client.* The family should be prepared for physical changes that might occur. The nurse can decide, with them, which activities the family can do or assist with, for example, feeding the client, turning, and positioning, shaving the client, adjusting oxygen equipment, etc. The family should be taught the appropriate techniques required in the caretaking activities. The nurse should encourage the participation of as many family members as necessary, or practical, in the care of the dying client.

4. *Maintaining the dying client's participation in the family.* The nurse should encourage the client to participate in family discussions and deci-

sions. Communication gaps that occur as the client and family are involved in the grieving process should be bridged. When denial is utilized as a method of coping with grief, the nurse should confront the family or client. The nurse should support expressions of grief and the realization of role and structure changes that will occur in the family.

5. *Attempting to reduce the guilt of family members.* Time should be provided for the family to privately discuss their grief and especially their "regrets" about the dying person. They should be actively involved in the planning and execution of client care. Family members should be allowed to express feelings of relief that are anticipated when the death actually occurs.

6. *Increasing resources available to the family.* The family should be assisted in obtaining the resources they will need, such as financial aid, transportation, child care services, etc., while they are involved in attending to the dying person. Long-range needs that are identified, such as housing needs, can also be presented to an appropriate referral agency.

7. *Preparing the family to deal with the practical realities surrounding the death of the client.* The nurse should encourage the family to discuss matters of burial arrangements with the client. Also, the nurse can encourage and support them in clarifying the location of and information about wills, deeds, life insurance, and other legal documents of the dying person.

Finally, the nurse should be available to support the family at the time the death actually occurs. They should be encouraged to express their grief and allowed to view the body and spend time saying "goodbye." The nurse should encourage the involvement of all of the family, including children, in the acknowledgement of the reality of the death.

If it is possible to have continuing contact with the family, the nurse can assist the family in the resolution of grief and the restoration of equilibrium in the family. Referrals to follow-up or self-help groups that are appropriate for individual family members, such as a widows group, can be made.

Postdeath Activities

Confirming the Death. When death does occur, the family must be notified immediately. If the death has been anticipated and the family is present, this generally does not cause a problem. When the family is not present, the announcement of death must be made to them. The form this announcement takes is generally dependent upon the family's awareness of the impending death. For instance, if the next-of-kin is a sister who has not seen the client for some time, some explanation of the situation or delaying of the actual statement until she is present may be warranted. On the other hand, if the sister was at home after a day spent with the client in full awareness of the impending event, verbal, telephone confirmation may be all that is necessary. In general, the statement of confirmation of death comes from the physician. Since it is the physician who legally declares the client dead and signs the death certificate, the family generally needs to have the physician make the statement. The physician's statement transmits a sense of authority and finality. This does not, in any way, absolve the nurse from either participating in the statement or doing it for the physician, if necessary. The stereotype of the silent nurse stating "the doctor will see you" is an absurdity in modern professional practice. It is frequently the nurse who has developed a close relationship with the client and family and can be there to acknowledge the event and support expressions of grief by the family.

Viewing the Body. There are varieties of opinions about the viewing of the body by the family in the hospital setting. Some say that the presence of a grieving family on a unit will disrupt things or disturb other patients, or that the family will be so overcome with grief, they will become hysterical and uncontrollable. There is no evidence to suggest this is a valid position. Glazer and Strauss (1968) point out that allowing a "last look," particularly in circumstances of a rapid dying trajectory gives the family an opportunity to recognize and acknowledge the reality of death. In the United States this "last look" typically only lasts a few minutes and takes place in the room where the client has died, although the client could be moved to a viewing room if circumstances seem to warrant this. It should be remembered, however, that in other cultures the "last look" can involve the entire extended family and last several hours. These customs, particularly of Japanese and Gypsy cultures, can present accommodation problems in the usual hospital setting and a private viewing room is generally suggested.

Touching the body is also an important action in closing the mystical gap of death. Most of the time touching is gentle and loving and should be allowed.

Rationale for Postmortem Care. The announcement of death, the last look, and last touch generally take place in a rapid time frame so that the nurse can complete postmortem care of the body and ready it for removal by a mortuary service. Pennington (1978) has pointed out the adaptations that provide the rationale for traditional postmortem care practices. Briefly, these are livor mortis with postmortem bruising, rigor mortis, and decomposition (autolysis). *Livor mortis* occurs as there is gravitational settling of blood cell hemoglobin into dilated capillaries. The tissues become stained with the hemoglobin and appear bruised. This color change usually occurs in dependent areas of the body, but not where pressure has prevented deposits into the capillaries. Livor mortis is usually perceptible within 2 hours after death and reaches a maximum 8 to 12 hours after death. It is important for the nurse to position the dead client so that bruising will not occur in those areas (face, neck, chest, hands) that will be seen in viewing situations. The nurse should also carefully pad any bindings that have been placed on the extremities for support.

During *rigor mortis,* the muscles of the body gradually become rigid due to the loss of adenosine triphosphate (ATP), and the accumulation of lactic acid within the muscle fibrils. Eventually (usually within 96 hours), there is complete exhaustion of chemical activity, the lactic acid decomposes and flaccidity returns. The process begins about 2 to 4 hours after death and generally begins in the involuntary muscles of the GI tract, bladder, and arteries. It then spreads to the muscle fibers of the face, neck, and hands, and eventually over the entire body. Rigor mortis is sometimes absent or very slight in the very old because of the paucity of muscle tissue. The onset of rigor mortis can be delayed by refrigeration. It is important that the nurse replace dentures and position the client before the onset of rigor. Also, if removal to the mortuary is to be delayed, it is helpful to place the body in a refrigerated unit to slow this process.

Decomposition leading to decay and bacterial infestation is subject to time variation, depending upon preexisting body conditions, environmental temperature, and the circumstances of death. Autolysis refers to action of the digestive enzymes in the body breaking down body tissues, and can result in the rupture of the stomach or bowel wall and the discharge of infected fluid though body orifices. Autolysis is delayed by refrigeration. The body should be refrigerated as quickly as possible until removal to a mortuary where the embalming process prevents autolysis. Generally, postmortem care is done after the family has had the opportunity for viewing. If their arrival will be delayed more than 1 hour, the body should be placed in a refrigeration unit and then moved to a viewing room upon their arrival.

The Funeral. Although the nurse is generally not involved in the funeral activities, it is important to see the funeral as part of the total dying process. The nurse may be involved by helping the client plan his or her funeral, by helping the family cope with the immediate postdeath practices, or by becoming one of the attending grievers. American culture has inherent within it the long-established practice of the burial of the dead with its attendant ceremonies. Burial of the dead is not, however, unique to this culture, and is practiced by most Western and some Eastern societies.

A funeral is an organized, purposeful, time-limited, flexible group-centered response to death (Lamers, 1969). The funeral allows acknowledgement of the death, expression of grief and feelings, as well as the reestablishment of family and social ties among the mourners. Raether and Slater (1977) suggest that there are phases the mourners experience:

1. *Removal* involves the separation of the dead from the living. Modern funeral practices permit the removal of the body from the place of death to a neutral place while the family returns to its home. After acknowledging that death has occurred, this removal phase reinforces to the mourners that they are the living.

2. *The visitation period* may simply be a time for individual and group socialization and expressions of grief, or it may take on a religious function. It is at this point that the survivors begin to reorder and readjust to life without the

dead person. The period of visitation varies, depending upon ethnic and local customs.

3. *The funeral rite* is that specific time period when rites and rituals concerning the dead are carried out. It is usually a ceremonial, often a religious rite, of relatively brief duration, 30 to 60 minutes. The funeral rite is part of the larger funeral observance and tends to become the focal point of the process.

4. *The procession* refers to the movement of the body from the place of the funeral services to the place of final disposition, the cemetery or crematorium. The procession adds to the impact of the movement of the dead away from the living. It also impacts on the living moving away toward a life without the deceased. Moving *to* the place of final disposition helps one to accept the finality of what has occurred. Moving *from* the place of final disposition helps one get back in the normal mainstream of life.

5. *The committal,* a simple act of committing the body to a final place, emphasizes the finality of what is experienced more than any of the other phases. It is important that some true act of finality takes place, i.e., the lowering of the body, or the placement of dirt into the grave, or the retrieval of the ashes after cremation.

The funeral process evokes strong emotions and people develop positive and negative attitudes. The experience can be seen as necessary, traditional, and useful, or it can be seen as an expensive ritual. This negative view has led to alternative practices such as memorial services without the body present, or donation of the body. Whichever postdeath activities are chosen, they should provide comfort and meaning in this immediate period of grieving.

SUMMARY

Assisting in the process of dying, caring for the dead and the bereaved is not an easy experience for the nurse. It is, however, an expected part of working with the elderly. The nurse can experience anxiety, frustration, and confusion from not knowing how to help, and suffer from overidentification—particularly in a long-term situation—and a feeling of being overwhelmed by the intensity, magnitude,

and scope of problems inherent in working with the dying client. These feelings should not be suppressed; rather, the expression of the feelings and continuing discussions of their causes and implications will better enable nurses to assist clients and families. The nurse can learn about life, its meaning, and its expression, and also gain satisfaction from being involved in the client's attainment of this final developmental task.

REFERENCES

Ad Hoc Committee of the Harvard Medical School to Examine the Definition of Brain Death: A definition of irreversible coma. Journal of the American Medical Association 205(6):337, 1968

Aires P: The Hour of Our Death. New York, Knopf, 1981

Benoliel JQ: Overview: Care, cure and the challenge of choice, in Earle A, et al (eds), The Nurse as Caretaker for the Dying Patient. New York, Columbia University Press, 1976

Butler RN: The life review: An interpretation of reminiscence in the aged. Psychiatry 26(1):65, 1963

Cohen K: Hospice Prescription for Terminal Care. Germantown MD, Aspen Systems Corporation, 1979

Dumont R, Foss D: The American View of Death: Acceptance or Denial? Cambridge, MA, Schenkman, 1972

Engle G: Psychological Development in Health and Disease. Philadelphia, Lippincott, 1962

Epstein C: Nursing the Dying Patient. Reston, VA, Reston, 1975

Erikson EH: Identity and the life cycle: Selected papers. Psychological Issues 1(1):18, 1959

Feifel H: The meaning of death in American society: Implications for education, in Green B, Irish D (eds), Death Education: Preparation for Living. Cambridge, MA, Schenkman, 1971

Gavey CJ: The Management of the Hopeless Case. London, Lewis, 1952

Glaser BG, Strauss AL: Time for Dying. Chicago, Aldine, 1968

Gullo S, Carin L, et al: Suggested stages and response styles in life threatening illness: A focus on the cancer patient, in Schoenberg B, et al (eds), Anticipatory Grief. New York, Columbia University Press, 1974

Hadjidimos AA, Brock M, Baum P, Schurmann K: Cessation of cerebral blood flow in total irreversible loss of brain function, in Brock M, et al (eds), Cerebral Blood Flow. Berlin, Springer, 1969

Jameton A: The nurse: When roles and rules conflict. Hastings Center Report 7(4):22, 1977

Kalish RA: The onset of the dying process. Omega 1(1):57, 1970

Kalish RA, Reynolds DK: Death and Ethnicity: A Psycho-Cultural Investigation. Los Angeles, University of Southern California Press, 1976

Kastenbaum R: Death and bereavement in later life, in Kutscher AH (ed), Death and Bereavement. Springfield, IL, Thomas, 1969

Kastenbaum R: Death and development through the life span, in Feifel H (ed), New Meanings of Death. New York, McGraw-Hill, 1977

Kirk JE: Premortal clinical biochemical changes, in Bodansky O, Steward CP (eds), Advances in Clinical Chemistry. New York, Academic, 1968, vol 2

Kübler-Ross E: On Death and Dying. New York, MacMillan, 1969

Lamers WM Jr: Funerals are good for people—MD's included. Medical Economics 46:104, 1969

Latner J: The Gestalt Therapy Book. New York, Julian, 1973

Lieberman MA, Coplan AS: Distance from death as a variable in the study of aging. Developmental Psychology 2(1):84, 1969

Lifton RJ: Death in Life: Survivors of Hiroshima. New York, Random House, 1968

Lindemann E: Symptomatology and management of acute grief. American Journal of Psychiatry 101:141, 1944

Marshall JR: The geriatric patients' fears about death. Postgraduate Medicine 57(4):144, 1975

Matse J: Reactions to death in residential homes for the aged. Omega 6(1):21, 1975

Mellerio F: Clinical and EEG study of a case of acute poisoning with cerebral electrical silence, followed by recovery. Electroencephalography Clinical Neurophysiology 30:254, 1971

Metropolitan Life Insurance Company: Decline in life expectancy. Statistical Bulletin 62(2)4, 1981

Pattison EM (ed): The Experience of Dying. Englewood Cliffs, NJ, Prentice-Hall, 1977

Pennington EA: Post mortem care: More than just ritual. American Journal of Nursing 78(5):846, 1978

Raether H, Slater R: Immediate postdeath activities in the United States, in Feifel H (ed), New Meanings of Death. New York, McGraw-Hill, 1977

Riley JW: Attitudes toward death. in Riley MW, Faner A (eds), Aging and Society Volume 1: An Inventory of Research Findings. New York, Russell Sage Foundation, 1968

Saul SR, Saul S: Old people talk about death. Omega 4(1):27, 1973

Toole JF: The neurologist and the concept of brain death. Perspectives in Biology and Medicine 14(4):599, 1971

Veatch RM: Models for ethical medicine in a revolutionary age. Hastings Center Report 2(3):25, 1972

Veatch RM: Death, Dying and the Biological Revolution. New Haven, CT, Yale University Press, 1976

Verwoerdt A: Communication with the Fatally Ill. Chicago, IL, Charles C. Thomas, 1966

Walker M: The last hour before death. American Journal of Nursing 73(9):1592, 1973

Wass H, Scott M: Aging without death? The Gerontologist 17:206, 1977

Weisman AD: The psychiatrist and the inexorable, in Feifel H (ed), New Meanings of Death. New York, McGraw-Hill, 1977

Walstenholme GEW, O'Connor M (eds): Ethics in Medical Progress: With Special Reference to Transplantation. Boston, Little Brown, 1966

Yearling RR: Ethical analysis of a nursing problem: The scope of nursing practice in disclosing the truth to terminal patients. Part I. Supervisor Nurse 9(5):93, 1978

Index